The Specialty Practice of Rehabilitation Nursing

A Core Curriculum
Fifth Edition

Editor
Kristen L. Mauk, PhD RN CRRN-A APRN BC
Professor of Nursing
Valparaiso University
Valparaiso, IN

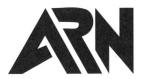

Association of Rehabilitation Nurses
4700 W. Lake Avenue
Glenview, IL
800/229-7530, 847/375-4710

E-mail, info@rehabnurse.org • Web site, http://www.rehabnurse.org
Copyright © 2007 Association of Rehabilitation Nurses
All rights reserved

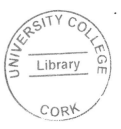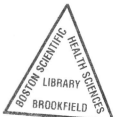

The Specialty Practice of Rehabilitation Nursing

A Core Curriculum
Fifth Edition

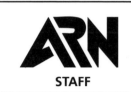

STAFF

Executive Director
Karen Nason, CAE

Editorial Director
Clay Baznik

Managing Editor
Larry A. Sawyer

Director of Sales
Kathryn M. Checea

Senior Sales Manager
Terri Berkowitz

Designer
LN Vaillancourt

ISBN 978-1-884278-13-6

Note. As new scientific information becomes available through basic and clinical research, recommended treatments and drug therapies undergo changes. The authors, editors, reviewers, and publisher have done everything possible to make this book accurate, up-to-date, and in accord with standards accepted at the time of publication. The authors, editors, reviewers, and publisher are not responsible for errors or omissions or for consequences from application of the book and make no warranty, expressed or implied, in regard to the contents of the book. Any practice described in this book should be applied by the healthcare practitioner in accordance with professional standards of care and used in regard to the unique circumstances that may apply in each situation. The reader is advised always to check product information (package inserts) for changes and new information regarding dose and contraindications before administering any drug. Caution is especially urged when using new or infrequently ordered drugs or treatments.

This volume contains many references and resources utilizing Internet addresses. Although these sites were current at the time of research, writing, and/or publication, many Internet postings are volatile and subject to expiration or deletion over time. Therefore, ARN cannot guarantee currency of electronic references. (Readers who wish to pursue the latest information on a cited topic are likely to find new or updated posting via online search engines.)

Table of Contents

Foreword

● ●

"There are two ways of spreading light: to be the candle or the mirror that reflects it."

—Edith Wharton

It is a pleasure to write the foreword for this important publication. This quote from Edith Wharton's poem, "Vesalius in Zante," symbolizes the potential influence of the fifth edition of the core curriculum. For the authors, it is a means to spread the light of new knowledge. Nurses who use the content will reflect that light to our patients, their families, our colleagues, and the community.

The fifth edition of the core curriculum stands on the shoulders of earlier versions and owes much to the editors and expert clinicians who contributed to those editions. The core curriculum captures the essence of rehabilitation nursing, yet it is broadly conceived to serve as a resource for nurses in diverse settings and at all levels of experience. The novice nurse as well as expert clinicians and researchers will find content to enhance their practice. The core curriculum is a critical resource not only for rehabilitation nurses, but for nurses in other settings. This book has played a key role in shaping the practice of rehabilitation nurses since 1981. The first edition, titled *Rehabilitation Nursing: Concepts and Practice, A Core Curriculum* and edited by Shannon Sayles, provided a solid framework for the future. Subsequent editions grew to include advances and breakthroughs in rehabilitation nursing. The second and third editions, edited by Christina M. Mumma, PhD RN CS CRRN, and Ann McCourt, RN MS, respectively, expanded the content to address advances in rehabilitation nursing. New content in the second edition included quality assurance, healthcare economics, and the Rehabilitation Standards of Nursing Practice. Examples of new content in the third edition were rehabilitation of aging individuals, ethics, healthcare legislation, health problems related to neuromuscular conditions, and the role of rehabilitation case managers.

The fourth edition, edited by Patricia Edwards, EDD RN CNAA, added important information on common chronic conditions, information technology and computer technology, and the delivery and evaluation of rehabilitation services, and updated the core content. The fifth edition, edited by Kristen Mauk, PhD RN CRRN-A APRN BC, builds on the last edition and incorporates best practice for topics from functional health problems through the delivery and evaluation of services. All the Core content for the fifth edition has been updated; a few chapters were almost entirely rewritten based on the current state of the science and practice. Two new chapters were added: case management and research in evidence based practice (EBP). The technology content was revised to reflect the explosion of knowledge in this area. Advanced practice content has been integrated into selected chapters. Although the evolution in practice is noted in each edition of the core curriculum, a sustaining principle in all editions has been the focus on improving the quality of life for the patient and family, no matter the setting for care delivery

The core curriculum addresses many of the changes in rehabilitation nursing practice and the healthcare system since the fourth edition was published. Examples of changes directly affecting rehabilitation nurses are managing care of persons with polytrauma and the need for innovative technology, an increase in the aging population with chronic illness and disability, an increased emphasis on EBP, and recognition of nursing excellence at Magnet organizations which provide rehabilitation services. Some of the changes in the healthcare system with implications for rehabilitation nurses include recognition of the importance of rehabilitation nursing as criteria for payment, explosion of knowledge in information technology, ever shorter lengths of acute rehabilitation stays, expansion in the need for and role of case managers, the emphasis on end-of-life decision making and palliative care, and disaster preparedness. There has been a marked increase in the numbers of doctorally prepared nurses, APNs, and nurse researchers to meet the demands of changing practice.

A vision of the future of ARN and its members has been created through the new strategic plan, with several supporting structures such as the revised research agenda and standards and scope of rehabilitation nursing practice. The revised core curriculum is a major tool in achieving this vision, providing a basis for action directed toward several of the goals. Clinicians often ask "what is the best way?", "why is this method better than that one?", or "how do I know what will work?". The authors of each chapter and section editors have integrated EBP content to address the "what", "why", and "how" of rehabilitation nursing practice. EBP is made more accessible with up-to-date supporting evidence grounding practice in science. The new section on evidence based practice (EBP) provides insights into current approaches to EBP that will further help nurses in the decision-making process in their day-to-day practice.

The fifth edition represents the work of many dedicated nurses who are committed to spreading the light of knowledge through their work as editor, section editor, author, or reviewer. I am confident that all who use this knowledge will make a difference in the lives of our patients and their families.

Wharton, E. (1902). Vesalius in zante. (1564). *North American Review, 175* (Nov.), 625–631. Retrieved July 30, 2007, from http://www.wsu.edu~campbell/wharton/whartpoe2.htm.

—Rosemarie King, PhD RN
July 2007

Preface

● ●

This most recent edition of the Association of Rehabilitation Nurses (ARN) core curriculum is a comprehensive guide to the current practice of the profession across multiple settings and age groups. The ARN Board of Directors charged us with updating the 2000 version of the core curriculum to reflect current practice while largely maintaining the previous format and outline. With no current plans to update the advanced practice core curriculum, the Board suggested that some advanced practice material also be incorporated into the new edition. While synthesizing some of this content into the new core curriculum, the main purpose of the core was kept in mind "to provide the essential information a nurse needs to know to practice rehabilitation nursing in any setting" (Edwards, 2000, iv).

This edition thus incorporates an emphasis on evidence-based practice and reflects current research trends. Two new chapters were added to discuss case management and the use of research in evidence-based practice. In addition, advanced practice content was included with many chapters to provide a holistic reference that should be useful to both general and advanced practice nurses.

This fifth edition builds on the excellent framework of the forth edition, completed by Pat Edwards and her chapter authors, by incorporating the knowledge and expertise of 40 chapter authors practicing in a variety of settings including inpatient rehabilitation, skilled care, clinics, long-term care, academics, research, case management, home health care, private consulting, and independent practice. These chapter authors and reviewers represent various educational and practice backgrounds, with most holding advanced degrees and certification in rehabilitation nursing as well as other related fields. A strength of the fifth edition of the core curriculum is the vast diversity and wealth of experience represented by the cohort of chapter authors.

Enhanced material on geriatrics, pediatrics, traumatic brain injury, sexuality, diabetes, and use of technology is included, as well as updates on health policy written by leaders in these respective areas. Popular features from the last edition such as "teaching topics" are still included, as well as numerous online references and resources that appear in each chapter. New case studies with discussion questions are included in an appendix to reflect several common diagnoses seen across a variety of settings, age groups, and levels of practice. Lastly, Pat Edwards provides a complete summary of the history of ARN including past presidents and *RNJ* editors, using interesting quotes from interviews with key ARN leaders who share direction for the future of rehabilitation nursing.

The conceptual framework from the fourth edition was built upon to complete this current work. **Section I** discusses general principles and concepts of the specialty of rehabilitation nursing. Theories and frameworks that help guide the profession are presented. Family-centered rehabilitation within the community is emphasized. Ethical, legal, and economic issues that impact persons with disabilities and chronic health alternations are presented. Health policy and legislative influences are also discussed, with guidance provided to rehabilitation nurses on how to take a proactive approach to advocating for our patients through legislation.

Section II provides information on functional health patterns related to rehabilitation nursing. Neuroanatomy is presented as a basis for understanding the underlying pathophysiology of common disorders discussed later. Essential information on physical problems such as maintaining skin integrity, promoting sleep, dealing with dysphagia, understanding the impact of chronicity on sexuality, and the effects of illness on mobility is included. Psychosocial health care patterns and intergenerational health promotion are discussed. Both chapters on physical and psychosocial health care patterns explore current research and provide recommendations for best rehabilitation nursing practice.

Section III contains updated material on stroke, traumatic brain injury, and spinal cord injury. Care of persons with musculoskeletal disorders such as osteoporosis, arthritis, and amputation is presented. These chapters also provide suggestions for advanced practice nurses wishing to enhance their roles of leader, educator, clinician, consultant, and researcher. Using Melnyk's protocol for finding and implementing evidence-based practice, several important clinical questions are explored in various chapters, with recommendations for best practice. The last edition of the core curriculum added new chapters on cardiovascular and pulmonary rehabilitation, pain management, and common diseases. These chapters were updated to reflect current best practices. New content on diabetes, HIV/AIDS, and cancer was added. Rehabilitation nursing management of Parkinson's disease, multiple sclerosis, and burns was also updated.

Section IV continues to present rehabilitation nursing across the continuum, beginning with a discussion of developmental theories across the lifespan for both individuals and families. The chapters on pediatric and geriatric rehabilitation nursing have been completely revised with much new content added. Nurses working in these specialties should find these chapters particularly informative.

In **Section V**, the delivery and evaluation of rehabilitation services is presented. Settings for care, outcomes measurements and performance improvements are discussed. Several excellent assessment and evaluation tools are included for nurses to reference. A new chapter on case management was added that includes both general knowledge and some advanced practice recommendations.

Section VI describes rehabilitation nursing in the 21st century. Changes in American health care and the rehabilitation nurse as a change agent are discussed. The chapter on technology and computer applications has been completely revised to reflect more current trends, software, and use. A new chapter introducing research and evidence-based practice and its use in rehabilitation has been added. The last chapter of this edition was expanded to provide a comprehensive summary of ARN's history including past presidents and past journal editors. Interviews with past and current ARN leaders provided quotes that help provide insight into the future of the profession. An appendix at the end of the book provides several case studies with discussion questions that cover a variety of settings, diagnoses, age groups, and practice levels of the rehab nurse.

—Kristen L. Mauk, PhD RN CRRN-A APRN BC

Acknowledgments

•

This fifth edition of the core curriculum builds on the excellent work of authors and reviewers from the prior edition, and their contributions are gratefully acknowledged.

Using the framework set forth by fourth edition editor Pat Edwards, this edition involved the dedicated energies and knowledge of 38 chapter authors and nearly 50 reviewers who updated content to reflect the current state of rehabilitation nursing with an emphasis on evidence-based practice. My most heartfelt thanks goes out to the chapter authors and reviewers for their commitment to sharing their expertise with others in the writing of this work, and to Larry Sawyer for his help in the timely completion of this project.

Dedication

•

To nurses everywhere who are committed to using their knowledge and expertise to make rehabilitation a part of all nursing practice, to lead the profession as global ambassadors for rehabilitation nursing, and to guide our patients toward a better quality of life.

Chapter Authors

Chapter 1
Janet Secrest, PhD RN

Chapter 2
Bonnie J. Parker, MSN RN CRRN; Leslie Neal-Boylan, PhD RNC CRRN FNP-C

Chapter 3
Pamela A. Masters-Farrell, MSN RN CRRN

Chapter 4
Anne Deutsch, PhD RN CRRN; Susan Dean-Baar, PhD RN CRRN FAAN

Chapter 5
Kelly Johnson, MSN RN CFNP CRRN; Jane Emanuelson, RN CRRN

Chapter 6
Kathy G. Dale, MS-HSA RN CRRN

Chapter 7
Michele Cournan, MS RN CNS CRRN APRN-BC; Donald D. Kautz, PhD RN CRRN-A; Brandy Conrad, BSN RN

Chapter 8
Barbara Brillhart, PhD RN CRRN

Chapter 9
Carla J. Howard, MS RN CRRN
Kristen L. Mauk, PhD RN CRRN-A APRN BC

Chapter 10
Linda Dufour, MSN RN CRRN; Joan Williams, MSN RN CRRN ARNP-C; Tiffany Lecroy, RN CMSN CCRC; Rachel Emery, BA; Kristen L. Mauk, PhD RN CRRN-A APRN BC

Chapter 11
Sue Pugh, MSN RN CRRN CNRN; Elizabeth Yetzer, MSN RN CRRN; Barbara Naden-Blucher, MSN RN CRRN GNP

Chapter 12
Lynn Carbone, RN CRRN

Chapter 13
Dalice Hertzberg, MSN RN ARNP BC

Chapter 14
Karen (Cervizzi) Manning, MSN RN CRRN CNA; Patricia A. Haldi, MN RN CRRN CDE

Chapter 15
Linda L. Pierce, PhD RN CNS CRRN FAHA

Chapter 16
Patricia A. Edwards, EdD RN CNAA; Dalice Hertzberg, MSN RN ARNP BC; Lyn Sapp, BSN RN CRRN

Chapter 17
Kristen L. Mauk, PhD RN CRRN-A APRN BC; Cheryl Lehman, PhD RN CRRN-A BC

Chapter 18
Patricia A. Quigley, PhD MPH ARNP CRRN FAAN

Chapter 19
Terrie Black, MBA BSN RN BC CRRN

Chapter 20
Donna Williams, MSN RN CRRN-A; Patricia L. McCollom, MS RN CRRN CDMS CCM CLCP

Chapter 21
Kathleen A. Stevens, PhD RN CRRN

Chapter 22
Elaine Tilka Miller, DNS RN CRRN FAHA FAAN; Carole Ann Bach, PhD RN CRRN

Chapter 23
Teresa L. Cervantez Thompson, PhD RN CRRN-A

Chapter 24
Patricia A. Edwards, EdD RN CNAA

Case Studies
Kristen L. Mauk, PhD RN CRRN-A APRN BC; Cindy Gatens, MN RN CRRN-A

Chapter Reviewers

Chapter 1
Rose Butler, MS RNC CCM CRRN
Cynthia Jacelon, PhD RN CRRN-A

Chapter 2
Leslie Neal-Boylan, PhD RNC CRRN FNP-C

Chapter 3
Rhonda Reed, MSN RN CRRN
Sherry Liske, MS RN CRRN

Chapter 4
Carol Gleason, RN CRRN CCM LRC
Aloma Gender, MSN RN CRRN

Chapter 5
Carole Ann Ottey, MSN RNC CRRN

Chapter 6
Marcia Potter, MS RN CRRN
Helen Carmine, MSN CRNP CRRN

Chapter 7
Marcia Grandstaff, RN CRRN
Barbara Ridley, MS RN CRRN FNP-C

Chapter 8
Pamala Larsen, PhD RN CRRN FNGNA
Kathleen Skrabut, EdD RN CRRN

Chapter 9
Cheryl Lehman, PhD RN CRRN-A
Ann Gunderson, MSN RN CRRN-A

Chapter 10
Barbara Ridley, MS RN CRRN FNP-C

Chapter 11
Kathy Dale, MS-HSA RN CRRN
Elizabeth Yetzer, MA MSN CRRN

Chapter 12
Donna Williams, MSN RN CRRN-A
Aleisa Kyper, BSN RN

Chapter 13
Kathy Dale, MS-HSA RN CRRN
Elizabeth Yetzer, MA MSN CRRN

Chapter 14
Rhonda Reed, MSN RN CRRN
Cindy Gatens, MN RN CRRN-A
Mary Pat Murphy, MSN RN CRRN

Chapter 15
Karen Preston, PHN MS CRRN FIALCP
Kathleen Skrabut, EdD RN CRRN

Chapter 16
Deirdre Jackson, MSN CRRN CNS C
Patricia A. Edwards, EdD RN CNAA
Lyn Sapp, BSN RN CRRN

Chapter 17
Cynthia Jacelon, PhD RN CRRN-A
Sherry Liske, MS RN CRRN

Chapter 18
Carol Gleason, RN CRRN CCM LRC
Ann Gunderson, MSN RN CRRN-A

Chapter 19
Rose Butler, MS RNC CCM CRRN
Kelly Johnson, MSN RN CFNP CRRN

Chapter 20
Karen Preston, PHN MS CRRN FIALCP
Kathleen Potempa, DNSc RN FAAN

Chapter 21
Dalice Hertzberg, MSN RN ARNP BC
Kathleen Potempa, DNSc RN FAAN

Chapter 22
Linda Pierce, PhD RN CNS CRRN FAHA

Chapter 23
Dalice Hertzberg, MSN RN ARNP BC

Chapter 24
Kelly Johnson, MSN RN CFNP CRRN
Marilyn Ter Maat, MSN RNC CNAA BC CRRN-A
Lois Schaetzle, MS RN CRRN

Section **I**

General Principles and Concepts of Rehabilitation Nursing as a Specialty

●●

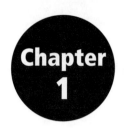

Rehabilitation and Rehabilitation Nursing

Janet Secrest, PhD RN

Advances in health care have enabled people to survive injuries and illnesses and to live longer than in the past. Over the next few decades, two trends will combine to increase the need for rehabilitation. First, the numbers of people with chronic illness and disability are expected to rise, and second, the number of older adults is increasing rapidly. Rehabilitation is a philosophy of practice and an attitude toward caring for people with disabilities and chronic health problems. The overall goal of rehabilitation is to improve quality of life and to help a person "who has a disability or chronic health problem in restoring, maintaining, and promoting his or her maximal health" (Association of Rehabilitation Nurses [ARN], 2000, p. 4). Rehabilitation is contingent on a team approach, and the discipline of nursing is integral to the team. Rehabilitation nursing is a specialty practice that offers a unique, holistic perspective to the care of clients with disabilities and chronic health problems.

The purpose of this chapter is to review rehabilitation philosophy, goals, and processes and examine the role of nursing, including nurses' values and philosophical perspectives. Nursing science—the relationship between theory, research, and practice—provides a basis for professional rehabilitation nursing. Included in this chapter is a description of the role responsibilities, educational preparation, competencies, certification, professional associations, and resources for the specialty practice of rehabilitation nursing.

The Evolution Of Rehabilitation
Historical Trends

Advances in health care over the past century have enabled people to live longer lives and to recover from injuries and illnesses that were previously fatal. With these advances have come disabilities and chronic illnesses that profoundly change the way a person lives in the world. The field of rehabilitation emerged to help individuals and families integrate the changes associated with disability and chronic health problems into their lives. Rehabilitation is a philosophy, an attitude, and an approach to caring for people with disabilities that improves the quality of their lives and provides a meaningful context in which to live.

The concept of rehabilitation as a philosophy and attitude is important. Attitudes toward people with disability, which arise from a philosophy, determine societal responsibilities and approaches. For example, in ancient Western civilization, disease and disability often were thought to be the result of evil spirits. Consequently, those so "possessed" were feared and shunned. Parents in ancient Rome could legally drown infants with congenital anomalies, and in Sparta such infants were left to die of exposure. This situation did not improve in the Middle Ages. Some people with disabilities were burned as witches, others were used as court jesters, and all who had disabilities were shunned from everyday societal functions (World Book, 1997). Even in more modern times, those living with disabilities or handicaps in World War II Germany were considered "flawed" and were among the first people exterminated in the Holocaust. Fortunately, philosophical approaches and attitudes have changed radically over time. [Refer to Chapter 24 for a historical overview of rehabilitation.]

Rehabilitation, as an interdisciplinary healthcare specialty, grew out of the wars of the 20th century. Many soldiers— young men for the most part—survived injury but faced serious disability. As a result, military hospitals established rehabilitation units that focused extensive efforts on returning these young men to society. Dr. Howard Rusk, head of the American Air Force Convalescent Training Program, was a strong leader in organizing rehabilitation programs (Lyons & Petrucelli, 1978). Soon, rehabilitation units and hospitals sprang up around the United States, and the interdisciplinary specialty of rehabilitation gained importance. By 1974, the Association of Rehabilitation Nurses (ARN) was formed, and nursing, which had always been involved in rehabilitation, formally became recognized as a rehabilitation specialty.

Legislative Initiatives

Legislation in the United States has been important in the development of the specialty of rehabilitation. The Rehabilitation Act of 1973 encouraged efforts to hire people with disabilities and prohibited unfair treatment of people with disabilities in activities supported in any way by federal funds. In 1975, the Education for All Handicapped Children Act required states to provide education free of cost to any school-age child. The Americans with Disabilities Act (ADA) of 1990 required that public buildings and transportation be made accessible to all (Watson, 2000). This act also prohibits discrimination against people with disabilities in the workplace. The result of these legislative acts has been to increase societal acceptance of people with disabilities and provide opportunities for them to maximize their potential. [Refer to Chapter 4 for more on legislation.]

Rehabilitation is a vital component of health care. Although the root causes of disability have changed over time, the need for rehabilitation today is greater than ever before.

Rehabilitation Across Disciplines
Philosophy and Goals

Rehabilitation is a philosophy that crosses the boundaries of practice disciplines. It has been defined as "a process of helping a person to reach the fullest physical, psychological, social, vocational, avocational and educational potential consistent with his or her physiologic or anatomic impairment, environmental limitations, and desires and life plans" (DeLisa, Currie, & Martin, 1998, p. 3). It is an inherently collaborative endeavor, and it places the client and family in the center of the healthcare team. Rehabilitation is contingent on a team approach. Indeed, most rehabilitation professionals would agree that the healthcare system would flourish if the ideals of rehabilitation permeated all aspects of health care.

In 1980, the World Health Organization (WHO) developed the International Classification of Impairment, Disability, and Handicap (cited in Kirby, 1998, pp. 55–57). This classification system has been translated into 13 languages and distinguishes between the following terms:

- **Impairment:** A loss or abnormality of a psychological, physiological, or anatomical structure and function
- **Disability:** A restriction or lack (resulting from an impairment) of ability to perform an activity in the manner or within the range considered normal for a human being
- **Handicap:** A disadvantage for a given person resulting from impairment or disability that limits or prevents fulfillment of a role that is normal for that person.

Thus, impairment occurs at the organ level, disability at the level of the person, and handicap at the societal level. These definitions provide a framework and a language that is not just for rehabilitation but for society as well.

Although many goals of rehabilitation have been articulated, improvement in quality of life is the ultimate goal (DeLisa et al., 1998). This goal can be accomplished through many avenues, and each member of the rehabilitation team contributes to this goal.

Process
Rehabilitation Team Models

The rehabilitation team consists of, first and foremost, the individual and his or her family. DeLisa et al. (1998) defined the team as "a group of healthcare professionals from different disciplines, who share common values and objectives" (p. 3). Team members contributing to a person's rehabilitation are varied and cross many disciplines (see Figure 1-1). Four models for team functioning have been described: medical, multidisciplinary, interdisciplinary (DeLisa et al., 1998), and transdisciplinary (Mumma &

Figure 1-1. Members of the Rehabilitation Team

Client and family

Nurses

Physiatrists

Other physicians

Physical therapists

Occupational therapists

Speech/language pathologists

Psychologists

Recreational therapists

Vocational therapists

Orthotists

Chaplains

Insurance case managers or representatives

Employers

Teachers

Audiologists

Nutritionists

Home health professionals

Nelson, 1996). In all models, nursing is an integral part of the rehabilitation team.

Medical model: The medical model is a physician-centered model of care in which all care is directed by the physician. This model is not consistent with rehabilitation philosophy or goals, and it is uncommon in rehabilitation practice.

Multidisciplinary model: The multidisciplinary team, which may be seen in rehabilitation, is one in which the professionals work in parallel; each discipline works toward particular client goals, with very little overlap between disciplines. Communication is more vertical than lateral, with the leader controlling team conferences. In a multidisciplinary model, the person working directly with the client does not always participate in team planning; rather, the department managers usually attend team conferences. This model is effective when the team membership is not stable (e.g., when there are different team members for different clients).

Interdisciplinary model: The interdisciplinary model is a matrix-like model in which lateral communication is predominant. This is an effective model when team membership is stable (e.g., in an inpatient rehabilitation unit). Decisions are determined by the group working directly with the client, which means that mutual trust must be established among team members, and conflict resolution is an important skill used by team members. Team goal setting is an important feature of this model.

Transdisciplinary model: A newer team model is the transdisciplinary model, in which the client has a primary provider from the team, who then is guided by the team in caring for the client. For example, the primary provider may be a nurse, who then provides physical, speech, and occupational therapy based on the advice and counsel he or she receives from team members in those disciplines.

Similarly, the primary therapist could be a physical therapist. Mumma and Nelson (1996) noted that this model requires flexibility and receptiveness on the part of team members because individual roles are less distinct. This model also raises many issues regarding licensure and accountability. It may be best suited for situations in which the client is stable and in need of long-term services.

Regardless of the rehabilitation team model, all team members can increase their effectiveness by understanding collaborative practice, group dynamics, conflict resolution, and team functioning. Components necessary for effective team function include trust, knowledge, shared responsibility, mutual respect, communication, cooperation and coordination, and optimism. Effective teams require a commitment from each member.

Provision of Services

The rehabilitation philosophy can infuse any healthcare setting. Collaboration between team members (through any of the team models) and the individual, family, and community is a vital aspect of rehabilitation. Mumma and Nelson (1996) offered a useful categorization of models for provision of services: client centered, setting centered, provider centered, and collaborative. For the purposes of this chapter, a collaborative model (i.e., a team concept) is assumed in all rehabilitation models.

Client-centered care: Client-centered models are those serving specialized populations. The focus may be on a specific developmental stage, such as children or older adults, or on a type of impairment, such as spinal cord or head injury. With a population-specific focus, providers can focus their resources and gain extensive expertise through experience.

Setting-centered care: Acute care, long-term care, outpatient care, home care, and community care are the traditional models focusing on settings. Each describes where rehabilitation takes place. The trend away from inpatient care has accelerated in recent years as a result of changing funding practices. A newer category of setting-focused rehabilitation is subacute care. Subacute/postacute care settings provide rehabilitation to people who continue to need substantial medical care and who are slower to progress. For adults, subacute/postacute care units usually are inpatient settings and often are housed in an acute care, traditional rehabilitation unit or long-term care facility. However, in the pediatric population, subacute/postacute rehabilitation is seen more often in day treatment programs, whereby the children return to home or residential settings at night (Hertzberg & Edwards, 1999).

Provider-centered care: Provider-centered models reflect how healthcare providers have decided to organize the provision of care. Many models have been used over the years, with the goal of maximizing the use of human resources. Within nursing, functional, team, and primary nursing and, more recently, case management have been the models. In functional nursing, the tasks are divided (e.g., one nurse delivers all the medications). In team nursing, a nurse oversees the care of a group of clients by providers of various skill levels. Primary nursing (not to be confused with primary care) became popular in the 1980s as a means of providing client-centered care. One nurse provides direct total care to a group of clients and is responsible for planning and coordinating that care when he or she is not on duty. This model spawned several variations. Primary nursing has coordinated, client-centered care as its goal, similar to case management.

Case management, though not a new concept in nursing and health care, is a common provider-centered model within rehabilitation. In this model, the goal is to provide high-quality, individualized, cost-effective care through an ongoing process of assessment, planning, implementing, coordinating, and evaluating care and services (Youngblood, 1999). Because of nursing's holistic focus, nurses are ideal case managers; however, they do not always assume this role. Although theoretically the case manager is the client advocate, it is important to recognize to whom the case manager is accountable (e.g., the insurance company, the hospital).

In the rehabilitation field, no single model dominates, and several models coexist. For example, a case management system may be operating within a subacute/postacute pediatric day treatment program. As health care continues to evolve, new models of providing services undoubtedly will emerge, and nurses are in an important position to lead the way.

Rehabilitation Nursing Perspectives
Nursing's Focus and Core Values

Nursing brings a unique, holistic focus to rehabilitation. Whereas members of other disciplines treat particular aspects of a person, nurses focus on the person as a whole, thus providing continuity and integrity to the client's rehabilitation experience.

Fawcett (1984) defined the central foci (or the metaparadigm) of nursing as person, health, environment, and nursing. The individual's philosophical view of these concepts is the foundation for how he or she approaches nursing care. The core values of rehabilitation as an interdisciplinary practice are congruent with those of nursing.

As a profession, nursing has stated its ethical foundation in the *Code of Ethics for Nurses* (American Nurses Association [ANA], 2001).

Rehabilitation nursing arises as a specialty practice from the nursing discipline. Values and assumptions for the discipline are explicated in *Nursing's Social Policy Statement* (ANA, 2003, p. 3):
- Humans manifest an essential unity of mind, body, and spirit.
- Human experience is contextually and culturally defined.
- Health and illness are human experiences. The presence of illness does not preclude health, nor does optimal health preclude illness.
- The relationship between nurse and patient involves both in the process of care.
- The interaction between the nurse and the patient occurs within the context of the values and beliefs of the patient and the nurse.

Rehabilitation nursing, as a specialty of the nursing discipline at large, embraces these values and further explicates its core values, which include the following (ARN, 2000, p. 4):

- Individuals with functional limitations have intrinsic worth that transcends their disability and/or chronic illness.
- Individuals are complex yet unified, whole persons who have the right and the responsibility to make informed decisions about their future.
- Individuals may benefit from rehabilitation nursing at any stage of the lifespan.

Definition of Rehabilitation Nursing

Rehabilitation nursing is defined as "the diagnosis and treatment of human responses of individuals and groups to actual or potential health problems relative to altered functional ability and lifestyle" (ARN, 2000, p. 4). This is congruent with the ANA (1980) definition of nursing: "the diagnosis and treatment of human responses to actual or potential health threats." Rehabilitation nursing interventions, in promoting maximal health, promote the client's quality of life. Explicitly essential and inherent in achieving this goal is collaboration with the client, his or her significant others, and other healthcare providers. Rehabilitation nursing is client centered, goal oriented, and outcome based.

Nursing Science as a Basis for Rehabilitation Nursing Practice: Philosophical Worldviews

Nursing's body of knowledge—its science—derives from the relationship between practice, theory, and research with respect to the focus of the discipline (i.e., the metaparadigm). The metaparadigm concepts provide the focus of nursing, and nursing models provide the context. These models or frameworks provide a lens through which nursing phenomena are viewed and thus reveal how to approach nursing care. What is common to all nursing models is the holistic view of human beings (see Table 1-1).

Whereas core values undergird all nursing models, philosophical worldviews shape the development of metaparadigm concepts in the models. They provide a broad understanding of the models in which the metaparadigm concepts are explicated. Although many categorizations of worldviews exist, Fawcett (1995) offered a synthesis of three categories:

- **Reaction:** The person is seen as the sum of parts (e.g., biological, psychological, sociological, spiritual) and responds to external stimuli in a linear, causal way. Change is predictable and necessary for survival. Nursing models do not mirror this view; however, it can be seen, for example, in B.F. Skinner's behaviorism model and in the germ theory model.
- **Reciprocal interaction:** Human beings are holistic, not reducible to parts, and in reciprocal interaction with the environment. Although the parts are not reducible, they are recognized and seen only in context of the whole. Change is the result of multiple factors in the person and the environment and is probabilistic, though not entirely predictable. Examples of this view in nursing theory include King's (1981, 1995) Systems Framework, Orem's (1995) Self-Care Framework, and Hall's (1964, 1969) Core, Cure, and Care Model.
- **Simultaneous action:** Human beings are more than and different from the sum of their parts. They are seen as unitary, irreducible, and known by patterns of behavior. Change is continuous, moving into an ever more complex organization, and is unpredictable. A nursing example of this worldview is Rogers's (1970, 1992) Science of Unitary Human Beings.

Table 1-1. Comparison of Selected Nursing Models

Principle	Hall	King	Orem	Rogers
Person	A unity of 3 interrelated parts: the person (core), disease and treatment (cure), and body (care); people strive for their own goals, and behavior is directed more by feelings than by knowledge.	An open system; a social, rational, and sentient being; major concepts include perception, self, growth and development, body image, time, and space.	A unity, functioning biologically, symbolically, and socially, who values self-care.	A unitary human being who cannot separate from environment knowledge.
Health	A behavior; achieves maximum potential through learning, particularly about oneself.	Dynamic life experiences, adjusting to stressors; ability to function in social roles.	A wholeness of body and mind; integrated.	Individually defined; an expression of the life process.
Nursing	A teacher and nurturer: By understanding the three aspects of a person, the nurse helps the client understand goals and motivation. Nursing should be provided by professional nurses.	An interactive endeavor in which the nurse and client share perceptions and mutually identify goals and means to reach those goals.	A helping profession in which nurses help others meet therapeutic self-care demands.	A learned profession; a science and art of promoting health.

Nursing Models That Guide Practice

Nursing models are frameworks that guide practice and research. Within the models are theories, which propose relationships between concepts. The nurses who developed the models and theories are called nursing theorists. These theorists drew from existing knowledge in nursing and other disciplines. For example, nursing theorists have drawn from general system theory (e.g., King), adaptation theory (e.g., Roy), learning and motivational theories (e.g., Hall), various developmental theories, and even physics (e.g., Rogers). Theorists incorporate their knowledge of existing theories with their nursing knowledge and perspectives to create models and theories that are unique to nursing. So whereas nursing is a discipline within the larger community of scientific disciplines in which knowledge is shared, this knowledge is applied in nursing situations with a nursing perspective.

One discipline with which nursing is intimately involved is medicine, and at times nurses may confuse nursing knowledge with medical knowledge. Of course, it is important for nurses to understand disease processes, but their goal is different from that of medical specialists. The question nurses must ask is, "Why do nurses need to know this?" The answer differs from that of the originating discipline. By using nursing models to guide practice, nurses can gain a clear understanding of their discipline and its unique contribution to health care in general and rehabilitation in particular. When nurses have a clear understanding of their discipline, its role, and the differences from other disciplines, they can confidently assume leadership roles in rehabilitation. Practicing nursing from a nursing model perspective provides that clear understanding.

In addition to grand theories that guide nursing practice globally, there are a group of theories that are known as mid-range theories. These theories are used to explain particular phenomena and are testable, including a limited number of variables, but are sufficiently general to be useful for practice and research (Walker & Avant, 1995, p. 11).

All of the nursing models have a holistic focus, and therefore all are appropriate to guide rehabilitation nursing practice. Nurses can make individual choices about their preferred nursing model, depending on their own philosophy of nursing. Rehabilitation nurses are encouraged to first consult an overview of nursing models and theories (e.g., Tomey & Alligood, 2001) to find one that resonates with their own philosophy and then consult the primary sources of the theory. Selected theorists have been included in this chapter as examples for nursing practice (see Table 1-1), although many others exist. These models were chosen because of their emphasis on interaction with clients and on the importance of setting goals from the client's perspective, both of which are of paramount importance in rehabilitation.

Lydia Hall

Lydia Hall is best known for her work at the Loeb Center at Montefiore Hospital in New York. This was a rehabilitation unit with a primary focus on nursing care. It was a nurse-run

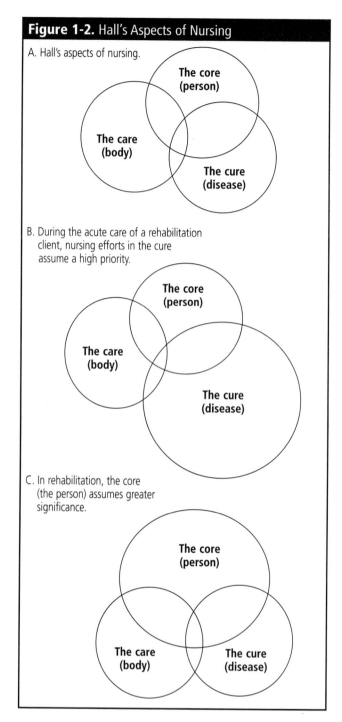

Figure 1-2. Hall's Aspects of Nursing

A. Hall's aspects of nursing.

The core (person)

The care (body)

The cure (disease)

B. During the acute care of a rehabilitation client, nursing efforts in the cure assume a high priority.

The core (person)

The care (body)

The cure (disease)

C. In rehabilitation, the core (the person) assumes greater significance.

The core (person)

The care (body)

The cure (disease)

center; members of other disciplines, including medicine, served in a consultant role to nursing (Alfano, 1988). Hall's theory of nursing provided the framework for the care. Research demonstrated that clients' length of stay was shortened and life satisfaction improved (Pearson, Durand, & Punton, 1988).

Three interlocking circles represent Hall's theory: the person (core), the body (care), and the disease (cure). She asserted that nurses provide different types of care in each circle and different types of care over the course of a person's illness (see Figure 1-2). She further asserted that wholly professional nursing care would hasten recovery.

Hall believed that nursing care should be provided only

by professional nurses. While the person is in the first stage of illness, medical specialists direct the care, with nurses in a supportive role. Nurses assume dominance in the second stage of illness, when the body and person assume greater importance. Her view of health can be inferred from her belief that people achieve their maximum potential through learning; however, because people behave according to their feelings, inattention to the person while teaching will not change his or her behavior. She specified that rehabilitation is a process of learning to live within limitations (Tomey & Alligood, 2001). Therefore, nursing intervenes to facilitate learning not only about physical and mental skills but also about self and one's feelings, behavior, and motivations. Hall was one of the first to assert that setting goals for clients that do not reflect the client's own goals is countertherapeutic.

Clinical application: When a stroke survivor, for example, enters the healthcare system, the cure circle assumes dominance. Nurses assist during the biological crisis, still attending to the person and body. During rehabilitation, the nurse attends to intimate body functions. Through communication, the nurse becomes the therapeutic modality in treating the person. By helping the person explore his or her feelings, behavior, and motivation, the nurse can work with the client to establish goals for rehabilitation. As rehabilitation progresses, the client assumes more responsibility for the body; in the diagrammatic representation of Hall's theory, the circles expand and contract to reflect nursing's relative role.

The nurse's approach to assessment is organized into three areas: the disease (cure), the body (care), and the person (core). The intervention approach, similarly, would be organized around the three aspects of the model. In the disease realm, interventions are primarily medically directed (e.g., administering medications, monitoring biological functions). In the body realm, nurses assist with the bodily functions the person is unable to manage (e.g., elimination). Finally, and most importantly in nursing, is the person. Nurses employ the therapeutic use of self to guide clients into a greater understanding of themselves and to help them achieve their maximal potential through learning. The nurse would focus teaching and learning on the client. For example, the nurse would help the stroke survivor set and continually evaluate goals.

Nurses who are developing a multidisciplinary, interdisciplinary, or transdisciplinary team could use Hall's model as a structure and a process. This, in fact, was how the Loeb Center functioned.

Imogene King

Imogene King (1981) developed a framework for nursing based on system theory and, within this framework, a theory of nursing. Her framework consists of three interacting systems: personal system (an individual), interpersonal system (two or more personal systems), and social systems (social forces) (see Figure 1-3). People, including nurses, function in all three systems. From the interpersonal system, she developed a theory of goal attainment. Mutual goal attainment results from transactions between nurse and client. Both must communicate and understand each other's role to understand each other's perspective of a situation (perceptual congruence). With this understanding, goals can be mutually set, and transactions can occur, resulting in mutual goal attainment (see Figure 1-3). Thus, mutuality achieved through perceptual congruence is the keystone. King's (1981) theory "focuses on goals to be attained in specific nursing situations through participative decision making by nurses and patients" (p. 155).

King (1981) views the person as an open system in interaction with the environment, who is unique, is holistic, and has intrinsic worth. Individuals are capable of making decisions in most situations, and they differ in their needs, wants, and goals. Health is defined as a dynamic life cycle that has different meanings for people and "implies continuous adjustment to stress in the internal and external environment through optimum use of one's resources to achieve maximum potential for daily living" (p. 5).

King (1981) sees nursing as an inherently interactive endeavor in which "nurse and client share information in the nursing situation" (p. 2). Nurses have special knowledge of nursing, and the client has special knowledge of himself or herself. By sharing this knowledge with each other, they can develop goals and the means to achieve those goals. The goal of nursing is "to help individuals maintain their health so they can function in their roles" (p. 4).

Clinical application: When a stroke survivor enters the healthcare system, the nursing assessment focuses on concepts in the personal, interpersonal, and social systems. Perceptual congruence in the assessment is crucial (e.g., does the nurse understand the client, and does the client

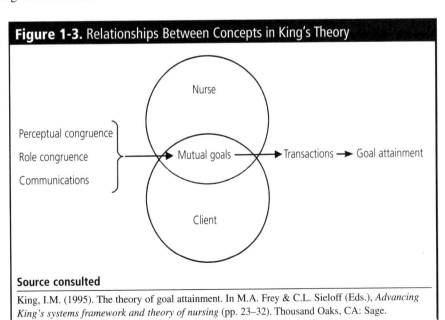

Figure 1-3. Relationships Between Concepts in King's Theory

Perceptual congruence
Role congruence
Communications

Nurse

Mutual goals → Transactions → Goal attainment

Client

Source consulted

King, I.M. (1995). The theory of goal attainment. In M.A. Frey & C.L. Sieloff (Eds.), *Advancing King's systems framework and theory of nursing* (pp. 23–32). Thousand Oaks, CA: Sage.

understand the nurse?). Unless there is communication, perceptual congruence will not occur, and goals will not be met. Communication occurs in many ways, and goal setting is not necessarily a formalized procedure. For example, the stroke survivor may communicate his or her fear of this bewildering event entirely nonverbally. The nurse validates his or her perception of the client's experience and uses special knowledge (of nursing) to reassure and comfort the client. The goal for the client is perhaps to receive reassurance, comfort, and information, whereas the nurse's goal is to provide that reassurance, comfort, and information. Because the client is a personal system embedded within interpersonal and social systems, the context of the client's life is vital. For many stroke survivors, explicit goals that extend beyond moment-to-moment care often are difficult to negotiate. In these cases, the nurse may set goals with the client's significant others, using the best data available. As the client progresses, he or she can be more active in setting goals. It is important to note that goal setting is not a one-time event but rather an ongoing process.

Goal attainment based on mutuality of all participants is process oriented. King's theory of goal attainment, though originally meant for nurse–client interactions, also provides a firm foundation on which nurses can build an effective interdisciplinary team.

Dorothea E. Orem

Dorothea Orem (1995) sees self-care as essential for health, well-being, and life itself. Orem's model focuses on individuals' self-care needs or demands (self-care requisites) and the ability of the person to meet those needs (self-care agency). The three groups of self-care requisites (universal, developmental, health deviation) are influenced by conditioning factors. Self-care agency is one's ability to meet these self-care requisites. When self-care requisites exceed self-care agency, nursing may intervene (see Figure 1-4).

Orem views health as a state of wholeness or integrity, and nurses design systems to facilitate this state. Nursing systems are action systems in which nurses design care. These include wholly compensatory, partly compensatory, and supportive–educative systems. Orem's theory specifically recognizes that clients may depend on others outside the healthcare system to meet self-care demands. Those who fulfill the responsibility to assist with the self-care agency of another are called dependent care agents.

Clinical application: When a stroke survivor enters the healthcare system, the nurse assesses the person's self-care requisites and self-care agency. The stroke increases the person's self-care requisites while decreasing the person's self-care agency. In the acute care

setting, a wholly compensatory nursing system may be most appropriate. As the person begins rehabilitation, the nurse uses a partially compensatory system and begins to form a supportive–educative system. As rehabilitation progresses, a supportive–educative system assumes primacy. During rehabilitation, the focus of the supportive–educative system may be a dependent care agent, such as a spouse.

Martha Rogers

Martha Rogers's Science of Unitary Human Beings theory focuses on "people and their worlds in a pandimensional universe" (Rogers, 1992, p. 29). Human beings are viewed as unified wholes, not parts. In this model, the human and the environment are energy fields that are inextricably intertwined and are irreducible—essentially, a unitary field. Rogers calls this concept integrality. People therefore are always viewed in the context of the environment, never separate from it. People are known by patterns, which are manifestations of the whole.

Change is fundamental to life; it is unidirectional, increasingly complex, and creative. This means that one never repeats patterns but rather continues to grow. "Each repatterning is a revision of the immediately preceding pattern" (Rogers, 1970, p. 98). For example, if a person vacations at the same location each year, and if all the elements of the vacation remain the same, it is still a different experience that has built on previous experience. In this model, the notion of a person returning to (as near as is possible) his or her previous existence is rejected because change is unidirectional and increasingly complex. After rehabilitation, the person has grown or developed into a more complex person than his or her previous existence.

Rogers's theory does not specifically define *health* but

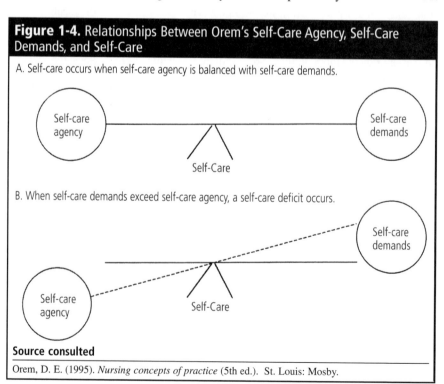

Figure 1-4. Relationships Between Orem's Self-Care Agency, Self-Care Demands, and Self-Care

A. Self-care occurs when self-care agency is balanced with self-care demands.

Self-care agency — Self-Care — Self-care demands

B. When self-care demands exceed self-care agency, a self-care deficit occurs.

Self-care agency — Self-Care — Self-care demands

Source consulted

Orem, D. E. (1995). *Nursing concepts of practice* (5th ed.). St. Louis: Mosby.

views *health* as a value-laden term imposed by society. It is not the opposite of illness, but as with illness, health is an expression of the life process. Rogers's view of nursing is that of knowing rather than doing; in other words, nursing is an abstract body of knowledge. She describes nursing as a learned profession, with the goal of promoting health and well-being. Human beings have the capacity to knowingly participate in change, which is creative and innovative, and nurses help people knowingly participate in change.

Clinical application: The nurse assesses the stroke survivor entering the healthcare system through a pattern appraisal. Gordon's (1987) functional health pattern model as a means of client assessment is particularly well suited to Rogers' model because it offers a holistic assessment of a person's interrelated patterns and therefore manifestations of the whole. Gordon's functional health patterns are useful for nursing assessments in most nursing models, and, in fact, all nursing diagnoses can be grouped under the various patterns (Carpenito-Monet, 2006). In Rogers's model, dissonance in patterns is identified. Nursing interventions focusing on the dissonance aim to help the person with patterning to achieve resonance. For example, if the pattern appraisal reveals a dissonance in urinary and bowel elimination, the nurse facilitates harmonious patterning in establishing new toileting routines, using data regarding past patterns.

Many nursing models and theories are useful in nursing practice. What distinguishes nursing models from those in other disciplines is their holistic focus. All of the models see clinical situations from a different perspective. It can be argued that if a clinical situation cannot be framed in a nursing model, then perhaps it is not a situation that is suited for nursing. Rehabilitation nurses are urged to explore nursing models (using primary sources) to find one that is congruent with their philosophy of nursing. Practicing from a conceptual or theoretical base is an important aspect of professional practice, and it reinforces nursing's unique contributions to health care.

In all nursing endeavors, the client is at the center. Nursing models and theories can be used not only in the direct provision of care but also in the design of nursing care delivery systems (e.g., Hall's model). Rehabilitation is inherently a team concept, and any model for care delivery systems must begin with this premise.

Nursing Research to Guide Practice

Research is necessary to provide a scientific foundation and to establish accountability for professional nursing practice. Health care in general, and nursing in particular, is becoming increasingly complex and costly; these trends place increasing demands on nursing care to be validated through systematic study.

The word *research* means simply "to search again." Scientific nursing research is the systematic study of phenomena that are of interest to nursing for the purposes of validating existing knowledge or developing new knowledge. Research allows nurses to understand phenomena (through qualitative research) and to describe, explain, predict, and ultimately control events (through quantitative research).

Nurses in all areas and levels of practice have an important role in research. The ANA (1989) delineated the levels of nurses' involvement in research. Nurses with associate degrees can help identify research problems, assist with data collection, and use findings in practice with supervision. Nurses who have baccalaureates must be able to access and evaluate research for use in practice. Master's-level nurses create the environment in which research and its use are fostered, collaborate with experienced investigators, and provide the clinical expertise needed for research. Doctoral and postdoctoral nurses develop nursing knowledge through research and theory development with funded research.

The Rehabilitation Nursing Foundation has developed the Rehabilitation Nursing Research Agenda (RNRA) (1995, 2005) to guide research in rehabilitation nursing. The RNRA is an outline of four areas of inquiry: nursing and nursing-led interdisciplinary interventions to promote function in people of all ages with disability or chronic health problems, experience of disability or chronic health problems for individuals and families across the lifespan, rehabilitation in the changing healthcare system, and the rehabilitation nursing profession. Evidence-based practice is an example of research-driven clinical practices.

ARN's *Standards and Scope of Rehabilitation Nursing Practice* (2000) reinforce the ANA's recommendations for professional rehabilitation nurses. These standards state that a research attitude (i.e., one of systematic searching) is important in all aspects of care. Whether by identifying particular problems in rehabilitation, using the research literature to determine practice approaches, or systematically evaluating nursing practices, nurses can use research to play an important role. Research should be considered an integral aspect of professional decision making.

A growing number of nurses practicing rehabilitation nursing are prepared at the doctoral level to be nurse researchers. These nurses are educated at universities and receive the doctorate of philosophy (PhD) or doctorate of nursing science (DNSc). These nurses are engaged in expanding and disseminating nursing knowledge through research and teaching.

The Specialty Practice Of Rehabilitation Nursing

The ARN and ANA both view rehabilitation nursing as a specialty practice. ARN's standards (2000) outline the scope of practice, standards of care, and standards of professional performance. The Rehabilitation Nursing Foundation (RNF, 1994) outlined specific competencies in a separate manual. ARN now offers a Competencies Assessment Tool (ARN-CAT) online that tests knowledge in 14 basic rehabilitation nursing competency areas and also includes both pediatric and geriatric questions.

Professional rehabilitation practice is guided by philosophy, theory, and research and therefore can be practiced in any setting. When the client is at the center of care, and the goals are to optimize health (however it is defined) and to improve the quality of life for those with disability or chronic disease, the boundaries of the healthcare system become less important. Instead, what assumes importance are the client's and his or her significant others' goals to reintegrate their lives. Practice settings for rehabilitation nursing may include the home, work settings, insurance companies, community centers, residential centers, day care centers, clinics, skilled care facilities, inpatient rehabilitation centers, subacute/postacute units, and acute care facilities.

Role Responsibilities
Professional Rehabilitation Nursing

The American Association of Colleges of Nursing (AACN, 1998) described the following role responsibilities for generalist nursing practice. They are discussed here in relation to rehabilitation nursing practice.

- **Provider of care:** The nurse "uses theory and research-based knowledge in the direct and indirect delivery of care . . . in the formation of partnerships with clients and the interdisciplinary health care team" (p. 16). Particular roles in rehabilitation with these responsibilities include caregiver, client advocate, client educator, counselor, nurse practitioner, expert witness, and researcher.

- **Designer, manager, and coordinator of care:** The nurse needs skills such as communication, collaboration, negotiation, delegation, coordination, and evaluation of interdisciplinary work. These are particularly important skills for rehabilitation nurses, who are team members or leaders. Rehabilitation roles fulfilling these responsibilities include care manager, case manager, consultant, administrator or manager, and clinical nurse specialist. Designing and coordinating care becomes increasingly important in nursing as healthcare systems use various skilled and semiskilled workers in direct care. Additionally, nurses are in a key position to provide leadership in the coordination of care across disciplines.

- **Member of a profession:** Professionals have a responsibility to value lifelong learning, identify with the profession's values, and incorporate professionalism into practice. Client advocacy is an important aspect of professional rehabilitation practice, and although this is an integral aspect of everyday practice, advocacy assumes a particularly important role in a larger societal sense. Rehabilitation nurses are responsible for helping shape public policy in such endeavors as dismantling societal barriers to people with disabilities and educating the public to prevent disease and trauma. Although many of these role opportunities already exist, many more roles could be developed by creative and entrepreneurial nurses. In today's dynamic healthcare system, nurses have the opportunity to develop unique nursing roles that will meet the goals of rehabilitation.

Advanced Practice Nursing

Advanced practice nursing is defined as "the application of an expanded range of practical, theoretical, and research-based competencies to phenomena experienced by patients within a specialized clinical area of the larger discipline of nursing" (Hamric, 2005, p. 89). There are four recognized types of advanced practice nurses: nurse practitioners (NPs), clinical nurse specialists (CNSs), certified nurse midwives (CMWs), and certified nurse anesthetists (CNAs). The AACN (1996) identified the essential focus of all advanced practice nurse roles as clinical. Although nurse educators and administrators may be educated at an advanced level, they do not meet the definition of advanced practice nursing because their primary focus is not clinical practice. According to Hamric (2005), the core competencies of advanced practice nurses include the following:

- Expert guidance and coaching of patients, families, and other care providers
- Consultation
- Research skills
- Clinical and professional leadership, including competence as a change agent
- Collaboration
- Ethical decision-making skills

Educational Preparation
Practical Nursing

Licensed practical nurses (LPNs) generally are educated in programs requiring 9 to 14 months of study. These nurses are taught many skills but do not have the same depth of knowledge as registered nurses. Under the supervision of a registered nurse, LPNs participate in direct and indirect nursing care, health maintenance, teaching, counseling, collaborative planning, and rehabilitation, to the extent of their basic and continuing education.

Professional Rehabilitation Nursing

Registered nurses (RNs) are prepared at the associate degree (AS) and bachelor's degree (BS) levels. Although both AS- and BS-prepared nurses are licensed as registered nurses, the BS has long been recommended as the entry level for professional practice. A baccalaureate degree better prepares practitioners for the high level of flexibility necessary as health care becomes increasingly sophisticated and provides a basis for practitioners to participate in, evaluate, and use research findings as greater evidence is needed to support practice. Therefore, a baccalaureate is important for specialty practice.

Advanced Practice Rehabilitation Nursing

Rehabilitation nurses in advanced practice usually are educated as CNSs and NPs. These people are prepared for advanced practice in programs offering either a master's degree or a doctorate. The master's degree has been the standard degree for the advanced practice nurse for many years. Recently a new degree, the doctorate of nursing practice (DNP), has been approved by the AACN as the entry level for advanced practice nurses as of 2015. The approval and subsequent guidelines for this degree are a result of the increasing complexity and required knowledge for advanced practice nurses (AACN, 2004).

Licensure

All nurses must be licensed by the state in which they practice. People who want to take the licensure exam for LPNs or RNs may do so after they have successfully completed an accredited nursing program. Licensure for advanced practice nurses varies from state to state. In general, a person wanting to obtain licensure as an advanced practice nurse must be an RN; have completed an approved educational program of advanced practice leading to an MS, DNP, or other approved degree; and meet the specific guidelines for licensure in the state in which they want to become licensed. Advanced practice licensure often relies on certification as an advanced practice nurse in the desired specialty area.

Certification

Certification is professional recognition of skills in a specialty practice. Certification programs are developed and maintained by professional nursing organizations such as the ANA or ARN. Certification in rehabilitation nursing is a means of validating specialized knowledge and skills and displays a sense of accountability to the public. Certification programs exist in many specialties for RNs and advanced practice nurses. There are no certification programs for LPNs.

Certified Rehabilitation Registered Nurse: At the RN level of practice, the ARN has developed and maintains a certification program in rehabilitation nursing. ARN's standards (2000) do not mandate which type of basic, professional nursing preparation (AS or BS) is necessary for generalist practice or certification. The Rehabilitation Nursing Certification Board (RNCB), a subsidiary of ARN, offered its first certification examination in 1984. Those who meet the criteria and pass the exam earn the certified rehabilitation registered nurse (CRRN) credential. As of 2007, nearly 10,000 nurses held the CRRN credential.

Advanced Certification

The RNCB offered certification at the advanced level for the first time in 2001. Because of changes in the certification standards and a very small number of people sitting for the examination, the advanced CRRN (CRRN-A) program was suspended in 2005. The CRRN-A credential will be phased out by 2009.

Advanced practice nurses working in rehabilitation setting are certified at the professional level as CRRNs and then advanced certification in a particular area of advanced practice as a clinical specialist or NP.

Competencies

The specialty practice of rehabilitation nursing has a defined area of competence within nursing. The ARN-CAT is offered free online and provides assessment of basic competencies in the following areas: autonomic dysfunction, bowel and bladder function, communication, disability/adjustment to disability/grieving, dysphagia, gerontology, musculoskeletal/body mechanics/functional transfer techniques, neuropathophysiology (CVA, SCI, TBI) and functional neuro assessment, pain, patient/family education, pediatrics, rehabilitation, sexuality and disability, skin and wound care. The ARN-CAT give multiple choice questions in each category and instant results of scoring, along with rationales for correct answers. Competencies provide accountability and standards of practice for the specialty. This new online tool can assist nurse managers and supervisors to evaluate the proficiency of staff nurses.

Professional Associations

Associations have played a crucial role in the development of nursing as a profession. They establish standards of practice and control policies and activities of nursing practice. To regulate its own practice is a hallmark of a profession, and professional nursing associations ensure that nurses control nursing practice. Being a member of a profession entails belonging to professional organizations. Associations provide nurses with a voice and with information in the form of newsletters, books, journals, educational conferences, and other resources.

The ANA is the primary voice for professional nurses. Professional rehabilitation nurses should also belong to the ARN, the specialty organization for rehabilitation nurses. The ARN's purpose is "to promote and advance professional rehabilitation nursing practice through education, advocacy, collaboration, and research to enhance the quality of life for those affected by disability and chronic illness" (ARN, 2007). Other professional associations that may be of interest to rehabilitation nurses include the American Association of Spinal Cord Injury Nurses, the National Geriatric Nursing Association (NGNA), the National Association of Directors of Nursing Administration (NADONA), the American Society of Pain Management Nurses, the Association of Nurses in AIDS Care, the Developmental Disabilities Nurses Association, and the National Association of Orthopedic Nurses.

Resources

In this information age, resources are readily available to all nurses. The Cumulative Index of Nursing and Allied Health Literature (CINAHL) can be accessed electronically through libraries that subscribe to the service. Interlibrary loans provide articles that are not locally available. Also, Medline is available, free of charge, through the Internet. Other electronic databases of interest to nurses are PsychLit and the Education Resources Information Center (ERIC). Nearly all professional associations have Web sites, and most have links to many other relevant sites. The ability to access information in a timely manner is a skill that all nurses must master in order to provide competent, evidence-based care to rehabilitation clients. [Refer to Chapter 21 for more on information technology and computer applications.]

References

Alfano, G. (1988). A different kind of nursing. *Nursing Outlook, 36*, 34–37.

American Association of Colleges of Nursing (AACN). (1996). *The essentials of master's education for advanced practice nursing.* Washington, DC: Author.

American Association of Colleges of Nursing (AACN). (1998). *The essentials of baccalaureate education for professional nursing practice.* Washington, DC: Author.

American Association of Colleges of Nursing (AACN). (2004). *AACN position statement on the practice doctorate in nursing.* Retrieved November 26, 2006, from http://www.aacn.nche.edu/DNP/pdf/DNP.pdf

American Nurses Association (ANA). (1989). *Education for participation in nursing research.* Kansas City, MO: Author.

American Nurses Association (ANA). (2001). *The code of ethics for nurses with interpretive statements.* Washington, DC: Author.

American Nurses Association (ANA). (2003). *Nursing's social policy statement.* Kansas City, MO: Author.

Association of Rehabilitation Nurses (ARN). (2000). *Standards and scope of rehabilitation nursing practice* (4th ed.). Skokie, IL: Author.

Association of Rehabilitation Nurses (ARN). (2007). *Mission statement.* Retrieved March 27, 2007, from http://www.rehabnurse.org/about/index.html

Carpenito-Monet, L.J. (2006). *Nursing diagnosis. Application to clinical practice* (11th ed.). Philadelphia: Lippincott Williams & Wilkins.

DeLisa, J.A., Currie, D.M., & Martin, G.M. (1998). *Rehabilitation medicine: Past, present, and future.* In J.A. DeLisa & B.M. Gans (Eds.), *Rehabilitation medicine: Principles and practice* (pp. 3–32). Philadelphia: Lippincott-Raven.

Fawcett, J. (1984). The metaparadigm of nursing: Current status and future refinements. *Image: The Journal of Nursing Scholarship, 16*, 84–87.

Fawcett, J. (1995). *Analysis and evaluation of conceptual models of nursing* (3rd ed.). Philadelphia: F.A. Davis.

Gordon, M. (1987). *Nursing diagnosis: Process and application* (2nd ed.). St. Louis: McGraw-Hill.

Hall, L.E. (1964). Nursing: What is it? *Canadian Nurse, 60*, 150–154.

Hall, L.E. (1969). The Loeb Center for Nursing Rehabilitation. *International Journal Nursing Studies, 6*, 81–95.

Hamric, A. (2005). A definition of advanced practice nursing. In A.B. Hamric, J.A. Spross, & C.M. Hanson (Eds.), *Advanced practice nursing: An integrative approach* (3rd ed., pp. 85–108). Philadelphia: Elsevier Saunders.

Hertzberg, D., & Edwards, P.A. (1999). Introduction to pediatric rehabilitation nursing. In P.A. Edwards, D.L. Hertzberg, S.R. Hays, & N.M. Youngblood (Eds.), *Pediatric rehabilitation nursing* (pp. 3–19). Philadelphia: W.B. Saunders.

King, I.M. (1981). *A theory for nursing: Systems, concepts, process.* Albany, NY: Delmar.

King, I.M. (1995). The theory of goal attainment. In M.A. Frey & C.L. Sieloff (Eds.), *Advancing King's systems framework and theory of nursing* (pp. 23–32). Thousand Oaks, CA: Sage.

Kirby, R.L. (1998). Impairment, disability and handicap. In J.A. DeLisa & B.M. Gans (Eds.), *Rehabilitation medicine: Principles and practice* (pp. 55–60). Philadelphia: Lippincott-Raven.

Lyons, A.S., & Petrucelli, R.J. (1978). *Medicine: An illustrated history.* New York: Harry N. Abrams, Inc.

Mumma, C.M., & Nelson, A. (1996). Models for theory-based practice of rehabilitation nursing. In S.P. Hoeman (Ed.), *Rehabilitation nursing. Process and application* (2nd ed., pp. 21–31). St. Louis: Mosby.

Orem, D.E. (1995). *Nursing concepts of practice* (5th ed.). St. Louis: Mosby.

Pearson, A., Durand, I., & Punton, S. (1988). The feasibility and effectiveness of nursing beds. *Nursing Times, 84*(47), 48–50.

Rehabilitation Nursing Foundation (RNF). (1994). *Basic competencies for rehabilitation nursing practice.* Skokie, IL: Author.

Rogers, M.E. (1970). *An introduction to the theoretical basis of nursing.* Philadelphia: F.A. Davis.

Rogers, M.E. (1992). Nursing science and the space age. *Nursing Science Quarterly, 5*, 27–34.

Tomey, A.M. & Alligood, M.R. (2001). *Nursing theorists and their work* (5th ed.). St. Louis: Mosby.

Walker, L.O., & Avant, K.C. (1995). *Strategies for theory construction in nursing* (3rd ed.). Appleton and Lange, Norwalk, CT.

Watson, P. G. (2000). The Americans with Disabilities Act: More rights for people with disabilities. *Rehabilitation Nursing, 25*(4), 145–149.

World Book. (1997). *World Book encyclopedia.* Chicago: Author.

Youngblood, N.M. (1999). Models for practice and service. In P.A. Edwards, D.L. Hertzberg, S. R. Hays, & N.M. Youngblood (Eds.), *Pediatric rehabilitation nursing* (pp. 113–126). Philadelphia: W.B. Saunders.

Suggested Resources

Alligood, M.R., & Marriner-Tomey, A. (Eds.). (2000). *Nursing theory: Utilization and application.* St. Louis: Mosby.

Davidson, A.W., & Young, C. (1985). Repatterning of stroke rehabilitation clients following return to life in the community. *Journal of Neurosurgical Nursing, 17*, 123–128.

Edwards, P.A., Hertzberg, D.L., Hays, S.R., & Youngblood, N.M. (Eds.). (1999). *Pediatric rehabilitation nursing.* Philadelphia: W.B. Saunders.

Folden, S.L. (1993). Effects of a supportive educative nursing intervention on older adults' perceptions of self-care after stroke. *Rehabilitation Nursing, 18*, 162–167.

Hoeman, S.P. (Ed.). (2002). *Rehabilitation nursing. Process and application, and outcomes* (3rd ed.). St. Louis: Mosby.

Smith, D.W. (1995). Power and spirituality in polio survivors: A study based on Rogers' science. *Nursing Science Quarterly, 8*, 133–139.

Taylor, S.G. (1990). Nursing practice applications of self-care deficit nursing theory. In M. Parker (Ed.), *Nursing theories in practice* (pp. 61–70). New York: National League for Nursing.

Temple, A., & Fawdry, K. (1992). King's theory of goal attainment: Resolving filial caregiving role strain. *Journal of Gerontological Nursing, 18*, 11–15.

Woods, E.C. (1994). King's theory in practice with elders. *Nursing Science Quarterly, 7*, 65–69.

Chapter 2

Community and Family-Centered Rehabilitation Nursing

Bonnie J. Parker, MSN RN CRRN • Leslie Neal-Boylan, PhD RNC CRRN FNP-C

As the healthcare profession continues to strive for a balance between quality of care and fiscal responsibility, the emphasis of care delivery will continue to move toward a community focus. Healthcare professionals are accepting this shift and recognizing that communities support and nurture the health of individuals. With this recognition comes the realization that structures must be in place to support these relationships. The family provides the nucleus of the community support structure. As a result, rehabilitation nurses must focus on understanding family and the relationships that exist for rehabilitation clients. Providing education and training to address weaknesses and maximize strengths is an integral part of the rehabilitation process. The rehabilitation team process draws on the expertise of many people to provide a plan to meet the needs of clients and families and to promote health in the community.

I. Overview

A. Definitions of Community

1. A community is a group of people living in the same area and under the same government (Webster's American Family Dictionary, 1999, p. 163).

2. Community is a complex concept that refers to individuals in the context of an environment and the relationships between them.

   a. A community is an ever-changing system that responds to input and output, which can occur at any time.

   b. The reciprocal nature of the relationships between individuals and their community greatly affects health. For example, just as family members function in specific roles to serve the family, a community functions in roles such as caregiver, nurturer, and sustainer (Klainberg, Holzemer, Leonard, & Arnold, 1998) to serve the people who reside within it.

   c. The needs of a healthy community can be viewed in terms of Maslow's hierarchy of individuals' needs (Table 2-1).

3. A community involves "people, location, and social systems" (Hunt, 2005).

B. Theory of Community Nursing

1. Margaret Newman's (1994) theory focuses on community and family-centered rehabilitation nursing.

2. Newman (1994) views the meaning of life and health in terms of "an evolving process

Table 2-1. Maslow's Hierarchy of Individuals' Needs as Compared to Community Needs	
Individual Needs	**Community Needs**
Self-actualization	Community actualization
Esteem	Community pride
Belongingness	Educational preparation
Safety	Security
Physiological needs	Life-sustaining activities
Source consulted	

Klainberg, M., Holzemer, S., Leonard, M., & Arnold, J. (1998). *Community health nursing: An alliance for health.* St. Louis: McGraw-Hill Nursing Core Series.

of expanding consciousness" (p. xxiv).

3. "The pattern of the whole contains the individual as an open system interacting with the family as an open system interacting with the community as an open system. The previous assumptions apply also when focusing on the community. Health of the community is conceptualized in terms of changing patterns of energy in the evolution of the system. A pattern of disease endemic to a community can be considered a manifestation of the pattern of the community health. The diversity and quality of interaction within the community and between the community and its larger environment are indicators of the level of consciousness and thus of the health of the community" (Newman, 1994, pp. 28–29).

   a. Health and illness are viewed as different patterns in the life of the individual as opposed to a dichotomy or continuum.

b. Disease and chronic illness are manifestations of health.

c. Changes in the health status of an individual or family result in changes in the pattern as related to the whole community.

d. The problem with trying to separate views of health and illness is that it becomes more than just a useful way of thinking; it becomes reality. For example, our language promotes the idea that one object can act on another (e.g., "the person had a stroke" or "the person sustained a spinal cord injury").

e. If health is viewed as encompassing disease and nondisease states, health can be considered just one of the underlying patterns of the person and environment.

4. Rehabilitation nursing as a specialty practice meshes with Newman's concept of community-based nursing practice.

5. The Neal theory of home health nursing practice (Neal, 1998, 1999)

a. In the practice of community-centered care, nurses proceed through a three-stage process toward autonomy in the role.

b. Nurses enter community care at Stage 1: dependence on others for help with the clinical and logistical aspects of community-centered care.

c. Nurses move into Stage 2 of community-centered nursing when they are moderately dependent. Nurses are able to manage clinical aspects of care but still need help with office procedures, reimbursement issues, and factors that restrict their autonomy.

d. After approximately 2 years, the nurse moves into Stage 3 and feels autonomous with regard to the logistical and clinical aspects of community-centered nursing.

e. The ability to adapt is necessary to move through the stages.

f. The nurse moves through the stages as time, experience, and confidence grow.

g. Factors that temporarily restrict the nurse's autonomy between Stage 2 and Stage 3 are office procedures, conflicts with the physician, unfamiliar clinical situations, and anyone or anything that affects the patient's care.

h. Factors that temporarily restrict the nurse's autonomy between Stage 1 and

Stage 3 are role changes and process changes.

C. Principles of Community-Based Rehabilitation Care

1. Self-care (client and family responsibility)

a. The client and family retain primary responsibility for healthcare decisions.

b. Empowering the client through education allows him or her to make informed healthcare choices about issues such as advance directives and living wills.

2. Emphasis on the client achieving goals to improve quality of life

a. Goal development may be short term, long term, or lifelong.

b. Importance is placed on goals being mutually developed by the client, the family, and the nurse.

c. Goals are developed in the context of the client's community.

3. Preventive care

a. "Treatment efficacy rather than technologic imperative promotes nursing care that emphasizes prevention" (Hunt & Zurek, 1997, p. 18).

b. Community-based rehabilitation primarily involves tertiary prevention (e.g., teaching a client with spinal cord injury [SCI] about skin care to prevent pressure ulcers).

4. Care in the context of the community

a. The nurse recognizes that the health of the client and family is linked to the health of the community.

b. Nursing care considers culture, values, and available resources.

c. The community's location and social systems influence care. Location often determines eligibility for healthcare resources; therefore, access to and availability of services can affect the health of the community (Hunt, 2005). For example, a client with a stroke may need outpatient rehabilitation services that he or she cannot continue to receive after discharge because the rehabilitation facility is located 150 miles from the client's home.

5. Continuity of care

a. Acute care nursing services typically are episodic (i.e., treatment is rendered for a specific disease or condition for a short period of time).

b. Community-based rehabilitation is marked by the continuity of care that the client experiences as he or she moves from one healthcare setting to another.

c. "Continuity is the glue that holds community-based nursing care together" (Hunt & Zurek, 1997, p. 20).

6. Collaborative care

a. Collaborative care, which is a hallmark of rehabilitation nursing, is a basic tenet of community-based care.

b. All members of the healthcare team should work with the client and family to achieve goals. Each team member should focus on the overall goals of the client and family.

c. The team may use an interdisciplinary model, a transdisciplinary model, or an interagency model. [Refer to Chapter 1 for more on rehabilitation team models.]

d. The nurse often is designated as the coordinator of communication.

7. Communication

a. Principles of interpersonal communication are applied in all interactions with clients, families, and healthcare professionals.

b. Interpersonal communication skills are essential to establish, maintain, and terminate therapeutic relationships (Hunt, 2005).

D. Levels of Community-Based Services

1. Health

a. The focus of community-based rehabilitation nursing

b. A pattern of wholeness that encompasses the client (as opposed to the opposite of illness)

c. Maximization of the client's potential in terms of independence and quality of life in the client's own environment

2. Preventive health care (Neal, 1999)

a. Primary prevention: interventions that promote optimal health and provide special protection to prevent illness, disabilities, or injuries

b. Secondary prevention: interventions that limit disabilities and are done primarily through early identification and prompt treatment

c. Tertiary prevention: interventions that decrease disabilities and impairments caused by illness or injury

3. Health maintenance

a. Maintaining the current status of one's health

b. Interventions directed at the client that facilitate sequential learning of health activities (e.g., teaching a client with SCI to perform active range-of-motion exercises to maintain flexibility)

c. Activities directed at achieving goals that are part of the client's community regardless of the setting

4. Health restoration

a. Interventions are aimed at maximizing the client's and family's level of health.

b. Interventions incorporate the client's values and culture (e.g., the nurse recognizes the client's Jewish faith and schedules visits accordingly), and goal setting takes place in active participatory fashion.

E. The Continuum of Community-Based Care

1. Care is delivered in many practice settings (Hoeman, 2002)(see Table 2-2).

a. Acute care (e.g., hospitals, freestanding rehabilitation facilities)

b. Long-term care (e.g., nursing homes, extended care facilities, subacute or postacute rehabilitation units or facilities)

c. Community-based settings (e.g., outpatient clinics, day treatment programs, independent living centers, community reentry programs, rural outreach programs)

d. Home care (i.e., continuing rehabilitation services that have been initiated in other settings)

e. Schools

2. The practice area or setting determines the primary focus of the nurse's role across the spectrum of health care (see Table 2-3).

II. Rehabilitation Nurses in Community-Based Care

A. Skills and Competencies That Healthcare Professionals Need to Practice in the Community (Pew Health Professions Commission, 1995)

1. Have an interest in community health

2. Expand access to effective care

3. Provide contemporary clinical care

4. Emphasize primary care

5. Participate in coordinated care

6. Ensure cost-effective, appropriate care

Table 2-2. Settings, Models, and Programs Where Community-Based Rehabilitation Is Used

Setting	Purpose	Types of Clients	Delivery System	Nursing Roles
Home health care	To provide health care to individuals and families in their place of residence for the purpose of prompting or restoring health, maximizing independence, and minimizing the effects of disability (Hankwitz, 1993)	All age levels Common conditions: • Fractures • Degenerative joint disease • Multiple sclerosis • Parkinson's disease • Cancer • Alterations in function secondary to neuropathy or myopathy • Amputations • Burns	Primary care Case management	Partner Teacher Resource manager Clinician (Neal, 1998)
Subacute care	To serve clients whose medical treatment does not allow for participation in acute rehabilitation programs or who are classified as slow to progress or who cannot qualify for a standard rehabilitation program (Mumma & Nelson, 1996)	Typically older than age 16, although specialty pediatric facilities are available Common conditions: • Closed head injury with quadriparesis • Anoxic encephalopathy secondary to cardiac arrest • Strokes • Aneurysms	Team nursing Primary care delivered by nursing assistants; LVNs provide unit supervision and treatments; RNs serve in the case management and coordination role	Planner Coordinator Evaluator of client outcomes Client advocate
Long-term care	To serve clients who are unable to live independently and meet their self-care needs	Primarily the geriatric population, as well as an unknown number of younger people with chronic disabilities Common conditions: • Joint fractures • Strokes • Closed head injury • Anoxia • Rheumatoid arthritis	Team nursing Primary care delivered by licensed vocational nurses (LVNs) and nursing assistants with RNs serving the case coordination and management role	Planner Coordinator Evaluator of client outcomes Client advocate
Independent living	To serve individuals who want to take control of their lives, participate in decision making, and achieve the highest level of independence possible	Primarily adults Common conditions: • SCI • Closed head injury	Care provided by personal care attendants RN serves as care manager	Partner Educator Client advocate

7. Practice prevention
8. Involve clients and families in decision-making process
9. Promote healthy lifestyles
10. Assess and use technology appropriately
11. Improve the healthcare system
12. Manage information
13. Understand the role of the physical environment
14. Provide counseling on ethical issues
15. Accommodate expanded accountability
16. Participate in a racially and culturally diverse society
17. Continue to learn (Hunt & Zurek, 1997, pp. 21–22)

B. Primary Nursing Roles in the Community
  1. Partner or physical caregiver (Neal, 1998)
    a. As clients and families become more educated consumers and take responsibility for making healthcare choices, the relationship between the nurse and client naturally shifts toward a partnership.
    b. The client takes primary responsibility for setting goals; the nurse's role varies depending on the client's degree of independence.
  2. Teacher
    a. The most important goal of teaching in community-based rehabilitation is to help the client and family achieve the highest level of independence possible.

Table 2-3. Role Differentiation of Nurses Based on Practice Setting Programs Where Community-Based Rehabilitation Is Used

Roles	Percentage of time on each role spent by hospital-based nurses	Percentage of time on each role spent by home care nurses	Percentage of time on each role spent by community-based nurses
Physical caregiver	84%	61%	63%
Manager, administrator	2%	10%	10%
Manager, supervisor	6%	12%	9%
Communicator, teacher, consultant	5%	14%	15%

Sources consulted

Hughes, K., Kostbade, K., & Marcantoinio, R. (1992). Practice patterns among home health, public health and hospital nurses. *Nursing and Health Care, 13*(10), 532–536.

Hunt, R., & Zurek, E. (1997). *Introduction to community-based nursing.* Philadelphia: Lippincott.

b. High-quality teaching results in positive outcomes.
   1) Improvements in care
   2) Facilitation of health promotion
   3) Reduction of complications
   4) Resumption of functional activities
c. Sharing knowledge about health care improves client and family satisfaction (Hunt, 2005).
d. Education increases the client's and family's sense of control by encouraging mutual participation in the planning of care (see Figure 2-1).

3. Resource or care manager
   a. The nurse maintains responsibility for tracking and directing the client's care and progress throughout the healthcare system.
   b. The nurse oversees the client's primary needs.
      1) Assesses the client appropriately
      2) Establishes the plan of care
      3) Delegates specific nursing care tasks to other qualified personnel
      4) Initiates interventions
      5) Coordinates and collaborates with the healthcare team
      6) Evaluates outcomes
   c. Collaboration and coordination are vital to the implementation of this role because rehabilitation clients and families interact with many healthcare professionals who have different areas of expertise and training.
   d. The care manager facilitates the client's treatment plan to ensure that it is consistent with the client's needs and is achieved in a timely manner.
   e. Culture is an important part of the client's environment.

Figure 2-1. Benefits of Client Education

Better Outcomes for Client and Family
- Improved care
- Reduction of complications
- Development of self-care skills
- Achievement of highest possible level of independence
- Provision for personal needs
- Resumption of functional activities

Improved Client and Family Satisfaction
- Acquisition of knowledge
- Acquisition of confidence
- Sense of control through participation
- Individual decision making

Improved Staff Satisfaction
- Satisfaction regarding safety to move through different types of healthcare services
- Positive results from discharge
- Client successfully manages care

Continuity of Care
- Identical plans and actions by all professionals
- Movement through different types of healthcare services that does not disrupt treatment

Cost Containment
- Efficient use of resources
- Prevention strategies incorporated into care

Source consulted

Hunt, R., & Zurek, E. (1997). *Introduction to community-based nursing.* Philadelphia: Lippincott.

1) Cultural norms influence the client's behavior.
2) Culture provides the foundation for the client's social behavior.
3) It is imperative that the nurse use knowledge of cultural diversity to positively affect the client's health (see Figure 2-2).

4. Advocate
   a. An advocate defends the cause of another person.
   b. In nursing, advocacy involves empowering clients, families, and client

Figure 2-3. Keys to Developing Advocacy Skills

Understanding and Knowledge of Self Personally and Professionally
- Knowledge of oneself: Awareness of personal goals and how these goals affect relationships with clients
- Realistic self-concept: Awareness of own limitations and abilities that will affect client care
- Value clarification: Awareness of personal bias and prejudices, moral and ethical values; knowledge of personal perceptions concerning what is fair and acceptable and how these perceptions may affect relationships with clients

Knowledge of Treatment and Intervention Options
- Development of a strong knowledge base about interventions and outcomes
- Awareness of rationale for interventions

Knowledge of the Healthcare System
- Awareness of how the healthcare system relates to clients, families, and the community
- Awareness of specific aspects of community (e.g., politics, economy) and how these factors affect the healthcare system

Knowledge of How to Put Advocacy into Action
- Assessment
  - What does the client identify as the problem?
  - What support or resources does the client already have?
  - What knowledge does the client have about health services and treatment options?
  - In what areas does the client feel a need for more personal control?
- Planning: Mobilizing resources, consulting, collaborating with the healthcare team
- Implementation: Educating and empowering the client (the nurse helps the client assert control over variables affecting the client's life)

populations through knowledge.

   c. Advocacy involves changing the system, collaborating with other professionals, role modeling, and maximizing the use of community resources (see Figure 2-3).

C. Types of Community-Based Nurses

   1. Nurses in outpatient rehabilitation clinics focus on integrating rehabilitation principles into the community.

   2. Nurses in assisted living environments focus on promoting health in a structured community living setting that is accessible for people with disabilities.

   3. Home healthcare nurses provide hands-on nursing care in the client's home.

   4. School nurses provide education, counseling, and referral services for health promotion and disease prevention and for meeting the needs of children with disabilities.

   5. Parish nurses act as health counselors, educators, and referral sources for meeting the needs of individuals, use a holistic focus with a foundation based on spiritual health, and usually provide care within a faith community.

   6. Case managers act as liaisons, health educators, health promoters, and referral sources.

      a. Facilitate return to work for workers with injuries

      b. Integrate workers with catastrophic injuries into the community

III. Community Reentry and Reintegration

A. Overview

   1. Focuses on transition from an acute care environment to the community through a gradual acquisition of community skills and training with active participation by the family

   2. Focuses on self-care, leisure, and vocational activities and psychosocial integration into the client's environment

   3. Focuses nursing services on education, resource management, and advocacy

   4. Threads structure and consistency throughout the interventions

   5. Focuses on acquiring skills through training and education, resulting in behavioral changes

   6. Involves addressing or overcoming community-based barriers and handicaps (handicap is defined as the result of an impairment or disability, a disadvantage that limits or prevents normal role performance [World Health Organization, 1980] and is measured by the interaction and adaptation of the client to his or her surroundings)

      a. Societal barriers (Kim & Fox, 2004; Neal-Boylan & Buchanan, in press)

         1) Ineligibility to receive services based on agency criteria

         2) Need for service not available from a community agency

         3) Cultural or attitudinal prejudices

         4) Invisibility of disability to others

         5) Violence and abuse of people with disabilities

6) Reimbursement practices
b. Personal barriers, which are controlled by the individual
   1) Negative attitude
   2) Poor self-esteem
   3) Lack of motivation
   4) Poor self-image
   5) Feelings of dependence
   6) Insecurity
   7) An inability to plan and meet goals
   8) Unrealistic expectations (Frieden, 1992)
c. Transportation issues, which greatly affect a client's environment and community reintegration efforts and can make the difference between community reintegration and reinstitutionalization
   1) Accessibility of healthcare services
   2) Ability to pursue vocational interests
   3) Accessibility of public facilities
   4) Participation in social and recreational activities
   5) Ability to pursue education
   6) Ability to achieve independence in high-level self-care skills
d. Issues related to quality of attendant care
   1) Attendant care often is linked with eligibility requirements and income.
   2) Waiting lists for programs can be lengthy.
   3) The types of services provided by attendants and homemaker services often are deemed custodial by third-party payers and may not be reimbursable.
   4) Responsibility for hiring, firing, and training is placed on the client and family.
   5) Training can be very costly and can involve limited staff retention.
   6) If an attendant is sick or unable to work for personal reasons, the client must have alternative resources to meet his or her needs.
e. Housing barriers
   1) Accessible housing in many communities is not adequate to meet the needs of the population.
   2) There are several causes of inadequate housing (Neal-Boylan & Buchanan, in press).
      a) Insufficient supply
      b) Inaccessibility
      c) Architectural barriers
      d) Long waiting lists
      e) Poor location and high cost

   3) "The individual's ability to make decisions about housing is severely hampered by the government view that everyone with a similar diagnosis has the same needs for services and that affordability and access can be acquired only by mandating that they have their living arrangements set up for them" (Neal-Boylan & Buchanan, in press).
f. Barriers to financial independence, identity, and life satisfaction through employment opportunities
   1) Budget restraints in federal and state agencies limit the access to vocational rehabilitation programs for people with disabilities.
   2) Job coaches to help train and supervise people with disabilities may be limited (Wehman, Targett, & Cifu, 2006).
   3) Return to work is affected by the client's level of disability, level of education, gender, age, and preinjury wages.
   4) New opportunities may exist for people with disabilities as the trends continue toward more home-based businesses and the use of computer technology.
g. The tremendous cost of health care and the client's inability to meet financial needs
   1) People with chronic illness or disability often face incredible financial burdens.
   2) Lost or reduced employment can lead to a loss of insurance benefits, which places further burdens on the client and family.
   3) Often, the client's spouse or caregiver must face additional stress in trying to meet the needs of the client in the home setting while balancing work and home obligations.
h. Issues related to appropriate caregiving at home (Neal-Boylan & Buchanan, in press)
   1) Caregiver and family needs must be assessed to identify potential handicaps for the client.
   2) When a person with a chronic illness or disability returns home, the entire family system is affected.
   3) Research has demonstrated that interventions that offer social support and help caregivers adapt while

problem solving may be helpful (Grant et al., 2006).

    4) Community-based rehabilitation nurses use their skills and training to identify needs regardless of the setting to help the client and family reduce their burdens as much as possible.

B. Life Skills and Independent Living

  1. Overview

    a. Early in the rehabilitation process, client expectations may be unrealistic and extreme.

    b. As the client and family gather more information and training and synthesize this knowledge into their personal environment, they can begin to adjust and readapt to the community.

  2. History: The concept of independent living began with a focus on quality-of-life issues in the late 1960s and early 1970s.

  3. The essence of independent living is the ability of individuals to have control over their lives based on choice.

    a. Minimizing dependence on other people for daily living needs

    b. Managing personal affairs

    c. Participating in community life

    d. Fulfilling social roles

    e. Having options

  4. Grassroots efforts: Lobby groups (including policy makers, politicians, healthcare professionals, community members, and family members) were formed to promote independent living programs.

    a. Developed new laws that protect the rights of people with disabilities

    b. Required the new construction of or adaptations to public buildings, housing, transportation, schools, and places of employment to ensure accessibility

    c. Worked to change public attitudes toward people with disabilities

    d. Provided new opportunities for people with disabilities to enjoy opportunities that enhance quality of life

C. A Conceptual Model for Nurses Working in Community Reentry and Independent Living Programs

  1. The client serves as manager of his or her life and care in a community-based or independent living setting.

    a. Based on the knowledge and skills that the client acquires during the acute phase of rehabilitation, options are considered and decisions are made.

    b. The nurse's role is one of an active participant to help the client through education, coordination of resources, and understanding of how the community's needs and resources will affect his or her health and the health of the family (see Figure 2-4).

  2. The client's lifestyle and needs are considered in terms of his or her environment and community.

    a. The nurse promotes health by determining accessibility for meeting self-care needs and by facilitating opportunities for community reintegration.

    b. The nurse's role is to facilitate communication and collaborate with other healthcare professionals so that the client's energy can be optimized during the transition period.

  3. Client and family education is an ongoing process.

    a. Initially, education is focused and goal directed to help the client and family meet the client's basic self-care needs.

    b. As the client reintegrates into the community, the focus of education changes to enhance the client's problem-solving skills and to teach strategies to maximize health by identifying resources.

    c. Preventive care is always emphasized, from the time of initial education through the rehabilitation process. Preventing complications is the simplest way to diminish handicaps and barriers that can

Figure 2-4. Rehabilitation Nursing Competencies for Helping Clients in Community Reintegration and Independent Living

- Identify the family's role in the rehabilitation process.
- Involve the client's family in the rehabilitation process.
- Discuss factors that influence community reentry of a person with a disability.
- Provide family with appropriate strategies to use and options to seek in the community to cope with the client's or the family's dysfunctional behavior.
- Collaborate with the team to develop a resource bank of supportive services for clients.
- Collaborate with the rehabilitation team to develop an appropriate home program that includes interventions to manage severe cognitive or physical deficits.
- Provide a resource list to help clients with community reintegration.

Source consulted

Rehabilitation Nursing Foundation (RNF). (1994). *Basic competencies for rehabilitation nursing practice.* Skokie, IL: Author.

increase the stress and burden on the client and family.

4. The management of attendant care training and services facilitates independent living and helps the client maintain community-based living.

5. Equipment and supplies should be evaluated before discharge from the acute rehabilitation setting.

   a. The nurse communicates with the family during acute care and the transition to the community to ensure that equipment and supplies meet the client's needs.

   b. The nurse establishes a partnership with the client and family and maintains the lines of communication.

   c. The nurse coordinates the equipment and monitors its effectiveness in meeting the client's needs while monitoring cost.

6. The client's and family's financial resources must be assessed in terms of current availability and future projections.

   a. As part of the educational process, the nurse helps the client and family identify options and make choices that will meet their future needs.

   b. Identifying barriers early in the community living process gives the client and family time to make calm, informed choices rather than having to make decisions during crises.

   c. By helping the client and family realistically appraise their financial needs and available resources, the nurse helps the client maintain ongoing success and health in the community setting.

7. Identifying barriers and options in the community helps the client and family make good healthcare and personal choices.

   a. In the management role, the nurse can help educate the client and family about housing alternatives and architectural designs that maximize independence.

   b. Through collaboration with other healthcare professionals and coordination of efforts within the healthcare system, the nurse can use community resources to help the client and family make the transition to independent living.

8. Independent living is fostered in environments where healthcare providers cooperate.

   a. Collaboration and coordination of services between agencies and healthcare

systems maximize clients' financial and self-care resources.

   b. Identification of resources and plans of action that address healthcare emergencies facilitate clients' transition to independent living and overall health.

D. Housing Issues

1. Components of an in-depth assessment of housing alternatives and the client's needs

   a. Awareness of the client's functional ability

   b. Family needs and support

   c. The client's goals

   d. Availability of resources

2. Considerations for the client's transition to the community

   a. Necessary modifications to the home environment (e.g., building ramps, widening doorways, making bathroom and kitchen modifications, and ensuring access to the community)

   b. Independent living environments that allow the client to maintain his or her own residence and provide support services in specific areas

      1) Communication techniques
      2) Homemaking skills
      3) Transportation skills
      4) Recreational opportunities
      5) Emergency procedures
      6) Management of attendants
      7) Advocacy services
      8) Peer counseling
      9) Personal business management

3. Residential living arrangements: housing in which a group of people with disabilities live in the same geographic area or building and share support services

4. Extended care facilities (e.g., subacute or postacute rehabilitation, neurobehavioral programs, skilled care facilities)

5. Laws that affect housing availability and accessibility

   a. The Housing Act (1959) provided funds for mortgage loans to developers to build housing for people who are disabled or elderly.

   b. The Architectural Barriers Act (1968) mandated that all federally funded buildings being constructed must be made accessible for people with disabilities.

   c. The Rehabilitation Act (1973) prohibited discrimination against people with disabilities when they purchase or rent federally subsidized housing. Incorporated in this law is the 504 plan. This plan provides a program of instructional services to assist students with special needs who are in a regular education setting.

d. The Housing and Community Development Act (1974) allowed families with low incomes to receive subsidized rent payments.

e. The Rehabilitation, Comprehensive Services, and Developmental Disabilities Amendment (1978) issued grants for housing.

f. The Americans with Disabilities Act (1990) established new laws concerning physical access to the community; the laws are evaluated in relation to access to services and ways to implement them in communities to ensure access for all people.

6. Components of a home assessment

a. Safety of the client in the home environment and the ability to maximize function while meeting healthcare needs

b. Availability of healthcare services to continue to meet the client's needs

c. Architectural design of the building and accessibility

d. Assistive devices to promote community living skills

e. Availability of support services, transportation, and recreational and leisure opportunities in the community

f. Furniture, floor surfaces, and clutter that can affect client safety

g. Adequacy of lighting, ventilation, and toileting facilities

h. Accessibility of parking to residence entrance

i. Availability of emergency services (e.g., telephone, fire alarms, emergency exits)

E. Financial Issues

1. People often have limited life skills or financial resources to deal with catastrophic illness.

2. Stress from financial burdens can reduce the client's ability to continue rehabilitation and ultimately prevent reaching his or her maximum health potential.

3. Rehabilitation nurses can help perform a realistic assessment of the client's financial resources and potential future burden to the client and family as a result of disability or chronic illness.

4. Rehabilitation nurses can enlist a representative from the client's payer or reimbursement source as part of the treatment team to facilitate communication and provide prompt justification of resources. [Refer to Chapter 4 for more information on economics and health plans.]

a. Group health

b. Self-insurance

c. Health maintenance organization (HMO) or preferred provider organization (PPO) plans

d. Third-party payers

e. Workers' compensation

f. Medicare

g. Medicaid

F. Transportation Issues

1. Legislation that guarantees basic rights for all people

a. Equal access to public transportation

b. Equal access to airplanes, terminals, buses, subways, and public railway systems

2. Roles of the rehabilitation nurse in facilitating transportation for rehabilitation clients

a. Provide education about the availability of community resources and how to problem solve when moving to other communities

b. Advocate to ensure that the transportation needs of clients are met in the community

c. Collaborate with other healthcare professionals to expand knowledge of available resources and support services

3. Considerations for assessing clients' transportation needs

a. Hand controls, lifts, transfer mechanisms, and seating in existing vehicles

b. Adaptive training with modified vehicles

c. Financial considerations for vehicle modifications

d. Travel programs or clubs for people with disabilities

G. Issues Concerning Care Providers

1. Making the choice to use care providers

a. Facilitation of the client and family's transition to the community must include in-depth consideration of the client's self-care needs.

b. The burden of care for the family attempting to meet the client's needs and the implications for home management and finances must be assessed.

   c. Sometimes the client's quest for independence increases the risk of self-harm, which may be demonstrated by various problems (e.g., shoulder joint damage, stress-related illnesses, psychological alterations).

   d. When the rehabilitation nurse helps maintain the lines of communication, provides education, and helps the client evaluate options, the client and family may decide that using care providers is a valid option.

2. Steps in using care providers
   a. Determine hiring strategy.
   b. Determine need for training (e.g., should care providers be competent upon hiring, or is training on the job an option?).
   c. Determine what support services are available to the client and care providers.
   d. Solidify the role of the family and consider the implications of having non–family members in the home setting.
   e. Address financial implications.
   f. Consider the philosophies and definitions of care providers, which vary from state to state (e.g., what can a care provider do in this client's community?).
   g. Address safety issues.
   h. Determine ways to terminate the relationship with a care provider.
   i. Establish emergency measures to meet personal needs in case a care provider is unable to meet work obligations.

3. Use of care providers to promote autonomy (Cardol, De Jong, & Ward, 2002)
   a. It is important for the client to feel in charge, especially involving an activity he or she cannot do for himself or herself.
   b. The client should determine which activities take priority.
   c. The ability to pay for caregiving services may promote autonomy, and the receipt of unpaid services may be perceived as dependency.

4. A three-pronged model for nurses who teach clients and care providers to work together (DeGraff, 1992)
   a. Instruct the client.
     1) Teach which skills qualify as self-care skills and which skills require attendant services.
     2) Teach safe and efficient methods to instruct others to provide self-care.
     3) Encourage self-advocacy when needs are not being met or the quality of care is unacceptable.
     4) Teach the client how to be assertive.
   b. Offer support services: Provide education about safe and efficient personal care methods and about how to find, manage, and work with care attendants (see Figure 2-5).
   c. Provide practical opportunities: Behavioral changes and integration of knowledge cannot occur without the ability to practice new skills.
     1) Allow practice time that addresses specific skill training and follows instruction.
     2) Encourage or require practice sessions, with the healthcare professional acting as the attendant in the client's room.
     3) Allow for mistakes without instilling a fear of punishment.
     4) Schedule additional practice opportunities with support when necessary (DeGraff, 1992).

H. Finding Support in the Client's Community
1. The foundation of community-based rehabilitation care involves using the options available in the community that support and facilitate the health of the client and enhance the client's options and opportunities for maintaining a gainful and healthy lifestyle.
2. Examples of community support systems.
   a. Churches
   b. Neighbors
   c. Friends
   d. Public or private services
3. Congregational (parish) nursing is an evolution of natural supports in the community.
   a. Parish nursing provides an alternative means for health care for those who might not be served otherwise.
   b. Parish nursing focuses on holistic health care and integrates spiritual health. It is practiced in the context of the values, beliefs, and practices of a faith community.
   c. Congregational nursing began in the 1970s in the Chicago area through the efforts of Reverend Granger Westburg.
     1) In his work as a hospital chaplain, Westburg found that nurses often took on the responsibility of

Figure 2-5. Topics with Which Clients and Families Who Will Be Using Care Providers Should Be Familiar

Teaching Topics

Management skills

Management situations

Qualities of a good manager

Styles of management

Training and ongoing management

Predicting and recognizing problems

Ways to maintain independent living

Rights of people with disabilities and care attendants

Settings in which people with disabilities may use help

Types of help and services that providers can perform

Job expectations

Work environments

Abusing help or taking advantage of assistance (e.g., not completing tasks that could be done independently because it is easier to have someone else do it)

Activities that qualify for attendant services

Making a master list of needs

Residence locations for attendants

Reasons why attendants quit and are fired

Paying salaries and taxes

Recruiting, interviewing, training, and parting with help

Creating a job description

Sources of recruiting

Methods of recruiting

Interviewing and screening

Parting ways with a care attendant

Source consulted

DeGraff, D. (1992). Teaching attendant management skills. In C.P. Zedjlik (Ed.), *Management of spinal cord injury* (2nd ed., pp. 661–671). Boston: Jones and Bartlett.

---

decoding medical terminology for clients, making it more understandable and often basing it in the context of faith and healing.

2) Westburg was impressed with the work of a nurse educator at the University of Arizona who served in the position of minister of health. As a health promoter in the local Lutheran church, this nurse spread her message through programs that were focused on health promotion and disease prevention. Westburg took these principles and started the first parish nursing program in the Chicago area.

d. The primary roles of parish nurses include health education, health counseling and referral, and health screening. Hands-on nursing is not a component of this role.

e. Congregational nurses believe that all human beings are sacred and deserve to be treated with respect and dignity and empower people to become active partners in their health by managing their healthcare resources. Congregational nurses recognize that spiritual health is fundamental to well-being and that health and illness can occur simultaneously. Therefore, using illness to evaluate life goals can mobilize untapped strengths. Healing may take place in the absence of cure because physical well-being is only one dimension of a person's health.

4. School nursing.

a. Initiated in Boston in 1894, with primary role of inspecting school children to evaluate for chronic and contagious diseases (Selekman, 2006).

b. Role has evolved to encompass
   1) Clinician
   2) Advocate
   3) Case manager
   4) Health educator

c. In clinician role, school nurse is the first responder to medical emergencies and provides first aid. Many children with chronic health conditions or special needs are mainstreamed into today's classrooms. The school nurse provides the link to assist and educate other staff members to ensure that the child's healthcare needs are met in the school setting.

d. As advocate, the school nurse is responsible for helping students maximize attendance and facilitating students' educational processes.
   1) Advocacy can include the recommendation for an independent healthcare plan, 504 plan, or individualized educational plan (IEP).
   2) The purpose of the independent healthcare plan is to meet the student's healthcare needs by optimizing functioning while maximizing learning opportunities (Selekman, 2006, p. 182).
   3) Typically, the 504 plan is developed for students in regular education with regular curriculum who have a physical or mental impairment that limits one or more major life activities. The plan provides accommodations to maximum educational experience. 504 plans are covered under the Rehabilitation Act of 1973, but no

funding is tied to this plan. Examples include students with diabetes, arthritis, or spinal cord injuries.

    4) The IEP is tied to funding and used for students who need specially designed instruction or related services to benefit from educational processes (e.g., students with traumatic brain injury, cerebral palsy, or mental retardation).

  e. As case manager, the nurse functions as communication hub and care planner with other members of the educational team and with members of the community who provide health services for the student.

  f. Health education provided by the nurse facilitates an understanding of the student's healthcare needs and how they might be affected by the educational setting. The nurse is also responsible for identifying and initiating contacts in the community who might improve the student's health care.

5. Telerehab [Refer to Chapter 21 for further discussion.]

  a. "The use of telecommunication and electronic technologies to provide rehabilitation and long-term support to people with disabilities in remote settings" (Case Management Advisor, 2000, p. 164)

  b. Provides extended postdischarge follow-up

  c. Provides a view of the home environment

  d. Offers monitoring of the client's condition form a remote site

  e. Eliminates transportation difficulties

  f. Allows consultation with experts

6. Research validating the need for rehabilita–tion nursing skills in community settings

  a. Neal (1999) evaluated the congruence between rehabilitation nursing principles and home health nursing practice.

  b. Neal's findings determined that rehabilitation principles are congruent with home health nursing principles and that educating and training home health nurses about rehabilitation principles may result in better health outcomes for clients.

IV. Employment Opportunities for People with Disabilities in the Community

A. Vocational Rehabilitation

1. Each state is required by federal law to have an office of vocational rehabilitation that provides vocational services for people with disabilities.

2. Funding is available to help people seek gainful or supported employment.

  a. To make home or vehicle modifications

  b. To participate in work-hardening programs or functional work capacity examinations Work-hardening programs are custom-designed programs formulated to address a client's specific needs based on his or her ability to perform activities of daily living. The goal is for the client to achieve the highest level of function, which will prepare him or her to return to work

  c. To determine the client's vocational strengths or weaknesses

  d. To identify abilities, previous work experiences, or vocational interests

  e. To assess the job market

  f. To educate and train employers

  g. To match the client's functional and cognitive abilities with job options

3. Supported employment allows people with disabilities to integrate into employment settings.

  a. In 1986, the amendments to the Rehabilitation Act described how supported employment programs would be implemented. Before this act, vocational rehabilitation programs met the needs of people with disabilities through sheltered workshops.

  b. The Workforce Investment Act of 1998 called for statewide workforce investment systems "that include, as integral components, comprehensive and coordinated state-of-the-art programs of vocational rehabilitation[:] i. independent living centers and services; ii. research; iii. training; iv. demonstration projects; and v. the guarantee of equal opportunity" (http://www.nationalrehab.org/website/history/98amendments.html).

  c. Key aspects of supported employment

    1) Meet the employment needs of people with severe disabilities

    2) Pay all workers

    3) Integrate the work environment by placing able-bodied workers with workers with disabilities

4) Provide support and job supervision

5) Provide training that includes job adaptations, money management, personal care, and social skills

6) Provide transportation

B. Rehabilitation Nurses' Role in Disability Management in the Workplace

1. Rehabilitation nurses are uniquely qualified to provide disability management in the workplace.

   a. By identifying potential sources of work-related injury

   b. By providing education and training on preventive techniques and health maintenance

   c. By recognizing that clients need to make informed choices (Hagen-Foley, Rosenthal, & Thomas, 2005)

2. When injuries occur, rehabilitation nurses serve as case managers and emphasize prompt assessment and intervention by using the healthcare team to facilitate return to work as soon as possible for the injured employee.

3. Rehabilitation nurses perform other case management tasks such as job analysis, job modification and training, and education for employers on job placement.

4. Rehabilitation nurses can provide training for employers in work-hardening programs.

5. Rehabilitation nurses facilitate positive outcomes by being involved in disability management.

   a. Lower workers' compensation costs

   b. Decreased absenteeism

   c. Decreased cost of rehabilitation services for injured employees

   d. Increased employee satisfaction

   e. Increased employee retention

References

Cardol, M., De Jong, B.A., & Ward, C.D. (2002). On autonomy and participation in rehabilitation. *Disability and Rehabilitation, 24*(18), 970–974.

Case Management Advisor. (2000). Telerehab supports community reentry: Technology eases gaps caused by shorter stays. *Case Management Advisor, 11*(10), 164–166.

DeGraff, D. (1992). Teaching attendant management skills. In C.P. Zedjlik (Ed.), *Management of spinal cord injury* (2nd ed., pp. 661–671). Boston: Jones and Bartlett.

Frieden, L. (1992). Is there life after rehabilitation? In C.P. Zedjlik (Ed.), *Management of spinal cord injury* (2nd ed., pp. 631–641). Boston: Jones and Bartlett.

Grant, J.S., Elliott, T.R., Weaver, M., Glandon, G.L., Raper, J.L., & Giger, J.N. (2006). Social support, social problem-solving abilities, and adjustment of family caregivers of stroke survivors. *Archives of Physical Medicine and Rehabilitation, 87*(3), 343–350.

Hagen-Foley, D.L., Rosenthal, D.A., & Thomas, D.F. (2005). Informed consumer choice in community rehabilitation programs. *Rehabilitation Counseling Bulletin, 48*(2), 110–117.

Hankwitz, P.E. (1993). Role of physician in home care. In B.J. May (Ed.), *Home health and rehabilitation concepts of care* (pp. 1-23). Philadelphia: F.A. Davis.

Hoeman, S. (Ed.). (2002). *Rehabilitation nursing: Process and application* (2nd ed.). St. Louis: Mosby.

Hunt, R. (2005). *Introduction to community-based nursing.* (3rd ed.). Philadelphia: Lippincott, Williams, & Wilkins.

Hunt, R., & Zurek, E. (1997). *Introduction to community-based nursing.* Philadelphia: Lippincott.

Kim, K., & Fox, M.H. (2004). Knocking on the door: The integration of emerging disability groups into independent living. *Journal of Vocational Rehabilitation, 20,* 91–98.

Klainberg, M., Holzemer, S., Leonard, M., & Arnold, J. (1998). *Community health nursing: An alliance for health.* St. Louis: McGraw-Hill Nursing Core Series.

Mumma, C., & Nelson, A. (1996). Models for theory-based practice of rehabilitation nursing. In S.P. Hoeman (Ed.), *Rehabilitation nursing: Process and application* (2nd ed., pp. 21-33). St. Louis: Mosby.

Neal, L. (Ed.). (1998). *Rehabilitation nursing in the home health setting.* Glenview, IL: Association of Rehabilitation Nurses.

Neal, L. (1999). Research supporting the congruence between rehabilitation principles and home health nursing practice. *Rehabilitation Nursing, 24*(3), 115–121.

Neal-Boylan, L.J., & Buchanan, L.C. (in press). Community-based rehabilitation. In S.P. Hoeman (Ed.), *Rehabilitation nursing.* St. Louis: Mosby.

Newman, M.A. (1994). *Health as expanding consciousness.* (2nd ed.). New York: National League for Nursing.

Pew Health Professions Commission. (1995). *Health America: Practitioners for 2005.* Durham, NC: Author.

Selekman, J. (Ed.). (2006). *School nursing: A comprehensive text.* Philadelphia: F.A. Davis.

Webster's American family dictionary. (1999). Springfield, MA: Merriam-Webster.

Wehman, P.H., Targett, P.S., & Cifu, D.X. (2006). Job coaches: A workplace support. *American Journal of Physical Medicine & Rehabilitation, 85*(8), 704.

World Health Organization (WHO). (1980). International classification of impairments, disabilities, and handicaps. Geneva: Author.

Suggested Resources

Hunt, R. (2005). *Introduction to community-based nursing* (3rd ed.). Philadelphia: Lippincott, Williams & Wilkins.

Maurer, F., & Smith, C. (2005). *Community/public health nursing practice* (3rd ed.). Philadelphia: Elsevier Saunders.

Porche, D. (2004). *Public and community health nursing practice: A population-based approach.* Thousand Oaks, CA: Sage.

Zedjlik, C.P. (Ed.). (1992). *Management of spinal cord injury* (2nd ed.). Boston: Jones and Bartlett.

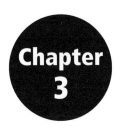

Chapter 3

Ethical, Moral, and Legal Considerations

Pamela A. Masters-Farrell, MSN RN CRRN

Rehabilitation nurses confront a variety of ethical and moral dilemmas in their practice settings. They often face the problem of working with clients and families whose decisions do not reflect their own values and beliefs about health, self-care, and independence and whose quality of life has been significantly affected by technological advances in medicine and health care. Dilemmas surrounding birth and death have been augmented by dilemmas related to whether health care is a right or a privilege, rationing of care, cost containment, quality of care, and the results and appropriateness of research, including the moral and ethical issues associated with gene therapy, stem cell research, and cloning (Ellis & Hartley, 2004).

A common problem facing rehabilitation providers today is that of access to services. This problem is compounded by issues of quality of life, advocacy, personal choice, financial capacity, ability to achieve self-sufficiency, and the needs of the community. Regulations, requirements of insurers, and personal choices influence development of and adherence to the recommended plan of care. Social pressures and technological development push for more services, often at a higher cost, at the same time that resource allocations have decreased and come under closer scrutiny. This leaves the client, family, and medical community struggling with decisions about who deserves what services at which level of care.

To help clients and families make informed decisions about care and treatment options, rehabilitation nurses should be careful to adhere to established parameters and to seek ethical and legal consultation when necessary to determine the most appropriate course of action. Rehabilitation nurses' participation in collaborative decision making with clients, families, and other health professionals should reflect the understanding that care should be ethical, legal, compassionate, and culturally sensitive and that those affected by the care should be well informed. This chapter provides an overview of the ethical and legal considerations that are common in rehabilitation nursing practice.

I. Ethical and Moral Considerations

A. Definitions
1. "Ethics: study of the nature and justification of general ethical principles that can apply to special areas where there are moral problems" (McCourt, 1993, p. 230)
2. "Morality: traditions of belief about right and wrong moral conduct" (McCourt, 1993, p. 230)
3. Moral decision making: use of ethical principles to guide decision making through a rational course (Hoeman & Duchene, 2002)
4. Bioethics: the study of the relationships between biology, medicine, technology, and scientific advancements as related to ethical issues. Universally, bioethical issues change with social changes (Ellis & Hartley, 2004).
5. Rehabilitation nursing ethics (see Figure 3-1): "judgments about decisions to act and subsequent actions based on the rules of conduct or precepts of rehabilitation nursing practice" (Graham-Eason, 1996, p. 35)

B. Ethical Models and Associated Theorists (Ellis & Hartley, 2004)
1. Deontology, also known as duty-based ethics (Immanuel Kant, 1724–1804): Decisions derive from moral rules and universal values that do not change; there is a categorical imperative. Consequences of decisions are less important than following the rules.
2. Utilitarianism, also known as situational ethics (Jeremy Bentham, 1748–1832, and John Stuart Mill, 1806–1873): Based on the assumption that actions lead to maximizing the overall good; the ends justify the means.
3. Objectivism (St. Thomas Aquinas, 1225–1274): Actions are considered morally right when they are in accord with our nature, promote good, and avoid evil.
4. Social equality and justice (John Rawls, 1921–2002): Supports justice and equal rights for all through development of positions that use a "veil of ignorance" so that decisions are not colored by the specific details of those involved, allowing the disadvantaged to receive the same social and economic benefits as others.
5. Ideal observer (Raymond W. Firth, 1901–2002): Decisions should be made by an impartial observer fully informed of the situation and the potential consequences of the decision.

C. Models of Ethical and Moral Decision Making

1. Nursing process: Identify the problem, gather data, identify options, make a decision, act, and assess (Ellis & Hartley, 2004).

2. Three-step ACT model (Graham-Eason, 1996)

   a. A: Anticipate obstacles to action

   b. C: Clarify position related to planning action

   c. T: Test choice

3. Savage model (Savage & Michalak, 1999) for facilitating ethical decision making (see Figure 3-1)

4. Josephson Institute of Ethics (Savage & Michalak, 1999) decision-making model

   a. All decisions must take into account and reflect a concern for the interest and well-being of stakeholders.

   b. Ethical values and principles always take precedence over nonethical ones.

   c. It is proper to violate an ethical principle only when it is clearly necessary to advance another true ethical principle, which, according to the decision maker's conscience, will produce the greatest balance of good in the long run.

5. Other ethical decision-making models (see Figure 3-2)

D. Factors Influencing Actions of the Individual Nurse (Hoeman & Duchene, 2002)

1. Choices are based on the person's philosophy of life, religious practice, secular habits, practice setting, political beliefs, and other factors.

2. Each nurse must have a clear understanding of his or her own values and a plan for critical assessment of situations in which there are conflicts with client beliefs, regulations, or professional codes.

3. There are few simple, final solutions to ethical dilemmas. Each situation must be assessed and acted on individually. There is no clear response to conflicts posed when sanctity of life conflicts with quality of life.

4. Cultural diversity has added new values and practices into healthcare, social, and political arenas.

5. In today's world, the burden of care placed on family members is for some an ethical dilemma.

6. Issues of euthanasia, assisted suicide, and suicide are not simply ethical dilemmas. They are under legal scrutiny and debate and addressed in professional codes of practice.

E. Moral Conflict

1. Conflict occurs when a choice must be made between two equal possibilities. Types of moral conflict as defined by Redman and Fry (1998):

   a. Moral dilemma: occurs when two or more clear moral principles apply, but they support mutually inconsistent courses of action

---

Figure 3-1. Savage Model for Facilitating Ethical Decision Making

1. Gather facts of the case and understandings of those parties involved.

2. Identify the questions and goals.

3. Organize a meeting with key players—parents, physicians, nurses, social workers, therapists, and others who might assist in the decision making.

   a. Pose questions, clarify information, set goals.
   b. Explore options and their consequences and ethical ramifications.
   c. Make plan for future management of case.

4. Provide information, referrals, education, and emotional support to family.

5. Participate in implementation of decision, if appropriate.

6. Review the process, evaluate your role, and revise process as needed.

Reprinted with permission of W.B. Saunders from Savage, T., & Michalak, D. (1999). Ethical, legal, and moral issues in pediatric rehabilitation. In P.A. Edwards, D.L., Hertzberg, S.R. Hays, & N.M. Youngblood (Eds.), *Pediatric rehabilitation nursing* (p. 67). Philadelphia: W.B. Saunders.

Figure 3-2. Two Models of Ethical Decision Making

Model 1 (Aiken & Catalano, 1994)	Model 2 (Blanchard & Peale, 1988)
1. Collect, analyze, and interpret data.	1. Ask "Is it legal?" If the answer is yes, then stop. If no, go on to Items 2 and 3.
2. State dilemma clearly.	2. Ask "Is it balanced?" This will help answer issues of fairness vs. giving advantages to one or more parties.
3. Consider choices for action.	
4. Consider and weigh choices	
5. Analyze advantages and disadvantages of each choice.	3. Ask "How will the decision make me feel?" This will help answer issues of personal standards of morality.
6. Make decision from choices.	

Primary Sources: Model 1: Adapted with permission of F.A. Davis Company from Aiken, T., & Catalano, J. (1994). *Legal, ethical, and political issues in nursing* (pp. 31–35). Philadelphia: F.A. Davis. Copyright 1994 by F.A. Davis Company. Model 2: Adapted with permission of William Morrow & Company, Inc., from Blanchard, K., & Peale, N. (1988). *The power of ethical management* (pp. 20–27). New York: William Morrow. Copyright 1988 by Blanchard Family Partnership and Norman Vincent Peale by William Morrow & Company, Inc.

Secondary Source: Armstrong, M. (Ed.). (1998). *Telecommunications for health professionals: Providing successful distance education and telehealth* (p. 247). New York: Springer.

b. Moral distress: occurs when a person knows the right thing to do, but institutional constraints make it nearly impossible to pursue the right course of action

c. Moral uncertainty: occurs when a person is unsure about which moral principles or values apply or even about what the moral problem is

2. Defining attributes of a dilemma (Ellis & Hartley, 2004):

a. Must make a choice

b. Equally unattractive alternatives

c. Awareness of alternatives

d. May have to defend a decision

e. Uncertainty of action

F. Ethical Principles and Rights

1. The ethical principles in Table 3-1 reflect issues common to rehabilitation settings (Hoeman & Duchene, 2002).

2. Rights are the basis of professional, regulatory, and legal codes and judgments; they reflect what society believes a person is entitled to. Rights can come into conflict with values (Ellis & Hartley, 2004; Masters-Farrell, 2006).

a. Self-determination rights: The Patient Self-Determination Act (1990) or the Danforth amendment requires that patients be given an opportunity to decide on life support options on admission to any healthcare service. Organizations must supply documentation and education to support informed choice.

b. Patient rights: The American Hospital Association published *A Patient's Bill of Rights* in 1973, focusing on confidentiality, privacy, and informed consent. Updated in 1992, it began to reflect the responsibilities of healthcare providers and to reinforce the concept of collaborative care. In 2003 the document was rewritten and titled *The Patient Care Partnership*, encouraging patients to get involved in their care and to ask questions. The Joint Commission (JC) and the Commission on Accreditation of Rehabilitation Facilities requires that patients receive information about their rights. JC has expanded these rights to include the right to effective pain management. A federally mandated patient rights program is also under consideration. It includes the following rights for patients:

1) The right to receive considerate and respectful care

2) The right to obtain relevant, current, and understandable information about diagnosis, treatment, and prognosis

3) The right to make decisions about the plan of care

4) The right to have advance directives about treatment

5) The right to privacy in all aspects of care

6) The right to expect that all communication and records will be treated confidentially

7) The right to review records pertaining to care

8) The right to expect reasonable responses to requests for appropriate and medically indicated care and services

9) The right to be informed about business relationships that may influence treatment and care

10) The right to consent to or decline participation in proposed research studies

11) The right to expect reasonable continuity of care

12) The right to be informed about hospital policies and practices that relate to patient care, treatment, and responsibility

G. Professional Ethics Codes, Standards, and Statements

1. The ethical standard for the profession of nursing is established in the Code of Ethics for Nurses: Provisions (American Nurses Association, 2006).

2. The Association of Rehabilitation Nurses (ARN, 2000) supported these standards and incorporated them into the Standards and Scope of Rehabilitation Nursing Practice (see Figure 3-3). ARN contributes additional comments about standards of ethical rehabilitation nursing practice in the ARN Position Statement on Ethical Issues (Pilkington & Strong, 2003). This statement presents concerns of rehabilitation nurses.

a. Patients' rights, including the rights of minors. (Minors may or may not be capable of understanding the decisions made in their name by their parents. If a minor was not involved in the decision-making process and does not agree with his or her parents' decision, the minor

Table 3-1. Assessment and Moral Principles*

Principle	Descriptor	Dilemma or Concern
Autonomy	Patient has right to choose; self-determination	1. Informed consent—related to research 2. Ventilator-dependent client feels he has no quality of life; lives in a nursing home, has no resources—financial or family. Wants to die. Questions to ask relate to whether the client has been informed of all resources.
Nonmaleficence	Do no harm	Should a client be sent home with family member if it appears as though the family member is not interested or just cannot follow through? Should a head-injured client be restrained? Is this protection?
Beneficence Advocacy (loyalty)	Doing good Standing for client	When dealing with adolescents or children who are comatose: Are parents always in the best position to make decisions? What is the nurse's role in the situation where the family or caregiver's decision is not consistent with philosophy of rehabilitation?
Veracity	Truth telling: Client needs information before he or she can consent	When a client is admitted to rehabilitation, how "honest is honest" when giving prognosis while "still offering hope"?
Client fiduciary responsibility	Recognize costs to client when provided or do not provide treatments	1. Is length of stay determined by insurance? 2. Who determines level of care?
Ethic of care	Gives rise to compassion, equity, fairness, envisions problem in context—framework of relationships, dignity	Dilemma is that nurses work in situations and institutions where policies and practices may be based on paternalistic views of what is right. Nurses in rehabilitation also work with other team members who are involved with client. Nurse-client relationship here is one that takes into consideration other relationships and available resources. Does not act on what is understood common right but looks at the unique rights of the client now.
Reciprocity	Develop one's talents, integrity—be true to one's self, impartial, consistent, having respect for client's goals and values	Setting contracts with clients. They need to behave in manner consistent with plan of care. Staff members need to be fair, impartial in contract setting, and be able to keep their end of the deal. Involves having relationship. Are staff members open to compromises with clients who want to tailor a trust contract?
Fidelity	Always keep promises	Promise to keep child from ever hurting again—find out client to be returned to family that caused injury. Need to consider promises in ethical dilemma, especially in light of legal consequences or long-term outcomes.
Concern for community as a whole	Costs to the community; values of the community	1. Who will take care of indigent rehabilitation clients? 2. Client has placement problem—will end up in nursing home. Do costs that allow independence in the nursing home balance with benefits? 3. Is rehabilitation necessary when many in community do not even have access to basic healthcare needs? Is rehabilitation a basic healthcare need?
Sanction for life	Maintaining life rather than intent to end life	Persons with Parkinson's disease and others may benefit from fetal transplant neuron tissue. Is it ethically responsible to end one life to benefit another? What if fetus will be aborted anyway? Who benefits from abortion?

Note. *Moral principles form bases for nursing practice. Dilemmas or concerns may arise for one or more principles, as with these examples from rehabilitation practice.

Source consulted

Hoeman, S. P. (Ed.), *Rehabilitation nursing: Process, application and outcomes* (3rd ed.). St. Louis: Mosby.

may have no recourse, which leads to an ethical and legal conflict.)

 b. The use of restraints

 c. Do-not-resuscitate orders

 d. Advance directives, which imply nursing intervention and responsibility regarding living wills and durable power of attorney

 e. Management of clients who are disposed to self-destructive behaviors or suicidal gestures

 f. Issues related to healthcare reform and changes in how health care is allocated and delivered, including providing access to health care and rehabilitation, containing costs, ensuring quality of health care, determining length of stay, defining who meets the criteria for rehabilitation, dealing with patients' noncompliance with treatment and rehabilitation, teaching the patient and family in preparation for discharge to home or another level of care, and discharging patients to a care level with appropriate skills for their needs

 g. Confidentiality, security, and privacy related to patient care

 h. Substance abuse

 i. Abused clients

 j. The nurse–client relationship (e.g., when does it become too intimate, and when is

Figure 3-3. ARN Standards Regarding Ethics

Standard V. Ethics: The rehabilitation nurse's decisions and actions on behalf of clients are determined in an ethical manner.

- The rehabilitation nurse's practice is guided by *Code for Nurses with Interpretive Statements* (ANA, 1985) and ARN's position statement on ethical issues.
- The rehabilitation nurse maintains a client's confidentiality.
- The rehabilitation nurse acts as a client advocate.
- The rehabilitation nurse delivers care in a nonjudgmental and nondiscriminatory manner that is sensitive to clients' diversity.
- The rehabilitation nurse delivers care in a manner that preserves and protects the client's autonomy, dignity, and rights.
- The rehabilitation nurse maintains an awareness of his or her beliefs and value systems and what effect they may have on care he or she provides to the client and client's significant others.
- The rehabilitation nurse supports the client's right to make decisions that may not be congruent with the values of the rehabilitation team.
- The rehabilitation nurse seeks available resources to help formulate ethical decisions.
- The rehabilitation nurse promotes the provision of information and discussion that allows the client to participate fully in decision making.
- The rehabilitation nurse participates in decision making regarding allocation of resources.

Source consulted

Association of Rehabilitation Nurses (2000). *Standards and scope of rehabilitation nursing practice* (3rd ed.). Glenview, IL: Author.

intimacy between the nurse and the client appropriate?)

H. Ethics Committee

1. Definition: a multidisciplinary group of healthcare professionals established specifically to address ethical dilemmas that occur in a particular setting. Often includes members of the community and an ethicist (Ellis & Hartley, 2004).

2. Pros (Savage & Michalak, 1999):

   a. Allows multidisciplinary perspectives to be considered

   b. Provides a forum for communication

   c. Allows anticipatory discussion of potential conflicts

   d. Has a clinical focus

   e. Allows objective, detached deliberation

   f. Fosters policy development

   g. Promotes awareness of ethical issues

3. Cons (Savage & Michalak, 1999):

   a. Can allow dominant members' opinions to prevail

   b. Can intrude on a physician–patient relationship

   c. Has potential for bureaucratic inefficiency

   d. Can become a "rubber stamp" for physician opinion

   e. Has potential to disfranchise interested

parties who are not included in the committee

4. Responsibilities of an ethics committee (McCourt, 1993):

   a. Address issues of informed consent

   b. Render decisions for incompetent or incapacitated patients when an emergency exists or an immediate decision is needed

   c. Rule on difficult decisions that present a compelling case

   d. Attempt resolution of treatment differences

   e. Serve as a forum for discussion of such concerns and act in an advisory capacity before judicial review

   f. Educate staff

5. Special responsibilities of a nursing ethics committee (Habel, 1999):

   a. Address unique concerns of nursing

   b. Help nurses identify, explore, and resolve ethical issues in practice

   c. Provide education and staff development

   d. Develop and follow a defined model of critical thinking

   e. Review department policies related to ethics

II. Legal Issues and Considerations (Ellis & Hartley, 2004)

A. Patient Self-Determination Act: Requires that people receiving medical care be given written information about their right to make decisions regarding end-of-life issues

B. Living Wills and Life-Prolonging Declarations: Allow people to make their wishes known before hospitalization regarding medical care, illness, or conditions resulting in incompetence

C. Durable Power of Attorney: Enables a competent person to appoint a surrogate decision maker who is empowered to act legally for the patient

D. Guardianship: A position of responsibility granted to a person by the court to make decisions for the incapacitated person's life

E. Incompetence: A court decision based on clinical opinion of the person's mental or cognitive fitness

F. Informed Consent: Full description of the risks and consequences of agreeing or refusing to have an operation or procedure

G. Estate Planning: Long-term planning for future care and expenses

H. Legal Death or Brain Death: Legal parameters defining when life ceases

I. Withholding or Withdrawing Treatment

J. Do-Not-Resuscitate Order

K. Research on Human Subjects (Hoeman & Duchene, 2002)

1. Basic rules and requirements for research studies can be found in various codes and regulations and focus on issues of informed consent.

2. Participants should understand the purpose of the research and what is expected of them.

3. Participants should be competent to decide to participate.

4. Participants have the right to have questions answered before participation.

5. Participants should be free to withdraw from the study at any time without fear of reprisal.

III. Ethical, Legal, and Moral Issues in Practice

A. Diagnosis and Prognosis

1. Involves withholding or withdrawing treatment

2. Entails consideration of the presence of chronic illness

3. Involves patients in treatment decisions

B. Collaborative Decision Making and Effective Communication

1. Involves discussing the intensity of medical care with the individual and family

2. Encourages a dialogue to determine cultural and socioeconomic attitudes related to defining an appropriate level of care

3. Identifies components of life support systems, policies of the healthcare setting, and support resources

4. Involves the entire rehabilitation team in communicating with the family and discussing their concerns about treatment

C. Acute Care Versus Long-Term Care: Involves making decisions in the best interest of the patient

D. Allocation of Resources

1. Microallocation: deciding what to spend on a specific patient's care

2. Macroallocation: deciding how to distribute spending across a patient population, including healthcare rationing

E. Ethical Rehabilitation (Hoeman & Duchene, 2002)

1. Client participates in the plan of care as fully as possible.

2. Client values independence and wellness.

3. Client regains self-worth and makes physical gains.

4. Nurse collaborates with other team members.

5. Nurse demonstrates caring, good judgment, and advocacy.

6. Rehabilitation helps a client regain his or her capabilities and self-worth.

7. Rehabilitation happens in the shortest possible time and is cost-effective.

F. Team Issues

1. Team members should be aware of the roles and core values of all team members.

2. Team members should show respect for relationships and functions.

3. Team members should consider self-care, independence, and client well-being the ultimate goals.

G. Ethical Issues Related to Alternative and Complementary Medicine and Therapies

1. The patient's right to choose alternative and complementary medicine and therapies

2. Possible interactions between alternative or complementary medicine and traditional Western medicine

H. Ethical Implications of Caring

1. Maintain the status of special relationships in a healthcare organization

2. Maintain personal and professional standards in a managed care environment

3. Maintain an administrative perspective on pursuing the good of the patient and the organization

I. Ethical Foundations of Healthcare Reform (Graham-Eason, 1996)

1. Universal access: Every American citizen and legal resident should have access to health care without financial or other barriers.

2. Comprehensive benefits: Guaranteed benefits should meet the full range of health needs, including primary, preventive, and specialized care.

3. Choice: Each consumer should have the opportunity to exercise choice about providers, plans, and treatments. Each consumer should be informed about what is known and not known about the risks and benefits of available treatments and should be free to choose between them according to his or her preferences.

4. Equity of care: The system should provide care based only on differences in need, not on individual or group characteristics.

5. Fair distribution of costs: The healthcare system should spread the costs and burdens of care across the entire community, basing the level of contribution required of consumers on ability to pay.

6. Personal responsibility: Under health reform, each individual and family should assume responsibility for protecting and promoting health and contributing to the cost of care.

7. Intergenerational justice: The healthcare system should respond to the unique needs of each stage of life, sharing benefits and burdens fairly across generations.

8. Wise allocation of resources: The nation should balance prudently what it spends on health care against other important national priorities.

9. Effectiveness: The new system should deliver care and innovations that work and that patients want. It should encourage the discovery of better treatments. It should enable the academic community and healthcare providers to exercise their responsibility to evaluate and improve health care by providing resources for the systematic study of healthcare outcomes.

10. Quality: The system should deliver high-quality care and provide people with the information necessary to make informed healthcare choices.

11. Effective management: By encouraging simplification and continuous improvement and making the system easier to use for patients and providers, the healthcare system should focus on care rather than administration.

12. Professional integrity and responsibility: The healthcare system should treat the clinical judgments of professionals with respect and protect the integrity of the provider-patient relationship while ensuring that health providers have the resources to fulfill their responsibilities for the effective delivery of high-quality care.

13. Fair procedures: To protect these values and principles, fair and open democratic procedures should underlie decisions about the operation of the healthcare system and the resolution of disputes that arise within it.

14. Local responsibility: Working within the framework of national reform, the new healthcare system should allow states and local communities to design effective, high-quality systems of care that serve all their citizens.

IV. Future Considerations and Directions

A. End-of-Life Issues
1. Making no-code decisions
2. Dying at home
3. Limiting treatment for those with dementia or terminal illness
4. Withholding nutrition and fluids
5. Using euthanasia, including assisted suicide

B. Genetic Research
1. Decoding genes that are responsible for specific diseases
2. Gene therapy
3. Genetic engineering
4. Use of genetic information
5. Cloning

C. Beginning-of-Life Issues
1. Abortion
2. Newborns with severe defects
3. Fetal tissue experimentation
4. Genetic counseling
5. Genetic manipulation
6. Surrogacy

D. Resource Allocation
1. Microallocation
2. Macroallocation
3. Cost containment
4. Individual access to services
5. Clinical decisions made by for-profit managed care organizations (Habel, 1999)

E. Issues That Rehabilitation Professionals Must Address
1. Balancing medical and rehabilitative needs that present moral quandaries
2. Team contributions to decision making with regard to services for clients and clients' progress and outcomes
3. Definitions of quality-of-life issues
4. Access to rehabilitative services regardless of the client's disability or funding level
5. Legal requirements for providing rehabilitation services
6. Meeting standards and regulations imposed by various entities
7. Client decisions to adhere or not to adhere to recommended regimens as defined by the rehabilitation team

References

Aiken, T., & Catalano, J. (1994). *Legal, ethical, and political issues in nursing.* Philadelphia: F.A. Davis.

American Hospital Association. (2005). *The patient care partnership: Understanding expectations, rights and responsibilities.* Retrieved January 12, 2007, from http://www.aha.org/aha/issues/Communicating-With-Patients/pt-care-partnership.html

American Nurses Association. (1985). *Code for nurses with interpretive statements.* Kansas City, MO: Author.

American Nurses Association. (2006). *Code of ethics for nurses: Provisions.* Washington, DC: Author. Retrieved January 12, 2007, from http://www.nursingworld.org/ethics/chcode.htm

Armstrong, M. (Ed.). (1998). *Telecommunications for health professionals: Providing successful distance education and telehealth.* New York: Springer.

Association of Rehabilitation Nurses (ARN). (2000). *Standards and scope of rehabilitation nursing practice* (4th ed.). Glenview, IL: Author.

Blanchard, K., & Peale, N. (1988). *The power of ethical management.* New York: William Morrow.

Ellis, J.R., & Hartley, C.L. (2004). *Nursing in today's world: Trends, issues & management* (8th ed.). Philadelphia: Lippincott, Williams & Wilkins.

Graham-Eason, C. (1996). Ethical considerations for rehabilitation nursing. In S. Hoeman (Ed.), *Rehabilitation nursing: Process and application* (2nd ed., pp. 34–46). St. Louis: Mosby.

Habel, M. (1999). Bioethics: Strengthening nursing's role. *Nurse Week* [Online]. Available: http://www.nurseweek.com/ce/ce420a

Hoeman, S.P., & Duchene, P.M. (2002). Ethical matters in rehabilitation. In S. Hoeman (Ed.), *Rehabilitation nursing: Process, application, and outcomes* (3rd ed., pp. 45–55). St. Louis: Mosby.

Masters-Farrell, P.A. (2006). Ethical/legal principles and issues. In K.L. Mauk (Ed.), *Gerontological nursing competencies for care* (pp. 589–618). Sudbury, MA: Jones and Bartlett.

McCourt, A.E. (Ed.). (1993). *The specialty practice of rehabilitation nursing: A core curriculum* (3rd ed.). Skokie, IL: Rehabilitation Nursing Foundation of the Association of Rehabilitation Nurses.

Pilkington, D., & Strong, S. (2003). *ARN position statement on ethical issues.* Skokie, IL: Association of Rehabilitation Nurses.

Redman, B., & Fry, S. (1998). Ethical conflicts reported by certified registered rehabilitation nurses. *Rehabilitation Nursing, 23,* 179–184.

Savage, T., & Michalak, D.R. (1999). Ethical, legal and moral issues in pediatric rehabilitation. In P.A. Edwards, D.L. Hertzberg, S.R. Hays, & N.M. Youngblood (Eds.), *Pediatric rehabilitation nursing* (pp. 62–83). Philadelphia: W.B. Saunders.

Suggested Resources

Andrews, M., Goldberg, K., & Kaplan, H. (2004). *Nurses' legal handbook* (5th ed.). Springhouse, PA: Springhouse.

Aveyard, H. (2005). Informed consent prior to nursing care procedures. *Nursing Ethics, 12*(1), 19–29.

Beauchamp, T.L. & Childress, J.F. (2001). *Principles of biomedical ethics.* New York: Oxford University Press.

Butler, K.A. (2004). Ethics paramount when patient lacks capacity. *Nursing Management, 35*(11), 18, 20, 52.

Coverston, D., & Rogers, S. (2000). Winding roads and faded signs: Ethical decision-making in a post-modern world. *The Journal of Perinatal & Neonatal Nursing, 14*(2), 1–11.

Ellis, J.R., & Hartley, C.L. (2004). *Nursing in today's world: Trends, issues & management* (8th ed.). Philadelphia: Lippincott, Williams & Wilkins.

Esterhuizen, P. (1996). Is the professional code still the cornerstone of clinical nursing practice? *Journal of Advanced Nursing, 23*(1), 25–31.

Hall, J. (1996). *Nursing ethics and the law.* Philadelphia: W.B. Saunders.

Rumbold, G. (1999). *Ethics in nursing practice* (3rd ed.). Philadelphia: W.B. Saunders.

Salladay, S. (1996). Rehabilitation ethics and managed care. *Rehab Management, 9*(6), 38–42.

Scanlon, C., & Fibison, W. (1995). *Managing genetic information: Implications for nursing practice.* Washington, DC: ANA.

Silva, M. (1995). *Ethical guidelines in the conduct, dissemination, and implementation of nursing research.* Washington, DC: ANA.

Sletteboe, A. (1997). Dilemma: A concept analysis. *Journal of Advanced Nursing, 26,* 449–454.

Trandel-Korenchuk, D., & Trandel, K. (1997). *Nursing and the law.* Gaithersburg, MD: Aspen.

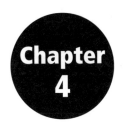

Chapter 4

Economics and Health Policy in Rehabilitation

Anne Deutsch, PhD RN CRRN • Susan Dean-Baar, PhD RN CRRN FAAN

The American healthcare system, including the delivery of rehabilitation services, is financed largely through federal and state programs and private health insurance. Rising healthcare costs, caused in part by an aging population and the high cost of new technology, have resulted in shifting the reimbursement of healthcare services by insurance and government agencies from a fee-for-service model to managed care and prospective payment models with shared financial risks. In addition to healthcare coverage, various income support programs (e.g., workers' compensation) are available for people with disabilities.

The rising cost of health care is only one of the many important themes in the development and modification of healthcare policy. Other important health policy issues are access to health care and the quality of health services.

The process of developing and modifying health policy provides opportunities for rehabilitation nurses to share their expertise with local, state, and federal government agencies and legislators. Rehabilitation nurses' unique knowledge and understanding of the needs of people with disabilities position them to advocate for health policy reform. A rehabilitation nurse's involvement may include a range of activities including educating the public about health issues (e.g., at schools or senior centers) or promoting letter-writing campaigns to garner support for a proposed bill.

The Association of Rehabilitation Nurses (ARN) Health Policy Committee represents ARN members and monitors pending legislation and regulation. In addition, the committee serves as a resource for individual members and ARN chapters to participate in local and state issues.

This chapter reviews the important issues related to the economics of healthcare delivery, including financing of health care, reimbursement (payment) models, and income support programs. It also describes how health policy is developed and modified and how rehabilitation nurses can influence policy.

I. **Economics: Financing the Delivery of Healthcare Services in the United States (see Table 4-1)**

A. Public Programs

1. Medicare: a federal health insurance program for people who are elderly or disabled under the authority of the U.S. Department of Health and Human Services (DHHS); began with the enactment of Title XVIII of the Social Security Act of 1965.

   a. Administration: managed by the Centers for Medicare and Medicaid Services (CMS), which designates fiscal intermediaries to process claims

   b. Coverage

      1) Original Medicare plan:

         a) Medicare Part A: hospital insurance plan that covers services provided by hospitals, skilled nursing facilities (SNFs), home health programs (skilled care only), hospice, and nursing homes; financed by employees and employers through the Social Security system.

         b) Medicare Part B: insurance plan that covers physicians' services; paid for by federal taxes and monthly premiums from beneficiaries.

         c) Medicare beneficiaries in the original plan may buy private Medicare supplemental insurance (i.e., Medigap) to cover the costs not covered under Part A and Part B.

      2) Medicare Part C: Medicare Advantage Plans that are offered through private insurance companies such as health maintenance organizations (HMOs) and preferred provider organizations (PPOs). Provides both hospital and physician coverage and is an alternative to original Part A and Part B coverage. Some plans include prescription drug coverage. Financed through Social Security system and monthly

Table 4-1. Funding Sources for Healthcare and Rehabilitation Programs

	Programs			
	Medicare (Federal)	**Medicaid (State)**	**Workers' compensation**	**Private health insurance**
Eligibility Requirements	Must be over the age of 65, have end-stage renal disease or have been disabled for 2 years	For people with low income	Workers injured in the course of employment	Policyholders
Benefits	Part A – hospital Part B - supplemental medical insurance Part C – Medicare Advantage Plans Part D – Prescription drug coverage	Hospital costs and visits to a physician Care in a skilled nursing facility	Medical care for a work-related injury Income support during period of disability	Hospital costs and outpatient treatment, as specified in policy Physician visits, as specified in policy May or may not cover rehabilitation care

Adapted with permission by ARN from McCourt, A.E. (Ed.). (1993). *The specialty practice of rehabilitation nursing: A core curriculum* (3rd ed., p. 227). Skokie, IL: Rehabilitation Nursing Foundation of the Association of Rehabilitation Nurses.

premiums from beneficiaries.
   a) PPO plans: These plans offer beneficiaries some choice of hospital and provider; additional costs may be incurred if services are furnished by a provider outside the network. Benefits can vary across plans and may include prescription drug coverage.
   b) HMO plans: These plans offer beneficiaries health services from within the plan network. Most plans charge a copayment each time a service is used. Benefits vary greatly by plan, but they usually include preventive care services and prescription drug coverage.
   c) Private fee-for-service: These plans offer the beneficiary a choice of hospital and provider. Benefits covered and costs per service vary according to the plan. The healthcare provider bills for every service rendered, based on previously established rates. Providers who accept Medicare assignment cannot charge the beneficiary for the difference between the charge and the established rate.
   3) Medicare Part D prescription drug coverage: Offered through private companies. Coverage varies depending on plan chosen. Financed through premiums from beneficiaries.
   c. Eligibility

   1) Upon reaching age 65, people who are eligible for Social Security are automatically enrolled in Medicare Part A whether or not they are retired. Medicare is a secondary payer if the person also has private health insurance.
   2) People younger than age 65 who are totally and permanently disabled may enroll in Medicare Part A after they have been receiving Social Security disability benefits for 24 months. People with chronic renal disease requiring dialysis or a transplant are eligible for Medicare Part A without the 2-year waiting period.
   3) All residents residing in a long-term care facility and are dual eligible will be automatically enrolled into plans by CMS, although these plans may not be the best for the individual. [Refer to Chapter 17 for more information.]
2. Medicaid: medical assistance program for certain individuals and families with low income and resources; began with the enactment of Title XIX of the Social Security Act of 1965.
   a. Administration: managed by each state; funded by federal, state, and (sometimes) local taxes.
   b. Coverage: Medicaid managed care and non–managed care options are available. Some states require enrollment in a managed care plan. The federal government requires states to provide hospital, physician, laboratory, X-ray, prenatal, and preventive care services;

nursing home and home health care; and medically necessary transportation. States can add services to this list and can place certain limitations on the federally mandated services.

   c. Eligibility:

     1) To be eligible for federal funds, states are required to provide Medicaid coverage for most people who get federally assisted income maintenance payments and for related groups not getting cash payments. Some examples of the mandatory Medicaid eligibility groups include the following:

      a) Limited-income families with children, who meet certain of the eligibility requirements in the state's Aid to Families with Dependent Children (AFDC) plan in effect on July 16, 1996

      b) Supplemental Security Income (SSI) recipients (or in states using more restrictive criteria, aged, blind, and disabled people who meet criteria that are more restrictive than those of the SSI program and were in place in the state's approved Medicaid plan as of January 1, 1972)

      c) Infants born to Medicaid-eligible pregnant women

      d) Children under age 6 and pregnant women whose family income is at or below 133% of the federal poverty level. States are required to extend Medicaid eligibility until age 19 to all children born after September 30, 1983 (or such earlier date as the state may choose) in families with incomes at or below the federal poverty level.

      e) Recipients of adoption assistance and foster care under Title IV-E of the Social Security Act

      f) Certain people with Medicare

      g) Special protected groups who may keep Medicaid for a period of time (e.g., people who lose SSI payments because of earnings from work or increased Social Security benefits and families who are provided 6–12 months of Medicaid coverage after loss of eligibility under Section 1931 because of earnings or 4 months of Medicaid coverage after loss of eligibility under Section 1931 because of an increase in child or spousal support)

     2) States have the option to provide Medicaid coverage for other "categorically needy" groups. These optional groups share characteristics of the mandatory groups, but the eligibility criteria are somewhat more liberally defined. Examples of the optional groups that states may cover as categorically needy (and for which they will get federal matching funds) under the Medicaid program include the following:

      a) Infants up to age 1 and pregnant women not covered under the mandatory rules whose family income is below 185% of the federal poverty level (the percentage to be set by each state)

      b) Optional targeted low-income children

      c) Certain aged, blind, or disabled adults who have incomes above those requiring mandatory coverage but below the federal poverty level

      d) Children under age 21 who meet income and resource requirements for the AFDC but who otherwise are not eligible for the AFDC

      e) Institutionalized people with limited income and resources

      f) People who would be eligible if institutionalized but are receiving care under home- and community-based service waivers

      g) Recipients of state supplementary payments

      h) Tuberculosis-infected people who would be financially eligible for Medicaid at the SSI level (only for tuberculosis-related ambulatory services and drugs)

      i) Low-income, uninsured women screened and diagnosed through a Centers for Disease Control and Prevention Breast and Cervical Cancer Early Detection Program and determined to be in need of treatment for breast or cervical cancer

3) States have the option to cover medically needy people, those who are poor but earn too much money to qualify for AFDC or SSI but who would otherwise be eligible for one of these programs by virtue of being in a family with dependent children, older than age 65, blind, or totally and permanently disabled.

   d. Program options: traditional or managed care plans

3. State Children's Health Insurance Plan: health insurance plan for children and working families who do not earn enough to afford coverage for their children.

   a. Administration:
      1) Jointly financed by the state and federal government. States are given broad flexibility in tailoring programs to meet their own circumstances.
      2) States can create or expand their own separate insurance programs, expand Medicaid, or combine both approaches.

   b. Eligibility: States have the opportunity to set eligibility criteria for age, income, resources, and residency within broad federal guidelines.

4. Workers' compensation: government-sponsored and employee-financed systems for compensating employees who incur an injury or illness in connection with their employment. Benefits provided include medical care, disability payments, rehabilitation services, survivor benefits, and funeral expenses.

   a. Administration: Each state, the District of Columbia, Puerto Rico, and the U.S. Virgin Islands designate an agency that will administer the program (e.g., state department of labor, independent workers' compensation agency, court administration).

   b. Eligibility: workers who are disabled by injury or families of a worker whose death arose out of and in the course of employment

   c. Coverage: provides both medical care related to the compensable injury and income benefits through the following sources:
      1) Private commercial insurance companies
      2) Self-insurance (corporations that are able to carry the risk)
      3) State funds
      4) State's second injury fund

   d. Medical care provisions:
      1) Treatment and rehabilitative programs for work-related injury
      2) Reimbursement in full or, in certain states, according to a medical fee guide

   e. Vocational rehabilitation benefits: Most states provide job retraining, education, and job placement.

B. Private Health Insurance

   1. Purchasing private health insurance plans

      a. Entities (e.g., an employer) may purchase private health insurance on behalf of a group of individuals. Purchasing groups often negotiate coverage, so benefits often vary by group. Group members (e.g., employees) contribute to the insurance premium.

      b. An individual may purchase private health insurance and pay the full premium.

   2. Types of health insurance and service plans

      a. Indemnity plans: provide comprehensive coverage for medical and hospital services
         1) The employer or subscriber pays a premium, and the subscriber agrees to pay any required deductible, copayments, and amounts over the insurer's usual and customary rate for specific services.
         2) The subscriber may receive services from physicians, hospitals, or other qualified providers of his or her choice for services that are medically necessary and meet accepted standards of medical practice.
         3) Preapproval for coverage may be required.
         4) Experimental and other noncovered services may be negotiable under certain circumstances.

      b. Managed care plans (Kongstvedt, 2001)
         1) Overview
            a) Managed care plans provide an identified set of medical or hospital care services for a fixed, predetermined premium.
            b) The managed care organization (MCO) may restrict the subscriber's choice of providers and control subscriber access.
            c) Subscribers often choose or are assigned a primary care

physician who is employed or under contract with the MCO. In many cases, the primary care physician acts as a gatekeeper for all other medical and hospital services.

d) The different types of insurance plans were reasonably distinct until the late 1980s. Since that time, the differences between traditional forms of health insurance (e.g., indemnity plans) and managed care plans have reduced substantially.

e) MCOs vary greatly in terms of their focus on controlling costs and quality (see Figure 4-1).
   (1) Less controlled: managed indemnity plans that may include precertification of elective admissions and case management of catastrophic cases
   (2) More controlled: group and staff model HMOs

2) Types of managed care plans
   a) HMOs: organized healthcare systems that are responsible for both the financing and the delivery of a broad range of healthcare services to an enrolled population. The original definition of HMO also included financing health care for a prepaid fixed fee. HMOs must ensure that their members have access to covered healthcare services and are responsible for the quality and appropriateness of these services.
      (1) Staff model (closed model): Physicians are employed by the HMO, typically are paid on a salary basis, and may receive bonus or incentive payments based on performance.
      (2) Group practice (closed model): The HMO contracts with a multispecialty physician group practice to

Figure 4-1. Continuum of Managed Care

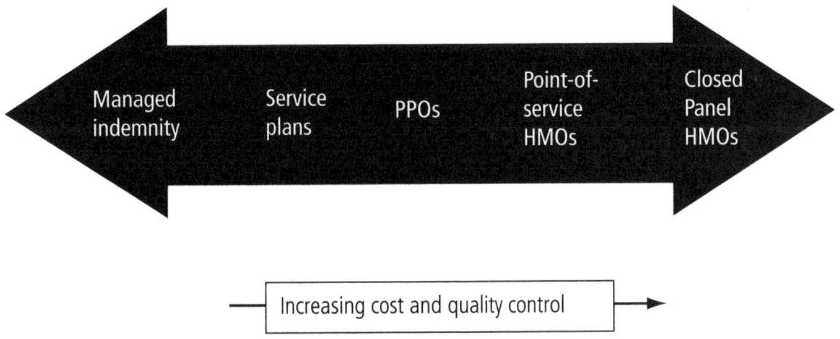

Managed indemnity — Service plans — PPOs — Point-of-service HMOs — Closed Panel HMOs

Increasing cost and quality control

Kongstvedt, P.R. (2001). *Essentials of managed health care* (4th ed., p. 19). Gaithersburg, MD: Aspen.

provide all physician services to members. The physicians are employed by the group practice, not the HMO.
      (3) Network (closed or open model): The HMO contracts with more than one group practice to provide physician services to members.
      (4) Independent Practice Association (IPA) (open model): The HMO contracts with an association of physicians to provide services to enrollees. The physicians are members of the IPA, a separate legal entity, but they remain as individual providers with their own offices and identities. Participation is open to all community physicians who meet the selection criteria. The HMO compensates the IPA on an all-inclusive physician capitation basis to provide services to enrollees. The IPA also compensates its participating physicians on a fee-for-service primary care capitation basis.
      (5) Direct contract: The HMO contracts directly with individual physicians to provide medical care to enrollees. Compensation to participating physicians may be on a fee-for-service or primary care capitation basis.

b) PPOs: Employer health benefit plans and insurance carriers contract with PPOs to purchase healthcare services for covered beneficiaries from a selected group of participating providers who typically agree to follow utilization management and other processes implemented by the PPO and agree to the reimbursement structure and payment models. PPOs offer incentives for enrollees to use the participating providers. Enrollees are permitted to use non-PPO providers, but they typically must pay higher coinsurance or deductible. Key attributes of a PPO include a selected provider panel, negotiated payment rates, rapid payment terms, utilization management, and consumer choice.

c) Point-of-service (POS) plans: POS plans offer enrollees some indemnity-type coverage but typically incorporate high deductibles and coinsurance to this coverage to encourage members to use the HMO-type services.

c. Medicare supplemental benefits plan (Medigap): purchased by Medicare beneficiaries to pay for expenses that are not covered by Medicare

d. Auto liability: covers medical care needed as a result of an auto accident

C. Programs for Special Groups

1. Benefits for veterans of the armed forces: coverage provided for treatment of a service-related illness or for needy veterans who have non–service-related medical problems; administered by the Department for Veterans Affairs.

2. Federal government civilian employee workers' compensation programs

3. Family and Medical Leave Act (Public Law [PL] 103-3): requires employers of 50 or more employees (and all public agencies) to provide up to 12 weeks of unpaid, job-protected leave to eligible employees for the health-related problems of the employee or a family member.

4. Indian Health Service: an agency of the U.S. DHHS that provides hospital care, dental and health benefits, substance abuse counseling, public health nursing, and other services to American Indians and Alaskan Natives.

5. Railroad Retirement Act Program

6. Black Lung Benefits Act of 1972

7. Longshoremen and Harbor Workers' Compensation Act

8. Life care planning: the process of mapping out short- and long-term care needs, expenses, and resources for patients with a debilitating, chronic illness or injury. A life care plan is created to ensure that the patient receives consistent, comprehensive, cost-effective care from present and future caregivers (Barker, 1999).

II. Reimbursement for Healthcare Services

A. Payment Units

1. Prospective payment system (PPS): The payment rate to the healthcare facility is predetermined based on the medical diagnosis, treatment, or other information, regardless of the cost for care for a specific patient.

2. Per discharge payment: The provider or hospital is paid one sum for all services delivered during one stay.

3. Per diem payments: The healthcare facility is paid one sum for all services delivered to a patient during one day.

B. Medicare Payment Systems

1. Acute care hospitals

a. Inpatient hospital acute care.

b. Medicare implemented a per-discharge inpatient PPS in acute care hospitals in 1983. PPS payments are expected to cover all operating and capital costs. PPS payments are determined based on patient and facility factors:

1) The patient classification system for the inpatient PPS is diagnosis-related groups (DRGs). Data from the bill are used to assign each patient into one of the 536 DRGs (payment groups).

2) Adjustments are made for a rural or urban location, indirect medical education, the proportion of low-income population, and the geographic differences in labor costs.

3) The base payment rate is updated each year.

2. Critical access hospitals (CAHs)

a. CAHs are small hospitals, limited to 25 beds, and operate primarily in rural areas. In addition to the 25 acute care beds, CAHs may have distinct part skilled nursing facilities, 10-bed psychiatric units, 10-bed rehabilitation units, and home health agencies.

b. Each CAH receives 101% of costs for outpatient, inpatient, laboratory, therapy services, and post–acute care in the hospital's swing beds.

3. SNFs

a. An SNF provides short-term skilled care (nursing or rehabilitation services) on an inpatient basis. Medicare beneficiaries must have a hospital stay of a least 3 days to be eligible for SNF services to be covered. The Medicare SNF benefit covers skilled nursing care, rehabilitation services, and other goods and services up to 100 days if the patient meets established criteria.

b. The SNF patient assessment instrument is the Minimum Data Set (MDS 2.0). Data collected using the MDS 2.0, such as treatments provided and patient characteristics, are used to categorize each patient into payment groups and to calculate facility-level quality indicators.

c. Medicare implemented a per diem SNF PPS in 1998. PPS payments are expected to cover all operating and capital costs, with certain high-cost, low-probability ancillary services paid separately. PPS payments are determined based on patient and facility factors:

   1) The patient classification system for the SNF PPS is Resource Utilization Groups (RUGs). Data from the MDS 2.0 are used to assign each patient into one of the 53 RUGs (payment groups).

   2) Adjustments are made for rural or urban location and geographic differences in labor costs.

   3) The base payment rates are updated each year.

4. Home health care

a. A home health agency provides skilled care (from a nurse or physical or occupational therapist) on a part-time or intermittent basis in the person's home. In order to qualify for this benefit, Medicare beneficiaries generally are restricted to their homes.

b. The home health agency patient assessment instrument is the Outcome and Assessment Information Set (OASIS). Data collected using the OASIS, such as clinical characteristics, functional status, and service use rates, are used to categorize each patient into a payment group and to calculate facility-level quality indicators.

c. Medicare implemented a PPS for home health in 2000 that pays a predetermined rate to the agency for each 60-day episode. PPS payments are determined based on patient and facility factors:

   1) The patient classification system for the home health agency PPS is the Home Health Resource Groups (HHRGs). Data from the OASIS are used to assign each patient into one of the 80 HHRGs (payment groups).

   2) Payments are adjusted if fewer than 5 visits are delivered during the 60-day episode and for other special circumstances, such as high-cost outliers.

   3) Adjustments are made for geographic differences in labor costs.

   4) The base payment rate is updated each year.

5. Inpatient rehabilitation facilities (IRFs)

a. IRFs, including freestanding rehabilitation hospitals and distinct part rehabilitation units within general (acute care) hospitals, provide intensive rehabilitation services, such as physical, occupational, or speech therapy to patients after an illness, injury, or surgical care. Patients must be able to tolerate and benefit from 3 hours of daily therapy. (Providing services no less than 5 days a week satisfies the requirement for "daily" services.)

b. The 75% rule requires that 75% of patients admitted to an IRF have one of 13 selected medical conditions.

c. The IRF patient assessment instrument is the Inpatient Rehabilitation Facility Patient Assessment Instrument (IRF-PAI). Data include demographic, diagnostic, and FIM™ instrument (functional status) data. Data are collected on admission and discharge, and admission data are used to categorize each patient into payment groups.

d. Medicare implemented a per-discharge IRF PPS in 2002. PPS payments are expected to cover all operating and capital costs, with certain high-cost, low-probability ancillary services paid separately. PPS payments are determined based on patient and facility factors:

    1) The patient classification system for the IRF PPS is Case-Mix Groups (CMGs). In addition, payments are adjusted for the presence of a tiered comorbidity. Data from the IRF-PAI are used to assign each patient into one of the 353 CMG comorbidity (payment) groups.

    2) A transfer rule aims to discourage IRFs from discharging patients to other institutional settings.

    3) Payments are adjusted for short-stay outliers and high-cost outliers.

    4) Adjustments are made for rural or urban location, treatment of low-income patients, teaching status, and geographic differences in labor costs.

    5) The base payment rate is updated each year.

  6. Long-term care hospitals (LTCHs)

    a. An LTCH provides care to patients with clinically complex problems, such as multiple acute or chronic conditions, who need hospital care for extended periods of time. On average, LTCH patients must have a length of stay of 25 days. LTCHs are not distributed evenly across the United States.

    b. The 25% rule for hospitals within hospitals limits the proportion of patients that can be admitted from a hospital within a host hospital during a cost reporting period.

    c. Medicare implemented a per-discharge LTCH PPS in 2002. PPS payments are expected to cover all operating and capital costs, with certain high-cost, low-probability ancillary services paid separately. PPS payments are determined based on patient and facility factors:

      1) The patient classification system for the LTCH PPS is the long-term care diagnosis related groups (LTC-DRGs). The LTC-DRGs are the same groupings used in the acute care inpatient PPS, but the relative weights for each group are different. Data from the hospital bill (e.g., diagnosis, procedures, patient characteristics) are used to assign each patient into one of the

more than 500 LTC-DRGs (payment groups).

    2) Payments are adjusted for short-stay outliers and high-cost outliers.

    3) Adjustments are made for indirect medical education and geographic differences in labor costs.

    4) Transfer policies aim to discourage transfers between an LTCH and a co-located acute care hospital and transfers to co-located SNFs, IRFs, and psychiatric facilities.

    5) The base payment rates are updated each year.

III. Economic Barriers to Care

  A. Lack of Health Insurance

    1. Overview

      a. The majority of Americans under the age of 65 receive health insurance coverage through their employers, and almost all older adults receive coverage through Medicare. Medicaid and the State Children's Health Insurance Program provide insurance for millions of nonelderly low-income people, especially children. However, program limits and gaps in employer coverage mean that many do not have health insurance.

      b. Approximately 46.1 million people, nearly 18% of nonelderly people, in the United States did not have health insurance in 2005 (Kaiser Commission on Medicaid and the Uninsured, 2006).

      c. The percentage of people without health insurance varies greatly across states because of the structure and health of local economies, the proportion of low-income families, and the scope of state Medicaid program coverage. For example, in 2004–2005, in Hawaii, Iowa, and Minnesota, less than 10% of the nonelderly population was uninsured, whereas in Florida, Texas, and New Mexico, the rate of uninsured people was higher than 20% (U.S. Census Bureau).

    2. Who does not have insurance

      a. Low-income Americans are likely to be uninsured. More than one-third of the poor (family incomes below 200% of the poverty level) and 30% of the near-poor (family incomes 100% to 199% of the poverty level) do not have health insurance.

      b. Approximately 81% of the uninsured are

in working families. Low-wage workers are likely to be uninsured, as are people employed in small businesses, the service industries, and blue-collar jobs.

    c. Medicaid covers low-income children; coverage for adults is more limited. Parent income eligibility levels are much lower than the levels for children. There are also enrollment hurdles and lack of outreach.

    d. The rate of uninsured among older adults is low (less than 2%) as a result of the Medicare program; however, underinsurance can be an economic barrier for older adults who must supplement their insurance coverage with out-of-pocket money. Black and Hispanic older adults are disproportionately uninsured (Okara, Young, Strine, Balluz, & Mokdad, 2005).

B. Underinsurance and Other Limitations of Access and Coverage

    1. Health insurance does not always ensure access to care. An estimated 16 million adults between 19 to 64 are underinsured. There are often limitations on coverage for special services, such as behavioral health care, preventive care, long-term care, catastrophic illnesses or accidents, and psychiatric care. Also, exclusions or waiting periods for illnesses or conditions may exist at the time the person enrolls in the health plan.

    2. Most health insurance plans also include copayments or deductibles to discourage overuse of services and to reduce premium costs. Copayments and high deductibles can discourage some patients from seeking preventive care (e.g., immunizations, mammograms) and effectively managing chronic conditions. This is particularly a problem for people with low incomes.

    3. Substantial gaps in cost-sharing provisions and coverage exist in the traditional Medicare program:

       a. There are large deductibles and copayments for hospital care and restrictions on long-term care coverage.

       b. It is estimated that Medicare pays less than 50% of the total costs of health care for older adults. To cover these expenses, many older adults have supplemental coverage (e.g., Medigap), which is offered through employer or retirement plans or may be purchased directly. More

than 20% of older adults and 35% of low-income older adults have no supplemental coverage (Jonas & Kovner, 2005).

    4. Low-income older adults may qualify for Medicaid in addition to Medicare. Although Medicaid is comprehensive, many physicians do not participate in the program because of its low level of payment. Therefore, barriers still exist for low-income older adults trying to access basic healthcare services.

C. Effects of Limited or No Health Insurance

    1. Limited or lack of health insurance creates substantial barriers to obtaining timely and appropriate health care:

       a. More than 40% of nonelderly uninsured adults have no regular source of health care, and many delay or go without needed care because of concerns about high medical bills.

       b. More than one-third of the uninsured have a serious problem paying medical bills, and one-quarter are contacted by collection agencies because of medical bills.

    2. Delaying or not receiving treatment can lead to more serious illness and avoidable health conditions:

       a. The uninsured are less likely to receive preventive care and are more likely to be admitted to a hospital for a preventable or avoidable condition than people with insurance.

       b. Researchers estimate that at least 18,000 Americans die prematurely each year because of lack of health insurance. A reduction in mortality of 5%–15% could be achieved if the uninsured had health insurance.

    3. Uninsured and underinsured patients typically receive care from a select group of providers (e.g., community clinics and public hospitals) that are willing to provide care regardless of a person's ability to pay, such as hospital-based outpatient departments, emergency rooms, and community-based clinics:

       a. Costs in these institutional-based settings often are high, increasing the total costs of delivering care.

       b. To cover the costs of caring for uninsured and underinsured people, providers must either shift fees to other payers or seek government or private subsidies.

       c. Current market forces, including managed

care and fixed-fee schedules, make cost shifting difficult, resulting in decreasing services provided to underinsured and uninsured people.

   4. At a societal level, limited and no health insurance leads to more disability, lower productivity, and a greater burden on the healthcare system.

D. Responses to the Lack of Health Insurance

   1. The Health Insurance Portability and Accountability Act prohibits group insurance plans from including eligibility criteria related to health status, medical history, genetic information, or disability and reduces exclusions for preexisting conditions when the person was previously covered by a group insurance plan.

   2. The Consolidated Omnibus Budget Reconciliation Act gives people in specific categories the right to continued health plan coverage for up to 18 months after voluntary or involuntary termination of employment or reduction in work hours. The person must pay the entire premium.

IV. Funding for Assistive Technology

A. Definition: *Assistive technology* refers to any item, piece of equipment, or product system—whether acquired commercially, off the shelf, modified, or customized—that is used to increase, maintain, or improve the functional capabilities of people with disabilities.

B. Why Funding for Assistive Technology Is a Significant Problem:

   1. Insurance or health programs do not pay for assistive devices if they are not considered medically necessary.

   2. The Technology Related Assistance for Individuals with Disabilities Act of 1988 (PL 100-407) provided grants to states:

      a. To increase the availability of assistive technology
      b. To conduct need assessments
      c. To develop innovative programs
      d. To manage public awareness
      e. To identify policies that promote the availability of assistive technology

   3. In 1994, an amendment (PL 103-218) expanded and strengthened the 1988 act.

V. Income Support Programs (see Table 4-2)

A. Social Security Programs

   1. Old-Age and Survivors Insurance

      a. Eligibility

         1) Must be a retired worker at least 65 years old (by 2009, the minimum age will be 66); reduced benefits are available to workers who retire at age 62 or to widow(er)s or surviving divorced spouses.
         2) Must have reached "fully insured" status (i.e., must have worked under the program for a minimum of 10 years [1 year = 4 quarters; 40 quarters are needed to be eligible]).

      b. Benefits

         1) No means test is required.
         2) Benefits are paid as an earned right.
         3) No minimum income amount is required during active working years.
         4) There is no limit on other sources of income, including savings, pensions, or insurance.

   2. Disability insurance

Table 4-2. Income Support Programs Pertinent to Rehabilitation

	Program		
	Social Security	**State Workers' Compensation**	**Private or Individual Disability Insurance**
Population	Workers disabled before the age of 65 years and "fully insured" under covered work	Injured workers who meet state criteria for work-related conditions	Injured workers with a nonoccupational disability who are defined as unable to perform either the work related to their own occupation or any reasonable occupation
Benefits	Amount payable in retirement	Temporary total benefits that are calculated by a state formula, which is usually two-thirds of salary	A percentage of previous earnings
Time period	For as long as person is disabled; trial work period may be stipulated	Variable; could be for person's lifetime; some states stipulate a maximum number of weeks (e.g., 500)	Policy may have a maximum benefit period (e.g., 2 years)

Sources consulted

Reprinted with permission from Edwards, P. (Ed.). (2000). *The specialty practice of rehabilitation nursing: A core curriculum* (4th ed., p. 52). Glenview, IL: Rehabilitation Nursing Foundation of the Association of Rehabilitation Nurses.

a. Eligibility:
    1) Must be a worker younger than age 65 with a disability: A disabling condition is one in which the worker is so severely impaired physically or mentally that he or she is not able to perform substantial gainful work.
    2) Must have "fully insured" status and have 20 quarters in the 40-quarter period, ending with the quarter in which the disability was sustained.

b. Benefits: Applicants are referred to state departments or agencies for vocational rehabilitation services, which vary by state.

B. State Income Support Programs
  1. Workers' compensation
    a. Eligibility: Condition must be work related.
    b. Benefits: Usually calculated as a percentage of the worker's weekly earnings at the time of the injury or death.
      1) Restrictions
        a) Each state designates maximum amount, often two-thirds of gross salary.
        b) There may be a waiting period.
        c) Some states stipulate a maximum number of weeks for benefits (e.g., 500 weeks).
      2) Types of benefits
        a) Temporary total disability: Worker is disabled for a temporary period but expected to recover.
        b) Permanent total disability: Worker is disabled permanently and unable to perform any type of work.
        c) Temporary partial disability: Worker is able to work but has diminished capacity.
        d) Permanent partial disability: Worker is able to work but has a partial impairment.
        e) Survivor (death): Payments are made to spouse until remarriage and to children until age 18.

  2. State or federal income programs
    a. Temporary Assistance for Needy Families
    b. Food stamps
    c. Supplemental food program for women, infants, and children
    d. Public housing and subsidized housing
    e. State general assistance or welfare programs

C. Private Insurance and Benefits
  1. Retirement plans (e.g., individual or group plans)
  2. Disability income insurance (e.g., individual or group plans)
  3. Automobile insurance benefits
    a. No fault
    b. Automobile liability
  4. General liability for personal injury or wrongful death
  5. Accidental death and dismemberment insurance
  6. Hospital indemnity insurance benefits
  7. Travel accident insurance benefits
  8. Mortgage and credit disability insurance benefits

VI. Economics of Prevention

A. Levels of Prevention
  1. Primary prevention focuses on supporting or protecting the health and well-being of society at large. Efforts are geared toward reducing susceptibility to illness and injury, controlling exposure to disease-causing agents, minimizing risky behaviors, and removing or reducing environmental factors that increase the risk of disease or injury.
  2. Secondary prevention consists of efforts directed to high-risk populations. These include early detection of potential health problems and, if appropriate, interventions to stop, reverse, or slow down the disease progress.
  3. Tertiary prevention is the effort to maximize function and minimize the sequelae of an injury or illness.

B. Statistics Related to Disability in Society
  1. Approximately 54 million American have some kind of disability that affects their ability to function (McNeil, 2001).
  2. In 1991, disability was estimated to cost the United States almost $200 billion annually in medical care and lost productivity (Institute of Medicine, 1991).
  3. The prevalence of disability increases dramatically with advancing age (Kassner & Bectel, 1998).
    a. Among people 50–64 years of age, approximately 1% receive help with two or more activities of daily living.
    b. Among people 85 years and older, approximately 11% receive help with two

or more activities of daily living.

4. Having an activity limitation more than doubles the average number of physician visits per year.

5. In addition to healthcare expenses, costs relate to lost productivity, lost taxes, and increased spending on expensive adaptations.

C. Shift from Responding to Medical Conditions to Promoting Health

1. Healthcare services that respond to medical conditions (e.g., trauma care, treatment of infection) have expanded at the expense of addressing causes or contributory factors of health problems.

2. National initiatives support disease prevention, health promotion, and a community focus for the healthcare system.

a. Healthy People 2010, a statement of national health objectives designed to identify the most significant preventable threats to health and to establish national goals to reduce these threats

b. The Centers for Disease Control and Prevention

1) National Center for Injury Prevention and Control focuses on preventing death and disability from nonoccupational injuries, including those that are unintentional and those that result from violence.

2) National Center on Birth Defects and Developmental Disabilities provides national leadership for preventing birth defects and developmental disabilities and for improving the health and wellness of people with disabilities.

3) National Center for Chronic Disease Prevention and Health Promotion focuses on preventing premature death and disability from chronic diseases and promotes healthy personal behaviors.

c. Health America: Practitioners for 2005, an agenda for action by U.S. schools for health professionals

d. Recommendations from the Institute of Medicine's Disability in America: Toward a National Agenda for Prevention (see Figure 4-2)

D. Challenges for Health Professionals, Including Rehabilitation Nurses

1. Determine the types of education programs that actually prevent illnesses or injuries and

how these programs should be implemented.

2. Meet increasing demands to make health promotion and disease prevention economically worthwhile by conducting cost-effectiveness analyses.

I. Health Policy: Overview

A. Definition: *Policy* refers to the choices that are made about goals and priorities and the ways in which resources are allocated to reach these goals. The choice of policies reflects the values, beliefs, and attitudes of those designing the policy. Health policy includes the decisions made to promote the health of individual citizens.

B. Stakeholders: The healthcare industry has a variety of stakeholders who may have common or conflicting concerns regarding policies.

1. Patients tend to favor comprehensive coverage, high-quality health care, and low out-of-pocket

---

Figure 4-2. Recommendations for a National Agenda for the Prevention of Disability

Organization and Coordination
• Develop leadership of National Disability Prevention Program at CDC
• Develop an enhanced role for the private sector
• Establish a national advisory committee
• Establish a federal interagency council
• Critically assess progress periodically

Surveillance
• Develop a conceptual framework and standard measures of disability
• Develop a national disability surveillance system
• Revise the National Health Interview Survey
• Conduct a comprehensive longitudinal survey of disability
• Develop disability indices

Research
• Develop a comprehensive research program
• Emphasize longitudinal research
• Conduct research on socioeconomic and psychological disadvantage
• Expand research on preventive and therapeutic interventions
• Upgrade training for research on disability prevention

Access to Care and Preventive Services
• Provide comprehensive health services to all mothers and children
• Provide effective family planning and prenatal services
• Develop new health service delivery strategies for people with disabilities
• Develop new health promotion models for people with disabilities
• Foster local capacity for building and demonstration projects
• Continue effective prevention programs
• Provide comprehensive vocational services

Professional and Public Education
• Upgrade medical education and training of physicians
• Upgrade the training of allied professionals
• Establish a program of grants for education and training
• Provide more public education on the prevention of disability
• Provide more training opportunities for family members and personal attendants of people with disabling conditions

Reprinted with permission from *Disability in America*. Copyright 1991 by the National Academy of Sciences. Courtesy of the National Academies Press, Washington, DC.

expenses and tend to oppose limited access to care and increased patient payments.

2. Providers (individual and entities) tend to favor income maintenance, autonomy, and comprehensive coverage and tend to oppose limits on provider payments.

3. Taxpayers tend to favor limits on provider payments and tend to oppose higher taxes.

4. Employers and payers tend to favor cost containment, administrative simplification, and elimination of cost shifting and tend to oppose government regulation.

5. Regulators (government) tend to favor disclosure and reporting by providers, cost containment, access to care, and high-quality health care and tend to oppose provider autonomy.

6. Vendors and suppliers tend to favor comprehensive coverage and tend to oppose limits on provider payments.

C. Reasons Why Nurses Should Get Involved in Developing Health Policy:

1. Enables participation in decisions relating to the future of the profession and health care

2. Has a positive effect on the healthcare delivery system

3. Promotes the ability to provide input at policy-making and health-planning levels

4. Shows a commitment to maintaining healthcare standards

D. Emerging Healthcare Policy Issues:

1. The delivery of healthcare services

   a. Access to care: Many people have a limited ability to obtain necessary health services for two reasons:
      1) Ability to pay: People have no health insurance or are underinsured.
      2) Location: People may not have healthcare personnel and facilities that are close to where they live, accessible by transportation, culturally acceptable, or capable of providing appropriate care using the language with which the patient is most familiar.

   b. Costs of care:
      1) In 1960, the national health expenditures represented 5.1% of the gross domestic product (GDP); expenditures per capita were $141.
      2) In 2006, health care represented 16% of the GDP (i.e., 16 cents of every dollar was spent on health care); average expenditures per capita were $7,110.

      3) As a result, various cost containment strategies (e.g., PPS, managed care) are now used.

   c. Quality of health care: Healthcare quality may be defined as the "degree to which patient care services increase the probability of desired patient outcomes and reduce the probability of undesired health outcomes given the current state of knowledge" (Institute of Medicine Committee on Clinical Practice Guidelines, 1992).

   d. Health disparities: Disparities in healthcare use and outcomes for people from racial and ethnic minorities and low-income people result in significantly higher rates of chronic illness and disability.

2. Nursing services and workforce

   a. Reimbursement for nursing services, including rehabilitation nurses

   b. Scope of practice (e.g., for advanced practice nurses), as defined by state licensure laws and regulatory bodies

   c. Emerging critical shortage of nurses and nursing faculty

   d. Funding for nursing education and research

3. Social issues related to populations that rehabilitation nurses serve

   a. Community accessibility

   b. Discrimination against people with disabilities in hiring practices or in the workplace

   c. Disincentives for people with disabilities to return to work

   d. Availability of vocational rehabilitation services

4. Environmental health issues

   a. Occupational health hazards (e.g., neurotoxicity from chemicals in the workplace)

   b. Testing of food and drugs

5. Prevention of catastrophic injuries and illness

   a. Mandating the use of seatbelts and inflatable restraints and helmet use while motorcycling, bicycling, skiing, and skating

   b. Providing education about substance abuse, particularly as a cause of accidents that can result in spinal cord injury or traumatic brain injury

c. Promoting smoke-free environments

6. Women's issues

a. Equal rights for women, including research on women's health concerns

b. Economic equity (including child support)

c. Child care and elder care

d. Employers' support of family health

e. Vocational training for women who are new or returning to the workplace because of circumstances such as divorce or death of a spouse

7. Men's issues

a. Research on men's health concerns (e.g., prostate cancer)

b. Child care and elder care

c. Employers' support of family health

8. Genetic testing (including privacy)

9. Privacy and confidentiality

a. Health Insurance Portability and Accountability Act privacy rule regulations on protected health information, effective April 2003

b. Development and implementation of electronic medical records

10. Telemedicine [Refer to Chapter 21 for more information.]

a. Strategy to improve access to health care for people in rural areas

b. Regulatory issues related to provider in one location and patient in another

c. Consumer-directed health care

11. Internet use by consumers to find healthcare information and receive support (Cudney, Winters, Weinert, & Anderson, 2005; Pierce et al., 2004; Hill, Schillo, & Weinert, 2004)

E. Rehabilitation Legislation (Watson, 1988):

1. Education amendments (1980, PL 96-374) provide centers, services, personnel, training, and research related to educational needs of children with disabilities.

2. Social Security Disability amendments (1980, PL 96-265) extend trial work periods for the disabled, enabling them to retain Social Security benefits; place gainfully employed people with disabilities in a special benefit category for needed services.

3. Surface Transportation Assistance Act (1982, PL 97-424) encourages removal of architectural barriers in transportation industry.

4. Individuals with Disabilities Education Act (IDEA) (1983, PL 98-199) ensures access to educational opportunities for children with disabilities.

5. Vocational Education Act (1984, PL 98-524) requires states to provide funds for people with disabilities to have access to available vocational educational opportunities.

6. Rehabilitation amendments (1984, PL 98-221) modify the definition of "severely disabled" and place a lower age limit at 16 years; extends provisions of 1973 Rehabilitation Act.

7. Rehabilitation amendments (1986, PL 99-506) emphasize rehabilitation needs of Native Americans with disabilities; provide funding for rehabilitation engineering to develop technologically current devices for people with disabilities; decrease federal share of the basic state rehabilitation program; expand influence of the National Council on the Handicapped.

8. Technology-Related Assistance for Individuals with Disabilities (1988, PL 100-407) provides grants to states in an effort to increase the availability of assistive technology, conduct need assessments, develop innovative programs, manage public awareness, and identify policies that promote the availability of assistive technology.

9. Americans with Disabilities Act of 1990 (PL 101-336) (see Figure 4-3) prohibits discrimination on the basis of disability in the areas of employment, public services, and public accommodations; addresses telecommunications and other miscellaneous provisions.

10. Technology-Related Assistance for Individuals with Disabilities amendments (1994, PL 103-218) expands and strengthens the 1988 act.

11. Health Insurance Portability and Insurance Act of 1996 (PL 104-191) improves portability and continuity of health insurance coverage.

12. Balanced Budget Act of 1997 (PL 105-33) mandates new Medicare PPS for SNFs, home care, inpatient rehabilitation facilities, and long-term care hospitals.

13. Balanced Budget Refinement Act of 1999 (PL 106-113) refines post–acute care payment policies.

14. Deficit Reduction Act of 2005 (PL 109-171) mandates that CMS develop a standardized patient assessment and implement a demonstration project for post–acute care payment reform.

F. Guidelines for Taking Political Action:

1. Register and vote for the candidates of your choice.

2. Be informed on issues.

3. Get involved in professional nursing associations and their health policy task forces.

4. Obtain lists of local, state, and national legislators (available from government offices, Web sites, or public libraries).

5. Join the ARN Health Policy Committee:

    a. Be informed about ARN's position on legislation by contacting the ARN office or the ARN Health Policy Committee Chair or by searching the ARN Web site (http://www.rehabnurse.org).

    b. Communicate with the ARN Health Policy Committee Chair about local and state issues and personal activities.

    c. Attend legislative conferences (e.g., Nurse-in-Washington Internship).

6. Do not act as a spokesperson for a national or local organization unless specifically authorized to do so.

7. Establish a relationship and communicate with federal, state, and local legislators to make them aware of positions on specific

issues (see Figure 4-4):

    a. Write letters.

    b. Make telephone calls.

    c. Send faxes.

    d. Send e-mail.

    e. Meet in person.

    f. Volunteer professional services or provide monetary support.

    g. Provide expert testimony.

II. Process of Making Health Policy

A. Phases of Health Policy Making (see Figure 4-5)

1. Policy formulation (Longest, 1996):

    a. Agenda setting

        1) This first stage of policy development refers to identifying problems and possible solutions given by diverse political interests.

        2) Once issues become prominent in the political agenda, they can proceed to

the next stage of policy formulation: the development of legislation. However, only a small percentage of issues reach that point.

  b. Development of legislation (see Figure 4-6)

    1) The legislative process begins with proposals (bills), which may be drafted by senators or representatives and their staff members, by members of the executive branch, by political or special interest groups, and by individual citizens.

      a) Only members of Congress can officially sponsor a bill.

      b) Occasionally, identical bills are simultaneously introduced in the Senate and the House of Representatives for consideration.

    2) Each bill is assigned to the appropriate committee(s) based on its content and the jurisdiction of the committees and subcommittees. Hearings are held, and the bill is marked up. Once it is approved by the full committee, the House or Senate receives the bill and places it on the legislative calendar for floor action. The bill may be further amended during debate on the floor.

    3) Once the bill passes either the House or the Senate, it is sent to the other chamber of Congress, where the process is repeated. If the second chamber passes the bill, any differences between the House and Senate versions must be resolved before the bill is sent to the White House for presidential action.

    4) The president has the option to sign the bill to make it a law or to veto the bill and return it to Congress with an explanation for the rejection. A presidential veto may be overridden by a two-thirds vote in both houses of Congress. If the president does not sign or veto the bill after 10 days, the bill automatically becomes law.

2. Policy implementation (includes rule making and policy operation):

  a. Once a law is enacted, implementation rests primarily with the executive branch of the government. Cabinet departments such as DHHS and agencies such as CMS and the Centers for Disease Control and Prevention oversee the implementation.

  b. Other agencies such as the Government Accountability Office, the Congressional Budget Office, the Congressional Research Office, and the Office of Technology and Assessment have oversight responsibility.

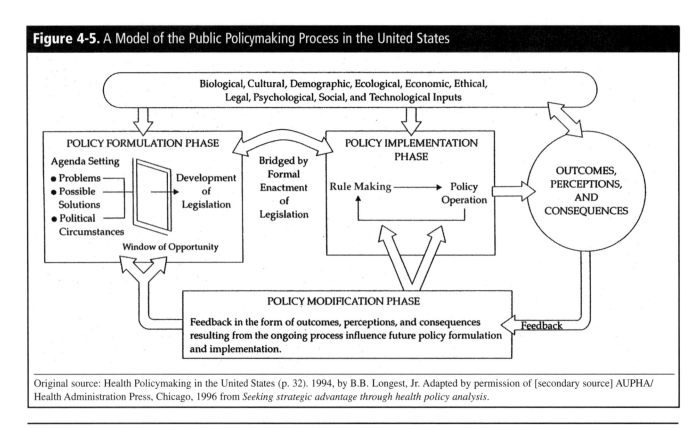

Figure 4-5. A Model of the Public Policymaking Process in the United States

Original source: Health Policymaking in the United States (p. 32). 1994, by B.B. Longest, Jr. Adapted by permission of [secondary source] AUPHA/ Health Administration Press, Chicago, 1996 from *Seeking strategic advantage through health policy analysis*.

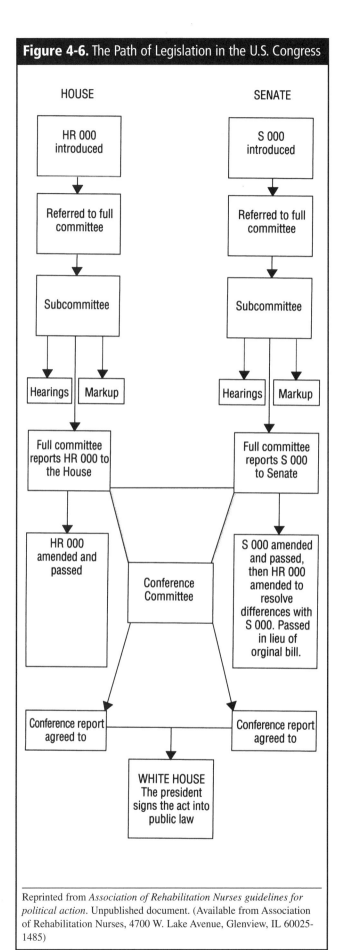

Figure 4-6. The Path of Legislation in the U.S. Congress

HOUSE

HR 000 introduced

Referred to full committee

Subcommittee

Hearings | Markup

Full committee reports HR 000 to the House

HR 000 amended and passed

SENATE

S 000 introduced

Referred to full committee

Subcommittee

Hearings | Markup

Full committee reports S 000 to Senate

S 000 amended and passed, then HR 000 amended to resolve differences with S 000. Passed in lieu of orginal bill.

Conference Committee

Conference report agreed to

Conference report agreed to

WHITE HOUSE
The president signs the act into public law

Reprinted from *Association of Rehabilitation Nurses guidelines for political action*. Unpublished document. (Available from Association of Rehabilitation Nurses, 4700 W. Lake Avenue, Glenview, IL 60025-1485)

c. Laws often are vague on implementation details, so the organization responsible for implementing the law publishes a "Notice of Proposed Rule Making" and "Final Rule" in the *Federal Register*.

d. Policy implementation involves the actual operation of programs that are described in the enacted legislation.

3. Policy modification: This stage allows all prior decisions to be modified once the outcomes, perceptions, and consequences of existing policies are discovered. Modifications to any legislation must begin with the agenda-setting stage.

B. Opportunities for Rehabilitation Nurses to Influence Health Policy Making

1. In policy formulation:

a. Agenda setting
1) Define and document problems.
2) Develop and evaluate solutions to problems.
3) Shape political circumstances by lobbying and working through the legal system.

b. Legislation development
1) Participate in drafting legislation.
2) Testify at legislative hearings.

2. In policy implementation or rule making:

a. Provide formal comments on proposed rules published in the *Federal Register*.

b. Serve on and provide input to rule-making advisory bodies.

c. Work on policy operation by interacting with policy operators.

3. In policy modification: Document cases for modification through operational experience and formal evaluations (i.e., research).

III. Healthcare System's Response to Health Policy (Nosse, Friberg, & Kovacek, 1999)

A. Growth and Development of the Healthcare Delivery System (1965–1980)

1. The structure of the delivery system included small independent physician group practices.

2. Larger multispecialty clinics were developing but were uncommon. Hospitals provided secondary and tertiary care.

3. The supply of and demand for healthcare services expanded in response to several factors:

a. Introduction of Medicare and Medicaid programs

b. An increased need for the capacity,

capabilities, and number and types of healthcare providers

   c. An increased number of people accessing the delivery system

   d. An increased amount of care provided

   e. New and improved treatments and technology

B. Cost Containment in the Delivery of Health Care (1981–1991)

   1. Cost containment was a concern for physicians, hospitals, and public and private insurers.

   2. Acute care PPS began in 1983 and helped reduce the costs of inpatient hospital care by:

      a. Decreasing the average length of stay

      b. Decreasing the use of routine diagnostic tests during inpatient hospitalizations

      c. Shifting care to outpatient settings

      d. Increasing the use of post–acute care services (e.g., home care, rehabilitation hospitals and units, SNFs)

   3. The decrease in inpatient hospital use resulted in excess acute care bed capacity, decreased profits for hospitals and physicians, and imposed financial limits on purchasing new technologies and upgrading facilities.

   4. These trends caused providers to compete for a larger share of the healthcare market and to react in many ways:

      a. Reduced costs through reorganization and staff layoffs

      b. Developed and modified alternative care options (e.g., rehabilitation services, home care, ambulatory care, long-term care)

      c. Restructured the organization through vertical and horizontal integration with other providers so that hospital networks cover larger geographic areas and provide a full continuum of services

      d. Focused new attention on marketing provider services

C. Managed Care and Assessment and Accountability (1990s and early 2000s)

   1. Managed care enrollment increased dramatically.

   2. National, publicly traded, for-profit healthcare corporations became more common.

   3. Small independent providers joined together to form specialty service networks to capture and hold market shares.

   4. Large physician groups joined with hospitals or contracted with managed care organizations.

   5. Disease management and standardizing care received increased emphasis.

   6. Interest in the quality of care and documenting the outcomes of health services, including publishing healthcare report cards, increased.

   7. Consumerism increased.

   8. Interest in evidence-based practice increased.

   9. PPSs developed for skilled nursing facilities, home health agencies, inpatient rehabilitation hospitals, and long-term care hospitals.

IV. **Key Forces Shaping the Future of Healthcare Delivery in the United States (Jonas & Kovner, 2005; Schultz, 2006; Shortell & Reinhardt, 1992)**

A. Changing Demographics:

   1. Aging of the population: Healthcare resource use and costs increase significantly with advancing age.

   2. Increasing ethnic diversity: Racial and ethnic minority groups in the United States have poorer health than the majority White population. If the current disparities continue, then the burden of illness will increase as the minority population increases.

B. Reduced Spending for the Medicare and Medicaid Programs: Changes to these programs will affect the entire healthcare marketplace because these two programs combined account for 36% of personal health expenditures, 48% of hospital expenditures, 33% of physician and professional expenditures, 61% of nursing home care, and 32% of home health care (Jonas & Kovner, 2005).

C. The Public's Beliefs That Their Own Behaviors Affect Their Health: There is increasing understanding that the determinants of health have little to do with the healthcare system and more to do with the way we lead our lives and the environment we live in.

D. Increasing Rates of Uninsured: State-level experiments are being proposed.

E. Adoption of Health Information Technology: Technology may facilitate accountability and increase productivity.

F. Genomics: the linking of human diseases with variations in specific genes.

G. Technological Growth and Innovation: New

diagnostic and treatment modalities are expected to further shift care into outpatient settings and prolong life.

H. Changing Professional Labor Supply: shortages of key health professionals, redefinition of professional roles.

I. Globalization of the Economy: increased scrutiny of healthcare costs.

References

American Nurses Association (ANA). (1999). *Hill basics: Communication tips.* Available: http://www.nursingworld. org/gova/RN/contact.html

Association of Rehabilitation Nurses (ARN). (1999). *Association of Rehabilitation Nurses guidelines for political action.* Unpublished document. Available from ARN, 4700 W. Lake Avenue, Glenview, IL 60025-1485.

AUPHA. (1996). *Seeking strategic advantage through health policy analysis.* Chicago: Health Administration Press.

Barker, E. (1999). Life care planning. *RN, 52*(3), 58–61.

Cudney, S., Winters, C., Weinert, C., & Anderson, K. (2005). Social support in cyberspace: Lessons learned. *Rehabilitation Nursing 30*, 25–29.

Hill, W., Schillo, L., & Weinert, C. (2004). Effect of a computer-based intervention on social support for chronically ill rural women. *Rehabilitation Nursing, 29*, 169–173.

Institute of Medicine. (1991). *Disability in America.* Washington, DC: National Academies Press.

Institute of Medicine Committee on Clinical Practice Guidelines. (1992). *Guidelines for clinical practice: From development to use.* Washington, DC: National Academies Press.

Jonas, S. & Kovner, A.R. (2005). *Jonas and Kovner's health care delivery in the United States.* New York: Springer.

Kaiser Commission on Medicaid and the Uninsured. (2006). *Health coverage for low-income Americans: An evidence-based approach to public policy.* Washington, DC: Henry J. Kaiser Family Foundation.

Kassner, E., & Bectel, R.W. (1998). *Midlife and older Americans with disabilities: Who gets help?* Washington, DC: Public Policy Institute.

Kongstvedt, P.R. (1997). *Essentials of managed health care* (2nd ed.). Gaithersburg, MD: Aspen.

Kongstvedt, P.R. (2001). *Essentials of managed health care* (4th ed.). Gaithersburg, MD: Aspen.

Longest, B.B., Jr. (1996). *Seeking strategic advantage through health policy analysis.* Chicago: Health Administration Press.

McCourt, A.E. (Ed.). (1993). *The specialty practice of rehabilitation nursing: A core curriculum* (3rd ed.). Skokie, IL: Rehabilitation Nursing Foundation of the Association of Rehabilitation Nurses.

McNeil, J. (2001). *Americans with disabilities. Current population reports.* Household Studies, no. 1997. Retrieved January 21, 2007, from http://www.census.gov/prod/2001pubs/p70-73.pdf

National Academy of Sciences. (1991). *Disability in America.* Washington, DC: National Academies Press.

Nosse, L.J., Friberg, D.G., & Kovacek, P.R. (1999). *Managerial and supervisory principles for physical therapists.* Baltimore, MD: Williams & Wilkins.

Okara, C.A., Young, S.L., Strine, T.W., Balluz, L.S., & Mokdad, A.H. (2005). Uninsured adults aged 65 years and older. Is their health at risk? *Journal of Health Care for the Poor and Underserved, 16*(3), 453–463.

Pierce, L.L., Steiner, V., Govoni, A.L., Hicks, B., Thompson, T.L.C., & Friedemann, M.L. (2004). Internet-based support for rural caregivers of persons with stroke shows promise. *Rehabilitation Nursing, 29*, 95–99, 103.

Shortell, S.M., & Reinhardt, U.E. (1992). *Improving health policy and management: Nine critical research issues.* Ann Arbor, MI: Academy of Health Services Researchers.

Watson, P. (1988). Rehabilitation legislation of the 1980s: Implications for nurses as health care providers. *Rehabilitation Nursing, 13*(3), 137.

Watson, P. (1990). The Americans with Disabilities Act: More rights for people with disabilities. *Rehabilitation Nursing, 15*(6), 326.

Suggested Resources

Bodenheimer, T.S., & Grumbach, K. (2005). *Understanding health policy: A clinical approach.* Norwalk, CT: Appleton & Lange.

Center for Medicare and Medicaid Services: http://www.cms.gov

Craven, G.T.A., & Gleason, C.A. (2002). Public policy and rehabilitation nursing. In S.P. Hoeman (Ed.), *Rehabilitation nursing: Process and application* (3rd ed.). St. Louis: Mosby.

Dean-Baar, S. (2000). Health policy and legislation in rehabilitation. In J.B. Derstine & S.D. Hargrove (Eds.), *Comprehensive rehabilitation nursing.* Philadelphia: Saunders.

Edwards, P.A. (1999). Financing health care. In P.A. Edwards (Ed.), *Pediatric rehabilitation nursing* (pp. 52–61). Philadelphia: W.B. Saunders.

Edwards, P.A. (1999). Legislation and public policy. In P.A. Edwards (Ed.), *Pediatric rehabilitation nursing* (pp. 40–51). Philadelphia: W.B. Saunders.

Mason, D.J., Leavitt, J.K., & Chaffee, M.W. (2006). *Policy and politics in nursing and health care* (5th ed.). Philadelphia: W.B. Saunders.

Milstead, J.A. (2004). *Health policy and politics: A nurse's guide* (2nd ed.). Gaithersburg, MD: Aspen.

Rothstein, J.M., Roy, S.H., & Wolf, S.L. (2005). *The rehabilitation specialist's handbook* (3rd ed.). Philadelphia: F.A. Davis.

Schoen, C., Doty, M.M., Collins, S.R., & Holmgren, A.L. (2005). Insured but not protected: How many adults are underinsured? *Health Affairs, 10.*

Schultz, H., & Young, K. (2006). *Health care USA: Understanding its organization and delivery* (5th ed.). Sudbury, MA: Jones and Bartlett.

Section **II**

Functional Health Patterns and Rehabilitation Nursing
· ·

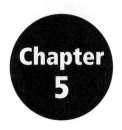

Neuroanatomy

Kelly Johnson, MSN RN CFNP CRRN • Jane Emanuelson, RN CRRN

Neurological injuries and illnesses are catastrophic events for patients and families. These patients need nurses experienced in rehabilitation and knowledgeable about neuroanatomy and pathophysiology to manage an array of complex needs. Solid understanding of neuroanatomy provides rehabilitation nurses with the foundation for providing optimal rehabilitation nursing interventions. Rehabilitation nurses can use their knowledge of neuroanatomy to help patients and their families set realistic, outcome-oriented goals based on expected functional and cognitive levels.

It is important for nurses who work with people with neurological illnesses and injuries to understand key anatomical and functional aspects of the central nervous system (CNS), peripheral nervous system (PNS), autonomic nervous system, and associated musculoskeletal system.. The value of this level of knowledge lies in the fact that the nature and location of injury to the nervous system affect the presentation of the patient, both acutely and in the long term.

I. Anatomy of the Brain

A. Meninges (Lewis, Heitkemper, & Dirksen, 2004)

1. Three layers of protective membranes that surround the brain and spinal cord (see Figure 5-1)

2. Composed of pia mater, arachnoid mater, and dura mater (PAD)

   a. Pia mater (P)
      1) The innermost layer, which adheres to the brain and spinal cord
      2) A highly vascularized layer that provides nourishment to the CNS

   b. Arachnoid mater (A): a thin, delicate, cobweb-like layer

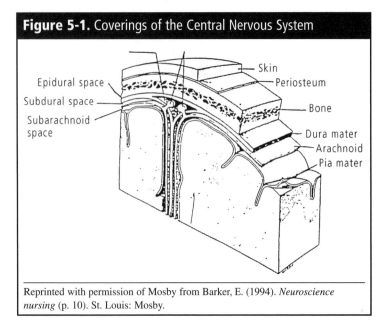

Figure 5-1. Coverings of the Central Nervous System

Epidural space
Subdural space
Subarachnoid space

Skin
Periosteum
Bone
Dura mater
Arachnoid
Pia mater

Reprinted with permission of Mosby from Barker, E. (1994). *Neuroscience nursing* (p. 10). St. Louis: Mosby.

c. Dura mater (D)
   1) The outermost layer that lies against the skull and vertebrae
   2) Composed of tough, white, fibrous tissue
   3) Includes the tentorium cerebelli, which is a fold of dura that separates the cerebellum from the cerebrum in the occipital lobe, and the falx cerebri, which is a fold of the dura that separates the two hemispheres and prevents expansion of brain tissue in situations such as the presence of a rapidly growing tumor or acute hemorrhage (Lewis et al., 2004)
   4) The location of a condition called tentorial herniation, which occurs when intracranial pressure causes the brain to push down through the tentorial notch, compressing the brainstem
   5) Creates spaces known as sinuses, through which cerebrospinal fluid (CSF) is reabsorbed into the bloodstream

B. Spaces (Mosby, 2006)
   1. Subarachnoid space
      a. Space between the pia mater and arachnoid mater that is filled with CSF.
      b. CSF flows from the ventricles to sinuses via the subarachnoid space.
      c. Subarachnoid hemorrhage occurs when bleeding occurs in this space. Caused by trauma, rupture of an aneurysm, or an arteriovenous anomaly.

2. Subdural space
   a. Space between the arachnoid and dura mater that is usually a potential (empty) space.
   b. Subdural hematoma occurs when venous blood leaks into this space, most commonly caused by injury (Mosby, 2006).
   c. Subdural hygroma occurs when CSF leaks into the subdural space. This is believed to be caused by a tear in the arachnoid mater.
3. Epidural space
   a. Space between the dura mater and the bone that is usually a potential (empty) space.
   b. Epidural hematoma results from bleeding between the dura and the inner surface of the skull, typically when the middle meningeal artery bleeds rapidly into the epidural space.
C. Ventricles (Barker, 1994)
   1. Spaces in the brain where CSF is found and produced.
   2. Two lateral ventricles (one in each hemisphere); CSF is formed here.
   3. The third and fourth ventricles are more centrally located and allow CSF to continually flow from the brain to the spinal cord.
D. CSF (Lewis et al., 2004)
   1. Cushions and protects the brain and spinal cord. Circulates within the subarachnoid space.
   2. Functions similarly to blood, carrying nutrients to the CNS and removing wastes.
   3. Intracranial pressure (ICP) is the hydrostatic force measured in the brain CSF compartment. Normal ICP is the pressure exerted by the total volume from the brain tissue, blood, and CSF (Lewis et al., 2004).
   4. Hydrocephalus is an abnormal accumulation of CSF in the cranial vault caused by an overproduction of CSF, obstruction of CSF flow, or defective reabsorption of CSF (Mosby, 2006).
E. Cerebrum (Cerebral Cortex) (Barker, 1994)
   1. Believed to contain approximately 14 billion neurons, which are the building blocks of the CNS.
      a. Composition of neurons
         1) A cell body (perikaryon) and elongated processes that come from the body
         2) Dendrites, which conduct impulses toward the perikaryon
         3) Axons, which conduct impulses away from the perikaryon
      b. Types of neurons
         1) Pseudounipolar
            a) Appear to have only one process originating from the perikaryon, which divides into two processes: One branch goes to the skin, and the other enters the CNS.
            b) Typically found in the sensory ganglia of peripheral nerves
         2) Bipolar
            a) Have two processes originating from the perikaryon: One functions as the dendrite, the other as an axon.
            b) Have limited distribution in the CNS
            c) Found primarily in the visual, auditory, and olfactory systems
         3) Multipolar
            a) Possess one axon and many dendrites
            b) Are the most plentiful type of neuron
            c) Can be found throughout the CNS and PNS
   2. Gyri, sulci, and fissures form the geography of the cerebral cortex: bumps (gyri) and grooves (small grooves are called sulci; large grooves are called fissures).
   3. Composed of myelinated white matter, which is located deep inside the brain, and gray matter, which is made up of cell bodies located on the outer portion of the brain
   4. Divided into two halves (hemispheres)
      a. Hemispheres are connected by nerve fibers called corpus callosum that allow communication between the two sides.
      b. One hemisphere usually is dominant.
         1) The dominant hemisphere is responsible for speech and is most often located in the left hemisphere.
         2) Dominance is also related to handedness.
            a) 90% of the population is right handed. 99% of these people have a dominant left hemisphere.
            b) 10% of the population is left handed. 60% of these people have a dominant left hemisphere; however, 80% of all left-handed people have some mixed dominance.

5. Contains the lobes of the brain (Hickey, 2002). (Figure 5-2)
   a. Frontal lobes
      1) The anterior portion controls emotions, personality, complex intelligence (i.e., executive functions such as problem solving and organizational skills), and cognition.
      2) The posterior portion controls voluntary motor movements.
      3) Broca's area, which is responsible for the motor component of speech, is located in the left hemisphere.
      4) Injury to this area may be indicated by emotional lability, difficulty with executive functions, personality changes, difficulty initiating voluntary movements, and Broca's aphasia. Broca's aphasia is characterized by nonfluent but understandable speech.
   b. Parietal lobes
      1) Receive and interpret sensory input (e.g., pain, temperature, pressure, size, shape, texture, body image, left–right discrimination, and spatial orientation)
      2) Injury to this area usually is indicated by difficulty with left–right discrimination, spatial orientation, and body image perception.
   c. Occipital lobes
      1) Receive and interpret visual stimuli
      2) Responsible for depth perception
      3) Injury to this area is indicated by difficulty interpreting visual clues or stimuli.
   d. Temporal lobes
      1) Control hearing, taste, and smell
      2) Include Wernicke's area, which enables speech reception (usually in left hemisphere) and interpretation of sounds as words
      3) Control memory functions
      4) Injury to this area involves loss of smell, hearing deficits, loss of taste, memory deficits, and Wernicke's aphasia. Wernicke's aphasia is

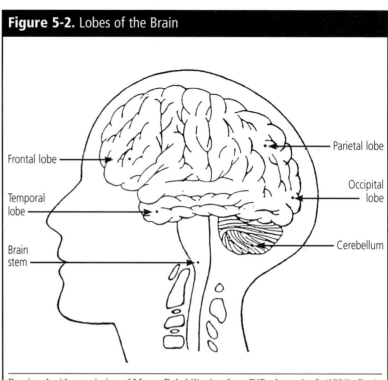

Figure 5-2. Lobes of the Brain

Reprinted with permission of Magee Rehabilitation from DiPaolantonio, J. (1996). *Brain injury: A family guide* (p. 8). Philadelphia: Magee Rehabilitation.

characterized by fluent speech that does not make sense.

6. Cerebral hemorrhages are classified by
   a. Location: subarachnoid, extradural, subdural
   b. Vessel type: arterial, venous, capillary
   c. Origin: traumatic, degenerative

F. Other Structures in the Brain (Figure 5-3)
   1. Limbic system includes structures in the brain involved in emotion, motivation, and emotional association with memory.
      a. Composed of a group of structures deep inside the brain associated with the hypothalamus
      b. Involved in primitive emotions (e.g., anger, rage, sexual arousal and behavior, pleasure, sadness) and the fight-or-flight response
      c. Affects motivation, attention, and biological rhythm
      d. Injury to this system usually results in a hyperarousal state, which is indicated by a person's disinhibited behaviors.
   2. Basal ganglia
      a. A mass of gray matter deep within the cerebrum
      b. A group of nuclei associated with motor and learning functions

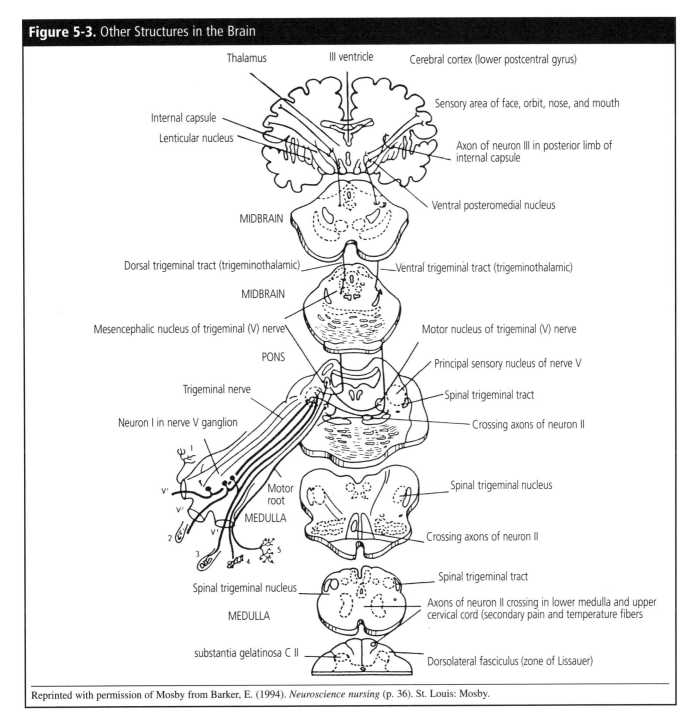

Thalamus

III ventricle

Cerebral cortex (lower postcentral gyrus)

Internal capsule

Lenticular nucleus

Sensory area of face, orbit, nose, and mouth

Axon of neuron III in posterior limb of internal capsule

MIDBRAIN

Ventral posteromedial nucleus

Dorsal trigeminal tract (trigeminothalamic)

Ventral trigeminal tract (trigeminothalamic)

MIDBRAIN

Mesencephalic nucleus of trigeminal (V) nerve

Motor nucleus of trigeminal (V) nerve

PONS

Principal sensory nucleus of nerve V

Trigeminal nerve

Spinal trigeminal tract

Neuron I in nerve V ganglion

Crossing axons of neuron II

Motor root

MEDULLA

Spinal trigeminal nucleus

Crossing axons of neuron II

Spinal trigeminal tract

Spinal trigeminal nucleus

MEDULLA

Axons of neuron II crossing in lower medulla and upper cervical cord (secondary pain and temperature fibers

substantia gelatinosa C II

Dorsolateral fasciculus (zone of Lissauer)

Reprinted with permission of Mosby from Barker, E. (1994). *Neuroscience nursing* (p. 36). St. Louis: Mosby.

c. The cerebellum is excitatory, and the basal ganglia are inhibitory, which allows steady voluntary movements and suppression of meaningless and unintentional movements.

d. Injury to this system usually results in dyskinesias (i.e., abnormal involuntary movements) and muscle tone alteration (i.e., rigidity and bradykinesia).

1) Tremors: rhythmic and purposeless movements that occur at rest and disappear during intentional movements

2) Athetosis: slow, snakelike, writhing movements of the extremities, face, and neck

3) Chorea: rapid, purposeless, jerky movements that often are associated with facial grimacing

3. Diencephalon: located between the cerebrum and the mesencephalon. Consists of the hypothalamus, thalamus, metathalamus, epithalamus and most of the third ventricle (Lewis et al., 2004).

a. Thalamus

1) Functions as a relay station for some sensory messages, particularly pain, touch, and pressure
2) Helps to distinguish pleasant feelings from unpleasant feelings
3) Lesions tend to be associated primarily with sensory loss.
4) Thalamic syndrome is a vascular disorder that causes disturbances of sensation and partial or complete paralysis of one side of the body (Mosby, 2006). Also characterized as a nonspecific, spontaneous, intolerable pain that cannot be relieved pharmaceutically.

b. Hypothalamus
1) Located below the thalamus
2) Is the master controller of both divisions (parasympathetic and sympathetic) of the autonomic nervous system
3) Plays a role in producing two hormones that are stored and released from the pituitary gland
   a) Antidiuretic hormone (ADH) enhances reabsorption of water in the kidneys.
      (1) Too much ADH leads to syndrome of inappropriate ADH secretion (SIADH), which leads to water retention. It is common to see this syndrome in trauma patients.
      (2) Too little ADH leads to diabetes insipidus and excessive water loss.
   b) Oxytocin stimulates uterine contractions.

4. Brainstem: includes the midbrain, pons, and medulla oblongata. The cell bodies of cranial nerves III through XII are in the brainstem (Lewis et al., 2004).
a. Midbrain
1) Approximately 2 cm long
2) Composed of two structures
   a) Substantia nigra: motor nuclei that are concerned with muscle tone. This area is impaired in patients with Parkinson's disease.
   b) Red nucleus: large motor nuclei associated with flexor rigidity
3) Injury to the midbrain is associated with decorticate posturing (i.e., abnormal flexion).
b. Pons

1) A bridge between the cerebellar hemispheres
2) Contains two areas that help control breathing
   a) Apneustic center initiates inspiration.
   b) Pneumotaxic center inhibits inspiration.
3) Injury to the pons usually involves abnormal breathing patterns.
   a) Central neurogenic hyperventilation: sustained regular, rapid, deep breaths
   b) Apneustic breathing: sustained, cramplike inspiratory efforts that pause when inspiration is complete; there also may be an expiratory pause.
4) Involves two reflexes that are tested in comatose patients to determine pontine and brainstem involvement
   a) Oculocephalic reflex (doll's eyes): In this reflex, the eyes move in sync with head movement. In normal pontine activity, movement of the eyes lags behind.
   b) Oculovestibular reflex (caloric test): To test for this reflex, water is placed in the ear canal. In pontine lesions, the eyes do not deviate toward the stimulated ear. In normal pontine function, the eyes deviate toward stimulated ear.
5) Pontine lesions produce a "locked-in" syndrome in which the person has no movement except for the eyelids, but the patient is conscious and has sensation, and cognition typically is intact.

c. Medulla oblongata
1) Houses the respiratory center
   a) Inspiratory dominant: The medulla senses the need to inspire; exhalation is a passive process.
   b) Produces rhythmic breathing
   c) Involves chemoreceptors that are sensitive to CO_2 levels in the blood and cause an increase in ventilation when CO_2 is elevated
   d) Injuries to this area result in ataxic breathing, in which breathing is irregular with both shallow and deep inspiratory efforts.
2) Controls temperature, regulates hunger, thirst, and sleep–wake patterns

3) Houses the vasodilation and vasopressor centers
4) Originates the swallowing and vomiting centers
d. Reticular formation
1) Located in the brainstem
2) Receives sensory input from all sensory organs and acts as a relay station to determine which area of the brain receives the input. Influences excitatory and inhibitory control of spinal motor neurons.
3) The reticular activating system is part of the reticular formation and usually is associated with controlling states of consciousness.
4) Particularly susceptible to trauma
5) Involves the following functions:
a) Motor control modulation: coordinates (but does not inhibit) movement and plays a role in the extrapyramidal system
b) Visceral functioning: controls the state of consciousness
c) Sensory filtering: plays an inhibitory role to prevent the brain from becoming overstimulated
d) Inhibition of stimuli: helps to narrow down stimuli to allow selective attention and plays a major role in attention and concentration
e) Arousal and alertness
6) Injury to this area may cause coma.
5. Cerebellum
a. Located below the cerebrum
b. Involves two hemispheres and a medial portion called the vermis
c. Contains gray matter on the outside of the cerebellar cortex and white matter on the inside of the cortex
d. Receives sensory and motor impulses
e. Responsible for the following functions:
1) Coordination of all reflex activity and voluntary motor activity
2) Regulation of muscle tone and trunk stability
3) Influence and maintenance of equilibrium
f. Injury to this area can produce a variety of signs of dysfunction.
1) Deficits on the same (ipsilateral) side of the body as the injury
2) Hypotonia: decreased resistance to passive movement

3) Postural changes and wide-based gait to compensate for loss of muscle tone
4) Ataxia: impaired ability to coordinate movement
a) Intentional tremors
b) Jerky movements
c) Dysmetria: inability to judge movement within space, thereby losing control of motor activity
d) Dysdiadochokinesis: inability to perform alternating movements rapidly or regularly
e) Nystagmus: disorders or ataxia of ocular movement
f) Ataxia of speech muscles (slurred speech)
G. Cranial Nerves (Barker, 1994)
1. Twelve cranial nerves (CNs) (Table 5-1)
a. CN I: Olfactory (smell)
b. CN II: Optic (vision)
c. CN III: Oculomotor (eye movement, e.g., elevating eyelids, moving eyes in and out, constricting pupil, accommodating for light)
d. CN IV: Trochlear (eye movement down and outward)
e. CN V: Trigeminal (chewing, sensations of face, scalp, and teeth)
f. CN VI: Abducens (outward eye movement)
g. CN VII: Facial (facial expression, taste [anterior two-thirds of tongue], salivation, crying)
h. CN VIII: Acoustic (hearing and sense of balance)
i. CN IX: Glossopharyngeal (secretes saliva, swallowing, controls gag reflex, sensation in the throat, and taste)
j. CN X: Vagus (swallowing, voice production, heart rate, rate of peristalsis, sensation of throat, thoracic and abdominal viscera)
k. CN XI: Spinal accessory (shoulder and head movement)
l. CN XII: Hypoglossal (tongue movement)
2. Mnemonic tip for remembering the cranial nerves: On Old Olympus' Towering Top, A Finn And German Viewed Some Hops.
H. Components That Provide the Vascular Supply to the Brain (Barker, 1994) (Figure 5-4)
1. Internal carotid arteries (right and left)
a. Supply 80% of the blood supply to the brain

Table 5-1. Cranial Nerves

Cranial Nerve	Origin and Course	Function
CN I: Olfactory		
Sensory	Mucosa of nasal cavity; only CN with cell body located in peripheral structure (nasal mucosa). Pass through cribriform plate of ethmoid bone and go on to olfactory bulbs at floor of frontal lobe. Final interpretation is in temporal lobe.	Smell. However, system is more than receptor and interpreter for odors; perception of smell also sensitizes other body systems and responses such as salivation, peristalsis, and even sexual stimulus. Loss of sense of smell is called anosmia.
CN II: Optic		
Sensory	Ganglion cells of retina converge on the optic disc and form optic nerve. Nerve fibers pass to optic chiasm, which is above pituitary gland. Some fibers decussate, others do not. The two tracts then go to the lateral geniculate body near the thalamus and then on to the end station for interpretation in the occipital lobe.	Vision.
CN III: Oculomotor		
Motor	Originates in midbrain and emerges from brainstem at upper pons.	Extraocular movement of eyes.
	Motor fibers to superior, medial, inferior recti, and inferior oblique for eye movement; levator muscle of the eyelid.	Raise eyelid.
Parasympathetic	Parasympathetic fibers to ciliary muscles and iris of eye.	Constrict pupil; change shape of lens.
CN IV: Trochlear		
Motor	Comes from lower midbrain area to innervate superior oblique eye muscle.	Allows eye to move down and inward.
CN V: Trigeminal		
Sensory	Originates in fourth ventricle and emerges at lateral parts of pons. Has three branches to face: ophthalmic, maxillary, and mandibular.	Ophthalmic branch: Sensation to cornea, ciliary body, iris, lacrimal gland, conjunctiva, nasal mucosal membranes, eyelids, eyebrows, forehead, and nose.
		Maxillary branch: Sensation to skin of cheek, lower lid, side of nose and upper jaw, teeth, mucosa of mouth, spheno-polative-pterygoid region, and maxillary sinus.
		Mandibular branch: Sensation to skin of lower lip, chin, ear, mucous membrane, teeth of lower jaw and tongue.
Motor	Goes to temporalis, masseter, pterygoid gland, anterior part of digastric muscles (all for mastication), and the tensor tympani and tensor veli palatin muscles (clench jaws).	Muscles of chewing and mastication and opening jaw.
CN VI: Abducens		
Motor	Arises from a nucleus in pons to innervate lateral rectus eye muscle.	Allows eye to move outward.
CN VII: Facial		
Sensory	Lower portion of pons goes to anterior two-thirds of tongue and soft palate.	Taste anterior two-thirds of tongue. Sensation to soft palate.
Motor	Pons to muscles of forehead, eyelids, cheeks, lips, ear, nose, and neck.	Movement of facial muscles to produce facial expressions, close eyes.
Parasympathetic	Pons to salivary gland and lacrimal glands.	Secretory for salivation and tears.
CN VIII: Acoustic		
Sensory	Cochlear division: Originates in spinal ganglia of the cochlea, with peripheral fibers to the organ of Corti in the internal ear. Goes to pons, and impulses transmitted to the temporal lobe.	Hearing.
	Vestibular division: Originates in otolith organs of the semicircular canals in the inner ear and in the vestibular ganglion. Terminates in pons, with some fibers continuing to cerebellum. Only cranial nerve originating wholly within a bone, petrous portion of temporal bone.	Equilibrium.

(Continued)

Table 5-1. Cranial Nerves *(Continued)*

Cranial Nerve	Origin and Course	Function
CN IX: Glossopharyngeal		
Sensory	Posterior one-third of tongue for taste sensation and sensations from soft palate, tonsils, and opening to mouth in back of oral pharynx (fauces). Fibers go to medulla and then to the temporal lobe for taste and sensory cortex for other sensations.	Taste in posterior one-third of tongue. Sensation in back of throat; stimulation elicits a gag reflex.
Motor	Medulla to constrictor muscles of pharynx and stylopharyngeal muscles.	Voluntary muscles for swallowing and phonation.
Parasympathetic	Medulla to parotid salivary gland via otic ganglia.	Secretory, salivary glands. Carotid reflex.
CN X: Vagus		
Sensory	Sensory fibers in back of ear and posterior wall of external ear go to medulla oblongata and on to sensory cortex.	Sensation behind ear and part of external ear meatus.
Motor	Fibers go from medulla oblongata through jugular foramen with glossopharyngeal nerve and on to pharynx, larynx, esophagus, bronchi, lungs, heart, stomach, small intestines, liver, pancreas, kidneys.	Voluntary muscles for phonation and swallowing. Involuntary activity of visceral muscles of heart, lungs, and digestive tract.
Parasympathetic	Medulla oblongata to larynx, trachea, lungs, aorta, esophagus, stomach, small intestines, and gall bladder.	Carotid reflex. Autonomic activity of respiratory tract, digestive tract including peristalsis and secretion from organs.
CN XI: Spinal Accessory		
Motor	This nerve has two roots, cranial and spinal. Cranial portion arises at several rootlets at side of medulla, runs below vagus, and is joined by spinal portion from motor cells in cervical cord. Some fibers go along with vagus nerve to supply motor impulse to pharynx, larynx, uvula, and palate. Major portion to sternomastoid and trapezius muscles, branches to cervical spinal nerves C2–C4.	Some fibers for swallowing and phonation. Turn head and shrug shoulders.
CN XII: Hypoglossal		
Motor	Arises in medulla oblongata and goes to muscles of tongue.	Movement of tongue necessary for swallowing and phonation.

Reprinted with permission of Mosby from Barker, E. (1994). *Neuroscience nursing* (pp. 78–79). St. Louis: Mosby.

b. Divide to form the anterior cerebral artery and the middle cerebral artery

2. Vertebral arteries (right and left)
   a. Supply 20% of the blood supply to the brain
   b. Join to form the basilar artery as it passes over the pons and then splits and becomes the posterior cerebral arteries at the level of the cerebrum

3. Communicating arteries
   a. Posterior: connects the posterior cerebral and middle cerebral arteries
   b. Anterior: connects the two anterior cerebral arteries

4. Circle of Willis
   a. Formed by the anastomosis of the two internal carotid arteries and the two vertebral arteries.
   b. Composed of the following arteries:
      1) Anterior cerebral
      2) Posterior cerebral
      3) Anterior communicating (supplies the medial portion of the frontal lobes)
      4) Posterior communicating
      5) Internal carotid
   c. Allows blood that enters either the internal carotid arteries or the vertebral arteries to be distributed to the brain and acts as a safety valve when differential pressures are present in these arteries. It may also function as an anastomotic pathway when occlusion of a major artery on one side of the brain occurs (Lewis et al., 2004).
   d. Located at the base of the skull in the subarachnoid space
      1) The site of many congenital aneurysms
      2) If an aneurysm bursts or vessels are sheared or torn, a subarachnoid hemorrhage occurs.

I. Skull (Lewis et al., 2004)

1. Composed of 8 cranial bones and 14 facial bones. The structure of the skull cavity often explains the physiology of head injuries because of the many ridges, prominences, and foramina.

2. Skull fractures often occur with head trauma.

   a. Linear: break in continuity of bone caused by low-velocity injuries

   b. Depressed: inward indentation of skull caused by powerful blow

   c. Simple: linear or depressed skull fracture without fragmentation or communicating lacerations, caused by low to moderate impact

   d. Comminuted: multiple linear fractures with fragmentation of bone into many pieces, caused by direct, high-momentum impact

   e. Compound: depressed skull fracture and scalp laceration with communicating pathway to intracranial activity, caused by severe head trauma

II. Anatomy of the Spinal Cord

A. Spinal Column: The Bony Structure That Surrounds and Protects the Delicate Nervous Tissue of the Spinal Cord (Figure 5-5)

1. Vertebrae

   a. 7 cervical vertebrae
      1) The C1 vertebra is called the atlas.
      2) The C2 vertebra, also called the axis, has a finger-like projection called the odontoid process (dens) that articulates with the anterior arch of the atlas.

   b. 12 thoracic vertebrae

   c. 5 lumbar vertebrae

   d. 5 fused sacral vertebrae

   e. 5 fused coccygeal vertebrae

   f. The anterior portion of the vertebra is the body.

   g. The posterior portion of the vertebra is the arch. The arch is formed from two transverse processes, one spinous process, and two superior and inferior facets. Two laminae form the roof of the arch, and

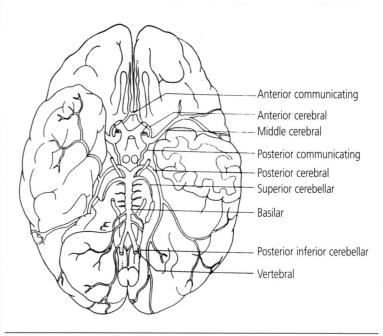

Figure 5-4. Vascular Supply to the Brain

Anterior communicating
Anterior cerebral
Middle cerebral
Posterior communicating
Posterior cerebral
Superior cerebellar
Basilar
Posterior inferior cerebellar
Vertebral

Reprinted with permission of Mosby from Barker, E. (1994). *Neuroscience nursing* (p. 31). St. Louis: Mosby.

two pedicles attach the arch to the body of the vertebra.

2. Intervertebral discs

   a. Situated between every two vertebral bodies and act as shock absorbers

   b. The disc is formed from an outer fibrous cartilage ring (annulus fibrosis) containing a spongy inner material (nucleus pulposus).

3. Ligaments

   a. Anterior and posterior longitudinal ligaments are the two main supporting ligaments that run from the atlas to the sacrum.

   b. Short, dense ligaments are located between the vertebral arches.

   c. Ligamenta flava run between the laminae.

   d. Supraspinal and interspinal ligaments run between the spinous processes.

   e. Transverse ligaments run between the transverse processes.

B. Spinal Cord

1. The spinal cord begins at the caudal end of the medulla oblongata and leaves the cranial vault by extending through the foramen magnum into the vertebral canal and in the adult usually terminates at the intervertebral disc between L1 and L2 (Goshgarian, 2003).

a. Conus medullaris: the cone-shaped area from T10 to T12

b. Cauda equina (horse's tail): the area at the end of the conus medullaris that is not actually a part of the spinal cord but is composed of peripheral spinal nerves

2. Neuroanatomic organization of the spinal gray and white matter: major afferent/ascending, sensory tracts (Figure 5-6)

a. In a transverse section of the spinal cord, the white matter is located peripherally, whereas gray matter (shaped like a butterfly) is centrally located: This is the opposite of the brain's makeup of white and gray matter.

b. White matter contains ascending and descending bundles of fibers contained in fiber tracts and glial cells and appears white because it contains myelin (Zejdlik, 1992; Goshgarian, 2003).

   1) Major afferent/ascending tracts
      a) Posterior spinocerebellar tract and posterior columns: proprioception from muscles, tendons, and joints. Sensations of deep touch, proprioception, and vibration and most bowel and bladder sensations.
      b) Lateral spinothalamic tract: transmission of pain and temperature sensations. The fibers cross at the level of the cord after ascending one or two segments and ascend on the contralateral side of the cord.
      c) Anterior spinothalamic tract: light touch and sensation and some pain transmission
   2) Major efferent/descending tracts
      a) Lateral corticospinal tracts: neurons found in the cerebral cortex. Most of these fibers cross at the medulla before traveling to their target muscles.
      b) Anterior (ventral) corticospinal: fine tuning of muscle tone

c. Gray matter consists predominantly of neurons, their processes, and glial cells and has an enriched blood supply (Goshgarian, 2003).

3. Spinal nerves (ASIA, 2002)

a. There are 31 pairs of spinal nerves: 8 cervical (C), 12 thoracic (T), 5 lumbar (L), 5 sacral (S), and 1 coccygeal (C) (Table 5-2).

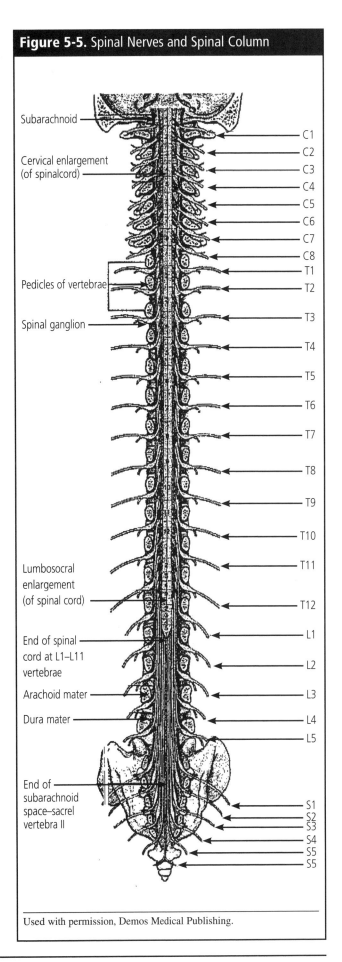

Figure 5-5. Spinal Nerves and Spinal Column

Subarachnoid

Cervical enlargement (of spinalcord)

Pedicles of vertebrae

Spinal ganglion

Lumbosocral enlargement (of spinal cord)

End of spinal cord at L1–L11 vertebrae

Arachoid mater

Dura mater

End of subarachnoid space–sacrel vertebra II

C1
C2
C3
C4
C5
C6
C7
C8
T1
T2
T3
T4
T5
T6
T7
T8
T9
T10
T11
T12
L1
L2
L3
L4
L5
S1
S2
S3
S4
S5
S5

Used with permission, Demos Medical Publishing.

b. Each root has a dorsal (posterior) sensory root that transmits afferent impulses to the cord and a ventral (anterior) motor root that transmits efferent impulses from the cord to target muscles and organs.

c. Cervical: The C1 nerve roots exit over the top of the body of C1. The C2 nerve root exits between C1 and C2. All other cervical nerve roots exit over the top of the caudal vertebrae until C8, which exits between C7 and T1.
   1) C1: Innervates the chin for sensation
   2) C2: Innervates the lateral neck muscles that provide head support
   3) C3: Innervates the anterior and posterior neck muscles that provide head support
   4) C4: Innervates the deltoids and diaphragm (C3–C5 form the phrenic nerve and innervate the diaphragm)
   5) C5: Elbow flexors (biceps, brachialis)
   6) C6: Wrist extensors (extensor carpi radialis longus and brevis)
   7) C7: Elbow extensors (triceps)
   8) C8: Finger flexors (flexor digitorum profundus) to the middle finger

d. Thoracic
   1) T1: Small finger abductors (abductor digiti minimi)
   2) T1–T6: Intercostal muscles
   3) T7–T12: Upper and lower abdominal muscles, thoracic muscles, quadratus lumborum flexors

e. Lumbar
   1) L1–L2: Hip flexors (iliopsoas)
   2) L3: Knee extensors (quadriceps)
   3) L4: Ankle dorsiflexors (tibialis anterior)
   4) L5: Long toe extensors (extensor hallucis longus)

f. Sacral
   1) S1: Ankle plantar flexors (gastrocnemius, soleus)
   2) S2–S4: Innervates specific motor and sensory functions, including anorectal muscles, perineal sensation, sphincter control, genitalia, and sexual function

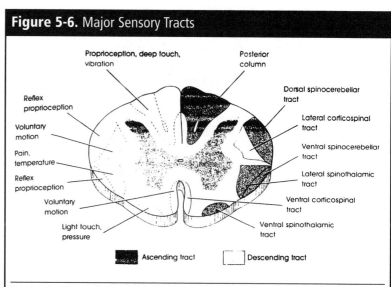

Figure 5-6. Major Sensory Tracts

Reprinted with permission of Mosby from Barker, E. (1994). *Neuroscience nursing* (p. 18) St. Louis: Mosby.

Table 5-2. Muscles and Functions Affected by Level of Spinal Cord Injury

Spinal Nerve	Muscle Group Movement	Assessment Technique
C4–C5	Shoulder abduction	Shoulders are shrugged against downward pressure of examiner's hands.
C5–C6	Elbow flexion (biceps)	Arm is pulled up from resting position against resistance.
C7	Elbow extension (triceps)	From flexed position, arm is straightened out against resistance.
C7	Thumb index pinch	Index finger is held firmly to thumb against resistance to pull apart.
C8	Hand grasp	Hand grasp strength is evaluated.
L2–L4	Hip flexion	Leg is lifted from bed against resistance.
L5–S1	Knee flexion	Knee is flexed against resistance.
L2–L4	Knee extension	From flexed position, knee is extended against resistance.
L5	Foot dorsiflexion	Foot is pulled up toward nose against resistance.
S1	Foot plantar flexion	Foot is pushed down (stepping on the gas) against resistance.

Reprinted with permission of Mosby from Barker, E. (1994). *Neuroscience nursing* (p. 88). St. Louis: Mosby.

4. Spinal reflexes, which are necessary for normal neurologic function (Barker, 1994) (Figure 5-7)
   a. The brain is able to inhibit approximately 80% of spinal reflexes to maintain voluntary control over posture and movement.
   b. A normal spinal cord reflex involves the following:
      1) Sensory input, which ascends to the cell body, where it synapses with a motor neuron
      2) The motor cell body, which sends an impulse down to initiate motor activity
   c. The brain is able to prevent or speed up a synapse if the stimulus is anticipated (i.e., the brain maintains ultimate control over the spinal cord).
   d. Sensory messages also reach the brain as a part of this process.
   e. When a person sustains a spinal cord injury (SCI), reflex activity resumes after spinal shock; however, the connection between the brain and spinal cord is missing and therefore the brain can no longer inhibit or facilitate spinal reflexes, which causes spasticity.
   f. If damage occurs to the peripheral nerves or the cauda equina, reflex activity does not occur. Reflex activity may not return at the level of injury because of damaged or destroyed neurons at the level of injury.
5. Blood supply to the spinal cord (Goshgarian, 2003) (Figure 5.8)

   a. The spinal cord is a highly vascularized organ that receives its blood supply from the vertebral arteries.
      1) Damage to the arteries can be a result of damage to the vertebrae or vertebral alignment.
      2) Damage can be caused by trauma, vascular anomalies, infarcts, or vascular surgery.
   b. The anterior spinal artery provides the blood supply to the anterior two-thirds of the spinal cord. Occlusion can cause anterior artery syndrome.
   c. The posterior spinal arteries provide the blood supply to the posterior one-third of the spinal cord: These arteries provide the needed blood supply to the posterior one-third of the white matter and some of the posterior portions of the meninges.
   d. Radicular arteries contribute to the anterior and posterior blood supply of the spinal cord.

C. Classifications of Incomplete SCI or Clinical Syndromes (ASIA, 2002)
   1. Central cord syndrome
      a. A lesion that occurs almost exclusively in the cervical region
      b. Central damage to the cord
      c. Produces sacral sensory sparing and greater weakness in the upper limbs than the lower limbs
   2. Brown–Sequard syndrome
      a. Damage to one side of the spinal cord
      b. Produces greater ipsilateral proprioceptive

Figure 5-7. Spinal Reflexes

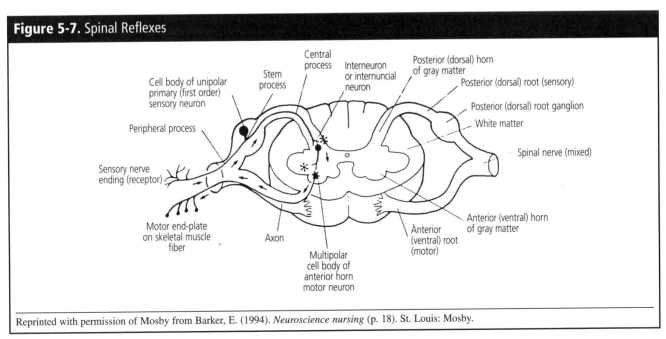

Reprinted with permission of Mosby from Barker, E. (1994). *Neuroscience nursing* (p. 18). St. Louis: Mosby.

and motor loss and contralateral loss of sensitivity to pain and temperature

3. Anterior cord syndrome
    a. Damage to or disruption of blood supply to the anterior two-thirds of the spinal cord
    b. Produces variable loss of motor function and of sensitivity to pain and temperature while preserving proprioception

4. Conus medullaris syndrome
    a. Injury of the sacral cord (conus) and lumbar nerve roots within the spinal canal
    b. Usually results in areflexic bladder, bowel, and lower limbs

5. Cauda equina syndrome
    a. Injury to lumbosacral nerve roots within the neural canal
    b. Results in areflexic bladder, bowel, and lower limbs

Figure 5-8. Blood Supply to the Spinal Cord

Used with permission, Demos Medical Publishing.

III. Autonomic Nervous System (Figure 5-9)

A. Overview (Barker, 1994)

1. The part of the peripheral nervous system that controls the viscera at an unconscious level

2. Involves major effector organs
    a. Smooth muscle
    b. Cardiac muscle
    c. Glands

3. Carries messages from the CNS to the peripheral effector organs

4. Includes two divisions: sympathetic and parasympathetic

5. Autonomic dysfunction can result in the following conditions:
    a. Autonomic dysreflexia
    b. Orthostatic hypotension
    c. Poikilothermia (inconsistent body temperature regulation)

B. Anatomy and Physiology (Barker, 1994)

1. Has two divisions that are parallel but act in an opposing manner
    a. Sympathetic division
        1) Prepares the body to meet crises
        2) Produces a "fight-or-flight" pattern, which is characterized by elevated heart rate and blood pressure and dilation of the pupil of the eye
        3) Slows peristalsis and closes the bladder neck
    b. Parasympathetic division
        1) Is more vegetative in action
        2) Operates in calm moments and allows the body to restore itself
        3) Slows the heart rate, lowers blood pressure, increases gastrointestinal activity, and shunts blood from the periphery to the internal organs

2. Functions independently of the hypothalamus and vasomotor centers in the brainstem.

3. Responds to local stimulation. Both inhibitory and facilitative influences from higher centers are blocked.

IV. The Neurological Assessment

A. Neurological Assessment: For the rehabilitation nurse this is a function of monitoring neurological status for changes and is a fundamental component of a comprehensive functional assessment.

B. Team Approach: A team approach provides the patient and the team with the data that will help them determine an appropriate plan of care. The treatment team varies by patient diagnosis but may include a physician, nurse, physical therapist, occupational therapist, speech therapist, recreational therapist, neuropsychologist, dietitian, respiratory therapist, chaplain, alternative medicine practitioner, or others.

C. Comprehensive Assessment: A comprehensive assessment of a patient with neurological needs includes multiple domains (Chin, 1998).

1. Cognitive, motor, and sensory function

2. Disability

3. Activities of daily living

4. Affective assessment such as depression

5. Learning needs

6. Quality of life

D. Spinal Shock: This is a result of the concussive effect of the primary SCI on the nervous system (Bader & Littlejohns, 2004). This concussive effect results in transient depression of all reflexes, including loss of deep tendon reflexes, paralysis, loss of sensation, loss of autonomic function, and loss of bowel and bladder control. The duration of spinal shock may range from days to months (Tator, 2000). It is not possible to determine completeness of SCI until spinal shock resolves (Bader & Littlejohns, 2004). Resolution of spinal shock is indicated by return of the bulbocavernosus reflex.

E. Classification of Spinal Cord Injury (ASIA, 2002).

1. Tetraplegia

a. Impairment or loss of motor and sensory function in the cervical segments of the cord

b. Results in loss of function in the upper and lower extremities and the trunk, including the pelvic organs

2. Paraplegia

a. Impairment or loss of motor and sensory function in the thoracic, lumbar, or sacral segments of the cord

b. Results in loss of function in the lower extremities and the trunk, including the pelvic organs

F. ASIA Impairment Scale (ASIA, 2002).

1. A = Complete. No sensory or motor function is preserved in the sacral segments S4–S5.

2. B = Incomplete. Sensory but not motor function is preserved below the neurological level and includes the sacral segments S4–S5.

3. C = Incomplete. Motor function is preserved

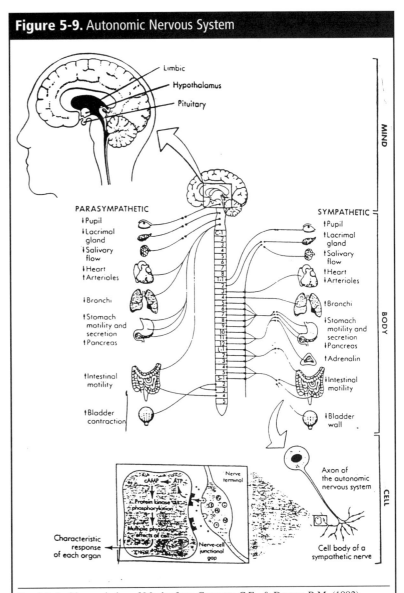

Figure 5-9. Autonomic Nervous System

Reprinted with permission of Mosby from Guzzetta, C.E., & Dassey, B.M. (1992). *Cardiovascular nursing: Holistic practice.* St. Louis: Mosby.

below the neurological level, and more than half of key muscles below the neurological level have a muscle grade less than 3.

4. D = Incomplete. Motor function is preserved below the neurological level, and at least half of key muscles below the neurological level have a muscle grade greater than or equal to 3.

5. E = Normal. Sensory and motor function are normal.

6. Motor examination: used to quantify degree of muscle using standard measurements of strength in key muscles (ASIA, 2002).

a. Grade 0 = Total paralysis

b. Grade 1 = Palpable or visible contraction

c. Grade 2 = Active movement, full range of motion (ROM) with gravity eliminated

d. Grade 3 = Active movement, full ROM against gravity

e. Grade 4 = Active movement, full ROM against moderate resistance

f. Grade 5 (normal) = Active movement, full ROM against full resistance

G. Classification of Neurogenic Function

1. Upper motor neurons (UMN): These neurons of the motor cortex contribute to formation of the corticospinal and corticonuclear tracts. Although not motor neurons in the strict sense, they are classified as motor neurons because their stimulation produces movement, and their destruction causes moderate to severe disorders of movement.

   a. Impairment occurs in SCI when the damage to the cord is above the conus medullaris and the reflex center remains intact (S2–S4).

   b. Often used to classify bladder, bowel, and sexual function

   c. SCI above T12 generally results in impaired bladder, bowel, and sexual organ function.

   d. Impairment is characterized by presence of muscle tone, spastic paralysis, positive reflexes, and sphincter tone.

2. Lower motor neurons (LMN): These are the final motor neurons that innervate the skeletal muscles.

   a. Impairment occurs in SCI of the sacral cord segments in the conus medullaris or the sacral nerve roots in the cauda equina.

   b. Impairment is characterized by flaccid paralysis, loss of muscle, absent reflexes, and loss of sphincter tone.

References

American Spinal Injury Association (ASIA). (2002). *Standards for neurological classification of spinal injury patients* (6th. ed.). Chicago: American Spinal Injury Association.

Bader, M.K., & Littlejohns, L.R. (2004). *AANN core curriculum for neuroscience nursing* (4th ed.). Philadelphia: Saunders.

Barker, E. (1994). *Neuroscience nursing*. St. Louis: Mosby.

Chin, P.A. (1998). Nursing process and nurse client relationship. In P.A. Chin, D. Finocchiaro, & A. Rosebrough (Eds.), *Rehabilitation nursing practice* (pp. 61–76). New York: McGraw-Hill.

Goshgarian, H.G. (2003). Anatomy and function of the spinal cord. In V.W. Lin (Ed.), *Spinal cord medicine: Principles and practice*. New York: Demos.

Hickey, J.V. (2002). *The clinical practice of neurological and neuroscience nursing* (5th ed.). Houston: J.B. Lippincott.

Lewis, S.M., Heitkemper, M.M., & Dirksen, S.R. (2004). *Medical–surgical nursing: Assessment and management of clinical problems* (6th ed.). St. Louis: Mosby.

Mosby. (2006). *Mosby's dictionary of medical, nursing and health professionals* (7th ed.). St. Louis: Mosby Elsevier.

Tator, C.H. (2000). Clinical manifestations of acute spinal cord injury. In C.H Tator & E.C. Benzel (Eds.), *Contemporary management of spinal cord injury: From impact to rehabilitation* (pp. 21–32). Park Ridge, IL: American Association of Neurological Surgeons.

Zejdlik, C.M. (1992). *Management of spinal cord injury*. Boston: Jones and Bartlett.

Suggested Resources

American Association of Neuroscience Nurses (AANN). (2004). *AANN core curriculum for neuroscience nursing* (4th ed.). Glenview, IL: Author.

Barker, E. (2007). *Neuroscience nursing*. St. Louis: Mosby.

Brain Injury Association of America. http://www.biausa.org/

Clayman, C. (1995). *The human body: An illustrated guide to its structure, function, and disorders*. New York: DK Publishing.

Netter, F. (2006). *Atlas of human anatomy* (4th ed.). Philadelphia: Saunders Elsevier.

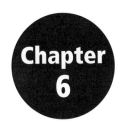

Chapter 6

Health Maintenance and Management of Therapeutic Regimens

Kathy G. Dale, MS RN-HSA CRRN

"The goal of rehabilitation nursing is to assist the individual who has a disability and/or chronic illness in restoring, maintaining, and promoting his or her maximal health" (Association of Rehabilitation Nurses [ARN], 1994, p. 3). Rehabilitation clients must have effective health management to achieve and maintain an optimal quality of life. Maintenance of optimal health includes both the prevention of further loss of function and the prevention of secondary conditions such as cardiovascular, cardiopulmonary, and psychosocial disorders. In addition, the impact falls and injuries can have on clients and families cannot be overstated.

All these conditions can prolong the rehabilitative process and increase the cost of health care. Certainly, pathological factors may contribute to the onset of these conditions. Very often they are caused by problems and changes in the healthcare system. For example, the average length of stay for a person with a spinal cord injury (SCI) has decreased in acute care units from 25 days in 1974 to 18 days in 2004 and in rehabilitation units from 115 to 39 days. In June 2006 approximately 253,000 SCI clients were alive in the United States, and there are 11,000 new cases each year (Foundation for Spinal Cord Injury Prevention, Care & Cure, 2006). An estimated 5.3 million Americans are living with disabilities resulting from traumatic brain injuries, with more than 1.4 million sustaining a traumatic brain injury each year (Brain Injury Association of America, 2005).

People with disabilities are living longer and need long-term health promotion interventions. Although health promotion and disease prevention interventions that focus on people with disabilities have received little attention in the past, now is the time for rehabilitation nurses to ensure that clients receive this vital information. Health promotion interventions for people with disabilities should be comprehensive and address personal and social factors. Access to needed health and community services will enable the client to maintain health, prevent disease, and manage the therapeutic regimen. With the passage of the Americans with Disabilities Act (ADA) of 1990 (PL 101-336), people with disabilities gained legal rights to equal access in the community.

Successful rehabilitation nursing includes the transfer of knowledge and accountability for healthcare needs from nurses to clients and their families and significant others in a manner that promotes health and wellness for the person with a disability (Viggiani, 2000). Self-empowerment is critical, and clients need to take an active role in attaining self-care goals. This is accomplished when all members of the team work together, including the client's primary care provider (Haines, Kuruvilla, & Borchert, 2004). The range of primary care providers has expanded to include nurse clinical specialists, nurse practitioners, and physician assistants who address the specialty and total health needs of people with disabilities. This chapter examines the concepts of health promotion and disease prevention and describes strategies to obtain access to needed services.

I. Overview of Health Promotion

A. Definitions
   1. Health
      a. In its constitution the World Health Organization describes health "as a state of complete physical, mental and social well-being and not merely the absence of disease or infirmity" (WHO Constitution, 2006, p. 1).
      b. Health describes a number of entities (Edelman & Mandle, 2006).
         1) A philosophy of care (e.g., health promotion, health maintenance)
         2) A system (e.g., the healthcare delivery system)
         3) Practice (e.g., good health practices)
         4) Behaviors (e.g. health behaviors)
         5) Costs (e.g., healthcare costs, insurance)
      c. Health relates to all aspects of a person's life, including physical well-being, social interactions, mental and emotional capacities, spiritual beliefs and practices, and cultural background.
      d. "Health is created and lived by people within the settings of their everyday life, where they learn, work, play, and love. Health is created by caring for oneself and others, by being able to make decisions and have control over one's life circumstances and by ensuring that the

Figure 6-1. Health Belief Model

Individual Perceptions or Readiness for Change	The value of health to the individual compared with other aspects of living	Perceived susceptibility to a disease level threatening the achievement of certain goals or aims	Perceived seriousness of the disease level threatening the achievement of certain goals or aims	Belief in the diagnosis and therapy plan			
Modifying Factors About the Person	Demographic variables (e.g., age, gender)	Socioeconomic variables (family and peer group characteristics, income and education) Advice from others	Previous experience with the disease	Risk factors to a disease attributed to heredity, race or culture, medical history, or other causes	Level of participation in and satisfaction with regular health care	Actual extent of change necessary	Personal aspirations in life and valued social and vocational activities
Motivating and Environmental Factors (Cues to Action)	Exposure to mass media	Perceived benefits of health action	Reminders from health professionals	Illness of a family member or friend	Perceived benefits of complying with a treatment plan	Previous success at changing behaviors	
Client–Nurse Transaction Factors *(assessing the likelihood of taking preventive health actions, the nurse compares this picture of "perceived threat of disease")*	Past use of health services		Perceived barriers to promotion action	Continued reassessment of the treatment plan by client and provider			

Adapted with permission of Mosby from Edelman, C., & Mandle, C. (1998). *Health promotion throughout the lifespan* (4th ed., p. 228). St. Louis: Mosby

society one lives in creates conditions that allow that attainment of health by its members" (Dines & Cribb, 1993, p. 209).

2. Wellness
   a. Wellness is dynamic. It is often conceptualized as a continuum, with illness at one end and wellness at the other end. The degrees of health span the entire spectrum.
   b. Wellness is a dynamic, evolving process that reflects physical, psychological, and social integration and growth within an individual and an enhanced quality of life (Edwards, Hertzberg, Hays, & Youngblood, 1999; Hanak, 1992).
   c. In the pursuit of health, a person seeks growth-producing challenges, positive and flexible relationships with others, and health-enhancing activities (Edwards et al., 1999).

B. Principles and Theories Related to Health and Wellness
   1. *Nursing's Agenda for Health Care Reform* called for consumers to assume more responsibility for their own care and become better informed about the range of providers and the options for services (American

Nurses Association [ANA], 1991).
2. Wellness requires active participation and is based on personal experience and observation (i.e., learning by experiencing the positive or negative consequences of behavioral choices made by self or others) (Ardell & Tager, 1982).
3. Health belief models help formulate a plan that will meet the needs and capabilities of the client in making health behavior changes. The health belief model (Rosenstock & Becker, 1988) helps assess a person's perceived state of health or threat of disease and guides nurses who are considering factors that contribute to a client's perceived state of health or risk for disease and to the probability of the client taking appropriate action (Edelman & Mandle, 2006) (see Figure 6-1).
4. The idea of self-efficacy is that behavior is determined by expectations and incentives (Bandura, 1977a, 1977b; Edelman & Mandle, 2006).
   a. There are three types of expectations and incentives (Edelman & Mandle, 2006).
      1) Environmental cues or beliefs about how events are connected

2) Outcome expectations or the consequences of personal actions
3) Efficacy expectations or personal competence to perform the behavior needed to influence outcomes

b. Incentives are defined as the values of a particular object or outcome.

5. The theory of hardiness is associated with health and wellness (Kobasa, Hilker, & Maddi, 1979; Kobasa, Maddi, & Zola, 1983).

a. People who have a high level of hardiness involve themselves in whatever they are doing (commitment), believe and act as if they can influence the events that form their lives (control), and consider change to be not only normal but also a stimulus to development (challenge) (Kobasa et al., 1983).

b. Characteristics of people with a low level of hardiness:
1) Alienation
2) Sense of powerlessness
3) Sense of threat in the dynamic, changing process of life

c. People with a high level of hardiness maintain and strive for wellness even in highly stressful situations. They cope and deal with stress by being more flexible to seek constructive solutions and are more tolerant, self-sufficient, and self-reliant.

6. The concept of person-centered planning is an approach for learning about people with disabilities and creating a lifestyle that can help people contribute in community life; it is an ongoing process of social change. Approaches include lifestyle planning, whole life planning, and essential lifestyle planning, focusing on moving from institutional living back into the community (Mount, 2002).

7. The concept of personal future planning, a consumer-driven request for support after traditional service delivery, focuses on the person's capabilities, interests, contributions, and right to choose and direct his or her care and goals (Mount, Riggs, Brown, & Hibbard, 2003).

8. Locus of control is also associated with health and wellness.

a. Locus of control is the "individual's beliefs about whether or not a contingency relationship exists between behavior (action) and reinforcements (outcomes)" (Shillinger, 1983, p. 59).

b. Types of control (Lefcourt, 1981):
1) Internal control: a person's belief

that his or her own actions influence outcomes
2) External control: a person's belief that external forces determine outcome
a) Chance: belief that events occur randomly and are divorced from individual action
b) Powerful others: belief that outcomes are dominated by powerful authority figures

II. Injury Prevention

A. Secondary Conditions

1. Adults with physical disabilities are at risk for a variety of secondary conditions that may reduce their health and independence. Whereas comorbidities consist of additional diseases after the primary disease diagnosis, secondary conditions are events not considered comorbidities, such as nonmedical events, conditions affecting the general population, and problems that arise later in one's lifetime. The National Council on Disability and the Centers for Disease Control and Prevention (CDC) are developing efforts to prevent these health problems and help consumers maintain their health and independence (White & Seekins, 1996).

2. There is a hopeful trend in disabilities among older people. Data reveal that 1.2 million fewer older Americans were disabled in 1994 than had been expected based on previous rates. Some researchers think that this decline in disabilities in older adults is accelerating, with secondary disabilities appearing to be less severe (World Health Organization, 2006).

3. White and Seekins (1996) described secondary conditions as being causally related to a disabling condition (e.g., pathology, impairment, functional limitation, additional disability).

4. Examples of secondary conditions (White & Seekins, 1996):
a. Urinary tract infections
b. Pressure sores
c. Psychosocial problems (e.g., depression, isolation)
d. Cardiovascular or cardiopulmonary conditions
e. Neuromusculoskeletal conditions
f. Obesity

5. A secondary condition can involve

environmental problems such as lack of access to the physician's office or diagnostic services.

6. A secondary condition can arise if the newly injured person has learned little about his or her disability and how to identify potential health risks. New strategies and outreach channels should be identified to provide information about prevention to people who need it.

B. Levels of Prevention (Edelman & Mandle, 2006)

1. Overview: Each level of prevention occurs at a distinct point in the development of the disease and entails specific nursing interventions.

2. There are three levels of prevention.

   a. Primary prevention

      1) Description: Generalized health promotion and specific protection against disease.

         a) O'Donnell (1987) defined health promotion as the science and art of helping people change their lifestyles to move toward a state of optimal health. Health promotion therefore is not just exercise and nutrition information; it is also proactive decision making at all levels of care.

         b) One aspect of health promotion is the prevention of secondary disabilities.

            (1) People with disabilities, particularly those who use wheelchairs or who are bedridden, are at great risk for acquiring other disabling conditions.

            (2) The health status of people with disabilities is affected by such factors as aging, traumatic injuries, debilitating illnesses, burns, deleterious lifestyle behaviors, and stress (Marge, 1988).

      2) Primary prevention strategies: These can also be considered wellness promotion activities for the general population, such as exercise, healthful eating, weight control, and substance abuse reduction (Marge, 1988).

   b. Secondary prevention

      1) Description: Emphasizes early diagnosis and prompt treatment to halt the pathological process, thereby reducing its duration and severity and enabling the person to return to a state of health as soon as possible.

      2) Secondary prevention strategies: Use screening and early detection measures (e.g., clinical screening protocol for pressure sore prevention) to limit or reverse the effect of the impairment and the development of secondary conditions (Marge, 1988).

   c. Tertiary prevention

      1) Description: Stops the disease process and prevents complete disability. The objective is to return the person to his or her maximum capacity of function in society within the constraints of the disability.

      2) Tertiary prevention strategies:

         a) Prevent disadvantages by incorporating goals of equal opportunity, full participation, independent living, and economic self-sufficiency.

         b) Build on partnerships that link the client with family, clinical healthcare providers, community service providers, friends, and peers (Patrick, 1997; Patrick, Richardson, Starks, Rose, & Kinne, 1997).

III. Falls and Restraints

A. Review of Research Related to Falls

1. Prevention of falls and related injuries is an essential aspect of secondary prevention for people with disabilities.

2. A number of factors can affect the risk for falling.

3. Numerous studies have assessed risk factors associated with falls in older adults, especially regarding risk management programs or nursing diagnoses (Hendrich, 1988a, 1988b; Porter, 1999; Robbins et al., 1989; Ross, Watson, Gyldenvand, & Reinboth, 1991). Many studies that are still cited in current fact sheets by the CDC were published in the 1990s (CDC, 2007).

4. A study by Mahoney (1999) produced strong evidence that older adults are at high risk for loss of independence in walking when they are hospitalized.

   a. This study determined that 1 in 8

hospitalized older adults lost the ability to walk independently, and one-fourth had not regained their walking ability 3 months later.

  b. Previous use of assistive devices, particularly walkers, placed clients at a higher risk, as did existing visual or cognitive impairments.

  c. The clients who were most frail before hospitalization were at the highest risk for falls.

  d. The use of assistive devices before hospitalization was a predictor for falls; it was related to a decline in functioning and a loss of walking independence with hospitalization.

5. Research that specifically addresses risk factors related to falls in rehabilitation settings has been minimal (Vlahov, Myers, & Al-Ibrahim, 1990) and reports various findings.

  a. A study by Mion et al. (1989) found that altered proprioception was the only major predictor of falling in medical rehabilitation clients.

  b. A study by Arbesman and Wright (1999) found that the risk of falling for hospitalized older people is highest soon after the client is placed in a mechanical restraint.

6. A study on medical, surgical, and nursing home units (Brians, Alexander, Grota, Chen, & Dumas, 1991) at a large veterans' hospital indicated that four variables were statistically related to client falls; clients with one or more of these four characteristics were at even greater risk if they used a wheelchair.

  a. Dizziness, unsteady gait, impaired balance

  b. Impaired memory or judgment

  c. Weakness

  d. A history of falling

7. More than 50% of all nursing facility residents fall each year, and more than 40% experience recurrent episodes (Tideiksaar, 2002).

8. The number of deaths caused by unintentional falls increased between 1988 and 2000, and death rates for men were 20% higher than for women (National Center for Injury Prevention and Control, 2006).

B. Use of Restraints

1. The final definition of physical restraint from the Department of Health and Human Services, Centers for Medicare and Medicaid

Service (CMS) (2006, p. 11) is "any manual method, physical or mechanical device, material or equipment that immobilizes or reduces the ability of a patient to move his or her arms, legs, body, or head freely." According to CMS regulations, the patient has the right to be free from restraints of any form that are not medically necessary or are used as a means of coercion, discipline, convenience, or retaliation by staff (JCAHO, 2003).

2. Chemical restraints:

  a. Defined as "a drug or medication used as a restriction to manage a patient's behavior or restrict the patient's freedom of movement and is not a standard treatment or dosage for the patient's condition" (Department of Health and Human Services, Centers for Medicare and Medicaid Service, 2006, p. 14)

  b. Associated with potential side effects in elderly people (Hendrich, 1988b)
     1) Oversedation
     2) Increased confusion
     3) Orthostatic hypotension
     4) Parkinsonian syndrome reactions

3. Caution for using restraints: Neither physical nor chemical restraints necessarily lessen agitated and confused behavior.

  a. Restraints can increase injury.

  b. Clients continue to fall by trying to climb over bedrails or getting tangled in restraints.

  c. An alternative is to create a restraint-free environment to maintain the client's safety by implementing specific interventions (Dochterman & Bulechek, 2004).

4. Regulatory agencies including OBRA have defined concerns about devices that serve multiple purposes, such as gerichairs or siderails, because they have the effect of restricting a patient's movement and cannot be easily removed by the patient (JCAHO, 2003).

C. Nursing Diagnosis: Risk for Injury and Falls

1. Definition (Doenges & Moorhouse, 1998): Risk of injury as a result of environmental conditions interacting with the person's adaptive and defensive resources

2. Risk factors

  a. Knowledge deficit regarding safety techniques and proper use of equipment

  b. Impaired mobility

  c. Neuromuscular deficit

  d. Cognitive deficit

e. Impaired sensation or perception
   1) Temperature (neuropathies)
   2) Touch (neuropathies)
   3) Positive sense (proprioception)
   4) Vision
   5) Hearing
f. Environmental hazards
g. Adverse effects of medication
h. Unmet elimination needs or urinary incontinence
i. Seizures, vertigo
j. Fatigue
k. Use of chemical or physical restraints
l. History of falling or osteoporosis

3. Interventions (see Figure 6-2)
   a. For use in institutions (Dochterman & Bulechek, 2004)
   b. For use in the home and community
      1) Evaluate the degree of risk by using a home safety assessment tool.
      2) Assess the client's and family's knowledge of safety needs and injury prevention and motivation to prevent injury in home, community, and work settings.
      3) Assess socioeconomic status and availability and use of resources.
      4) Identify interventions and safety devices to promote a safe physical environment and individual safety.
      5) Make referrals to occupational or physical therapists as appropriate (Doenges & Moorhouse, 1998).
      6) If covered by client's health insurance plan, arrange a home safety evaluation by a home health agency.
      7) Teach the client and family to monitor environmental hazards and recommend changes to promote the highest level of safety.
         a) Install secured grab bars or handrails.
         b) Use mobility devices.
         c) Unclutter the floors (e.g., get rid of scatter rugs).
         d) Place frequently used items in easily accessible places (e.g., small kitchen appliances, pots, and pans).
         e) Ensure adequate lighting, especially at night; most falls occur at night en route to the bathroom.
         f) Place the bed in a low position.

8) Help the client meet self-care needs until independence can be achieved or until the care attendant or caregiver has received appropriate education.
9) Teach the client, family, and significant others about the potential side effects of medications and alcohol.
10) Ensure safety for the client who has deficits in cognitive or thought processes by changing the environment to meet safety needs.
    a) Provide methods to communicate with caregivers.
    b) Establish a toileting program.
    c) Install door locks or an escape alarm.
    d) Provide an organized, consistent, uncluttered environment.
    e) Install a large bell on the door of a room where entrance is restricted; the noise may stop the patient and alert others to wandering (JCAHO, 2003).
    f) Install bright yellow tape strips on the floor in front of doors (JCAHO, 2003).
    g) Place a traffic stop sign on exit doors or restricted areas to prevent wandering and falls (JCAHO, 2003).
11) Teach mechanisms to compensate for sensory–perceptual deficits.
    a) Test water before bathing.
    b) Use compensatory strategies for visual field deficits.
    c) Prevent burns, frostbite, and skin integrity penetrations.
12) Teach the client and family the signs and symptoms of seizure activity and ways to maintain safety during and after a seizure.
13) Teach safety factors associated with transfer techniques, gait training, and mobility devices.
14) Provide proper, well-maintained footwear with adequate toe box and keep the client from going barefoot.
15) Ensure that the toileting program is adequate to meet nighttime needs.
16) Teach the client and family how to decrease the effects of orthostatic hypotension (e.g., sit on edge of bed for several seconds before transferring).
17) Provide appropriate information

Figure 6-2. Fall Prevention

Definition

Instituting special precautions with patient at risk for injury from falling

Activities

Identify cognitive or physical deficits of the patient that may increase risk of falling in a particular environment

Identify characteristics of environment that may increase potential for falls (e.g., slippery floors and open stairways)

Monitor gait, balance, and fatigue level with ambulation

Assist unsteady patient with ambulation

Provide assistive devices (e.g., cane, walker) to steady gait

Maintain assistive devices in good working order

Lock wheels of wheelchair, bed, or gurney during transfer of patient

Place articles within easy reach of the patient

Instruct patient to call for assistance with movement, as appropriate

Teach patient how to fall so as to minimize injury

Post signs to remind patient to call for help when getting out of bed, as appropriate

Use proper technique to transfer patient to and from wheelchair, bed, toilet, and so on

Provide elevated toilet seat for easy transfer

Provide chairs of proper height, with backrests and armrests for easy transfer

Provide bed mattress with firm edges for easy transfer

Use physical restraints to limit potentially unsafe movement, as appropriate

Use siderails of appropriate length and height to prevent falls from bed, as needed

Place a mechanical bed in lowest position

Provide a sleeping surface close to the floor, as needed

Provide seating on bean bag chair to limit mobility, as appropriate

Place a foam wedge in seat of chair to prevent patient from arising, as appropriate

Use partially filled water mattress on bed to limit mobility, as appropriate

Provide the dependent patient with a means of summoning help (e.g., bell or call light) when caregiver is not present

Answer call light immediately

Assist with toileting at frequent, scheduled intervals

Use a bed alarm to alert caretaker that patient is getting out of bed, as appropriate

Mark doorway thresholds and edges of steps, as needed

Remove low-lying furniture (e.g., footstools and tables) that present a tripping hazard

Avoid clutter on floor surface

Provide adequate lighting for increased visibility

Provide nightlight at bedside

Provide visible handrails and grab bars

Place gates in open doorways leading to stairways

Provide nonslip, nontrip floor surfaces

Provide a nonslip surface in bathtub or shower

Provide sturdy, nonslip step stools to facilitate easy reaches

Provide storage areas that are within easy reach

Provide heavy furniture that will not tip if used for support

Orient patient to physical setup of room

Avoid unnecessary rearrangement of physical environment

Ensure the patient wears shoes that fit properly, fasten securely, and have nonskid soles

Instruct patient to wear prescription glasses, as appropriate, when out of bed

Educate family members about risk factors that contribute to falls and how they can decrease these risks

Instruct family on importance of handrails for stairs, bathrooms, and walkways

Assist family in identifying hazards in the home and modifying them

Instruct patient to avoid ice and other slippery outdoor surfaces

Institute a routine physical exercise program that includes walking

Post signs to alert staff that patient is at high risk for falls

Collaborate with other healthcare team members to minimize side effects of medications that contribute to falling (e.g., orthostatic hypotension and unsteady gait)

(Continued)

Figure 6-2. Fall Prevention *(continued)*

Provide close supervision or a restraining device (e.g., infant seat with seat belt) when placing infants or young children on elevated surfaces (e.g., table and highchair)

Remove objects that provide young child with climbing access to elevated surfaces

Maintain crib siderails in elevated position when caregiver is not present, as appropriate

Provide a bubble top on hospital cribs of pediatric patients who may climb over elevated siderails, as appropriate

Fasten the latches securely on access panel of incubator when leaving bedside of infant in incubator, as appropriate

Reprinted with permission of Mosby from McCloskey, J., & Bulechek, G. (Eds.). (1996). *Nursing interventions classification (NIC)* (2nd ed., pp. 272–273). St. Louis: Mosby.

on community resources (e.g., emergency call devices for outside assistance when the client is alone).

18) Use distraction, redirection, humor, and quiet areas to decrease agitated behavior and avoid the use of restraints.

19) If available, put telephone within easy reach.

4. Expected outcomes
   a. General
      1) Client is free of physical injury.
      2) Client, family, and significant others verbalize or demonstrate an awareness of risk factors related to the client's specific deficits.
      3) Client, family, and significant others know how to seek assistance if an injury occurs.
   b. Safety behavior: self-care assistance (Dochterman & Bulechek, 2004) (see Figure 6-3)
   c. Safety behavior: home maintenance assistance (Dochterman & Bulechek, 2004) (see Figure 6-4)

IV. Nursing Management of Therapeutic Regimens for Individuals

A. Effective Management Techniques
   1. A pattern of regulating and integrating into daily living a program for treatment of illness and its sequelae that is satisfactory for meeting specific health goals (Doenges & Moorhouse, 1998)
   2. Major defining characteristics
      a. Verbalized desire to manage treatment of illness and prevent sequelae
      b. Verbalized intent to reduce risk factors for progression of illness and sequelae

B. Nursing Assessment
   1. Client's coping status regarding responsibility for and access to health care
      a. Health and lifestyle before injury or illness
      b. Interest in a health management program: Does the client's health insurance plan cover ongoing telephonic disease management by nurses?
      c. Ability and motivation to take responsibility for health, including knowledge of nutritional needs
      d. Access to and availability of healthcare providers and facilities
      e. Knowledge of prescribed medications and their effects
      f. Knowledge of medical status and related treatment program: written action plans developed by client and primary care practitioner (physician, nurse practitioner, physician assistant, clinical specialist)
   2. Client's emotional status
      a. Resolution of grieving process related to injury or disease
      b. Grief stages (Maddox, 2006)
      c. Chemical dependency
      d. Methods of coping
   3. Client's spirituality: A spiritual assessment extends beyond merely ascertaining religious affiliation, church attendance, or dietary restrictions (Hoeman, 1996).
      a. Assess four specific areas (Hoeman, 1996).
         1) Sources of hope and strength (support system)
         2) Concept of God or other deity
         3) Relationships between spiritual beliefs and health
         4) Religious practices
      b. Use the spiritual well-being scale as an assessment tool (Ellison, 1982, as cited in Hoeman, 1996).
   4. Client's social support is an important predictor of coping effectiveness and stress tolerance (Hoeman, 1996).

Figure 6-3. Fall Prevention Behavior

Domain-Health Knowledge and Behavior   Care Recipient:

Class-Risk Control and Safety (T)   Data Source:

Scales(s)-Never demonstrated to Consistently demonstrated (m)

Definition: Personal or family caregiver actions to minimize risk factors that might precipitate falls in the personal environment

Outcome Target Rating: Maintain at_____Increase to _____

Fall Prevention Behavior Overall Rating		Never demonstrated 1	Rarely demonstrated 2	Sometimes demonstrated 3	Often demonstrated 4	Consistently demonstrated 5	
Indicators:							
190903	Places barriers to prevent falls	1	2	3	4	5	NA
190905	Uses handrails as needed	1	2	3	4	5	NA
190915	Uses grab bars as needed	1	2	3	4	5	NA
190914	Uses rubber mats in tub/shower	1	2	3	4	5	NA
190910	Uses well-fitting tied shoes	1	2	3	4	5	NA
190901	Uses assistive devices correctly	1	2	3	4	5	NA
190918	Uses vision-correcting devices	1	2	3	4	5	NA
190902	Provides assistance with mobility	1	2	3	4	5	NA NA
190919	Uses safe transfer procedure	1	2	3	4	5	NA
190922	Provides adequate lighting	1	2	3	4	5	NA
190909	Uses stools/ladders appropriately	1	2	3	4	5	NA
190906	Eliminates clutter, spills, glare from floors	1	2	3	4	5	NA
190907	Removes rugs	1	2	3	4	5	NA
190908	Arranges for removal of snow and ice from walking surfaces	1	2	3	4	5	NA
190911	Adjusts toilet height as needed	1	2	3	4	5	NA
190912	Adjusts chair height as needed	1	2	3	4	5	NA
190913	Adjusts bed height as needed	1	2	3	4	5	NA
190916	Controls agitation and restlessness	1	2	3	4	5	NA
190917	Uses precautions when taking medications that increase risk for falls	1	2	3	4	5	NA

From Moorhead, S., Johnson, M., & Maas, M. (2004). *Nursing outcomes classification (NOC).* St. Louis: Mosby.

Figure 6-4. Safe Home Environment

Domain-Health Knowledge and Behavior   Care Recipient:

Class-Risk Control and Safety (T)   Data Source:

Scales(s)-Not adequate to Totally adequate (f)

Definition: Physical arrangements to minimize environmental factors that might cause physical harm or injury in the home.

Outcome Target Rating: Maintain at_____Increase to _____

Safe Home Environment Overall Rating		Not adequate 1	Slightly adequate 2	Moderately adequate 3	Substantially adequate 4	Totally adequate 5	
Indicators:							
191001	Provision of lighting	1	2	3	4	5	NA
191002	Placement of handrails	1	2	3	4	5	NA
191023	Carbon monoxide detector maintenance	1	2	3	4	5	NA
191003	Smoke detector maintenance	1	2	3	4	5	NA
191004	Use of personal alarm system	1	2	3	4	5	NA
191005	Provision of accessible telephone	1	2	3	4	5	NA
191006	Placement of appropriate hazard warning labels	1	2	3	4	5	NA
191024	Safe storage of medication to prevent accidental use	1	2	3	4	5	NA
191007	Disposal of unused medications	1	2	3	4	5	NA
191008	Provision of assistive devices in accessible location	1	2	3	4	5	NA
191009	Provision of equipment that meets safety standards	1	2	3	4	5	NA
191010	Safe storage of firearms to prevent accidents	1	2	3	4	5	NA
191011	Safe storage of hazardous materials to prevent injury	1	2	3	4	5	NA
191012	Safe disposal of hazardous materials	1	2	3	4	5	NA
191025	Safe storage of matches/lighters	1	2	3	4	5	NA
191013	Arrangement of furniture to reduce risks	1	2	3	4	5	NA
191014	Provision of safe play area	1	2	3	4	5	NA
191015	Removal of unused refrigerator and freezer doors	1	2	3	4	5	NA
191016	Correction of lead hazard risks	1	2	3	4	5	NA
191017	Provision of age-appropriate toys	1	2	3	4	5	NA
191018	Use of electrical outlet covers	1	2	3	4	5	NA
191019	Room temperature regulation	1	2	3	4	5	NA
191020	Elimination of harmful noise levels	1	2	3	4	5	NA
191021	Placement of window guards as needed	1	2	3	4	5	NA

From Moorhead, S., Johnson, M., & Maas, M. (2004). *Nursing outcomes classification (NOC)*. St. Louis: Mosby.

    a. Amount, kind, and level of supportive contact

    b. Social support provided by people the client counts on, cares about, or loves

    c. Social facilitative support (e.g., service organizations or agencies or the client's church)

    d. Cultural or ethnic values, traditions, beliefs, and expectations

5. Client's functional status

    a. Strength and endurance

    b. Self-care needs (e.g., feeding, bathing, dressing, toileting)

    c. Mobility status: use of adaptive equipment or devices

d. Continence and elimination needs

e. Communication abilities

f. Ability to monitor environment

6. Client's general health and medical status

   a. History of falls, seizures, or orthostatic hypotension

   b. Perception and sensation (including vision and proprioception)

   c. Sleep (restorative) and planned rest needs

   d. Comorbid health problems, client's participation in self-management

   e. Prescription medications

   f. Over-the-counter medications

   g. Holistic, naturalistic, and alternative therapies (e.g., acupuncture, herbs, vitamins)

   h. Ethnic remedies

   i. Nutrition; appropriate consistency and texture of foods as necessitated by disease processes

   j. Weight control

   k. Smoking status

   l. Sexual health

7. Client's cognitive status

   a. Memory

   b. Judgment

   c. Reasoning

   d. Problem-solving ability

8. Pain [Refer to Chapter 13 for more information about pain.]

   a. Pain rating as the 5th vital sign. Record pain history, including the maximum, minimum, and typical amount of pain experienced (Hoeman, 1996).

   b. Determine what exacerbates the pain.

   c. Determine what alleviates the pain; use standardized scales (e.g., McGill–Melzack Pain Questionnaire).

   d. Assess chronic pain, including effects on premorbid and postmorbid lifestyle.

   e. Use the Agency for Healthcare Research and Quality standards for pain control.

C. Related Factors

1. Physical

   a. Loss of a body part

   b. Sensory deficits

   c. Motor skill deficits

   d. Chemical dependency

   e. Debilitating disease or injury

   f. Pain

2. Emotional and maturational

   a. Depression or prolonged or dysfunctional grieving

   b. Decreased self-esteem

   c. Lack of experience in managing wellness

   d. Lack of motivation

   e. Decisional conflicts

   f. Family conflicts

3. Cognitive

   a. Perceptual deficits

   b. Communication deficits

   c. Inexperience with or inability to comprehend or follow a complex treatment regimen

   d. Lack of education or intellectual development

4. Social and economic

   a. Inability to gain access to the healthcare system

   b. Nontherapeutic relationships with healthcare providers (e.g., healthcare professionals, personal care attendants)

   c. Language differences that interfere with ability to gain access to or use healthcare or self-care resources

   d. Funding resources inadequate to obtain and maintain needed equipment, supplies, and services

   e. Complexity of the healthcare system and the therapeutic regimen

   f. Inability to pay for prescribed medications (e.g., Medicare Part D and the "donut hole" effect)

D. Interventions

1. Identify and designate people responsible for the therapeutic regimen (e.g., client, parent, spouse, or significant others).

   a. Direct interventions toward all responsible people to help them develop strategies to improve management of therapeutic regimen.

   b. Direct responsible people to act on behalf of the client to promote the client's wellness and health management.

2. Educate the client at his or her learning level using age-specific adult learning principles to facilitate health maintenance.

   a. Determine readiness to learn: Lack of readiness occurs when physical endurance is poor or emotional limitations exist (Viggiani, 1997).

   b. Education environment may require

controlled stimulation to help the client to focus on the learning task.

   c. Use teaching tools (e.g., written materials, audiotapes or videotapes, lectures, models).

   d. Use demonstrations and return demonstrations.

   e. Use memory aids (e.g., written reminders [large print when necessary], medication dispensers, consistent location of supplies, software for life skills).

   f. Provide progressive sequential learning experiences that build on skills without overwhelming the learner (e.g., help the client take on progressive responsibility for bladder management).

3. Design a physical environment that minimizes dependency and the sick role, especially for clients living in institutions.

   a. Allow clients and healthcare providers to wear street clothes.

   b. Make the environment and activities as realistic or homelike as possible.
     1) Encourage the client to eat meals in the dining room with other people.
     2) Allow the client to have access to food and beverages between meals.

   c. Help the client identify and begin to resume family role responsibilities.

   d. Provide privacy when the client is performing physical care and interacting with others and allow time for the client to be alone.

   e. Introduce the client to role models (e.g., other clients who competently manage their health and wellness).

4. Establish a milieu that fosters self-reliance and wellness.

   a. Encourage the client to set realistic and achievable goals with the help of healthcare providers.

   b. Encourage the client to become involved in all phases of care planning; promote the client's control of the process.

   c. Negotiate to simplify or alter client behaviors and outcomes; adapt program methods or schedules to the client's preferred routine.

   d. Avoid assuming a "powerful other" role that reinforces external control.

   e. Create a contract with the client to define agreed-upon responsibilities, conditions, and goals for program participation.

5. Help the client and caregivers manage desired

health practices and promote wellness.

   a. Provide anticipatory guidance to maintain and manage effective health practices during periods of wellness.

   b. Identify adaptation strategies to use when progressive illness or long-term health problems occur (e.g., diabetes sick day rules).

   c. Monitor adherence to prescribed medical regimen.

   d. Help the client and family develop stress management skills.

   e. Identify ways to adapt an exercise program to meet the client's changing needs, abilities, and environmental concerns.

6. Refer the client to community resources and support groups.

7. Involve the client's case manager (e.g., home health agency nurse, insurance nurse case manager) in long-term follow-up and assessment of transition from inpatient to outpatient settings.

E. Expected Outcomes

1. Client will be free of physical injury.

2. Client, family, and significant others verbalize or demonstrate an awareness of risk factors related to client's specific deficits.

3. Client, family, and significant others are aware of how to seek assistance if an injury does occur.

4. Client, family, and significant others can identify necessary health maintenance activities.

5. Client assumes responsibility for healthcare needs within his or her level of ability.

6. Client adapts to lifestyle changes that support healthcare goals.

V. Nursing Management of Therapeutic Regimens in the Community

A. Overview

1. Access to health care historically has been a challenge for those with disabilities.

2. Healthcare providers must be able to define strategies for obtaining healthcare services, identify available financial resources, understand public laws governing access to healthcare services, and help people with disabilities in securing and using healthcare services.

B. Ineffective Management Techniques

1. Community programs for treatment of

illness and the sequelae of illness may be unsatisfactory for meeting health-related goals.

2. Major defining characteristics: Community members and agencies verbalize an inability to meet the therapeutic needs of all members (Doenges & Moorhouse, 1998).

C. Nursing Assessment

1. Obstacles to gaining access to healthcare services

    a. Geographic location
        1) Availability and transportation problems related to access to healthcare facilities and community resources
        2) Limited access to home-based care services
        3) Prohibitive cost of transportation services
        4) Limited public funds for assistance to obtain vehicle modifications or purchase a vehicle (e.g., a van with hand controls), which decreases access to healthcare services, especially in rural areas

    b. Architectural problems related to accessibility (including buildings and grounds)
        1) Limited parking lot accessibility and poor design
        2) Limited sidewalk accessibility
        3) Limited office building accessibility and poor design
        4) Limited healthcare facility accessibility and poor design

    c. Discrimination, stigma, negative attitudes

    d. Lack of information about the care needs of people with disabilities

2. Economic constraints

    a. Personal finances
        1) Loss of medical benefits, Supplemental Security Income (SSI), or Social Security Disability Insurance (SSDI) for people younger than age 65 if the person with the disability is employed and earns more than the allowable amount
        2) Possible reduction in Social Security benefits
        3) Medical benefits that are tied to income criteria, which encourage people with disabilities to be dependent on the system

    b. Unavailability of medical benefits for people with disabilities under Medicare until 2 years after the onset of disability

        1) Discourages people with disabilities who are younger than age 65 from seeking healthcare services
        2) Raises the possibility of people with disabilities being without medical benefits if they do not qualify for state assistance or Medicaid and thus increases the numbers of indigent people seeking healthcare services
        3) Raises the possibility that people with disabilities will seek healthcare services only when their illnesses or injuries are advanced and necessitate hospitalization
        4) Begins a cycle that increases the burden on healthcare providers to supply free care, which increases the overall cost of healthcare services

    c. Limited eligibility for funding for attendant care (see also Chapter 2)
        1) Funding that is usually tied to eligibility for income assistance
        2) Long waiting periods that often last 1–2 years
        3) Minimal reimbursement for care attendants, which makes it difficult to recruit and retain qualified people
        4) Programs that require clients to manage their own workers independently and to handle training and payroll, which may not be possible for older adults or people with severe disabilities
        5) Strict definitions of what constitutes a disability that may disqualify many people who need services

    d. Limited funding for independent living arrangements (residential and nonresidential models)
        1) Continued limitation of funds for independent living centers despite the fact that funding is mandated by the Rehabilitation, Comprehensive Services, and Developmental Disabilities Amendments of 1978 (PL 95-602)
        2) Some state support through Medicaid Title XIX funding for attendant assistance and community support services
        3) Scarcity of independent living programs in rural areas

3. Problems in attendant training

    a. On-the-job training

    b. Lack of regulations regarding worker qualifications

c. No supervision of work performance

d. Lack of public funding that would allow control over workers' qualifications and performance

e. Lack of availability of care attendants who can meet the specialized needs of the pediatric population

4. Limited ability to obtain needed equipment, supplies, and medications

   a. Dependence on insurance coverage

   b. Possible requirement of a downpayment (in cash) or full responsibility for repair of equipment once it is obtained

   c. Frequent limits on additional equipment covered by insurance

   d. Possible inability to obtain the necessary equipment (e.g., padded commode chair with removable arms for a person with SCI, power wheelchair)

5. Limitations on healthcare services caused by negative attitudes, flawed architectural designs, or reimbursement limits

   a. Limited counseling services

1) Medical social worker services, which usually are available only through home care agencies

2) The low number of mental health workers, psychiatrists, and psychologists who make home visits

3) Limited reimbursement for counseling

b. Special healthcare needs of people with disabilities

   1) Accessibility of medical offices, diagnostic services (mammography, scanners)

   2) Obstetric and gynecological services

      a) Exam tables that are accessible for women with disabilities

      b) Healthcare providers who are knowledgeable in obstetrics and gynecology

      c) Specialized training for personnel (e.g., how to care for a person with SCI who has had a baby)

   3) Dental services

      a) Offices that are architecturally accessible

      b) Accessible, comfortable office chairs

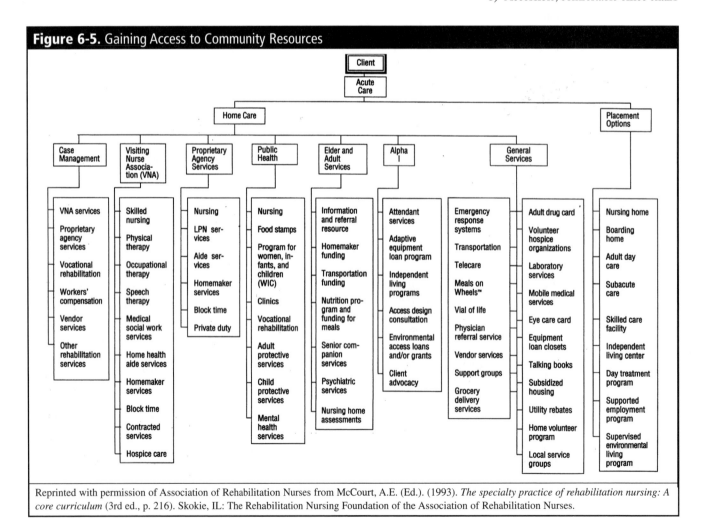

Figure 6-5. Gaining Access to Community Resources

Reprinted with permission of Association of Rehabilitation Nurses from McCourt, A.E. (Ed.). (1993). *The specialty practice of rehabilitation nursing: A core curriculum* (3rd ed., p. 216). Skokie, IL: The Rehabilitation Nursing Foundation of the Association of Rehabilitation Nurses.

c) Elimination of financial obstacles to preventive care (e.g., insurance such as Medicare or Medicaid that does not cover preventive care)

d) Education for staff and dentists in assisting people with physical and cognitive disabilities

D. Interventions

1. Obtain access to community resources and healthcare services (see Figure 6-5).

   a. Provide for communication and coordination between the healthcare facility team and community healthcare providers.

   b. Contact local government disability offices, city commissions, or city departments to determine public services available to people with disabilities.

   c. Involve comprehensive specialty teams when available.

   d. Make referrals as needed for community support services (e.g., Meals on Wheels, local churches with parish nursing programs, senior service organizations, councils on aging).

   e. Make referrals to organizations with support groups as appropriate (e.g., National Spinal Cord Injury Association, American Heart Association).

2. Identify barriers to community reentry.

   a. Accessible housing
      1) Established referral system
      2) Technical assistance
      3) Development, design, and building assistance
      4) Home mortgage loans
      5) Availability of accessible public housing
      6) Funding for adaptations in private residences
      7) "Medical home" (Sia, 1992), an integrated system of services that focuses on the well-being of the whole child in the context of the family; primary health care is continuous and comprehensive and provides coordinated care that is family centered and community based.

   b. Transportation
      1) Designated parking
      2) Private transportation services
      3) Public transportation (e.g., availability, accessibility)
      4) Reduced-price bus passes
      5) Paratransit services
      6) Parking stickers

7) Client's health insurance plan may provide transportation at reduced rates or free to assigned locations (e.g., physician offices).

   c. Advocacy
      1) Established advisory council
      2) Involvement of advocacy groups with communication agencies
      3) Funding for programs
      4) Information exchange regarding disability issues (e.g., legislation)
      5) Appointment of people with disabilities to government boards and commissions
      6) Legal assistance
      7) Public education on disability issues

   d. Employment
      1) Affirmative action for hiring people with disabilities
      2) Training and placement assistance; supported employment services
      3) Funding for environmental modifications

   e. Recreation
      1) Accessible community centers and leisure programs
      2) Special events focused on people with disabilities (e.g., wheelchair division of marathons)

   f. Supportive services
      1) Information and referral
      2) Counseling
      3) Personal care assistance programs
      4) Telecommunication devices for people who are deaf; sign language interpreters (e.g., at public hearings)
      5) Homemaker services
      6) Augmentative communication aids, adaptive toys, assistive technology
      7) Health screening services
      8) Funding for rehabilitation technology services and adaptive equipment
      9) Technology access, adaptive computers [Refer to Chapter 21 for more information about technology and computers for people with disabilities.]
      10) Telephonic ongoing disease or condition education by nurses

   g. Education
      1) Availability of educational opportunities
      2) Funding
      3) Building accessibility
      4) Programs for disadvantaged children
      5) Therapy services (e.g., occupational,

physical, speech and language) available in school systems

    6) Head Start program and early intervention programs

    7) Bilingual education

    8) Acquisition of equipment to supplement special education and related services; training in computer technology

    9) Self-help groups

    10) Playground accessibility and school environment modifications

    11) Specialized buses, vans, and cars to meet the needs of schoolchildren

  h. Availability of adequate financial resources to meet healthcare needs

VI. Gaining Access to Rehabilitation and Supportive Services in the Community

A. Funding Sources

  1. Agencies and sectors that receive state funding through appropriation of monies, grants, or direct reimbursement

    a. Visiting nursing associations (VNAs) and private not-for-profit home care agencies

    b. Alpha I agencies (members of National Council on Independent Living)

      1) Funded through state and federal monies

      2) Provide services to people with disabilities

        a) Peer support, attendant services, client advocacy

        b) Design consultation

          (1) Educate design professionals and the public about legal requirements for creating accessible environments.

          (2) Provide building product information.

          (3) Review designs.

          (4) Assess homes after occupancy.

        c) Grants and loans for environmental access

        d) Loan programs for adaptive equipment

          (1) Low-interest loans

          (2) Loans for citizens and businesses to purchase technological aids that enhance independence in the home, workplace, or other environments

        e) Independent living programs that provide instruction and hands-on

experience in transitional living skills

        f) Evaluation and education for adapted vehicle driving

        g) Monitoring of access issues

          (1) Have a watchdog project to correct building code violations and publicize standards for accessible design.

          (2) Mobilize statewide networks for grassroots advocacy.

          (3) Inform the design and construction industries about legal requirements for building or remodeling public buildings and housing.

          (4) File complaints or litigation if corrective action is not taken.

  2. Proprietary (for-profit) agencies

  3. Public health services

    a. Nursing services

      1) Home visits for health teaching and screening

      2) Clinics for blood pressure, screening, immunizations, and flu vaccines

    b. Vocational rehabilitation

    c. Adult and child protective services

  4. Elder and adult services

  5. Transportation resources

    a. Public transportation

    b. Private organizations receiving state funds to purchase vans with lifts and to serve people who are elderly, have disabilities, or receive state benefits (e.g., Medicaid, Paratransit)

  6. Independent living programs

    a. Services vary according to the locality and program.

      1) Referral to housing and training in independent living skills

      2) Permanent residential, transitional residential, or temporary housing

      3) Attendant referrals, training, or management training

      4) Client and system advocacy

      5) Disability awareness in community

      6) Equipment repairs and referrals

      7) Reduction of environmental barriers

      8) Promotion of consumer involvement in community activities and information and referral services

    b. Program components vary with each

independent living program.

7. Subacute and postacute care services, skilled nursing facilities, boarding homes, telemedicine

8. Vendor services
   a. Durable medical equipment
   b. Intravenous therapy (e.g., hydration, total parenteral nutrition, antibiotics, blood and blood products, pain management)
   c. Chemotherapy
   d. Medical supplies
   e. Oxygen and ventilator services
   f. Nutritional services (e.g., Meals on Wheels, community ministries)
   g. Enteral feedings

9. Selective professional services
   a. Physicians (office and home)
   b. Inpatient and outpatient hospital services
   c. Counseling
   d. Outpatient phlebotomy services
   e. Mobile medical services (e.g., radiography, electrocardiograms)
   f. Eye care cards (e.g., funding for eye exams, glasses)

10. Programs
    a. Adult day service programs and community-based care
    b. Day treatment programs (e.g., for people with head injuries or Alzheimer's disease)
    c. Person-centered long-term care community programs
    d. Supervised environmental living programs
    e. Stroke specialty programs (e.g., multiple sclerosis specialty programs, amyotrophic lateral sclerosis programs)
    f. Aging service networks
    g. Hospice care
    h. Specialty clinics (e.g., augmentative communication device clinics, assistive technology clinics)
    i. Prosthetic and orthotic services

B. Agencies and Sectors That Receive Federal Funding
   1. VNAs and private not-for-profit agencies providing home care services
   2. Vendor services
   3. Some independent living programs
   4. Outpatient phlebotomy services
   5. Physicians (office and home)

6. Extended rehabilitation facilities

7. Hospice care (expanded scope in 2006 for admission timeframe and duration of treatment, not just for terminal cancer but for terminal renal disease, heart failure)

8. Prosthetic and orthotic devices

9. Mobile medical services

10. Inpatient and outpatient hospital services (acute and rehabilitation)

11. Outpatient rehabilitation services (e.g., hospital based, VNA, private)

C. Department of Veterans Affairs Services
   1. Inpatient and outpatient hospital services
   2. Pharmacy services
   3. Vocational rehabilitation services
   4. Nursing home care
   5. Home health care
   6. Orthotic and prosthetic devices
   7. Durable medical and adaptive equipment
   8. Services for people with visual impairments
   9. Home modifications for people with disabilities
   10. Mortgage loans

D. Federal or State-Subsidized Assistance Programs Based on Income, Age, or Disability
   1. Adult drug cards
   2. Subsidized housing
   3. Utility and telephone rebates
   4. Eye care cards
      a. Provide reimbursement for eye examinations and glasses
      b. Are unavailable for those who have state medical cards because the card would duplicate some coverage
   5. Healthcare services at public clinics (e.g., immunizations, flu vaccines)
   6. Meals on Wheels programs
   7. Books on audiotape

E. Services for Older Adults
   1. Services are funded primarily for people older than age 62.
   2. Age and income are the two main criteria for determining eligibility for programs.
   3. Services may be provided by senior companion programs.
      a. Providing respite care
      b. Running errands
      c. Taking clients out to do errands

d. Doing light housekeeping

F. Preventive Healthcare Medicare Coverage

1. Flu shots

2. Screening mammogram every 12 months for all women aged 40 and older

3. Screening Pap smear and pelvic exam every 3 years or annually for women at high risk for cervical or vaginal cancer

4. Colorectal cancer screening

5. Blood glucose monitors, test strips, and lancets for all people with diabetes

6. Prostate screening for all men aged 50 and older

7. Coverage of diabetes outpatient self-management training services

8. Pneumococcal pneumonia vaccinations

G. Rehabilitation Nursing Interventions to Help Clients Gain Access to Healthcare Resources

1. Coordinate referrals to not-for-profit and private home care agencies.

2. Identify agencies that provide free care or sliding scale fees for services based on income and the duration of needed services.

3. Arrange for social work services to help gain access to community systems that can help provide subsidized housing, Medicaid applications, SSI, SSDI, counseling services, advocacy assistance, equipment, and transportation and that can help find organizations that provide services.

4. Contact the local department of human services about services available for rehabilitation care.

5. Contact legislators to support funding for transferring clients to independent living centers and for training care attendants and supplemental funding that allows people with disabilities to work without a drastic reduction in or termination of medical benefits.

6. Attend public hearings on issues that affect people with disabilities.

7. Act as a community advocate to promote increased environmental accessibility, decreased architectural barriers, increased access to public transportation, decreased cost of services to older adults on fixed incomes, and increased access to healthcare services.

8. Make referrals to rehabilitation counselors, peer counselors, and those providing psychological services.

9. Contact state disability offices, commissions, or departments for assistance.

10. Promote the education of healthcare providers and caregivers within facilities and the community.

a. Provide in-service education.

b. Consult one-on-one with providers regarding healthcare issues, ways to manage individual clients' healthcare needs, and ways to promote access to healthcare services.

c. Encourage family involvement early in the rehabilitation process and teach family members about equipment, procedures, medications, and ways to manage emergencies.

d. Coordinate a home visit by the rehabilitation team to evaluate the need for modifications, equipment, and ways to improve safety.

e. Promote interagency communication about rehabilitation needs, follow-up teaching needs, and previous nursing interventions in the event of a transfer to a different environment.

f. Periodically reassess and evaluate the client's ability to perform activities of daily living, changes in levels of independence, healthcare needs, and barriers to required services.

g. Contact healthcare providers in the community to determine access to buildings, cost of services, insurance coverage, ways to modify the office environment, and availability of transportation.

11. Speak at service club meetings.

12. Actively participate in professional organizations that support legislation and advocacy activities for people with disabilities (see Figure 6-6 for a list of laws governing access to rehabilitation services).

13. Promote the appointment of people with disabilities to public office and commissions and to private-sector industry and business boards.

14. Help clients with disabilities prepare testimony for legislative hearings.

15. Participate in health planning endeavors and advocate for services that meet the needs of children and adults.

Figure 6-6. Laws Governing Access to Rehabilitation Services

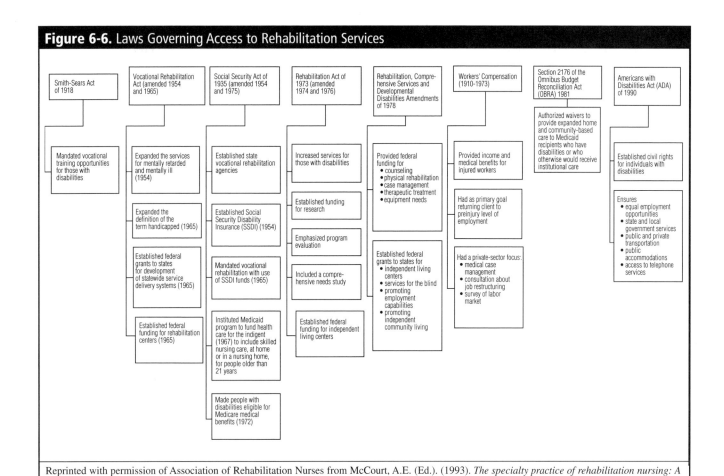

Reprinted with permission of Association of Rehabilitation Nurses from McCourt, A.E. (Ed.). (1993). *The specialty practice of rehabilitation nursing: A core curriculum* (3rd ed., p. 219). Skokie, IL: The Rehabilitation Nursing Foundation of the Association of Rehabilitation Nurses.

References

American Nurses Association (ANA). (1991). *Nursing's agenda for health care reform.* Kansas City, MO: Author.

Arbesman, M., & Wright, C. (1999). Mechanical restraints, rehabilitation therapies, and staffing adequacy as risk factors for falls in an elderly hospitalized population. *Rehabilitation Nursing, 24*(3), 122–128.

Ardell, D.B., & Tager, M.J. (1982). *Planning for wellness: A guide book for achieving optimal health* (2nd ed.). Dubuque, IA: Kendall/Hunt.

Association of Rehabilitation Nurses (ARN). (1994). *Standards and scope of rehabilitation nursing practice.* Skokie, IL: Author.

Bandura, A. (1977a). Self-efficacy: Toward a unifying theory of behavioral changes. *Psychological Review, 84*(2), 191–215.

Bandura, A. (1977b). *Social learning theory.* Englewood Cliffs, NJ: Prentice Hall.

Brain Injury Association of America. (2005, August). *Facts about traumatic brain injury.* McLean, VA: Author. Retrieved May 15, 2007, from www.biausa.org/aboutbi.htm

Brians, L., Alexander, K., Grota, P., Chen, R., & Dumas, V. (1991). The development of the risk tool for fall prevention. *Rehabilitation Nursing, 16,* 67–69.

Centers for Disease Control and Prevention. (2007). *Falls in nursing homes: Fact sheet.* Atlanta, GA: Author. Retrieved May 5, 2007, from http://www.cdc.gov/ncipc/factsheets/nursing.htm

Department of Health and Human Services, Centers for Medicare and Medicaid Service. (2006). Medicare and Medicaid Programs: Hospital conditions of participation—Patients' rights; Final rule. *Federal Register, 71*(236) 1–52.

Dines, A., & Cribb, A. (Eds.). (1993). *Health promotion concepts and practice.* Boston: Blackwell Scientific.

Dochterman, J., & Bulechek, G. (Eds.). (2004). *Nursing interventions classification (NIC)* (4th ed.). St. Louis: Mosby.

Doenges, M., & Moorhouse, M. (1998). Nurse's pocket guide: *Diagnoses, interventions, and rationales* (6th ed.). Philadelphia: F.A. Davis.

Edelman, C., & Mandle, C. (2006). *Health promotion throughout the lifespan* (5th ed.). St. Louis: Mosby.

Edwards, P., Hertzberg, D., Hays, S., & Youngblood, N. (Eds.). (1999). *Pediatric rehabilitation nursing.* Philadelphia: Saunders.

Foundation for Spinal Cord Injury Prevention, Care & Cure (FSCIP). (2006, June). *Spinal cord injury facts.* Fenton, MI: Author. Retrieved May 15, 2007, from http://www.fscip.org/facts.htm

Haines, A., Kuruvilla, S., & Borchert, M. (2004). Bridging the implementation gap between knowledge and action for health. *Bulletin of the World Health Organization, 82*(10), 724–732.

Hanak, M. (1992). *Rehabilitation nursing for the neurological patient.* New York: Springer.

Health Care Financing Administration (HCFA). (1999). *Medicare, preventive benefits: Empire Medicare Services answer your questions.* Syracuse, NY: Empire Medicare Services.

Hendrich, A. (1988a). An effective unit-based fall prevention program. *Journal of Nursing Quality Assurance, 3*(1), 28–36.

Hendrich, A. (1988b). *Patient fall prevention.* Greencastle, IN: Ann Hendrich & Associates.

Hoeman, S. (Ed.). (1996). *Rehabilitation nursing: Process and application* (2nd ed.). St. Louis: Mosby.

JCAHO. (2003). Alternatives to restraint and seclusion. In *Complying with Joint Commission standards* (Chapter 3). Oak Brook, IL: Joint Commission Resources.

Kobasa, S.C., Hilker, R.R., & Maddi, S.R. (1979). Who stays healthy under stress. *Journal of Occupational Medicine, 21,* 595–598.

Kobasa, S.C., Maddi, S.R., & Zola, M.A. (1983). Type A and hardiness. *Journal of Behavioral Medicine, 6*(1), 41–49.

Lefcourt, H. (Ed.). (1981). *Research with locus of control construct.* New York: Academic Press.

Maddox, S. (2006). *Paralysis resource guide.* Short Hills, NJ: Christopher and Dana Reeve Paralysis Resource Center.

Mahoney, J. (1999, August 31). *Assessment of falls risk after hospitalization: Interventions to decrease the risk of falls and improve mobility* [Online]. Madison, WI: UW–Madison Institute on Aging. Available: http://aging.wisc.edu/research/affil.php?Ident=38

Marge, M. (1988). Health promotion for persons with disabilities: Moving beyond rehabilitation. *American Journal of Health Promotion, 2*(4), 29–35.

Mion, L., Gregor, S., Buettner, M., Chwirchak, D., Lee, O., & Paras, W. (1989). Falls in the rehabilitation setting: Incidence and characteristics. *Rehabilitation Nursing, 14,* 17–22.

Mount, B. (2002). In S. Holburn & P. Vietze (Eds.), *Person centered planning applications of research to practice.* New York: Mount Sinai School of Medicine.

Mount, B., Riggs, D., Brown, M., & Hibbard, M. (2003). *Moving On: A Personal Futures Planning Workbook for Individuals with Brain Injury.* New York: Mt. Sinai Medical Center.

National Center for Injury Prevention and Control. (2006). *A toolkit to prevent senior falls: Figures.* Atlanta, GA: Author. Retrieved May 5, 2007, from http://www.cdc.gov/ncipc/pub-res/toolkit/figures.htm

O'Donnell, M. (1987). Definition of health promotion. *Journal of Health Promotion, 1*(1), 4, 14.

Patrick, D. (1997). Rethinking prevention for people with disabilities, Part I: A conceptual model for promoting health. *American Journal of Health Promotion, 11*(4), 251–260.

Patrick, D., Richardson, M., Starks, E., Rose, A., & Kinne, S. (1997). Rethinking prevention for people with disabilities, Part II: A framework for designing interventions. *American Journal of Health Promotion, 11*(4), 261–263.

Porter, E. (1999). Getting up from here: Frail older women's experiences after falling. *Rehabilitation Nursing, 24*(5), 201–206.

Robbins, A., Rubenstein, L., Josephson, K., Schulman, B., Osterweil, D., & Fine, G. (1989). Predictors of falls among elderly people. *Archives of Internal Medicine, 149,* 1628–1633.

Rosenstock, I.M., & Becker, M.H. (1988). The social learning theory and health belief model. *Health Education Quarterly, 15*(2), 175–183.

Ross, J., Watson, C., Gyldenvand, T., & Reinboth, J. (1991). Potential for trauma: Falls. In M. Maas, K. Buckwalter, & M. Hardy (Eds.), *Nursing diagnoses and interventions in the elderly* (pp. 18–31). Redwood City, CA: Addison-Wesley Nursing.

Shillinger, F. (1983). Locus of control: Implications for clinical practice. *Image: The Journal of Nursing Scholarship, 15*(2), 58–63.

Sia, C. (1992). The medical home: Pediatric practice and child advocacy in the 1990s. *Pediatrics, 90*(3), 1419–1423.

Tideiksaar, R. (2002). *Falls in older persons: Prevention and management* (2nd ed.). Health Professions Press.

Viggiani, K. (1997). Special populations. In S. Bastable (Ed.), *Nurse as educator: Principles of teaching and learning* (pp. 204–233). Boston: Jones and Bartlett.

Viggiani, K. (2000). Health maintenance and management of therapeutic regimen. In P. Edwards (Ed.), *The specialty practice of rehabilitation nursing* (pp. 80–101). Glenview, IL: Association of Rehabilitation Nurses.

Vlahov, D., Myers, A., & Al-Ibrahim, M. (1990). Epidemiology of falls among patients in a rehabilitation hospital. *Archives of Physical Medicine and Rehabilitation, 71,* 8–12.

White, G., & Seekins, T. (1996). Preventing and managing secondary conditions: A proposed role for independent living centers. *Journal of Rehabilitation*, pp. 14–21.

WHO Constitution. (2006, October). *Basic documents* (45th ed., suppl.).

Suggested Resources

Alston, R., & Leung, P. (1997). Reform laws and health care coverage: Combating exclusion of persons with disabilities. *Journal of Rehabilitation,* pp. 15–19.

Buchanan, R., & Alston, R. (1997). Medical policies and home health care provisions for persons with disabilities. *Journal of Rehabilitation,* pp. 20–23.

Fullmer, S., & Majumder, R.K. (1991). Increased access and use of disability related information for consumers. *Journal of Rehabilitation, 57*(3), 17–22.

Hagner, D., Helm, D., & Buttersworth, J. (1996). "This is your meeting": A qualitative study of person centered planning. *Mental Retardation, 34*(3), 159–171.

Huntt, D., & Growick, B. (1997). Managed care for people with disabilities. *Journal of Rehabilitation,* pp. 10–14.

Kennedy, J. (1997). Personal assistance benefits and federal health care reforms: Who is eligible on the basis of ADL assistance criteria? *Journal of Rehabilitation,* pp. 40–45.

Mahoney, J., Sager, M., Danham, N., & Johnson, J. (1994). Risk of falls after hospital discharge. *Journal of the American Geriatrics Society, 42*(3), 269–274.

McCourt, A.E. (Ed.). (1993). *The specialty practice of rehabilitation nursing: A core curriculum* (3rd ed.). Skokie, IL: The Rehabilitation Nursing Foundation of the Association of Rehabilitation Nurses.

Teague, M.L., Cipriano, R.E., & McGhee, V.L. (1990). Health promotion as a rehabilitation service for people with disabilities. *Journal of Rehabilitation, 56*(1), 52–56.

U.S. Census Bureau. (1990). *National Health Interview Survey on Assistive Services (NHIS-AD)*. Washington, DC: U.S. Government Printing Office.

Web Sites

Brain Injury Association of America: http://www.biausa.org

Centers for Disease Control and Prevention: http://www.cdc.gov/

Centers for Medicare and Medicaid Services: http://www.cms.hhs.gov/

Commission on Accreditation of Rehabilitation Facilities: http://www.carf.org

National Council on Disability: http://www.ncd.gov/

National Organization of Social Security Claimants' Representatives (NOSSCR): http://www.nosscr.org

Social Security Administration (SSA): http://www.ssa.gov/disability

World Health Organization: http://www.who.int/en/

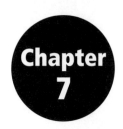

Chapter 7

Physical Healthcare Patterns and Nursing Interventions

Michele Cournan, MS RN CRRN APRN-BC
Donald D. Kautz, PhD RN CRRN-A • Brandy Conrad, BSN RN

The physical patterns of health form the basis of rehabilitation nursing. Nutrition, elimination, sleep and rest, activity and exercise, and sexual and reproductive patterns are all affected by the major illnesses, impairments, and disabilities seen in rehabilitation practice. Rehabilitation nurses must be experts in identifying actual problems and potential problems that result from the disruption of these health patterns. Nurses also must be able to collaborate with patients in setting realistic, appropriate goals and must be astute when selecting interventions to reach these goals in a timely and cost-effective manner.

The nursing process provides the framework, the functional health patterns provide the substance, and the nurse's professional philosophy guides nursing practice. Nurses must always begin with what the patient needs, expects, or wants. They must value growth, independence, interaction with others, and self-actualization. Nurses must always seek ways to integrate nursing practice into the interdisciplinary team's work of restoration and rehabilitation. Although all rehabilitation professionals work together to provide interdisciplinary care, nurses coordinate the care, interact with family and other community supports, and advocate for the patient across disciplines when services must be added, adapted, or revised.

In this chapter, the functional patterns of health have been revised slightly to focus particular attention on the assessment and care of skin and sleep habits as necessary precursors to activity. Also, the content of this chapter makes distinctions between mobility, self-care, and the physical aspects of sexuality and reproduction for people who have permanent health problems.

The topics of this chapter have allowed us to use current clinical guidelines in order to provide a level of evidence (LOE) for the major interventions listed. Throughout the chapter, rehabilitation nurses are encouraged to obtain these guidelines for more information about the topics listed. In addition, many of the interventions have not been systematically tested for their effectiveness. Rehabilitation nurses should be at the forefront of research to test these interventions.

LOEs are defined as follows:

LOE 1: evidence obtained from meta-analysis or systematic review of randomized controlled trials

LOE 2: evidence obtained from controlled studies or randomized controlled trials

LOE 3: evidence obtained from quasiexperimental or descriptive studies

LOE 4: evidence obtained from expert committee reports or respected authorities

I. Nutrition: Eating, Swallowing, and Feeding

A. Overview

1. Adequate nutrition is of particular importance for people with disabilities, chronic illness, or developmental difficulties.

2. Participation in therapeutic exercises and in relearning daily activities requires energy, strength, and endurance.

3. Inadequate intake of food or fluid or consumption that exceeds body demands places the patient at significant risk for multiple complications.

4. Impaired swallowing and risk for aspiration, often seen in patients with neurological injuries, warrants prompt and accurate identification to minimize the risk of aspiration.

5. Rehabilitation nurses must assess nutritional adequacy and select appropriate interventions to restore nutritional health.

B. Nutritional Needs (summarized from Porth, 2005): The body needs more than 40 nutrients each day, including carbohydrates, fats, proteins, vitamins, and minerals. Nutritional status is assessed by evaluating dietary intake, height and weight, health history and physical exam, and laboratory tests. Dietary preferences vary widely. The goal is for rehabilitation patients to have adequate intake to meet metabolic demands and to modify the diet as needed during acute and chronic illnesses.

1. Nursing assessment of nutritional adequacy

a. Body weight and height

b. Dietary history and preferences, including recent and remote past

c. Cultural and religious patterns, interests and choices, ability to select and prepare food

d. Apparent muscle wasting and absence of body fat stores (e.g., use of triceps measurement)
   1) Acute illness
   2) Comorbidities
   3) Depression

e. Presence of excessive body fat stores: The patient who is morbidly obese may have severe underlying nutritional deficiencies.
   1) Energy demands of body weight
   2) Inactivity
   3) Greater reliance for energy on fats, simple carbohydrates, and glucose
   4) Lower dietary fiber intake

f. Diagnostic laboratory data
   1) Serum albumin indicates available protein stores.
   2) Hemoglobin indicates ability to transport oxygen.
   3) Glycohemoglobin indicates blood glucose control over the past 3 months.
   4) Prealbumin level indicates nutritional status and protein synthesis and catabolism.

2. Nursing interventions to promote nutritional adequacy

a. Help the patient select balanced meals.
   1) Adequate calories, protein, and essential nutrients
   2) Select from what is available and acceptable and meets nutritional demands.

b. Teach about daily recommended intake of essential nutrients.

c. Pay attention to possible food–drug interactions.

d. Encourage and support efforts to improve intake for desired weight loss or maintenance.

e. Monitor weight and albumin and hemoglobin levels.

f. Use nutritional supplements, vitamins, and fluids as needed.

g. Institute small, frequent meals to meet calorie and vitamin needs when indicated.

h. Encourage sufficient fiber intake to promote bowel peristalsis.

i. Increase fluid intake for nutritional balance and elimination, if not contraindicated (e.g., in congestive heart failure).

j. Adjust food consistency for ease of chewing, for patient safety, and to compensate for swallowing impairment.

k. Teach patient to read food labels.

l. Teach patient about correct and adequate portion control of food.

m. Assess need for medications such as oxandrolone (Oxandrin) or megestrol (Megace) to stimulate appetite.

C. Frazier Rehab Center's Free Water Protocol: The Frazier Rehab Center, in Louisville, Kentucky, developed the following protocol in 1984 for water between meals for patients who are NPO or on a dysphagia diet (Palmer, 1999). The rationale is that water, even when aspirated, does not contribute to aspiration pneumonia. The protocol evidently is used in several rehabilitation facilities, and multiple Web sites contain information on this protocol. However, at the time of publication, chapter authors could not locate sources documenting the LOE in using this protocol. Rehabilitation nurses are encouraged to work with speech and language pathologists (SLPs) in their own facility when implementing this protocol. Further information on the protocol can be obtained from the American Speech–Language–Hearing Association Web site (http://www.asha.org) (Suiter, 2005).

1. All patients are screened with water. Impulsive patients or those with excessive coughing and discomfort are restricted to drinking water only under supervision. The physical stress of coughing may prevent oral intake of water in those with extreme coughing.

2. For patients on oral diets, water is permitted between meals. The intake of water is unrestricted before all meals and allowed 30 minutes after a meal. The 30-minute timeframe appears arbitrary but is used in several facilities to allow spontaneous swallows to clear food residues.

3. Medications are never given with water in the protocol but instead are administered with a spoonful of applesauce, pudding, yogurt, or thickened liquid.

4. Staff in all departments and families are educated on the rationale for encouraging water between meals, the guidelines for the intake of free water, and any restrictions. In some facilities, patients on the protocol wear armbands that indicate "no thin liquids except water between meals."

5. In all cases, recommendations given by the speech therapist for safe swallowing in each patient should be followed.

D. Typical Causes of Impaired Nutrition That Have Implications for Rehabilitation Nursing: The American Medical Directors Association has published the excellent guideline "Altered Nutritional Status" (available at http://www.guideline.gov), which provides evidence-based guidelines nurses can use with patients who have nutritional deficiencies caused by any of these problems.

1. Loss of teeth
2. Loss of sense of smell
3. Diminished saliva production
4. Impaired swallowing (e.g., excessive drooling, pocketing of food)
5. Risk of aspiration or silent aspiration
6. Impaired digestive ability caused by hiatal hernia, flattened diaphragm, or gastroesophageal reflux
7. Impaired gastric motility
8. Hyperglycemia (e.g., diabetes, steroids)
9. Hypoglycemia (e.g., diminished intake, insulin or other medications, exercise, vomiting)
10. Ineffective absorption of nutrients
11. Inattention to hunger from depression or isolation
12. Inability to initiate self-feeding patterns
13. Altered self-image (e.g., bulimia, anorexia)
14. Intake of food exceeding body's caloric demands
15. Altered demands for nutrients in periodic stages of childhood growth and development
16. Exacerbated metabolic demand for nutrients resulting from trauma or disease
17. History of underlying poor nutrition, vitamin deficiencies, and dehydration
18. Medication interactions and side effects
19. Effect of comorbidities (e.g., chronic respiratory disease, cardiac disease, diabetes)
20. Impaired mobility, limiting ability to obtain or prepare well-balanced meals
21. Impaired ability to perform activities of daily living (ADLs), limiting ability to prepare well-balanced meals
22. Financial impact of disability, limiting ability to purchase nutritious foods

E. Swallowing and Aspiration (adapted from Smith Hammond & Goldstein, 2006): Rehabilitation nurses are encouraged to obtain this evidence-based guideline. The LOEs for interventions 1–5 were determined by Smith Hammond and Goldstein.

1. Normal anatomy and physiology of swallowing (see Figure 7-1).
2. Clinical manifestations that indicate a high risk of aspiration and the need for a swallowing evaluation, preferably by an SLP, include need for oral pharyngeal suctioning, dysarthria, dysphonia, weak voluntary cough, drooling, cough, or wet voice or nasal regurgitation after water bolus (LOE 2).
3. Patients with a reduced level of consciousness should not be fed orally until the level of consciousness has improved (LOE 2).
4. Alert patients with cough and a high risk of aspiration should be observed drinking 3 oz of water; if the patient coughs or shows clinical manifestations of aspiration, refer to an SLP for further evaluation before further oral intake (LOE 2).
5. Patients with dysphagia should be managed by an interdisciplinary team, which may include an SLP, nurse, physician, dietitian, and physical and occupational therapists (LOE 2).
6. Patients with intractable aspiration may be considered for surgical intervention.
7. Patients may also have difficulty swallowing medications. See Griffith and Tengnah (2007) for a consensus guideline for patients who have difficulty swallowing medications.
8. The following nursing interventions may be recommended by the SLP for specific patients to assist in swallowing (Morris, 2006). (At the time of this printing, a guideline indicating the LOE for these interventions was not found; however, none of these interventions appear to be harmful. Deane, Whurr, Clarke, Playford, & Ben-Shlomo (2001) recommend that randomized controlled trials be conducted to test their effectiveness.)
   a. Seat patient upright, preferably in a chair.
   b. Select foods of appropriate consistency and texture.
      1) Progress over time from pureed to ground to regular food.
      2) With ground food, only gradually add food that fragments easily.
      3) Stay with one food and texture at a time.
      4) Do not mix solids and liquids.
   c. Progress liquid intake from pudding thick to honey thick to nectar thick to thin. If

Figure 7-1. Normal Swallow

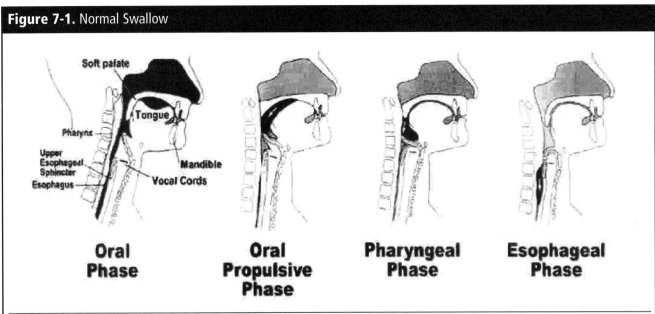

Soft palate
Tongue
Pharynx
Upper Esophageal Sphincter
Esophagus
Mandible
Vocal Cords

Oral Phase

Oral Propulsive Phase

Pharyngeal Phase

Esophageal Phase

Illustration reprinted with permission from the American College of Chest Physicians from Smith Hammond, C.A., & Goldstein, L. (2006). Cough and aspiration of foods and liquids due to oral–pharyngeal dysphagia: ACCP evidence-based clinical practice guidelines. *Chest, 129,* 156S.

necessary, use a commercial thickener to achieve the appropriate consistency.

d. Place food on unaffected side of mouth and use small mouthfuls; encourage the patient to turn his or her head to the unaffected side to bring food into the midline.

e. Teach patient to concentrate fully on chewing each small mouthful, forming a food bolus, and swallowing it before taking another mouthful.

f. Use the chin tuck method to protect the airway.
   1) Encourage patient to do a tongue sweep of mouth to self-check for food.
   2) Use compensatory strategies such as a double swallow between mouthfuls to prevent aspiration.
   3) Instruct patient to take small sips of water between mouthfuls or to alternate liquid and solid mouthfuls, as appropriate.

g. Visually inspect the oral cavity and use wide-mouth drinking vessels to allow visualization of progress of liquids into oral cavity.

h. Provide enough time and appropriate supervision.
   1) Use adaptive devices for self-feeding and independence.
   2) Give patients with impulsivity one item of food or drink at a time and limit distractions.

i. Eliminate distractions, give cues for strategies, and discourage the patient from conversing while eating.

j. Provide a calm, unhurried atmosphere.

k. Ensure that the patient remains upright for 20–30 minutes after eating a meal.

F. The National Dysphagia Diet (NDD) provides guidelines for progressive diets for those with dysphagia (Cowley, Diebold, Gross, & Hardin-Fanning, 2006).
   1. NDD1: dysphagia pureed
      a) Pudding-like consistencies
      b) No chunks
      c) Avoid lumpy foods and small pieces.
   2. NDD2: dysphagia mechanically altered
      a) Soft, moist foods
      b) Ground meats, soft vegetables
      c) No bread, peas, or corn
      d) Avoid skins and seeds.
      e) Mechanical soft (same as above but can have bread, cakes, rice)
   3. NDD3: dysphagia advanced
      a) Regular foods except very hard, sticky, or crunchy foods
      b) Avoid hard fruits and vegetables, corn, skins, nuts, seeds.
   4. Liquid consistencies are described as spoon thick, honey-like, nectar-like, or thin.

G. Administration of Specialized Nutritional Support
   1. Rehabilitation nurses may care for patients

who need either enteral (feeding tube) or parental (intravenous) nutritional support. The American Society for Parenteral and Enteral Nutrition regularly updates its clinical guidelines for assessing patients in need of specialized nutritional support, access, and administration of nutritional supplements though the enteral and parenteral routes. Rehabilitation nurses are encouraged to search for current guidelines through http://www.guideline.gov.

2. Patients who are fed by gastrostomy tube (G-tube) to provide temporary or permanent access to the gut when oral intake is not possible.

   a. Ensure adequate fluid intake by assessing hydration status.

   b. Monitor body weight and serum albumin.

   c. Regularly check gastric contents for residual.

   d. Maintain head of bed at 30 degrees or higher during feeding and do not lay patient flat for at least 30 minutes after meals.

   e. Time feedings to be either continuous or bolus. If caloric needs can be met, bolus is preferred, with gradual return to normal patterns of intake.

   f. Use portable equipment to allow participation in therapy regimen.

   g. Protect and routinely cleanse skin around gastrostomy site and use skin shields.

3. Patients who are fed by hyperalimentation via central intravenous catheters when use of the gut is not possible.

   a. Provide special care for access site, tubing, and solution.

   b. Ensure adequate caloric intake through periodic use of lipid solutions.

   c. Regularly monitor body chemistries to help in the adjustment of solution electrolytes and lipids.

   d. Gradually introduce oral intake and taper hyperalimentation.

II. Skin Integrity, Impairments, and Interventions

A. Overview

   1. Preservation and restoration of intact skin is a major focus of rehabilitation nursing because patients present with multiple risk factors and major disruptions in health.

   2. Prevention of skin breakdown is key to emphasize with the patient and family and must be the focus of the entire rehabilitation team.

   3. Pressure ulcers can seriously impede the recovery of health.

   4. Several groups have published practice guidelines based on extensive critique of research literature and expert review on the prevention of pressure ulcers (e.g., Institute for Clinical Improvement [2006], Wound, Ostomy and Continence Nurses Society [2003], Paralyzed Veterans of America [published in 2000 then reviewed and considered current as of December 2005]). The Registered Nurses Association of Ontario (RNAO) 2005 guideline was used to provide the LOEs for each of the interventions listed. Rehabilitation nurses are encouraged to develop a set of practice guidelines that focus specifically on standards of rehabilitation practice.

   5. Rehabilitation nurses need to be skilled in maintaining intact skin and in identifying and treating pressure ulcers.

   6. Rehabilitation nurses' major concern in skin care is to prevent and, when necessary, heal pressure wounds. All wounds should be treated with appropriate sterile techniques and dressings.

B. Anatomy and Function of the Skin (Porth, 2005)

   1. Epidermis: the outermost layer, which contains keratin that protects deeper layers of the skin and is constantly being replaced by newer cells from the dermis

      a. Protects against ultraviolet radiation

      b. Protects from environmental antigens

      c. Protects the body from injury

      e. Retains moisture

      f. Excretes waste products

      g. Assists in regulating body temperature

   2. Dermal layer: fibrous connective tissue

      a. Allows elasticity of skin

      b. Permits motion

      c. Supports healing

3. Subcutaneous layer
   a. Contains sweat glands, oil glands, and hair follicles
   b. Provides blood supply to the skin
   c. Contains neuron receptors for touch, pain, and vasomotor response
   d. Is sustained by a layer of fat
4. Circulation
   a. Provides nutrients, oxygenation, and moisture
   b. Promotes healing through increased blood supply, phagocytosis, and tissue rebuilding
   c. Provides support and healing in response to tissue load damage
5. Nerve supply: provides response to environment and supports homeostasis

C. Risk Factors for Loss of Skin Integrity
1. Physiological factors
   a. Altered metabolic states that increase the body's need for nutrients and may cause cellular level impairment
   b. Underlying medical conditions (e.g., diabetes, cardiopulmonary or renal disease) or disease treatment (e.g., high-dose steroids after spinal cord injury)
   c. Low serum protein, albumin, and hemoglobin, which impair the body's cellular rebuilding activity
   d. Impaired circulation from peripheral neuropathies, anemia, atherosclerosis, or hypertension
   e. Prolonged pressure and immobility, which lead to pressure ulcer formation
   f. Neurological injuries that result in impaired sensation (e.g., proprioception, temperature, touch), resulting in the inability to perceive the need to move the body
   g. Medications that suppress the immune response
   h. Smoking, which decreases the effectiveness of the vascular bed by increasing vasoconstriction
   i. Poor nutrition, especially inadequate intake of protein, vitamin C, thiamine, and zinc
   j. Bladder and bowel incontinence
   k. Increased age: Older adults have diminished effectiveness of skin protection and slowed healing ability and are more likely to have comorbidities and mobility problems.

2. Mechanical factors
   a. Sustained pressure: resting surfaces that are hard and unyielding and maintain constant pressure in one direction, particularly over bony prominences when repositioning is infrequent
   b. Shearing: the movement of muscle, subcutaneous, and fat tissues downward and compression against the bony skeleton while the epidermis does not slide (as occurs when the patient is sitting up in bed and slides down in response to gravity)
   c. Friction: rubbing of tissue across a rough surface (as occurs with incomplete lifting or dragging of a patient to pull him or her up in bed)
   d. Body moisture: incontinence, diuresis, or sweating, especially in the skin folds of an obese patient
   e. Particular problems associated with stomas (e.g., G-tube, tracheostomy, colostomy, urostomy)
   f. Incorrect fit of prostheses, braces, or orthoses and shoes, especially in the presence of neuropathy (e.g., diabetes)
3. Psychosocial factors
   a. Nonconformance with recommended healthcare practices
   b. Substance abuse that impairs nutrition, mobility, and sensation
   c. Impaired cognitive or intellectual ability
   d. Depression
   e. Social isolation, particularly when the patient needs assistance in daily care

D. Nursing Assessment of Patients at Risk for Impaired Skin Integrity: Assess all of the following when a patient is admitted to a rehabilitation facility and daily for those identified at risk for skin breakdown (LOE 4) (RNAO, 2005)
1. General assessment components
   a. Underlying medical conditions
   b. Nutrition: protein, albumin and prealbumin, hemoglobin, transferrin, and white blood cell count; hemoglobin A1c if diabetic
   c. Circulatory support
   d. Presence of neurological injury
   e. Bladder and bowel function and body moisture
   f. Sensory–perceptual ability
   g. Mobility, activity and exercise, body positioning

h. Pressure, shearing, and friction, which may occur in the course of bedside care

i. Age: Older adults are at particular risk for developing pressure ulcers because they are most likely to have problems in all of these categories.

2. Use of assessment scales. Assessment scales are routinely used in all inpatient care settings. However, note that the LOE is rated as 4 (RNAO, 2005). Rehabilitation nurses need to gather these data every day in order to show whether completing a risk assessment scale actually prevents skin breakdown.

    a. Braden scale: Contains six weighted elements, each of which is graded from 1 (*very poor or very limited*) to 4 (*excellent, normal*) and summed across all elements for a total score for person's risk status.

    b. Norton scale: Contains a simpler list of four weighted elements, scored from 1 (*immobile or poor*) to 4 (*excellent*) and summed across all elements for a total score for the person's risk status.

    c. For both scoring systems, areas of low score should prompt specific interventions to maintain or restore skin integrity. Scoring can be repeated over time to demonstrate improvement.

E. Expected Patient Outcomes Related to Potential Impaired Skin Integrity

1. Intact skin

2. Appropriate self-efficacy measures in the management of skin integrity

F. Nursing Interventions to Maintain Skin Integrity: Except when indicated otherwise, the LOE for all of the following interventions is 4 (RNAO, 2005)

1. Ensure good nutritional support and use supplements if needed. Consult dietitian.

2. Manage tissue loads.

    a. Turn and reposition the patient frequently.
        1) Every 2 hours in bed
        2) Every hour in chair
        3) Weight shift every 15 minutes in chair if independent

    b. Use good lifting, transfer, and turning techniques. Consult occupational or physical therapist as needed.

    c. Cushion bony prominences.

    d. Protect skin against friction and shearing.

    e. Position the patient with adequate support.

    f. Increase the patient's efforts toward mobility and activity.

g. Provide pressure redistribution mattress and chair cushion.

h. Involve interdisciplinary team.

3. Care for the skin

    a. Inspect skin daily and pay special attention to all bony prominences.

    b. Cleanse skin at regular intervals and use a mild cleansing agent to preserve the neutral pH of skin.

    c. Apply nonsensitizing, pH-balanced emollients to help retain or maintain skin moisture.

    d. Avoid massaging bony prominences to prevent tissue damage (LOE 2).

    e. Minimize exposure to incontinence, perspiration, or wound drainage.
        1) Use wicking materials to draw moisture away from the skin.
        2) Use topical agents as protective barriers.
        3) Institute bladder and bowel training regimens whenever possible.

4. Teach patients about the importance of self-efficacy in nutrition, management of tissue loads, skin inspection, and general skin care (LOE 3).

G. Normal Phases of Wound Healing

1. Vascular supply and wound stabilization (i.e., the wound bleeds and then clots)

2. Inflammation of the tissues with influx of phagocytes to remove dead tissue

3. Proliferation of fibrin and formation of a loose matrix within the wound, which supports additional tissue formation and retention

4. Maturation of the fibrin matrix into intact skin

H. Essential Elements for Planning Nursing Care for Pressure Ulcers and Expected Patient Outcomes

1. Nutritional assessment and support: Nutritional support provides sufficient protein to produce serum albumin values of at least 3.5, and the patient's weight will be more than 80% of ideal. Several weeks of intensive therapy is needed to increase serum albumin. Prealbumin testing shows a rise in 3–5 days.

2. Management of tissue loads: Resting surfaces and positioning provide adequate protection for tissue load to encourage healing and prevent further loss (LOE 4).

3. Care of the ulcer itself: Ulcer care will promote wound cleansing and healing. Response to treatment may be slow

because of underlying vascular damage, comorbidities, and immobility.

I. General Nursing Interventions for Pressure Ulcers

1. Promote increased protein intake, vitamin supplement, and adequate hydration. Correct any nutritional deficiencies (LOE 4).

2. Keep the patient off the wound as much as possible (LOE 3).

3. Turn and reposition the patient at least every 2 hours (while in bed, every hour in chair) using sheets to lift (not drag) the patient; if possible, use an over-the-bed trapeze to encourage the patient to assist with lifting (LOE 3).

4. Use positioning pillows and blocks to maintain pressure relief; consider using pressure-reducing devices (e.g., air mattresses, specialty foam surfaces, gel pads, low air-loss mattresses, and wheelchair cushions). Float heels off bed, if necessary, using pillows or other flotation devices (LOE 3).

5. Encourage mobility (LOE 3).

6. Assess circulatory status. Wounds must receive adequate circulation to heal (LOE 4).

7. Keep the skin clean, dry, and lubricated; do not massage reddened bony prominences because this may increase capillary destruction (LOE 3).

8. Change linens promptly and clean the skin after any episodes of bladder or bowel incontinence; ensure that wrinkles are removed to prevent further pressure. Provide a moisture barrier lotion for further protection (LOE 3).

9. Provide consistent, timely treatments and document progress (LOE 3). Pressure ulcers become visible quickly, worsen quickly, and heal slowly.

10. Focus treatment approaches on the whole person and the environment; pressure ulcers tend to be multivariate in cause (LOE 4).

11. Assess and reassess pressure ulcers using standard staging guidelines. Pressure ulcers are staged according to depth, characteristics of wound bed, and potential involvement of deep fascia (see Table 7-1). In some states, inpatient healthcare facilities are required to report all stage III and stage IV pressure ulcers. Therefore, some facilities allow only specially trained nurses to document the stage of ulcers.

J. Nursing Interventions for Pressure Ulcers (see Table 7-2).

K. Documentation of Wound Healing (LOE 4)

1. Describe location and measure (in centimeters) length (head to toe), width (side to side), and depth of the wound; use transparent grids for accuracy in measurement if needed. Measure wounds each week to determine effectiveness of treatments and healing.

2. Describe wound base (e.g., color, presence or absence of moisture, slough, eschar).

3. Evaluate undermining or sinus tract formation by gently probing the wound with sterile gauze swabs to determine the depth of these pockets or tracts. Use the clock method to describe the location of the undermine or tract (e.g., 2-cm tunnel at 2 o'clock).

4. Evaluate the amount and type of drainage. Note any odor from the wound.

5. Evaluate the peri-wound skin. Note any erythema, maceration, or callus formation.

6. Note evidence of pain, induration, or inflammation and remember that redness, hardness, or discoloration around pressure areas that have poor blood supply (e.g., heels, sacrum) can mask major tissue necrosis behind apparently intact skin.

7. Include present and planned treatment regimen.

8. Take pictures of the wound for baseline and repeat at periodic intervals (generally every 2 weeks) until the wound is healed. This is a helpful measure of the effectiveness of therapy; however, remember that patient consent may be needed, and each nurse should review the facility's policy on photographic documentation before taking pictures.

9. Document pressure wounds that are healing by retaining the label of the original stage with "healing" added; do not revert to lesser staging as the wound heals. However, with the Minimum Data Set and Inpatient Rehabilitation Facility Patient Assessment Instrument, staff are required to revert to lesser staging. The authors recognize that this advice is confusing.

III. Elimination: Bladder and Bowel Function

A. Overview

1. The human body eliminates the waste of metabolism through urine and stool.

2. Normal function depends on several factors.

   a. Anatomical integrity

Table 7-1. Stages of Pressure Ulcers

Suspected Deep Tissue Injury: Purple or maroon localized area of discolored intact skin or a blood-filled blister caused by damage to the underlying soft tissue. Area may be painful, boggy, mushy, firm, and warmer or cooler than adjacent skin. Evolution may be rapid, exposing additional layers of tissue even with optimal treatment.

Stage I Ulcer: Skin temperature, tissue consistency, and sensation differ from those of an adjacent or opposite area on the body. In lightly pigmented skin, the ulcer appears as a defined area of persistent redness that continues even after pressure to the area is removed. In darker skin, the ulcer may display persistent red, blue, or purple hues.

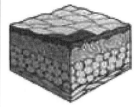

Underlying muscle and subcutaneous tissue are more susceptible to pressure injury than skin, so ulcers often are more severe than they appear.

Stage II Ulcer: Superficial and presents clinically as an abrasion, blister, or shallow crater.

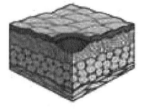

Stage III Ulcer: Deep crater with or without undermining of adjacent tissue.

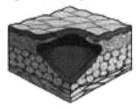

Involving damage to or necrosis of subcutaneous (fat) tissue that may extend down to, but not through, underlying fascia. If there is slough, then it is a stage III because slough is dead fat.

Stage IV Ulcer: Extensive destruction, tissue necrosis, or damage to muscle, bone, or supporting structures. Undermining and sinus tracts may also be associated with stage IV ulcers.

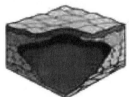

Unstageable: Base of the ulcer is covered by slough (yellow, tan, gray, green, or brown) or eschar (tan, brown, or black). Until enough slough or eschar is removed to expose the base of the wound, the true depth and stage cannot be determined.

This staging system was adopted by the National Pressure Ulcer Advisory Panel in February 2007. Please visit their Web site for additional resources (http://www.npuap.org).

---

b. Intact neurological components for both voluntary control and synergistic emptying

c. A predictable pattern of waste production

d. Physical and mental ability and the willingness to carry out toileting-related tasks

3. Patients in rehabilitation facilities often need management of neurogenic bowel or neurogenic bladder, treatment of urinary incontinence, or treatment of constipation.

4. Bowel and bladder disorders are major barriers to community living, employment, and social activity.

5. Rehabilitation nurses must be knowledgeable about the normal physiology of bladder and bowel function, clinically astute in identifying disruptions that produce incontinence and dysfunction, and expert in selecting interventions that will help

Table 7-2. Nursing Interventions for Pressure Ulcers

NOTE: The authors have included skin care products that are frequently recommended for use with different stages of ulcers. Nurses are encouraged to check with manufacturers and expert panels for current information on the use of these products.

Stage I

Provide pressure redistribution for reddened areas where skin is still intact.

Protect the skin from potential abrasion by applying barrier lotion.

Protect skin from friction and shearing forces by keeping head of bed below 30 degrees, padding bony prominences.

Keep skin clean and dry.

Stage II

Keep the wound moist and clean to promote healing from the base up for open areas that have a granulation base (clean, moist, red tissue bases, no drainage, no slough [i.e., yellow, thready] or eschar [i.e., black, hard, leathery]).

Use dressings that promote moist wound healing (i.e., hydrogels, hydrofibers).

Cleanse the wound with each dressing change, using either normal saline or a commercial wound cleanser. Irrigation should be strong enough to clean nonadherent particles but not so strong as to cause damage to new tissue. Pressure resulting from irrigation with an 18- or 19-gauge Angiocath on a 30-ml syringe meets this criterion.

Adjust frequency of dressing changes to allow assessment of improvement without disrupting fibroblastic activity and introducing additional pathogens into the wound. In the absence of symptoms of active infection, changing the dressing every 2–3 days may be sufficient. As healing is evidenced, less frequent dressing changes are indicated.

Potential products: hydrofibers, hydrocolloids, hydrogels

Stage III

Irrigate the wound with each dressing change as described in stage II, because stage III wounds usually have slough or drainage and may have tunnels and undermining.

Choose dressings based on the wound base and the amount of drainage. If the base is granulation tissue, select a dressing that promotes moist wound healing (see stage II) or consider use of vacuum-assisted closure. If the base is slough, debridement is needed (enzymatic). Nonselective debridement (e.g., normal saline wet-to-dry dressings) should be avoided because it can remove new granulating tissue. If the base is eschar, sharp debridement may be needed. Eschar must be cross-hatched to allow enzymes to be effective. Gently but thoroughly pack any dead space, making sure to include any tunnels and pockets of undermine. Select a packing material that will absorb any excess exudate (i.e., foam, alginate). Apply a secondary dressing. Change dressings according to the amount of drainage absorbed.

Protect the periulcer area from maceration by applying barrier cream.

Potential products: enzymatic debriding agents (if debridement necessary), hydrogels, hydrofibers, alginates, vacuum-assisted closure

Stage IV

See stage III ulcers. Consider use of vacuum-assisted closure. Stage IV wounds may warrant surgical closure with grafts or flaps once a clean margin is obtained.

Potential products: enzymatic debriding agents (if debridement necessary), hydrogels, hydrofibers, alginates, vacuum-assisted closure

Adapted from National Pressure Ulcer Advisory Panel (NPUAP). (2001). *Pressure ulcer treatment: A competency based curriculum for RNs.* Available: http://www.npuap.org

Wound, Ostomy and Continence Nurses Society (WOCN). (2001). *Guideline for prevention and management of pressure ulcers.* Available: http://www.guideline.gov

the patient develop predictable, effective elimination patterns.

6. Management of bowel and bladder function is a key aspect of rehabilitation nursing; however, bowel and bladder goals are best achieved through interdisciplinary team goals because cognitive ability, communication ability, hand function, and level of independence in ADLs and transfers are key factors in the choice of appropriate bowel and bladder management strategies.

7. Desired outcomes of bladder management are to remain continent, empty bladder completely, and avoid recurrent urinary tract infections and other complications of bladder dysfunction.

8. Desired outcomes of bowel management are to remain continent, have a formed bowel movement on a regular schedule, prevent diarrhea and constipation, and prevent complications such as hemorrhoids, abdominal distention, autonomic dysreflexia, and fecal impaction.

B. Physiology of Bladder Elimination (Porth, 2005, p. 856)

1. Purpose of the bladder is to store and control the elimination of urine.

2. Urination is a function of the peripheral autonomic nervous system.

3. Inhibition or facilitation of urination is controlled by spinal cord reflex centers,

micturition center in the pons, and cortical and subcortical centers in the brain.

4. Bladder filling control originates in the T11–L2 segments of the spinal cord, which cause the detrusor muscle to relax and the internal sphincter to contract.

5. Micturition occurs when the bladder detrusor muscle contracts while the external urinary sphincter relaxes.

6. Skeletal muscle in the external sphincter and pelvic muscles that support the bladder are controlled by the pudendal nerve, which exits the spinal cord from the S2–S4 segments.

C. Neurogenic Bladder and Neurogenic Bladder Management: The content for this section is adapted from Consortium for Spinal Cord Medicine (2006). This is an excellent guideline that rehabilitation nurses will find useful.

1. Neurogenic bladder disorders are classified in several different ways. Traditionally, nurses are taught to classify bladder dysfunction as primarily spastic bladder dysfunction, or failure to store urine (often associated with upper motor neuron spinal cord injuries), and flaccid bladder, or failure to empty urine (often associated with lower motor neuron spinal cord injuries). Head injury may accompany spinal cord injury, complicating bladder function and choice of bladder management strategy. A suprapontine lesion from other cerebrovascular diseases may lead to detrusor hyperreflexia (overactive bladder) without detrusor sphincter dyssynergia. Urologic evaluation is necessary to detect and manage spinal shock, uninhibited bladder contractions, autonomic dysreflexia, or detrusor–external sphincter dyssynergia during the acute phase of rehabilitation when choosing a management strategy.

2. Specific bladder management strategies (Consortium for Spinal Cord Medicine, 2006; see the guideline for contraindications for each of these strategies). The Consortium for Spinal Cord Medicine intentionally presented the indications, advantages and disadvantages, and nursing considerations for the most commonly used bladder management strategies. The consortium notes that there is no strong evidence that one method is superior to another. Recommended goals of any bladder management program are to prevent upper urinary tract damage, minimize lower urinary tract complications (stones, fistulas, chronic

effects of infections), and be compatible with the patient and caregiver lifestyles.

a. Intermittent catheterization may be effective for those who have sufficient hand skills to perform the catheterization or a caregiver willing to perform the intermittent catheterization (LOE 3).

1) Paralyzed Veterans of America recommends keeping bladder volumes below 500 ml by catheterizing every 4–6 hours in order to prevent overdistention of the bladder; the patient may need to wake during the night for catheterization. Keeping bladder volumes below 400 ml has been recommended in the past by many sources.

2) Train the patient or caregiver and institute clean intermittent catheterization before discharge.

3) Consider sterile catheterization in those with recurring symptomatic infections.

4) Treat urine leakage between catheterizations.

5) Catheter selection is made considering economic considerations and latex sensitivity.

6) Hands should be washed or aseptic towelettes used both before and after catheterization.

7) Catheters should be washed with mild soap, air dried, and kept in a paper bag until reused.

b. Credé and Valsalva: Applying suprapubic pressure to express urine from the bladder may be effective for those with lower motor neuron injuries and low outlet resistance or who have had a sphincterotomy (LOE 3).

c. Indwelling catheters inserted through the urethra or suprapubic catheters are used for those with high fluid intake, poor hand skills, cognitive impairment, vesicoureteral reflux, lack of success with less invasive methods, or limited assistance from a caregiver (LOE 3).

1) Suprapubic catheterization has several benefits over urethral catheterization.

2) Surveillance for urinary tract infections and bladder stones is recommended.

3) Urethral catheters (14–16 Fr) are recommended, with balloon filled

to 5–10 ml. Replace catheter every 2–4 weeks or weekly in those prone to catheter encrustation or bladder stones.

    4) Suprapubic catheters (22–24 Fr) are recommended, changed every 4 weeks by a trained healthcare provider, more often in those with catheter encrustation or stones.

    5) Anchor catheter with a belt, tape, or other device to abdomen or thigh.

    6) Daily irrigation is not recommended.

    7) If daytime and nighttime collection devices are reused, clean daily with a 1:10 bleach solution.

  d. Reflex voiding with a condom catheter is appropriate for males who have adequate hand skills, poor compliance with fluid restriction, and small bladder capacity (LOE 4).

    1) Apply condom catheter securely to avoid constriction and leakage for 24 hours.

    2) To avoid skin breakdown, wash glans daily when condom is changed and air skin for 20–30 minutes. Alternate the leg each day to anchor tubing to prevent skin breakdown.

    3) Clean daytime and nighttime urinary collection devices daily with a 1:10 bleach solution.

    4) Choose the appropriate size and length self-adhesive condom. Those with allergies to the adhesive can use nonadhesive condoms.

  e. Additional management strategies. Consortium for Spinal Cord Medicine (2006) outlines recommendations for the following additional bladder management strategies. Nurses are referred to the bladder management guideline for recommendations about those who might benefit from each strategy, advice about potential complications, and nursing considerations about each strategy.

    1) Alpha blockers

    2) Botulinum toxin injection

    3) Urethral stents

    4) Transurethral sphincterotomy

    5) Electrical stimulation and posterior sacral rhizotomy

    6) Bladder augmentation

    7) Continent urinary diversion

    8) Urinary diversion

    9) Cutaneous ileovesicostomy

D. Urinary Incontinence: Content for this section is adapted from two of the most current guidelines at the time of this publication: Bengtson et al. (2004) and University of Texas at Austin, School of Nursing, Family Nurse Practitioner Program (2002). Both are available from http://www.guideline.gov. Neither of these guidelines provides LOEs for any of the following interventions. Rehabilitation nurses are encouraged to search for guidelines that provide LOEs at http://www.guideline.gov.

Urinary incontinence is the involuntary loss of urine resulting from pathological, anatomical, or physiological factors. Postmenopausal women and men with prostatic hyperplasia, cognitive dysfunction, neurological movement disorders (e.g., multiple sclerosis, Parkinson's disease), or stroke are at risk for incontinence. Incontinence often is classified into the following types, determined by patient history, physical exam, and urologic workup:

  1. Stress: small losses of urine that occur when intraabdominal pressure is increased by activities such as coughing, laughing, exercising, or sneezing.

  2. Urge: loss of urine caused by abnormal detrusor contractions and sometimes associated with urinary retention; characterized as a strong urge to void; major component of overactive bladder syndrome.

  3. Mixed: clinical manifestations of both urge and stress incontinence.

  4. Overflow: loss of urine caused by bladder overdistention; clinical manifestations include urgency, frequent urination, dribbling, and both stress and urge incontinence.

  5. Total: continuous loss of urine, even with minimal activity.

  6. Functional: urine loss caused by acute or chronic physical and cognitive dysfunction. May or may not include urinary tract pathophysiology.

  7. Rehabilitation nurses should refer all patients who dribble or leak urine for diagnosis and treatment. Treatment decisions for incontinence are best made by physicians, advanced practice nurses, or specialty nurses trained to manage urinary incontinence after completing a detailed history, physical exam, and possibly one or more diagnostic tests, including voiding diary, postvoid residual measurement, and urodynamic testing.

  8. General, nonpharmacologic treatment for all types of incontinence (see University of Texas at Austin, School of Nursing, Family Nurse Practitioner Program, 2002):

    a. Diet counseling to limit caffeine intake,

ensure fluid intake is 1,500–2,400 ml/day, and limit fluids at bedtime for nocturia.

  b. Make environmental modifications to ensure ease in getting to toilet; consider bedside commode.

  9. Treatment of incontinence (see Table 7-3): If the nurse has any questions about these interventions, he or she should seek the advice of a physician or advanced practice nurse with specialized training in treating incontinence.

  10. CMS regulations (2005; F315, 483.25d) require that:

  a. Residents entering a facility without an indwelling urinary catheter not receive one unless medically necessary.

  b. Residents with urinary incontinence receive appropriate services and treatment to prevent urinary tract infections and restore as much bladder control as possible.

E. Bowel Function

1. Normal anatomy and physiology of bowel elimination

  a. Small and ascending large intestines absorb nutrients from liquid stool.

  b. Transverse component of the large intestines absorbs some of the fluid, and stool begins to be more formed.

  c. Descending large intestines and rectum absorb additional water, and kidney waste is added. Stool is compacted into a more solid form.

  d. Internal sphincter retains stool in the rectum.

  e. External sphincter expands to allow the passage of stool from the rectum.

  f. Abdominal wall musculature assists with evacuation.

  g. Peristalsis moves the stool along the gut.

  h. Bowel function continues with cerebral or spinal cord impairment.

   1) Voluntary and involuntary innervation occurs at the reflex,

---

Table 7-3. Treatment of Incontinence

Type of Incontinence	Recommended Treatment
Urge incontinence	Adjust urine output to approximately 1.5 L/day.
	Urge suppression training, bladder retraining, or prompted voiding
	Pelvic muscle (Kegel) exercises (see below)
	Pharmacological treatment: oxybutynin, tolterodine, propantheline, dicyclomine
Overflow incontinence	Medication changes, clean catheterizations, or decreasing postvoid residual
Stress incontinence	Urethral compression, pelvic muscle exercises (Kegel), pessary
	Surgical intervention: strongly recommended even in older women; includes bladder neck procedures, slide procedures, needle vaginal suspensions
	Pharmacological treatment: estrogen cream or ring, imipramine, pseudoephedrine
Functional incontinence	Environmental adaptations to increase ability to get to toilet. May need modifications in clothes to make it easier to manage clothing. Those who are aphasic may need nonverbal ways to communicate need to void.
Mixed incontinence	Combination of above methods.

Kegel Pelvic Floor Exercises (Engberg, Bender, & Stilley, 2003)

1. Tighten or contract your pelvic floor muscles by tightening your rectum as if you are trying to keep from passing gas. Tighten for 3 seconds (count "1 and-2-and-3") and then relax for 3 seconds. Do not hold your breath; breathe as you normally do.

2. Women may also feel their vaginal muscles tighten. Put your hand on your abdomen to be sure you are not tightening your abdominal muscles.

3. Repeat this exercise 15 times. Do two more sets of 15, spread out over the course of each day, for a total of 45 exercises each day. Do one set while standing, one set while sitting, and one set while lying down.

4. Gradually increase the amount of time spent contracting and relaxing your muscles, working up to 10 seconds for each contraction and 10 seconds relaxing.

Sources consulted

University of Texas at Austin, School of Nursing, Family Nurse Practitioner Program. (2002). *Recommendations for the management of stress and urge urinary incontinence in women.* Austin, TX: Author. Summary available at http://www.guideline.gov

Bengtson, J., Chapin, M.D., Kohli, N., Loughlin, K.R., Seligson, J., & Gharib, S. (2004). *Urinary incontinence: Guide to diagnosis and management.* Available: http://www.brighamandwomens.org; (*Note:* Diane K. Newman, RN MSN CRNP FAAN, is a nationally recognized expert on incontinence, and her work is frequently cited in health-related Web sites. Rehabilitation nurses are encouraged to search for her most current recommendations.)

segmental, and cortical level.

2) Parasympathetic and sympathetic innervation occurs from the autonomic nervous system.

3) Enteric nervous system influences the intrinsic neural control of the mobility, absorption, and secretion activities of the gut; it is influenced by the autonomic nervous system but is independent of it.

4) Like the bladder, the bowel is capable of emptying at a reflex level, when stretch fibers in the descending large colon stimulate the reflex arc.

2. Requirements for stool formation and normal bowel function

a. Adequate fiber in the diet to produce bulk so that water is trapped in the stool and enough solid matter exists to allow peristalsis to move the stool and to allow the body to defecate in an organized, effective manner

b. Adequate fluid intake to limit the amount of liquid reabsorbed from the descending colon

c. General activity and mobility to support and enhance peristalsis

d. Upright posture to allow gravity to assist in stool formation and passage

3. Patterns of defecation through the lifespan

a. Infants: Gut functions at the reflex level.

b. Children: As the child matures, he or she develops cortical control over the time and place of defecation.

c. Adults: Middle age is a time of intense activity and relative regularity, which may vary slightly with diet changes, infrequent bouts of illness, or activity; however, the bowel generally responds to simple interventions.

d. Older adults:

1) Changes occur in striated and smooth muscle strength.

2) Activity gradually lessens.

3) Older adults generally consume less roughage and have poorer dentition.

4) Self-limiting hydration may be present secondary to concerns about urinary incontinence.

5) Comorbidities may begin, along with increased medication use. These give rise to problems of constipation and help explain the focus on bowel regularity by many older adults.

F. Neurogenic Bowel Management: The following guidelines for nursing care are adapted from Consortium for Spinal Cord Medicine (1998) (last reviewed by the consortium in 2005 and considered current at that time; rehabilitation nurses are encouraged to check for a more current version of the guideline) and Rehabilitation Nursing Foundation (2002).

1. Assessment of bowel function is essential before a neurogenic bowel program is established or interventions to prevent or treat constipation are planned (LOE 4).

a. Patient history and prior bowel patterns, usual time-of-day pattern, frequency of stool, past reliance on laxatives or other aids

b. Present status and pattern, including time and characteristics of last stool

c. Oozing or small hard stool alternating with watery discharge, which may indicate impaction

d. Abdominal palpation to determine abdominal discomfort or palpable obstruction; rectal exam

e. Medications that may affect bowel function (e.g., sedatives, diuretics, antihistamines)

f. Infection, trauma, or stress that may affect stool formation

g. Medical problems that may affect interventions

1) Cardiac conditions, which would preclude the use of digital stimulation or the Valsalva maneuver

2) Renal impairment, which would preclude the use of milk of magnesia

2. Types of impaired bowel function

a. Chronic constipation: infrequent, small, hard stool or none at all in several days

1) Chronic constipation enlarges the descending colon and produces dependency on laxatives and cathartics or enemas.

2) Severe constipation and impaction cause sympathetic system problems (e.g., sweating, nausea, irritability, acute abdominal discomfort, and rise in blood pressure).

b. Diarrhea: highly frequent liquid stool with accompanying cramping

1) May be explosive, generally related to excessive caffeine ingestion, infection, irritability of the gut, or the possibility of food poisoning

2) May be associated with ulcerative colitis if it is not self-limiting

c. Upper motor neuron (reflexic neurogenic) bowel
   1) Like the bladder, the bowel is capable of reflexive emptying of the rectum without cortical awareness of the need to defecate.
   2) This condition is produced by damage to the spinal cord above T12–S1 or by damage to the cerebral cortex.
   3) Because of the innervation of the sympathetic nervous system, the patient may be aware of defecation and nervous system activity but have no conscious control over it.
d. Lower motor neuron (autonomous, areflexic, flaccid, atonal) bowel
   1) Subsequent to spinal cord damage at or below T12–S1
   2) No cortical control
   3) A lack of tone in the internal and external sphincters and a frequent oozing of stool, caused by damage to the reflex arc
e. Sensory paralytic (afferent nerve root loss or damage)
   1) Occurs subsequent to diabetes or tabes dorsalis
   2) Produces diminished or absent ability to distinguish the need or time of defecation but rarely produces incontinence because the motor function of the rectum is intact
f. Motor paralytic (efferent nerve root loss or damage)
   1) Occurs subsequent to poliomyelitis, intervertebral disc disease, tumor, or trauma
   2) Results in the inability to assist with defecation
   3) Is associated with incontinence only if there is widespread disease (because of the innervation of the intestines)
g. Colostomies and ileostomies: artificial openings on the abdominal wall to provide an exit for stool. (To obtain the current guidelines on ostomy care, consult the Wound, Ostomy and Continence Nurses Society (http://www.wocn.org.)
   1) Used when the colon has become obstructed and the rectum cannot be used (malignant tumors)
   2) Used when the gut is irritated beyond repair (ulcerative colitis)
   3) Used when it is necessary to rest the colon while it repairs (major abdominal resections)

G. Expected Patient Outcomes Related to Bowel Elimination
   1. Establish a regular bowel regimen with complete emptying of soft stool from the rectum every 1–3 days, using the least medication possible.
   2. Maintain a consistent habit and time.
   3. Have no incontinent episodes.
   4. Absence of complications: hemorrhoids, abdominal distention, autonomic dysreflexia, or fecal impaction

H. General Nursing Interventions: Because it is possible to use existing neural pathways to establish a regular bowel program, interventions for impaired bowel elimination are similar, although patients may have different clinical pictures.

I. Prevention of Constipation (adapted from RNAO 2005 guideline) (LOE 4): Rehabilitation nurses need to conduct clinical trials to determine the true effectiveness of these standards of practice.
   1. Toileting habits should include promptly responding to nurse to defecate, providing a consistent time for defecation, and providing privacy.
   2. Upright position for defecating if possible. If unable to sit, a left-side-lying position is recommended.
   3. Use a toilet for defecation.
   4. Eat 20–35 grams of fiber per day and drink 2 L of fluid per day.
   5. An exercise program should be a component of plans to prevent or treat constipation.
   6. Pharmacologic treatment of constipation should be short term, until bowel patterns are reestablished.

J. Neurogenic Bowel Management (adapted from Consortium for Spinal Cord Medicine, 1998, last reviewed by the consortium in 2005 and considered current at that time; rehabilitation nurses are encouraged to check for a more current version of the guideline). Those with neurogenic bowel also need to follow the guidelines for preventing constipation. (The LOE of these interventions is 4; rehabilitation nurses need to conduct clinical trials testing these standards of practice.)
   1. Reflexic bowel management includes the use of an appropriate chemical or mechanical rectal stimulant, a consistent personalized schedule, and the use of appropriate adaptive equipment.

2. Areflexic bowel management includes an appropriate manual evacuation technique, a consistent personalized schedule, and the use of appropriate adaptive equipment.

IV. Sleep and Rest

A. Overview

1. Adequate and restful sleep is essential to maintaining health, strength, endurance, and cognitive functioning.

2. Illness, particularly neurologic injury, deep pain, the effects of medications such as sedatives and hypnotics, the comorbidities of aging, and recent intensive care hospitalization all affect sleep patterns.

3. Rehabilitation nurses often care for people who have suffered major illnesses and subsequent disruption of normal sleep cycles.

4. To promote healing and endurance, rehabilitation nurses should assess disruptions in patients' sleep and apply specific interventions to restore restful sleep patterns.

5. There is a great need for nursing research to identify level 1 evidence for effective nursing interventions to promote sleep for patients admitted to rehabilitation facilities.

B. Normal Sleep Patterns (adapted from Porth, 2005)

1. Sleep is part of the sleep–wake cycle. The inactivity of sleep appears to restore mental and physical function. Melatonin, a hormone produced by the pineal gland, is generally believed to have a role in regulating the sleep–wake cycle.

2. There are two types of sleep: rapid eye movement (REM) and non-REM sleep.

   a. REM sleep is characterized by rapid eye movements, a lack of muscle movement, and vivid dreaming. The person is responding to internal auditory and visual sensory circuits.

   b. Non-REM sleep is characterized as quiet sleep, with a fully regulating brain and fully movable but inactive body. Non-REM sleep is divided into 4 stages, each deeper than the previous stage.

      1) Stage 1: brief transitional stage, occurs at the onset of sleep. The person appears asleep but is easily aroused and if asked later may deny being asleep.

      2) Stage 2: deeper sleep, lasts 10–25 minutes. Slowed respiration and

heart rate, metabolic rate, and muscle tone continue into stages 3 and 4.

      3) Stages 3 and 4: deep sleep. Muscles of the body relax, and gastrointestinal activity is slowed.

3. The sleep–wake cycle is integrated into a 24-hour circadian rhythm, apparently controlled by the hypothalamus.

C. Changes in Sleep Throughout the Lifespan (adapted from Porth, 2005).

1. In the newborn, REM sleep occurs at sleep onset, and periods of sleep and waking are distributed throughout the day.

2. By 8 months of age, an infant sleeps an average of 13 hours a day, and REM is approximately one-third of that time.

3. At 12–15 years of age, sleep is approximately 8 hours a day, with one-quarter in REM sleep.

4. Children usually do not complain of sleep disorders; common complaints of parents about their children include irregular sleep habits, too little or too much sleep, nightmares, sleep terrors, sleepwalking, and bedwetting.

5. Sleep changes in aging include fragmented sleep, shorter duration of stage 3 and 4 sleep, and reduced REM sleep. Older adults are also likely to have health problems and take medications that interfere with sleep.

D. Disruptions to Sleep Patterns Related to Illness and Disability: Managing the clinical manifestations of these illnesses and disability will assist in restoring the sleep–wake cycle.

1. Traumatic brain injury and stroke: disrupted normal patterns and initial reversal of day–night cycles, usually temporary

2. Myasthenia gravis: sleep apnea caused by skeletal muscle weakness

3. Multiple sclerosis, spinal cord injury, and uremia caused by renal disease: muscle twitching (clonus) or restless legs syndrome (RLS)

4. Rheumatoid arthritis: stiff, aching joints that make comfortable positioning difficult and frequent repositioning necessary

5. Cardiac disease: treatment with diuretics, necessitating nighttime toileting and disruption of sleep

6. Pulmonary disease: orthopnea, dyspnea, disrupted ability to breathe deeply

7. Morbid obesity: potentially partially occluded trachea caused by the compressing

effect on neck and jaw from facial and neck fat when supine

8. Permanent lifestyle changes resulting from injury and body image disruption: depression that causes disruption of adequate restful sleep

9. Medications (particularly sedatives, hypnotics, tranquilizers, and antidepressants): disrupted normal sleep, primarily through depression of delta wave sleep. Barbiturates depress delta and REM sleep, decrease consolidated sleep, and leave the person feeling less rested.

The following sections on sleep are summarized and adapted from University of Texas at Austin, School of Nursing, Family Nurse Practitioner Program (2005) and Umlauf et al. (2003). Rehabilitation nurses are encouraged to review these guidelines for more information.

E. Interdisciplinary Management of Chronic Primary Insomnia or Excessive Sleepiness.

1. Patients in acute rehabilitation settings are likely to have difficulty sleeping because of noise, being woken during the night for procedures, and a loss of usual sleep routines. Evidence-based guidelines for promoting sleep of inpatients were not found. This is a key area for rehabilitation nursing research. Once the patient is discharged home, clinical manifestations of his or her disability or chronic illness may continue to impair sleep. If so, the nursing interventions recommended in section H may be effective if implemented.

2. If nursing interventions do not correct these sleeping problems, the patient may need a comprehensive evaluation by sleep medicine specialists and includes the following (adapted from Umlauf et al., 2003) (LOE 3):

   a. Sleep history
   b. Clinical measures to assess excessive sleepiness:
      1) Epworth Sleepiness Scale
      2) Multivariable Apnea Prediction Index
      3) Functional Outcomes of Sleep questionnaire
      4) Pittsburgh Sleep Quality Scale
   c. Overnight sleep studies (polysomnography)
   d. Evaluation of patient's knowledge and use of sleep hygiene measures
   e. Assessment for clinical manifestations of disorders causing excessive sleepiness, including obstructive sleep apnea (OSA), insomnia, RLS, and narcolepsy

F. Interdisciplinary Interventions (LOE 3)

1. Adjust medications that cause drowsiness and sleep impairment.

2. Ensure that positive airway pressure devices are being used appropriately; educate patient and family as needed.

G. Nursing Interventions to Promote Sleep in Those with Chronic Insomnia or Excessive Sleepiness (adapted from Umlauf et al., 2003).

1. Manage problems that interfere with sleep (see section D).

2. Refer patient to sleep specialist for OSA and RLS (LOE 2).

3. Help the patient implement sleep hygiene measures (LOE 4).

H. Sleep Hygiene Measures (LOE 4) (adapted from Umlauf et al., 2003, and University of Texas at Austin, School of Nursing, Family Nurse Practitioner Program, 2005). Sleep hygiene measures are effective only when OSA, RLS, and other sleep disorders have been treated.

1. Use the bed and bedroom only for sleeping and sex.

2. Adopt consistent and rest-promoting bedtime routines, including maintaining the same bedtime and waking time every day.

3. Get out of bed slowly upon awakening.

4. If awakening during the night, avoid looking at the clock because this heightens anxiety and makes sleep onset more difficult. For those with insomnia, remove clocks from bedroom.

5. Avoid naps entirely or limit naps to 10–15 minutes.

6. Sleep in a quiet, cool, and dark environment. Sleep with earplugs or mask if necessary.

7. If unable to fall asleep after 15–20 minutes, get up, go to another room, and read or do a quiet activity using dim lighting until sleepy again. Don't watch television, which emits too bright a light. Low-impact activities, including board games and gentle stretching, have been shown to improve daytime performance and sleep quality.

8. Before bedtime avoid the following:

   a. Tobacco, stimulants, caffeine, or alcohol 4–6 hours before bedtime
   b. Large meals or exercise 3–4 hours before bedtime
   c. Emotionally charged, upsetting, unpleasant, or stimulating activities right before bedtime

9. If sleeping with pets or another person contributes to sleeping problems, moving to another bed or couch for a few nights or keeping pets from sharing the bed may be helpful.

I. Short-Term Use of Medications to Treat Insomnia in Patients Admitted to Rehabilitation Units. (At the time of this writing, the LOE has not been established; the following recommendations are based on the literature review of management of insomnia in hospitalized patients by Lenhart & Buysse, 2001.)

1. Nonpharmacologic approaches are the first line of treatment. If they are ineffective, short-term use of the following agents may be effective.

   a. Intermediate-acting benzodiazepines (e.g., lorazepam, temazepam) are good first-line agents.

   b. Zaleplon, zolpidem, and zopiclone are also excellent agents but often are used as second-line agents because of their cost. (See the National Institute for Clinical Excellence [2004] guideline, available at http://www.nice.org.uk, for more information)

2. Note that patients taking medications for sleep are at greater risk of falls.

J. Nonpharmacologic Nursing Interventions for Patients Admitted to Rehabilitation Units. (These are common practices that cannot cause harm; however, the authors have not identified sources that establish the LOE for these interventions.)

1. Use aspects of the patient's prior bedtime routines (e.g., unwinding, relaxing activities).

2. Play low music with gentle rhythm patterns (e.g., classical or chamber music).

3. Provide milk or herbal decaffeinated teas and low-sugar snacks.

4. Provide skin care or massage, especially using backrubs or lotions.

5. Ensure toileting before lights out.

6. Provide warmth (e.g., light blanket, bath blanket, socks).

7. Use comfort measures (e.g., hand holding, touch therapy, prayer, guided imagery, relaxation).

8. Ensure a quiet environment.

9. Ensure low levels of light, sound, and voices during the night.

10. Provide pain medication if indicated.

11. Use sleep medication only as a last resort because it produces artificial sleep.

12. Use available waking time whenever that occurs to consolidate nursing activities (e.g., repositioning, toileting, skin care, medications, vital signs) in ways that encourage returning to sleep.

13. Maintain a calm, unhurried demeanor that calms the patient; keep the lights low and voices hushed unless absolutely necessary.

14. Express confidence that sleep will come if the patient rests calmly.

K. Interventions for Common Sleep-Related Problems. (These are common practices that do not cause harm; however, the authors have not identified sources that establish the LOE for these interventions.)

1. Nightmares and night terrors: Use low lights to reorient the person, offer reassurance, and reestablish sleep-inducing interventions.

2. Snoring and sleep apnea: Reposition the person to a side-lying position and use pillows to retain that position.

3. Restlessness and irritability: Provide the person with a quiet, private opportunity to discuss what is troubling, offer comfort and reassurance, and then redirect to sleep.

4. Sleepwalking: Gently guide the person back to bed; it is not necessary to wake the patient.

5. Loud talking in sleep: Reposition the patient; it is not necessary to wake the patient.

L. Expected Patient Outcomes Related to Sleep Patterns

1. An established pattern that provides high-quality sleep and restoration of energy and comfort

2. Knowledge of effective sleep-enhancing modalities

V. Mobility and Immobility

At the time of publication, the authors were unable to locate specific clinical practice guidelines that focus on the following aspects of mobility and immobility for those with disability. However, the guideline by the Finnish Medical Society Duodecium (2004) (available from http://www.guideline.gov) provides the evidence justifying the need for physical activity. A large body of research shows the benefit of physical activity, especially in older adults. A great source is National Institute on Aging, available free from http://www.nia.nih.gov.

A. Overview

1. The desire to maximize mobility and independence in ADLs through physical and occupational therapy is the key reason

patients are admitted for rehabilitation. Nurses have a key role in ensuring that patients are able to participate in therapy and that they follow through with goals on the inpatient unit and at home.

2. Mobility allows patients to care for themselves, to interact with the environment, and to carry out purposeful activities.

3. Balance, strength, and endurance are all components of mobility.

4. Mobility may be lost suddenly through disease or trauma or more gradually through inactivity or illness.

5. Prolonged immobility produces marked diminution of all body functions and places the patient in a life-threatening situation. Adverse effects of immobility include decreased cardiac output, orthostatic hypotension and inability to sit or stand, dehydration, and increased risk of deep vein thrombosis, pneumonia, renal calculi, pressure ulcers, sensory deprivation, and impaired thought processes (Porth, 2005).

6. Rehabilitation nurses identify problems of impaired mobility, set realistic goals, and collaborate with patients, families, and therapy team members to achieve these goals.

B. Nursing Assessment for Mobility

1. Assessment of functional mobility traditionally includes four major areas.

   a. Bed mobility

   b. Transfers, including toilet transfers

   c. Wheelchair mobility

   d. Ambulation

2. All interdisciplinary team members evaluate levels of assist by using rankings and descriptive tools that are reliable and valid. These tools identify the amount of help or supervision needed or a device that the person needs to perform a specific activity safely, over the required distance, and in a timely fashion. The Functional Independence Measurement (FIM™) instrument, for use with adults, and the WeeFIM™, for pediatric populations, are the most common instruments used in rehabilitation facilities. In order to subscribe to the Uniform Data System, FIM™ System, and WeeFIM™ system and for the most current versions of the FIM™ and WeeFIM™, instructions in their use, and other related topics, see http://www.udsmr.org.

   a. FIM™ instrument (UDSMR, 1997) is scored as follows for 18 domains (e.g., eating, grooming, dressing upper, dressing lower, bathing):

      1) 7 = Independent

      2) 6 = Modified independence (device)

      3) 5 = Supervision or setup

      4) 4 = Minimal assistance (patient is able to do 75% or more of task)

      5) 3 = Moderate assistance (patient is able to do 50%–74% of task)

      6) 2 = Maximal assistance (patient is able to do 25%–49% of task)

      7) 1 = Total assistance (patient is able to do less than 25% of task)

   b. The FIM™ is required in acute rehabilitation facilities by Prospective Payment System.

   c. WeeFIM™ (UDSMR, 1997): The FIM™ instrument, adapted for pediatric populations, is scored as follows for three domains (16 motor, 14 cognitive, 6 behavioral):

      1) 0 = Never

      2) 1 = Rarely

      3) 2 = Sometimes

      4) 3 = Usually

   d. Other functional scales (e.g., Barthel, Katz, LORS, NANDA)

3. Nurses assess the components of mobility.

   a. Range of motion (ROM): Evaluate range of unassisted active motion of both sides (see Figure 7-2) and distinguish between active, assisted, and passive ROM. Rehabilitation nurses who use these ROM terms will be better able to communicate with physical therapists, occupational therapists, and physiatrists when discussing patient's mobility goals.

   b. Balance: sitting, standing, moving, amount of assistance needed, and distance involved

   c. Bed mobility: ability to turn side to side, move up in bed, move to the side of the bed, sit up in the bed, and bridge (i.e., raise hips while in the supine position)

   d. Transfer ability: ability to move between wheelchair and bed, toilet, bath bench or shower chair, standard seating (or automobile)

   e. Wheelchair mobility

   f. Ambulation

   g. Neuromuscular problems (e.g., spasticity, rigidity, resting tremors, intention tremors, flaccidity)

   h. Coordination and proprioception

   i. Ability to follow and remember instructions

   j. Patient's expectations and past level of

mobility, both recent and remote

k. Age-appropriate growth and development and behaviors

l. Comorbidities and general endurance

C. Expected Patient Outcomes Related to Impaired Mobility.

1. Attain optimal functional mobility using the simplest level of assistance possible.

2. Demonstrate the safe use of any needed device.

D. Injury Prevention: Nurses are at risk for injury to themselves when transferring patients, assisting patients with ADLs, and helping patients ambulate. Nurse researchers at Veterans Administration hospitals have been researching the best way to prevent caregiver injuries. An excellent source for rehabilitation nurses is Nelson and Baptiste (2004).

E. Nursing Interventions. (At the time of publication no guidelines are available to determine the LOEs for the following interventions; rehabilitation nurses need to develop EBP guidelines for all of these interventions.)

1. For bed mobility:
   a. Provide adequate changes in position and encourage patient's active participation.
   b. Use assistive devices (e.g., siderails, trapeze, overhead frame).

2. For transfers:
   a. Provide amount of assistance needed, using a consistent approach and verbal cues.
   b. Use assistive devices (e.g., slide board, sit to stand lift, total/mechanical lift).
   c. Make adaptations for impaired transfer mobility.
      1) For impaired weight-bearing mobility of one side of the body (e.g., hemiplegia, total hip precautions, fractures of the leg, unilateral leg amputation). The patient's physical therapist may make recommendations for assisting patients to transfer other than the steps outlined below. Follow the therapist's recommendations.

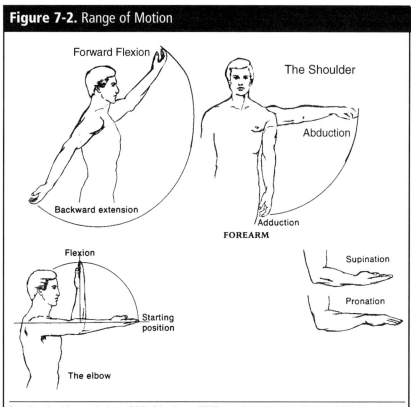

Figure 7-2. Range of Motion

Reprinted with permission of J.B. Lippincott Williams & Watkins, S. (Ed.). (2006). *Lippincott manual of nursing practice*. Philadelphia: J.B. Lippincott.

a) Nurse places wheelchair on patient's strong or unaffected side (nearest armrest may need to be removed if patient is unable to come to a standing position), locks the brakes, and moves foot pedals out of the way.

b) Patient comes to a standing position and places strong or unaffected foot forward toward chair.

c) Patient places unaffected arm on armrest of opposite side of chair.

d) Patient rotates body around on the ball of the unaffected foot so that body is square to the chair.

e) Patient lowers himself or herself into chair.

f) When another person helps the patient, the nurse explains the planned moves and encourages the patient to take sufficient time to complete each move and maintain as much weight over his or her own feet as possible. The helper should stand in front of the patient and use his or her own knees to control the patient's

Figure 7-2. Range of Motion (Continued)

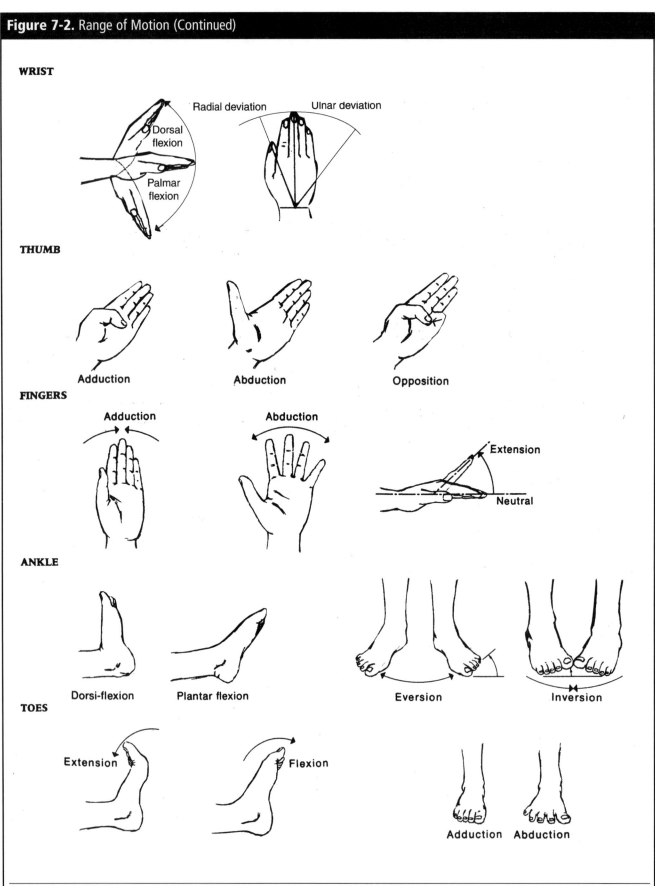

WRIST

Radial deviation   Ulnar deviation

Dorsal flexion

Palmar flexion

THUMB

Adduction   Abduction   Opposition

FINGERS

Adduction   Abduction

Extension

Neutral

ANKLE

Dorsi-flexion   Plantar flexion   Eversion   Inversion

TOES

Extension   Flexion

Adduction   Abduction

Reprinted with permission of J.B. Lippincott Williams & Watkins, S. (Ed.). (2006). *Lippincott manual of nursing practice.* Philadelphia: J.B. Lippincott.

descent into the chair seat while keeping one foot in front of the patient's feet to guard against slipping.

2) For impaired weight-bearing mobility of both legs (e.g., paraplegia, bilateral amputation):
   a) Nurse places wheelchair perpendicular to the middle of the bed in the locked position.
   b) Patient raises himself or herself to sit on the bed with legs and back to the chair.
   c) Patient lifts trunk by pushing down on the mattress and hitching trunk backward.
   d) Patient grasps arms of the wheelchair and lifts self into the chair.

3) For impaired weight-bearing mobility due to poor balance or low strength (using a slide board):
   a) Nurse places wheelchair next to the bed in the locked position and removes the armrest nearest to the bed.
   b) Patient comes to a sitting position at the side of the bed.
   c) Nurse places one end of the slide board just under the patient's buttocks and the other end on the chair.
   d) Patient hitches himself or herself toward the chair along the board by pushing down with the arms and raising the trunk or by pulling on the armrest of the wheelchair. The legs and feet follow.
   e) Once in the chair, the patient tilts away from the bed so that the slide board can be removed.

4) For impaired weight-bearing mobility due to poor balance or low strength (e.g., sliding board, sit to stand lift, or total/mechanical lift):
   a) Nurse positions slings under the patient either in one piece or under the arms and the thighs.

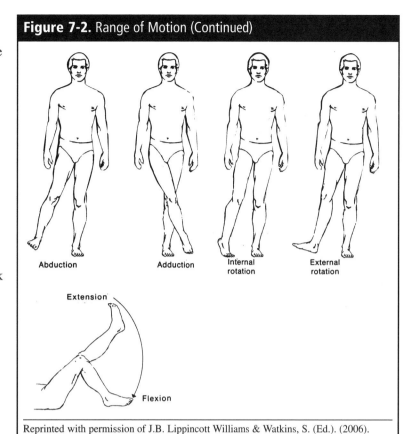

Figure 7-2. Range of Motion (Continued)

Abduction   Adduction   Internal rotation   External rotation

Extension

Flexion

Reprinted with permission of J.B. Lippincott Williams & Watkins, S. (Ed.). (2006). *Lippincott manual of nursing practice*. Philadelphia: J.B. Lippincott.

b) Nurse positions the lift over the patient and lowers it so that the crossbar is accessible.
c) Nurse uses the chains to attach the slings to the crossbar, taking care to have equal length on each side and the hooks facing away from the patient.
d) With a second person available to guide the legs and torso, the nurse pumps up the lift until the patient's body clears the bed.
e) Nurse slowly moves the lift away from the bed and over the chair, which is in the locked position.
f) Nurse slowly releases the lift, allowing the patient to descend into the chair.
g) Nurse removes the chains and may leave the slings in place for ease in returning the patient to bed.

3. For impaired wheelchair mobility: Wheelchairs may be used as a primary means of locomotion or for energy conservation and may be adapted to meet individual needs.
   a. May be powered manually or electrically

with rechargeable batteries

b. May have frame adaptations for sport participation, pediatric sizes, or body positioning needs

c. May be controlled by one or two hands, extensions to wheel spokes or brake levers, joysticks, pneumatic (sip and puff) switches, or voice activation

d. Wheelchair safety requires locking and unlocking brakes, controlling speed, changing direction, and having appropriate body support and seating surface.

4. For impaired ability to ambulate:

a. Requirements for ambulation: balance, strength, endurance, and ability to navigate various walking surfaces (e.g., floor, carpet, stairs, grass, pavement, uneven surfaces, hills)

b. Components of a normal gait: erect balance, foot lift, push off with alternate foot, heel strike, ride-over, and heel strike of opposite foot; contralateral arms may swing to provide stability and balance.

c. Protective assistance (e.g., gait belt, hands-on supervision, verbal cues)

d. Quadriceps strengthening exercises for knee and hip strength (e.g., isometric tightening of the knee and gluteus muscles, holding the contraction for 3–5 seconds and then relaxing; repeated in sets of 5–10 and increased in frequency as strength returns), bicep and tricep exercises for crutch weight bearing

e. Devices used to assist with ambulation:

1) Walkers for help with balance and forward gait: Height can be adjusted so that hands can bear some weight with elbows bent at about 30 degrees; the walker may be fitted with or without wheels; slit tennis balls may be placed over the base of the walker legs to encourage a smooth forward gait and a more normal forward progression.

2) Hemi-walkers and platform canes for increased balance are used with the platform extending away from the body.

3) Canes to provide stability and strength to one leg are adjusted for fit so that the wrist can bear some weight with the elbow slightly bent, used by placing ahead of and with the movement of the weak leg. Base

tip should have a secure gripping rubber base.

4) Crutches for protected or partial weight bearing (two- or four-point gait) or for non–weight bearing (three-point gait):

a) Proper fit for standard crutches should extend from three fingers below the axilla to a point 6–8 in. to the side and out from the heel, with the handpiece allowing a 30-degree bend at the elbow and the wrist to rest on the handpiece.

b) Base tip should have a secure wide rubber grip.

c) Proper gait instruction includes non–weight bearing on the axilla, careful placement of crutch tips, and caution on uneven surfaces, ice, or debris (see Table 7-4).

d) Forearm, Canadian, or Lofstrand crutches use the forearm for weight and are used when it is necessary to protect all joints in ambulation.

e) Specially fitted orthoses, prostheses, and braces for support and protection: It is imperative to do skin checks before and after use.

5. For all patients:

a. Encourage functioning at the maximally independent level that is safe.

b. Use verbal cues, reinforce learning, provide sufficient rest periods, and

---

Table 7-4. Crutch Walking Gaits

Four-Point Gait: Protected weight bearing on both feet
Right crutch followed by left foot
Left crutch followed by right foot
Repeat the pattern

Two-Point Gait: A faster version of the four-point gait
Right crutch and left foot move forward together
Left crutch and right foot move forward together
Repeat the pattern

Three-Point Gait: Full weight bearing on only one foot
Both crutches and the non-weight-bearing foot move forward together
Full weight bearing on the remaining foot
Repeat the pattern

Swing-Through Gait: A faster version of the three-point gait, also used with weight on both feet
Both crutches move forward together
Both legs are brought up to the crutches
Repeat the pattern

encourage adequate nutrition.

c. The University of Texas at Austin, School of Nursing, Family Nurse Practitioner Program (2004) has published a guideline that gives specific recommendations. The guideline is available at http://www.guideline.gov.

F. Disuse: The Hazards of Immobility: In 1967 Olson published a landmark article documenting the hazards of immobility. The following is an update of Olson's work, adapted from Porth (2005).

1. Overview

   a. Research continues to describe the deleterious consequences to all body systems from immobility and prolonged bed rest.

   b. Affects all body systems, not just limbs affected by disease
      1) Decreased cardiac output
      2) Orthostatic intolerance
      3) Dehydration
      4) Thrombophlebitis
      5) Muscle atrophy from disuse, especially in quadriceps
      6) Bone demineralization from decreased stress on bones
      7) Pneumonia from lowered tidal volume and decreased ability to clear bronchial secretions
      8) Formation of renal calculi, urinary retention, and urinary reflux
      9) Skin breakdown and the development of pressure ulcers from compromised circulation and pressure
      10) Bowel constipation from lowered peristalsis and inactivity
      11) Sensory deprivation
      12) Impaired thought processes, feelings of isolation, and depression

2. Expected patient outcomes related to actual or potential hazards of immobility

   a. Prevention of as many of the sequelae of immobility as possible

   b. Early identification of impairments related to disuse

   c. Self-advocacy regarding the need to include preventive measures in daily self-care

3. Nursing interventions to prevent or limit the effects of disuse

   a. Provide frequent turning and skin care to relieve pressure and restore circulation.

   b. Use pressure-relieving surfaces (e.g., air mattresses, seat cushions).

c. Pay careful attention to skin to ensure early recognition of reddened areas, wash skin gently with neutral pH soap, use lotions to lubricate skin and protect from moisture.

d. Pay attention to incontinent episodes; provide frequent checks, thorough cleaning, and protective barrier creams; and adjust bowel and bladder training regimens.

e. Encourage adequate fluid intake by mouth, by G-tube, or intravenously; monitor regularly for symptoms of dehydration.

f. Establish an effective bowel program without creating long-term dependence on laxatives, cathartics, or enemas.

g. Monitor lung sounds and encourage frequent deep breathing and coughing to move and clear bronchial secretions.

h. Provide regular gentle exercise such as ROM exercises (e.g., quadriceps-setting exercises).

i. Ensure early identification of venous thrombus (e.g., fever, pain, calf redness or warmth; positive Homan's sign often is used as an indication of deep vein thrombosis although there is no evidence to support its use).

j. Show concern for postural hypotension (e.g., quadriceps-setting exercises, elastic stockings, sitting before standing).

k. Use weight-bearing exercises to encourage retention of calcium in bones (e.g., tilt table, supported transfers).

l. Use recreational and diversional therapy to stimulate social interaction.

VI. Self-Care and Activities of Daily Living

A. Overview

1. The functional pattern of activity and exercise includes the basic elements of self-care (e.g., feeding, toileting).

   a. ADLs include eating, bathing, dressing, and grooming.

   b. Instrumental activities of daily living (IADLs), or more complex aspects of independence, include meal preparation, household management, finances, transportation, and outdoor and community-based activities.

2. Payer sources have a major role in determining the extent of services provided and the setting in which these services are

provided.

3. Rehabilitation nurses are the link between therapies, expected outcomes, and the realities of returning to community living.

B. Nursing Assessment of Self-Care Ability

1. Assess ability to independently perform basic ADLs (bathing, dressing, grooming, and eating), IADLs (e.g., meal preparation, shopping, housework), social activities, and the assistance needed to accomplish these tasks.

2. Kresevic and Mezey's (2003) guideline supports the following recommendations. However, Kresevic and Mezey do not provide an LOE for their recommendations.

3. Use rating scales to measure the level of independence or burden of care:

   a. FIM™ and WeeFIM™ systems

   b. North American Nursing Diagnosis Association International (NANDA International, 2007; http://www.nanda. org) scores for self-care and mobility: 0 = *fully independent*, 4 = *dependent and unable* (note that scoring is opposite of the FIM™ instrument)

   c. Mini-Mental State Exam: a short test of cognitive functions including orientation, registration, recall, calculation, language, and visual constructs

4. Assess specific motor impairments:

   a. Spasticity, paralysis, flaccidity, tremors (e.g., constant, resting, intention), rigidity, contractures

   b. Energy, endurance, strength, and safety

   c. Balance while sitting and standing and the ability to self-correct alone or if pushed gently

5. Assess specific sensory impairments:

   a. Visual field and acuity: diminished or lost visual field and acuity, hemianopia, peripheral field loss, macular degeneration, use of corrective lenses

   b. Tactile loss: paresthesia, proprioception, temperature discrimination (needed for bathing and meal preparation)

   c. Hearing: diminished or lost hearing, use of hearing aids

6. Assess cognitive ability, which can affect ability to perform ADLs.

7. Assess level of pain, which can interfere with learning and create additional body splinting:

   a. Assess location, intensity, possible causes of pain.

   b. Treat pain before planned therapy.

C. Expected Patient Outcomes Related to Impaired Self-Care Ability

1. Complete basic self-care activities as safely and independently as possible with or without devices as appropriate.

2. Demonstrate ability to use and care for assistive devices if appropriate.

3. Perform IADLs as independently as possible.

4. Demonstrate the ability to direct self-care when unable to perform independently.

D. Nursing Interventions for Impaired Self-Care Ability

1. Use general teaching strategies:

   a. Use the patient's preferred method of learning as much as possible.

   b. Begin with simple tasks that are familiar and meaningful to the patient.

   c. Repeat sequential tasks consistently.

   d. Use demonstration, hand-over-hand, verbal, and written instruction.

   e. Select the time of day at which the patient's attention span and energy are highest.

   f. Collaborate in teaching with other disciplines so that patient receives consistent, reinforcing instruction.

2. Use available devices for specific losses:

   a. Feeding: plate guards, rocker knives, hand braces for utensils, nonskid placemats for stability, drinking cups with weighted bases and wide mouths

   b. Bathing and hygiene: face cloths, mitts, soap-on-a-rope, long-handled sponges, nailbrushes with suction cups, hand braces for toothbrush, freestanding mirrors, shower mats, grab bars, shower seats

   c. Dressing: long-handled shoe horns, reachers, Velcro closures for clothes, elastic shoelaces, Sock Aide

   d. Grooming: long-handled combs, adapted holders for razor, long-handled mirrors for skin inspection

   e. Toileting: raised toilet seats, transfer bars

3. Adapt care to manage impaired energy and endurance:

   a. Teach pacing techniques.

   b. Provide work simplification strategies.

   c. Ensure changes in workplace environment to accommodate height and sitting needs.

d. Recruit assistance.

e. Gradually increase tasks when the patient's skills and strength return.

4. Provide strategies for household management and use of community resources.

VII. Sexuality and Reproduction

In this section the reader is referred to specific evidence-based guidelines for the treatment of some problems of sexuality and reproduction. However, much of the literature on sexuality and reproduction is based on the personal experiences of patients and their partners. What is effective for one couple may not be generalizable to others.

A. Overview

1. Sexuality and reproduction are important issues for rehabilitation patients.

2. Disability and major illnesses affect sexual function, self-esteem, body image, and social relationships. It is likely that all patients with new disabilities will have sexual changes. Some will want information on overcoming these changes; others will not care. However, it is best to ask all patients whether they have questions.

3. Rehabilitation nurses play a major role in educating patients about the effects of injury or illness on sexual function and reproduction.

4. To promote an atmosphere of permission and acceptance, rehabilitation nurses should separate their own values and attitudes in the area of sexuality in order to address the issue objectively.

5. Rehabilitation nurses should know about available methods and aids to enhance sexual expression and conception after disability. A key intervention is to provide patients and their partners with educational materials. For information for patients and their partners on specific chronic illnesses or disabilities, use a search engine and type in "sex and arthritis" or "sex and head injury," for example. For more information on sex after stroke, see Kautz (2007) and the resources listed in Table 7-5.

B. Kaplan's (1990) Stages and Descriptions of Human Sexual Response Cycle: common problems, changes with aging, and recommendations (see Table 7-6)

C. Normal Physiology of Sexual Response

1. Men

a. Penis is innervated by sympathetic (T10–L2), parasympathetic (S2–S4), and somatic (pudendal nerve) fibers.

b. Erection is under parasympathetic, sympathetic, and somatic control.

c. Psychogenic response is initiated by cortical input, including visual and tactile senses, and mediated by sympathetic pathways (T10–L2).

d. Reflex is initiated by internal or external tactile stimulation and mediated by sacral spinal reflex (S2–S4).

e. Emission is under sympathetic control (T10–L2), and ejaculation is under sympathetic and somatic control (S2–S4).

f. Fertility depends on endocrine regulation, ejaculatory ability, and semen quality.

2. Women

a. Genitalia are innervated by sympathetic (pudendal nerve and perineal nerve) and parasympathetic (splanchnic nerve) fibers.

b. Orgasm is thought to be under parasympathetic (S2–S4) and somatic control.

c. Fertility depends on endocrine regulation of ovulation cycles.

D. Expected Patient Outcomes Related to Sexual Function

1. Personal satisfaction with sexual function

2. Avoidance of sexually transmitted diseases

3. Pregnancy, if desired and possible; avoidance of pregnancy if not desired

4. Ability to plan and carry out parenting roles if appropriate

E. PLISSIT Model for Sexual Counseling (Annon, 1976).

1. Permission: process of allowing questions or fears to be raised and giving permission to talk about the subject

2. Limited Information: providing some specific information related to questions raised or concerns expressed and allowing the person to pursue the issue further if he or she is comfortable

3. Specific Suggestions: assisting people with problem identification, providing specific suggestions to resolve a problem (e.g., suggestions to deal with erectile dysfunction, bowel and bladder concerns, positioning, contraception). For more information on erectile dysfunction, see the guideline by the American Urological Association (2005), available at http://www.guideline.gov.

4. Intensive Therapy: providing expert assistance for intensive discussion and

Table 7-5. Sex Education Resources for Patients and Their Partners

The Web addresses and publications listed in this table were active and available at the time of publication; however, titles of publications and Web addresses often change.

Resources for Information and Comfortable Positions for Intercourse

Being Close: COPD and Intimacy: Available from http://lungline.njc.org

Chronic Low Back Pain and How It May Affect Sexuality: Available from http://ukhealthcare.uky.edu/patiented/booklets.htm

Sex and Arthritis: Available from http://www.orthop.washington.edu

Sex After Stroke: Our Guide to Intimacy After Stroke: Available from http://www.strokeassociation.org

Sex and cancer (several Web articles by the American Cancer Society): Available from http://www.cancer.org

Intimacy and Diabetes: Available from http://www.netdoctor.co.uk

Diabetes and Men's Sexual Health and Diabetes and Women's Sexual Health: Available from http://www.diabetes.org

Sex Education Web Sites

The following are professional Web sites that are highly recommended for those with chronic illness and disabilities. These are legitimate sex education Web sites, not pornography sites.

http://www.womenshealth.org

http://www.erectile-dysfunction-impotence.org

http://marriage.about.com

http://www.4woman.gov (sexuality and disability for women)

interventions (e.g., psychotherapy for marriage and relationship counseling, medical management of impotence, infertility, childbirth).

F. Common Classes of Medications and Their Effects on Sexual Functioning (see Table 7-7)

G. Functional Problems and Their Potential Effects on Sexual Relationships (Table 7-8)

H. Sex and Intimacy Problems with Chronic Illnesses and Disability (Table 7-9)

I. Comfortable Intercourse Positions for Those with Chronic Illness or Disability. Finding a comfortable position for sex can be very difficult for those with chronic obstructive pulmonary disease or back, hip, or knee pain or are hemiparetic after a head injury or stroke (Figure 7-3)

J. Additional Issues Surrounding Reproduction

1. Contraception: The method should be based on the patient's physical ability, cognitive ability to comply, potential medical risks of oral contraceptive use, and personal preferences. The Faculty of Family Planning and Reproductive Health Care Clinical Effectiveness Unit (2005) has published an excellent guideline.

2. Pregnancy, childbirth, and parenting: Options vary according to the disability, available resources, and medical issues.

3. Fertility:

Table 7-6. Kaplan's Phases of the Human Sexual Response, Common Problems, and Common Changes with Aging

Kaplan (1990), building on early work by Masters and Johnson, identified a triphasic model of human sexual response. The three phases are desire, excitement, and orgasm. Kaplan's model is more useful to the rehabilitation nurse than Masters and Johnson's because it helps the nurse understand why neurological impairment leads to the sexual problems. Typically sexual problems can be classified as desire, excitement, or orgasm phase disorders or combinations of the three. For decades changes in sexual response have been considered normal consequences of aging.

Phase and Physiological Response	Neurological Control	Common Problems in All Adults	Changes with Aging
The **desire phase** includes the sensations that move one to seek sexual pleasure. Love is a powerful stimulus to sexual desire.	Sexual desire probably is stimulated by endorphins, and the pleasure centers in the brain are stimulated by sex, whereas pain inhibits sexual desire.	Fatigue, pain, relationship problems, and lack of intimacy all lead to decreases in desire.	Desire may or may not change with aging; levels of desire may remain the same throughout life.
The **excitement phase** results primarily from myotonia, or increased muscle tone and vasodilation of the genital blood vessels. In men the penis becomes erect. In women the vagina becomes lubricated, the clitoris and vagina become longer and wider, and the labia minora extend outward.	Sexual excitement is controlled by the sympathetic nervous system, and fear inhibits sexual excitement.	Occasional difficulty in achieving an erection or vaginal lubrication occurs in most adults throughout the lifespan.	Erections may require more direct stimulation and may be softer. Vaginal lubrication may be decreased, and more direct stimulation may be needed.
The **orgasm phase** is a climactic release of the genital vasodilation and myotonia of the excitement phase.	Orgasm is an automatic spinal reflex response.	Premature ejaculation is common in men. Anorgasmia is common in women.	Ejaculation may not be as forceful. Women's orgasms may feel different.

a. Causes of infertility: anejaculation, impaired semen quality, impaired endocrine regulation

b. For men with spinal cord injury, the American Society for Reproductive Medicine (http://www.asrm.org) publishes the patient fact sheet "Sperm Recovery After Spinal Cord Injury in Men." The fact sheet includes causes of reproductive problems and discusses the techniques of vibratory stimulation, electroejaculation, and surgical sperm retrieval (ASRM, 2005).

K. Safety Issues Related to Sexuality

1. Sexually transmitted diseases

a. Syphilis, gonorrhea

b. AIDS

c. Hepatitis

2. Sexual abuse

L. Age-Specific Issues

1. Pediatric: injury and congenital disorders

2. Adolescence: concerns about acceptance, roles, and relationships. The American Academy of Pediatrics (2001) has published an excellent guideline on sexuality education for children and adolescents.

3. Adults: concerns about fertility, biological parenthood, pregnancy, and parenting

4. Older adults: consideration of the normal effects of aging and their relationship to disability or availability of a partner (see Kautz, 2006, for more information)

VIII. Example of Evidence-Based Practice

A. Evidence-Based Practice Related to Bladder Management

1. Facilities are practicing bladder management strategies without evidence to support their effectiveness.

2. Bladder management is a key aspect of rehabilitation nursing.

B. Clinical Question: Where is the research on strategies for bladder management in the rehabilitation patient?

C. Appraisal of Evidence

1. *Bladder management for adults with spinal cord injury* (Consortium for Spinal Cord Medicine, 2006) is based on level 3 evidence only.

Table 7-7. Medications and Sexual Functioning

The following groups of medications have been shown to cause sexual dysfunction by decreasing sexual desire or promoting vaginal dryness in women and erectile dysfunction in men. These sexual side effects may lessen 6–8 weeks after the medication is started. If the sexual dysfunction persists, a general recommendation for those experiencing sexual dysfunction is to contact the healthcare provider who prescribed the medication and ask whether a different medication from the same class or another class can be prescribed. Sometimes, despite changing medications, the side effects persist, and the person taking the medication will need to seek treatment for the sexual dysfunction.

Antidepressants, including tricyclics, monoamine oxidase inhibitors, and selective serotonin reuptake inhibitors, especially in women.

Antihypertensives, especially thiazide diuretics and beta blockers. Centrally acting alpha receptor blockers and peripherally acting anti-adrenergics can also cause problems.

Anticholinergics: propantheline and atropine.

Anticonvulsants: phenytoin, phenobarbital, carbamazepine.

H_2-blocking agents: cimetidine, ranitidine.

Lipid-lowering agents: niacin, clofibrate.

Digoxin.

Opioids.

Sources consulted

Hayes, A., & Kochar, M.S. (2004). Erectile dysfunction in patients with hypertension: Management tactics. *Consultant, 44*(12), 1534–1536.

Walsh, K.E., & Berman, J.R. (2004). Sexual dysfunction in the older woman: An overview of the current understanding and management. *Drugs & Aging, 21*(10), 655–675.

Wise, T.N., & Crone, C. (2006). Sexual function in the geriatric patient. *Clinical Geriatrics, 14*(12), 17–26.

Wooten, J.M. (2004). Erectile dysfunction. *RN, 67*(10), 40–46.

---

2. Two guidelines are available: Bengtson et al. (2004) and University of Texas at Austin, School of Nursing, Family Nurse Practitioner Program (2002). Neither contains LOEs.

D. Recommendation for Best Rehabilitation Nursing Practice

1. The evidence must be based on research to validate its effectiveness.

2. Nurses should participate in research specific to their specialty areas to validate current practice.

Table 7-8. Functional Problems and Their Potential Effects on Sexual Relationships

Functional Problem	Potential Effect	Suggestion
Sensory/Perception		
Vision	Decreased ability to appreciate visual stimuli, difficulties with depth perception.	If unilateral, uninjured partner should lie on unaffected side; use other senses (e.g., verbal, touch).
Sensation	Increased sensitivity or decreased or absent tactile sensation.	Define areas of tactile loss, modify stimuli to that part, modify touch to areas of hypersensitivity.
Proprioception (position sense)	Injured partner may not know where body parts are without visualizing, making sexual play clumsy or uncomfortable.	Allow enough light for visualization; use positioning supports for comfort.
Right–left discrimination	Injured partner may not be able to follow through with directions from partner.	Direct injured partner by using terms other than *right or left;* use hand-over-hand guidance.
Neglect or denial of deficits	Injured partner may have difficulty recognizing limitation and overstate abilities; may cause embarrassment for both partners if overstated abilities are acted out.	Uninjured partner take more active role and gently redirect partner; use positioning with pillows; alternate positions.
Communication		
Aphasia or dysarthria	Injured partner may have difficulty correctly interpreting affect of partner or expressing own desires.	Use nonverbal communication (touching, gestures).
Concrete thinking	Injured partner may miss subtle cues; sexual play may be concretely focused and one sided.	Uninjured partner may need to be very direct with sexual communication and give more specific directions to focus on mutual pleasure.
Disinhibition or impulse control	Injured partner may make inappropriate or offending statement to partner; may increase number of sexual partners as a result of impulse control; may show inappropriate public display of sexual impulses or activity.	Uninjured partner should give feedback to partner about responses and provide suggestions for better alternatives; enforce privacy and a consistent routine; do not reinforce inappropriate behaviors; may need to implement social skill retraining in matters related to sexual behaviors with the opposite sex.
Cognition		
Attention or concentration	Injured partner may be restless, unable to focus on sexual play; may affect ability to sustain an erection.	Decrease external distractions during sexual play; use relaxation, imagery, or guided fantasy by uninjured partner.
Memory or judgment	If short-term memory is impaired, injured partner may persevere on a sexual activity or request or pressure partner for frequent sex; contraceptive use should not rely on memory of injured partner.	Log sexual activity; discuss contraceptive options with physician; uninjured partner may need to take responsibility for contraception.
Initiative	Injured partner may lack ability to take active role in creating a supportive environment.	Uninjured partner may need to initiate, provide romantic environment, encourage
Mobility Impairment		
Paralysis	Inability to move body or a body part to position self or to respond to moves by the uninjured partner.	Use pillows, alternate positioning strategies; uninjured partner may need to take more active role.
Spasticity	Involuntary muscle contractions of affected parts of body; may interfere with attempts to position or reposition.	Use positions that place less stress on muscles that tend to spasm; select positions so that if spasms occur, they will not disrupt activity; use reminders to tend to bowel and bladder needs before initiating foreplay; be aware that pain in another part of the body may set off spasms; pay attention to positioning.
Elimination		
Bladder dysfunction	Bladder accidents decrease the appeal of sexual activity; presence of Foley catheter may hinder sexual activity; presence of urostomy may hinder sexual enjoyment.	Restrict fluids before sexual activity; complete toileting; keep towel or urinal nearby for potential accidents; if Foley catheter present, can be taped to the side (for women to the thigh, for men to the abdomen or place a condom over the shaft of penis); avoid positions that place pressure on the bladder; cover urostomy or tape to abdomen.
Bowel dysfunction	Bowel accidents decrease the appeal of sexual activity; presence of colostomy or ileostomy may hinder sexual activity.	Complete bowel regime before sexual activity; avoid positions that place pressure on the bowels; cover ostomy, tape to the side or remove and use an ostomy cap over stoma.

Table 7-8. Functional Problems and Their Potential Effects on Sexual Relationships *(Continued)*

Functional Problem	Potential Effect	Suggestion
Erectile Dysfunction or Anorgasm		
Man is unable to establish or maintain an erection	Decreased ability for penile–vaginal intercourse.	Explore alternative forms of sexual satisfaction, stuffing method, exploration of erogenous zones; seek psychological counseling; get referrals for erectile dysfunction assessment; use impotence treatments and medications (e.g., topical, intraurethral, oral, injectable); use external vacuum therapy; use penile implants (e.g., semirigid, inflatable).
Woman is unable to achieve orgasm	Decreased ability to reach climax.	Explore alternative forms of sexual satisfaction; seek psychological counseling; educate about potential to have orgasm; encourage use of clitoral stimulation.

Sources consulted

Rehabilitation Nursing Foundation (RNF). (1995). *Rehabilitation nursing: Directions for practice—a basic rehabilitation nursing course* (3rd ed., pp. 164–170). Glenview, IL: Rehabilitation Nursing Foundation of the Association of Rehabilitation Nurses.

Sipski, M.L., & Alexander, C.J. (1998). Sexuality and disability. In J.A. DeLisa & B.M. Gans (Eds.), *Rehabilitation medicine: Principles and practice* (3rd ed.). Philadelphia: Lippincott-Raven.

Table 7-9. Sex and Intimacy Problems with Chronic Illnesses

Chronic Illness	Common Changes in Sex and Intimacy	Recommendations for Overcoming the Problems
Heart disease Hypertension Peripheral vascular disease	Atherosclerosis and some medications may lead to erectile dysfunction in men and vaginal dryness (dyspareunia) in women. Both men and women may have fear of chest pain during sex. Fatigue may interfere with desire and lead to sexual dysfunction.	Smoking cessation, weight loss, and a consistent exercise program may increase genital circulation and reverse sexual dysfunction. Encourage couples to walk together to increase intimacy and endurance. If medications are leading to vaginal dryness or erectile dysfunction, ask physician to switch to a different medication in the same drug class.
Diabetes	Peripheral and autonomic neuropathy cause decreased genital sensation, erectile dysfunction, and vaginal dryness. Gastroparesis leads to flatulence. Ketosis leads to bad breath. Fatigue may lead to sexual dysfunction.	Smoking cessation, weight loss, and exercise all may assist in overcoming problems. Keeping the hemoglobin A1c below 7 may reverse clinical manifestations of neuropathy, atherosclerosis, gastroparesis, and ketosis. Explain that clinical manifestations vary over time.
Chronic lung disease	Loss of stamina, fatigue, and chronic cough all may lead to decreased desire and sexual dysfunction. Chronic cough often leads to stress incontinence in older women.	Smoking cessation, weight loss, and exercise all may improve breathing, reduce fatigue, and increase desire and sexual function. Adopt positions that prevent shortness of breath (see Figure 7-3). Wear oxygen cannula during sexual activity.
Arthritis (degenerative joint disease, rheumatoid arthritis, gout)	Impaired mobility and joint pain may limit sexual activity. Chronic pain will decrease sexual desire.	Plan for sex at a time of day when pain is less, often midmorning, when pain medications are at peak effect. Adopt sexual positions that don't cause pain (see Figure 7-3). Plan time for intimacy to combat feelings of worthlessness and depression.

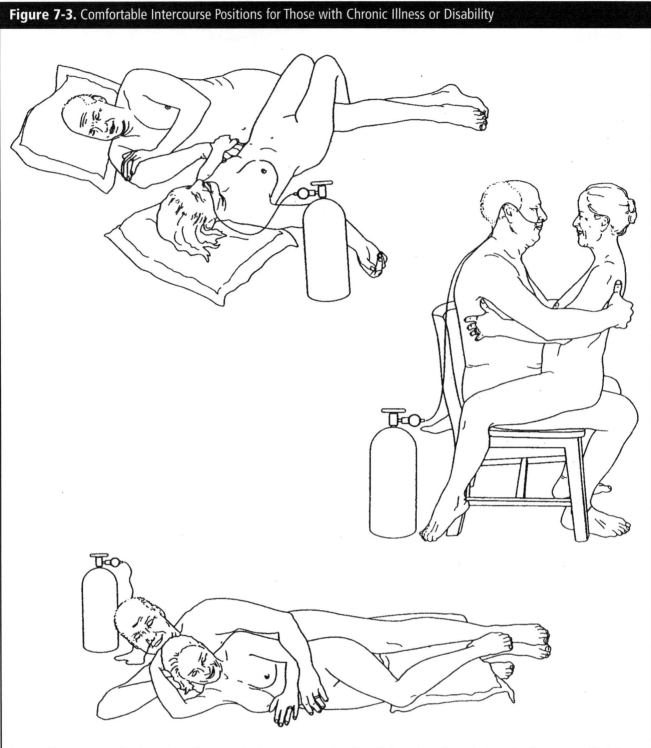

These positions are appropriate for couples when one or both partners cannot breathe well due to lung disease (or is restricted by oxygen tubing), have hip or knee pain due to arthritis, have back pain, or have limitations after a hip or knee replacement. These positions also work well when one or both partners have hemiparesis after a stroke. When side lying, lie on the affected side.

Adapted with permission from Mauk, K.L. (Ed). (2006). *Gerontological nursing: Competencies for care* (pp. 636–638). Sudbury, MA: Jones and Bartlett. http://www.jbpub.com.

References

American Academy of Pediatrics. (2001). Sexuality education for children and adolescents. *Pediatrics, 108*(2), 498–502.

American Society for Reproductive Medicine (ASRM). (2005) *Sperm recovery after spinal cord injury in men.* Birmingham, AL: Author

Annon, J.S. (1976). The PLISSIT model: A proposed conceptual scheme for behavioral treatment of sexual problems. *Journal of Sex Education Therapy, 2,* 1–15.

Bengtson, J., Chapin, M.D., Kohli, N., Loughlin, K.R., Seligson, J., & Gharib, S. (2004). *Urinary incontinence: Guide to diagnosis and management.* Available: http://www.brighamandwomens.org

Consortium for Spinal Cord Medicine. (1998). *Neurogenic bowel management in adults with spinal cord injury.* Washington, DC: Paralyzed Veterans of America. Available: http://www.pva.org

Consortium for Spinal Cord Medicine. (2006). *Bladder management for adults with spinal cord injury: A clinical practice guideline for health care providers.* Washington, DC: Paralyzed Veterans of America. Available: http://www.pva.org

Cowley, J., Diebold, C., Gross, J.C., & Hardin-Fanning, F. (2006). Management of common problems. In K.L. Mauk (Ed.), *Gerontological nursing: Competencies for care* (pp. 475–560). Sudbury, MA: Jones and Bartlett.

Deane, K.H. Whurr, R., Playford, E.D., Ben Shlomo,Y., & Clarke, C.E. (2001). A comparison of speech and language therapy techniques for dysarthria in Parkinson's Disease. Cochrane Database of Systematic Reviews, Online, CD002814.

Department of Health and Human Services, Department of Medicare and Medicaid Services (CMS). (2005). *CMS manual system.* Retrieved May 20, 2007, from http://www.cms.hhs.gov/transmittals/downloads/R8SOM.pdf

Engberg, S.J., Bender, M.A., & Stilley, C.S. (2003). Bladder matters. Kegels and communication: Home-based behavior modification is effective for treating UI in the elderly. *American Journal of Nursing, 103*(7), 93–94.

Griffith, R., & Tengnah, R. (2007). Consensus guideline on the management of medication related dysphagia. *Nurse Prescribing, 5*(1), 34–36.

Hayes, A., & Kochar, M.S. (2004). Erectile dysfunction in patients with hypertension: Management tactics. *Consultant, 44*(12), 1534–1536.

Kaplan, H.S. (1990). Sex, intimacy, and the aging process. *Journal of the American Academy of Psychoanalysis. 18,* 185–205.

Kautz, D.D. (2006). Appreciating diversity and enhancing intimacy. In K. Mauk (Ed.), *Gerontological nursing: Competencies for care* (pp. 619–643). Sudbury, MA: Jones and Bartlett.

Kautz, D.D. (2007). Hope for love: Practical advice for intimacy and sex after stroke. *Rehabilitation Nursing, 32*(3), 95–103.

Kresevic, D.M., & Mezey, M. (2003). Assessment of function. In M. Mezey, T. Fulmer, I. Abraham, & D.A. Zwicker (Eds.), *Geriatric protocols for best practice* (2nd ed., pp. 31–46). New York: Springer.

Lenhart, S.E., & Buysse, D.J. (2001). Treatment of insomnia in hospitalized patients. *Annals of Pharmacotherapy, 35*(11), 1449–1457.

Lippincott Manual of Nursing Practice. (2006). (8th ed.). Philadelphia: Lippincott Williams & Wilkins.

Mauk, K.L. (Ed). (2006). *Gerontological nursing: Competencies for care* (pp. 636–638). Sudbury, MA: Jones and Bartlett. Available: http://www.jbpub.com.

Morris, H. (2006). Dysphagia in the elderly: A management challenge for nurses. *British Journal of Nursing, 15,* 558–562.

NANDA International. (2007). *Nursing diagnoses: Definitions & classification: 2007–2008.* Available: http://www.nanda.org

National Pressure Ulcer Advisory Panel (NPUAP). (2001). *Pressure ulcer treatment: A competency based curriculum for RNs.* Available: http://www.npuap.org

Nelson, A., & Baptiste, A.S. (2004, September 30). Evidence-based practices for safe patient handling and movement. *Online Journal of Issues in Nursing, 9*(3), Manuscript #3. Available: http://www.nursingworld.org/ojin/topic25/tpc25_3.htm

Palmer, P.M. (1999). *Frazier free water protocol.* Retrieved March 27, 2007, from http://dysphagia.com/forum/showthread.html

Porth, C.M. (2005). *Pathophysiology: Concepts of altered health states* (7th ed.). Philadelphia: Lippincott Williams & Wilkins.

Registered Nurses Association of Ontario (RNAO). (2005). *Risk assessment and prevention of pressure ulcers.* Toronto: Author. Summary available at http://www.guideline.gov

Rehabilitation Nursing Foundation. (1995). *Rehabilitation nursing: Directions for practice—a basic nursing rehabilitation course* (3rd ed., pp. 164–170). Glenview, IL: Author.

Rehabilitation Nursing Foundation. (2002). *Practice guidelines for the management of constipation in adults.* Glenview, IL: Author. Available: http://www.rehabnurse.org

Sipski, M.L., & Alexander, C.J. (1998). Sexuality and disability. In J.A. DeLisa and B.M. Gans (Eds.), *Rehabilitation medicine: Principles and practice* (3rd ed.). Philadelphia: Lippincott-Raven.

Smith Hammond, C.A., & Goldstein, L. (2006). Cough and aspiration of foods and liquids due to oral–pharyngeal dysphagia: ACCP evidence-based clinical practice guidelines. *Chest, 129,* 154–168.

Suiter, D. (Ed.). (2005). *Frazier free water protocol: Evidence and ethics.* Available: http://www.asha.org

Umlauf, M.G., Chasens, E.R., & Weaver, T.E. (2003). *Evaluating excessive sleepiness in the older adult.* Summary available at http://www.guideline.gov

Uniform Data System for Medical Rehabilitation. (1997a). *Functional independence measure.* Buffalo, NY: University of Buffalo.

Uniform Data System for Medical Rehabilitation. (1997b). *Functional independence measure for children.* Buffalo, NY: University of Buffalo.

University of Texas at Austin, School of Nursing, Family Nurse Practitioner Program. (2002). *Recommendations for the management of stress and urge urinary incontinence in women.* Austin, TX: Author. Summary available at http://www.guideline.gov

University of Texas at Austin, School of Nursing, Family Nurse Practitioner Program. (2005). *Practice parameters for the nonpharmacologic treatment of chronic primary insomnia in the elderly.* Austin, TX: Author. Summary available at http://www.guideline.gov

Walsh, K.E., & Berman, J.R. (2004). Sexual dysfunction in the older woman: An overview of the current understanding and management. *Drugs & Aging, 21*(10), 655–675.

Wise, T.N., & Crone, C. (2006). Sexual function in the geriatric patient. *Clinical Geriatrics, 14*(12), 17–26.

Wooten, J.M. (2004). Erectile dysfunction. *RN, 67*(10), 40–46.

Wound, Ostomy and Continence Nurses Society (WOCN). (2001). *Guideline for prevention and management of pressure ulcers.* Available: http://www.guideline.gov

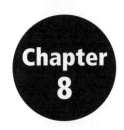

Chapter 8

Psychosocial Healthcare Patterns and Nursing Interventions

Barbara Brillhart, PhD RN CRRN

Rehabilitation nurses must understand the concept of psychosocial health, which involves the influence of mental processes and social interactions on behavior. Theories of development, learning, and chronic illness support psychosocial healthcare patterns. Psychosocial health incorporates cognition, behaviors, sensations, perceptions, self-concept, and role attainment. Rehabilitation nurses promote psychosocial health through professional assessment and interventions. The theories and concepts presented in this chapter provide a foundation for rehabilitation nurses to promote psychosocial health over the lifespan.

I. Developmental Considerations Related to Psychosocial Health

A. Cognitive Maturation in Children

1. Cognitive deficits can have a profound influence on the life of a developing child; these deficits impair the input, reasoning, and thinking processes needed for normal development.

   a. Children with brain injuries can have impaired cognitive development.

   b. Delays in speech and language development related to deafness, mental deficits, or emotional disturbances can affect the child's psychosocial development.

2. Piaget's (1952) and Erikson's (1963) levels of cognitive development for children provide a theoretical basis for normal development. [Refer to Chapter 15 for additional information on developmental stages.]

   a. Sensorimotor period (0–2 years)
      1) Description
         a) The psychosocial development of trust vs. mistrust: Disruptions in cognitive achievement during this period impair the psychosocial development of infants and toddlers (Piaget, 1952).
         b) Examples:
            (1) An 8-month-old child demonstrates goal-directed activities.
            (2) A 12-month-old child understands means-to-end relationships.
            (3) A 2-year-old child has the beginnings of symbolic thinking.
      2) Nursing interventions: Promote sensory stimulation, security by caregivers, motor coordination, consistent personal attention, and parental education about growth and development.

   b. Preoperative period (2–7 years)
      1) Description: the development of autonomy vs. shame, initiative vs. guilt, and the beginning of industry vs. inferiority (Erikson, 1963; Piaget, 1952)
         a) Children use representative thought to recall past events, represent the present, and anticipate the future.
         b) Children ages 4–7 years use increased symbolic functioning.
      2) Nursing interventions
         a) Conduct initial and ongoing cognitive and physical assessment.
         b) Encourage exploration of the environment.
         c) Encourage participation in age-appropriate activities.
         d) Promote consistent, affectionate caregiving.
         e) Diversify environmental stimuli.
         f) Provide intellectual stimulation.
         g) Promote peer interaction.
         h) Continue parental education about age-appropriate growth and development.

   c. Concrete operative period (7–11 years)

1) Description
   a) The continued development of industry vs. inferiority, characterized by cognitive, concrete operations
   b) Children use logical approaches to solve concrete problems.
2) Nursing interventions
   a) Promote peer interaction and socialization.
   b) Encourage formal education with peers.
   c) Promote creativity.
   d) Continue parental education about growth and development.
   e) Continue consistent interaction with parents, family, caregivers, and teachers.
d. Formal operative period (11–15 years)
   1) Description: the development of identity vs. role confusion
      a) Adolescents are capable of logical thought and abstract thinking.
      b) Role expectations include increasing independence, being socially successful and more mature, increasing autonomy, and increasing responsibilities (Satir, 1988).
   2) Research study findings
      a) A study of 14 children between the ages of 5 and 13 years with spinal cord injury (SCI) indicated that the children's scores for quality of life (QOL) were higher than their parents' scores. One explanation was that the children focused on current life expectations, whereas their parents also considered the long-term picture and future prospects (Johnston, Lauer, & Smith, 2006).
      b) A study that surveyed the coping strategies of adolescents with and without disabilities indicated that there was a continuing need to cope with life stressors. There was no difference in the types of coping used between the two groups of adolescents. There was a negative relationship between severity of mobility and both cognitive avoidance and emotional discharge. There was a moderately high correlation between level of involvement and both seeking guidance and solving problems. Finally, there was a moderately high correlation between self-esteem levels and the 8 methods of coping (Smith, Cook, Frost, Jones, & Wright, 2006).
      c) Adolescents who already have negative life experiences have higher stress levels. Common stressful situations for adolescents include body changes with puberty, new relationships with peers and family, sexual and moral dilemmas, and school expectations (Dacey & Margolis, 2006).
3) Assessment
   a) Conduct initial and ongoing psychosocial and physical assessment.
   b) Assess QOL with the PedsQL instrument, which contains the factors of total well-being, physical well-being, psychosocial well-being, and emotional, social, and school functioning (Johnston et al., 2006).
4) Nursing interventions
   a) Treat the adolescent with disability as a normal person.
   b) Allow time for the adolescent to adjust to changes caused by injury.
   c) Encourage the adolescent to have close bonds with family and nurses.
   d) Provide information to reduce fears and misconceptions about the injury.
   e) Provide encouragement, peer support, and motivation.
   f) Foster the adolescent's friendships with peers.
   g) Give the adolescent age- and ability-appropriate responsibilities.
   h) Ensure appropriate parental protectiveness.
   i) Ensure that the adolescent is involved with decision making.
   j) Use problem-focused coping approaches (Dacey & Margolis, 2006).
   k) Allow verbalization of frustrations (Dacey & Margolis, 2006).

B. Cognitive Maturation in Adults
1. Description of social learning theory (Bandura, 1977)
   a. This theory explains human behaviors in terms of active, dynamic interactions of behaviors, personal factors, and environmental influences.
   b. Personal interactions include the person's ability to symbolize behavioral meanings, foresee the outcomes of behaviors, learn through observations and experiences, and self-determine and self-regulate his or her life.
   c. Adults reflect and analyze to give meaning to experiences.
   d. Young and middle-aged adult development fulfills the psychosocial phases of intimacy vs. role confusion and generativity vs. stagnation (Erikson, 1963).
   e. Cognitive and physical disability can affect the potential and motivation to fulfill developmental phases.
   f. The roles of young adults can include positive pairing.
      1) Positive pairing is characterized by willing, knowledgeable, respectful support within the pair and includes relationships based on equality of value of the couple.
      2) Successful pairing depends on personal autonomy, emotional honesty, expression of needs, responsibility, accountability, freedom of choice, and cooperation (Satir, 1988).
   g. The adult faces developmental stresses of career, family, and independence. The adult environment contains stressors that are unavoidable because adults are more aware of the realities of life situations and are more aware of responsibilities (Dacey & Fiori, 2006).
   h. Middle-aged adults face unique stressors such as children living at home; children leaving home for marriage, college, or the military; the responsibilities associated with older relatives; and changes in their personal health (Dacey & Fiori, 2006).
2. Nursing interventions
   a. Encourage protective measures of coping such as supportive family environment, supportive networks, and personal control (Dacey & Fiori, 2006).
   b. Promote trust and balance of decision making.
   c. Promote the ability to adapt and cope with change.
   d. Promote recreational therapy.
   e. Encourage socialization with family and peers.
   f. Ensure access to vocational and academic counseling and education.
   g. Provide family counseling.
   h. Foster autonomy, independence, and personal responsibility.

C. Cognitive Maturation in Older Adults
1. The last psychosocial developmental phase of ego identity vs. despair
   a. Older adults reflect on their lives and remember worthwhile and unique experiences.
   b. Disability and chronic illness can profoundly affect QOL and psychosocial satisfaction.
   c. Transition is needed to progress from middle age to older adulthood.
      1) Transitional steps start with acknowledging changes that occur with aging.
      2) Mixed feelings are present with changes in work status and lifestyle.
      3) Life reflection can be positive or negative. Some resent that there may be no opportunity to change poor life decisions (Dacey & Fiori, 2006).
      4) Care of the older adult in poor health is considered one of the most stressful situations in a family, especially for the spouse (Dacey & Fiori, 2006).
      5) Older adults often experience multiple changes in mobility, cognition, social opportunities, financial stability, level of independence, and physical health.
      6) A successful transition is characterized by recognition of the positive aspects of aging and moving toward new challenges.
      7) A successful transition must incorporate positive attitudes, feelings of worth, flexibility, feelings of purpose, positive relationships, and being part of the family and community (Satir, 1988).
2. Assessment
   a. Conduct initial and ongoing assessment

of cognitive, social, functional, and physical health.

b. Assess the relationship and responsibilities of caregivers and the older adult.

c. Assess the change of role behaviors and responsibilities of spouses (Clark, 2000).

d. Investigate alternatives in caregiving such as adult care, in-home care providers, and respite care.

3. Nursing interventions

a. Promote recreational therapy and leisure.

b. Encourage socialization.

c. Provide family counseling.

d. Allow the client to reflect and reminisce.

e. Foster autonomy, independence, respect, and personal responsibility.

II. Family-Focused Care Model for Clients with Chronic Illness

A. Overview

1. Psychosocial adjustment for people with disability or chronic illness occurs in a recurrent, longitudinal sequence of stages that involve the person with disability or illness and his or her family and friends.

2. A conceptual model, Family-Focused Care of the Chronically Ill (Anderson & Tomlinson, 1992) (see Figure 8-1), can be applied to the complexity of psychosocial healthcare patterns.

B. Concepts Associated with the Model (Butcher, 1994)

1. Optimal family health: the core of the model. The concepts of development, integrity, coping, health, and interaction influence the core and all the other concepts in an interlocking pattern.

2. Development: composed of developmental stages, developmental tasks, and family transitions. Disability can have a profound effect on the developmental capacity of the client and family.

3. Coping: composed of managing resources,

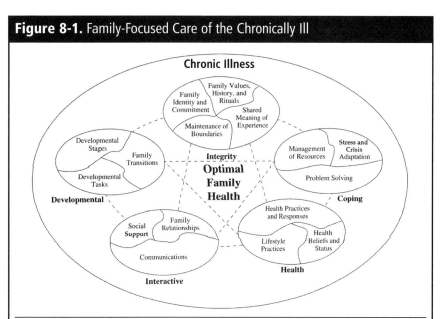

Figure 8-1. Family-Focused Care of the Chronically Ill

Anderson, K.H., & Tomlinson, P.S. (1992). The family health system as an emerging paradigmatic view for nursing. *Image: The Journal of Nursing Scholarship, 24*(1), 57–63. Reprinted with permission of Blackwell Publishing.

solving problems, and adapting to stress and crisis. Effective coping combines family members' coping abilities in an individual and collective manner.

4. Integrity: composed of family identity and commitment; family values, history, and rituals; shared meaning of experiences; and maintenance of boundaries.

5. Interaction: contains social support, communication, and family relationships Communication is the key factor, which forms the basis of the quality of social and family relationships.

6. Health: contains health practices, health beliefs and status, and lifestyle practices, which are modified, adapted, and reformatted to meet the needs of the individual and family related to disability or chronic illness.

III. Theories of Learning

A. Classical or Pavlovian Conditioning (Pavlov, 1927)

1. Initially, a neutral response is associated with another stimulus that elicits an unconditioned response.

2. Eventually, the neutral stimulus elicits the response.

3. Emotions are partially subject to classical learning (e.g., fear of an object or pet).

B. Operant Conditioning (Skinner, 1974)

1. Operant conditioning involves changing a child's behavior by providing a reward or

reinforcement for the consequence of the child's responses.

2. Reinforcement is the key element in operative learning theory.

   a. People tend to repeat behaviors that have desirable outcomes.

   b. Systematic reinforcement with positive reinforcers affects the rate at which responses occur.

   c. Reinforcers can also be negative if they are being used to terminate an aversive behavior.

   d. A conditioned behavior can be extinguished (undone) by repeated failure to reinforce it.

   e. Behaviors can be inhibited (counteracted) through punishment avoidance.

   f. Behaviors can be partially reinforced by inconsistent or random responses.

C. Social Learning Theory (Bandura, 1977)

   1. Positive reinforcement (e.g., food, care, attention) shapes behaviors.

   2. Learning occurs when behaviors are modified in response to physical rewards (e.g., food) and indirect rewards (e.g., a smile).

   3. Negative reinforcement (e.g., punishment) can be used to modify behaviors.

   4. Social learning theory is initiated within the family and later is influenced by the values and customs of those outside the family (e.g., peers and role models at school).

   5. Desired behaviors are obtained through direct observation and imitation of another's performance.

D. Gestalt Learning Theory (Wertheimer, 1959)

   1. This theory defines learning as a reorganization of the person's perceptual or psychological world.

   2. The focus is on motivation, perception, and transference of learning.

   3. A person's perception is related to the total situation and involves the interactions of many factors. The interaction of the person and environment is simultaneous and mutual.

   4. Learning occurs when the person tries to give meaning to the environment and successfully uses objects in the environment.

E. Andragogical Model of Adult Learning (Knowles, 1984)

   1. Adult learners are self-directed and responsible for their own learning.

2. Learners assess their own needs for learning and form their own objectives.

3. Learners possess a wide range of experiences; therefore, individualized learning plans are stressed.

4. Readiness to learn is determined by the need to know something in order to achieve a task.

5. Positive andragogy includes the presence of interactive environments, mutual respect, collaboration, mutual trust, support, openness, authenticity, pleasure, and mutual planning.

6. Learners evaluate their own level of learning by evaluating whether they have achieved their personal goals.

IV. Cognitive Influences on Psychosocial Health

A. Cognition

   1. Description:

      a. Cognition is defined as the concept of thinking and consists of attention, memory, abstract reasoning, generalization, concept formation, problem solving, and executive function (Grzankowski, 1997); cognitive deficits may involve one or more of these components.

      b. Cognitive development allows the processing of information through decoding, encoding, transferring, combining, storage, and retrieval (Travers, 2006).

      c. Cognition depends on sensory input, prior experiences, learning, and recall and memory.

      d. An injury to the cortex of the brain or the neural pathways interferes with sensory input, cognitive integration, and planning of appropriate responses.

      e. The cerebral cortex, internal nuclei, basal ganglia, and the cerebellum process and integrate sensory input and motor planning (see Table 8-1).

      f. Recovery depends on the extent, quality (e.g., edema vs. destruction), and area of the injury.

   2. Assessment:

      a. Conduct initial and ongoing cognitive assessment.

      b. Evaluate the client's ability to determine pertinent and irrelevant stimuli, to learn, to understand situations or conversations, to problem solve, and to follow a plan of action.

c. Obtain a symptom history from the person and family (Shah & Bennett, 2006)

d. Review the medical history and current medications, including alternative medications and treatments.

e. Assess the ability to conduct activities of daily living (Shah & Bennett, 2006).

f. Use the Rancho Los Amigos Scale as an assessment tool (Flannery, 1998).

g. Assess attention abilities, short- and long-term memory for processing information, recall and retrieval, and problem solving (Travers, 2006).

Table 8-1. Cognitive Functions Affected by Brain Injury

Area of Brain	Function	Results of Injury
Frontal lobe	Controls higher intellectual and social processing	Loss of intellect and inappropriate social behaviors
Temporal lobe	Controls new memory and learning	Impaired learning
Temporal lobe (hippocampus)	—	Temporary memory loss, lack of contralateral orientation, distractibility, hyperactivity, attention deficits, perseveration
Right hemisphere	Controls recognition of geometric patterns, faces, environmental sounds, a second language, music, sense of direction, and memory for pictures	Learning impairments, memory impairments
Left hemisphere	Controls memory for language, letters, works, verbal memory (e.g., reading, writing, speech), arithmetic	Deficits with math and communication
Limbic lobe of right and left hemispheres	Controls attention that affects socialization	Deficits with socialization

3. Nursing interventions

a. Use helpful cues (e.g., the client's name, pictures of familiar people or pets) to help the client identify locations.

b. Encourage the client to use daily logs, written schedules, and patterns for activities of daily living (ADLs).

c. Use sensory stimulation programs (e.g., visual, auditory, olfactory, cutaneous, taste, motion) that focus on short-term interventions several times a day to increase cognition.

d. Make materials meaningful for each person (Travers, 2006).

e. Use optimal timing when the person is not tired, rushed, hungry, or distracted.

f. Simplify the situation and repeat it for understanding.

g. Ensure a consistent schedule, staff, and environment.

h. Recommend a power of attorney for financial and health decisions (Shah & Bennett, 2006).

4. Research study findings: Ponsford et al. (1999) investigated outcomes in children with mild traumatic head injury. The children were evaluated for postinjury symptoms and behaviors and underwent neuropsychological testing. Findings indicated that the children with mild head injury had headaches, dizziness, and fatigue 1 week after injury.

17% of these children showed ongoing problems such as learning difficulties, neurological or psychiatric problems, and family stress by 3 months after trauma. Children with congenital heart disease are at risk for neurological damage related to hypoxia. The impact of neurological damage may include global cognitive deficits, memory deficits, and gross and fine motor delays and deficits (Townsend, Lohr, & Nelson, 2006).

B. Orientation

1. Definition: the ability to know about oneself (e.g., name, age, date of birth, home), the time (e.g., current date, month, year), and facts about the environment

2. Assessment

a. Conduct initial and ongoing assessment of orientation.

b. Distinguish between confusion, disorientation, physical conditions (e.g., electrolyte imbalance, medications, fluid imbalance, fatigue), and sensory deficits (Shah & Bennett, 2006).

c. Use the Mini–Mental State Examination (Newton, 2006).

3. Nursing interventions

a. Use cues to orient the client (e.g., familiar photographs of the client, family, or pets; familiar furniture; calendars; holiday decorations; clocks with large, clear numbers; schedules of daily events).

b. Clearly identify family, relatives, friends, and staff when interacting with the client.

c. Ensure that the client uses intact, functional sensory aids (e.g., glasses, hearing aids) (Remington, Abdallah, Melillo, & Flanagan, 2006).

d. Provide consistent environment and staff.

C. Attention

1. Definition: the ability to respond to and prioritize relevant information and to ignore or put aside irrelevant information.

   a. Older adults are vulnerable for attentional fatigue caused by age-related physiological changes in vision, hearing, touch, and taste.

   b. Attentional capacity is influenced by the capacity to direct attention, attentional demands, attentional fatigue, and restorative activities.

   c. Attention works through global neural inhibitory mechanisms that allow the focusing that is needed for prolonged or intense directed attention (Jansen & Keller, 1998).

2. Research study findings: Findings of a qualitative study of perceptions after closed head injury found that there were problems in thinking sequentially and conceptually. The participants also had problems dealing with multiple stimuli. These problems affected their ability to concentrate and process thoughts (Paterson & Stewart, 2002).

3. Assessment

   a. Assess short-term memory, planning, problem solving, incidence of accidents, irritability, impulsiveness, and frustration (Jansen & Keller, 1998).

   b. Use standard questions to assess attention:
      1) Inquire about home activities that require more or new effort (e.g., physical or environmental factors).
      2) Discern the feelings that the client experiences most often.
      3) Identify times the client would like to but cannot express feelings and share experiences.

   c. Assess changes in the person's feelings, emotions, anger, and frustration, which may accompany loss of motivation (Paterson & Stewart, 2002).

4. Nursing interventions

   a. Use conservation and restoration measures to reduce neurological fatigue.
      1) Conservation measures: Reduce or limit the extent and number of attentional demands in the internal and external environments; help the client complete necessary and desired activities in a controlled, stable environment.
      2) Restoration measures: Allow rest and recovery by changing activities (e.g., taking a walk in a park, gardening, bird watching).

   b. Prioritize activities for attention.

   c. Break the task into parts, focusing on step-by-step instructions.

   d. Encourage daily physical activity.

   e. Advise the client to avoid alcohol and drugs.

   f. Individualize music selections and avoid stressful selections.

   g. Modify expectations to fit the reality of the client's status.

   h. Provide growth and development opportunities.

   i. Allow for variance in the client's attention throughout the day.

   j. Identify triggers (e.g., situations, people, places, events) that contribute to intellectual or emotional conflict.

   k. Provide client and family education.

   l. Avoid denial, devaluation, or demeaning of the client.

   m. Participate in group therapy (Paterson & Stewart, 2002).

   n. Allow rest to recover from the overwhelming fatigue of dealing with loss of cognitive abilities (Paterson & Stewart, 2002).

D. Judgment

1. Description: remembering, planning, foresight, abstraction, transference of information, and evaluating the appropriateness of an action

2. Assessment

   a. Observe the client's accuracy with managing money, learning new skills, applying old knowledge in new situations, solving problems, and creating and following through with realistic plans.

   b. Periodically reassess the client's judgment deficits to meet his or her increasing or decreasing needs.

3. Nursing interventions: Tailor interventions to match the client's level of cognition.

   a. For clients with high cognitive

functioning: Coordinate counseling, education, crisis management, vocational assessment and planning, and individualized self-care.

   b. For clients with moderate cognitive functioning: Provide or coordinate scheduled routines, a structured environment, counseling, individualized education, and vocational assessment and planning.

   c. For clients with lower cognitive functioning: Help coordinate supervised living situations, a protective environment, sheltered vocational opportunities, case management, and legal guardians.

E. Problem Solving

   1. Definition: a high-level cognitive function that involves considering, recalling, and analyzing factors and selecting appropriate choices from various alternatives

   2. Research study findings

      a. A study of people surviving stroke for 6 months to 8 years indicated that confusion and errors in decision making were noted by both family members and caregivers. Regardless of levels of education, subjects exhibited behaviors of inertia, indifference, cognitive deficits, problems with interpersonal communication, and emotional instability such as panic (Williams & Dahl, 2002).

      b. Spalding (2005) described a mentoring situation for a professional person who had sustained a head injury. The head injury resulted in a high level of cognitive impairment for this person. The problem-solving deficits noted during the mentoring experience included lack of focus and direction, fragmented documentation, impaired memory, anxiety, lack of organization, distraction, impulsivity, lack of flexibility, and lack of appropriate priority judgments. The cognitive impairments severely affected this person's ability to problem solve in the working environment.

   3. Assessment

      a. Assess the ability to problem solve initially and in an ongoing manner.

      b. Assess the ability to plan and organize thoughts and behaviors.

      c. Assess the ability to formulate alternative solutions for a problem.

      d. Assess the ability to comprehend potential consequences of choices.

   4. Nursing interventions

      a. Help the client approach problems by taking one step at a time.

      b. Encourage the client to differentiate between solutions to a problem and examine the consequences of solutions.

      c. Encourage successful problem-solving plans and build on successes.

      d. Examine unsuccessful problem-solving plans and discuss ways to select positive action plans.

      e. Plan family and caregiver education with a focus on brain function and strategies for dealing with the lack of decision-making skills after stroke (Williams & Dahl, 2002).

      f. Involve the family and caregivers with discharge planning decisions after stroke or head injury.

F. Motivation

   1. Description

      a. Motivation is the external, internal, or combined forces that influence behavior to satisfy needs and achieve goals.

      b. Motivation can be influenced by needs and wants, the cost and rewards of participating in an activity, and personal beliefs about the ability to participate and succeed (Bandura, 1977).

   2. Assessment

      a. Assess the amount and persistence of the client's activities toward achieving goals.

      b. Assess the barriers to client motivation (e.g., memory impairment, problem-solving deficits).

      c. Use the Apathy Evaluation Scale, an 18-item instrument that measures thoughts, actions, and emotions during the previous month. This instrument helps determine motivation that affects discharge function and functional levels after rehabilitation (Resnick, Zimmerman, Magaziner, & Adelman, 1998).

   3. Nursing interventions

      a. Help the client establish immediate and long-term goals.

      b. Help the client and family set a realistic plan to achieve goals.

      c. Break long-term goals into small, attainable goals.

      d. Reward successes with family and peer recognition.

---

e. Provide resources that lead to the successful achievement of goals.

G. Coping

1. Description
   a. Coping is defined as cognitive and behavioral efforts directed at managing demanding and stressful situations.
      1) Problem-focused coping efforts are directed at lowering or eliminating threats.
      2) Emotion-focused coping efforts are directed at decreasing negative emotions.
   b. Personal competence with coping includes many factors (Satir, 1988):
      1) The components of relationships (being content with self and others)
      2) Differentiation (distinguishing between self and others)
      3) Autonomy (relying on self, separate and distinct from others)
      4) Self-esteem (feeling worthy about self)
      5) Power (using energy to initiate and guide behaviors)
      6) Productivity (manifesting competence)
      7) Love (being compassionate, accepting, and giving as well as receiving affection)
   c. Antecedents of stress require coping skills:
      1) Personal and environmental demands that exceed resources
      2) Ambiguity and uncertainty
      3) Loss of control
      4) Loss of social support
   d. Many variables influence coping efforts:
      1) Developmental age
      2) Severity of disability
      3) Visibility of disability
      4) Threat of chronicity
      5) Sense of control
      6) Prior coping abilities
      7) Self-esteem
      8) Values
      9) Perceived social support

2. Research study findings
   a. Polio survivors have been known for positive coping, resulting in achievements in family, social, and professional lives. Postpolio syndrome presents new challenges to independence and functional abilities. Life satisfaction scores of polio survivors are high, but postpolio syndrome is associated with declining scores.

People with postpolio syndrome have new challenges such as muscle weakness, scoliosis, elimination problems, fatigue, and pain (Stuifbergen, 2005).

   b. A survey of 230 people with SCI indicated that there was a significantly positive correlation between life satisfaction and spirituality. This study supported prior research that levels of life satisfaction correlated with levels of spirituality. Spirituality included the concepts of faith, submission, and peace of mind (Brillhart, 2005).

   c. A qualitative study of 10 people with chronic illness who lived in rural areas indicated that spiritual coping helped them cope with despair. The themes of spirituality included feeling that one is not alone, putting on a happy face, recognizing that others are worse off, transcending despair, and letting go. Participants stated that praying with friends brought inner peace and helped them find positive meaning to the chronic illness experience (Walton, Craig, Derwinski-Robinson, & Weinert, 2004).

   d. Parents of school-aged children with disabilities indicated by survey that parental coping was enhanced most often by spiritual support, passive appraisal, reframing, and mobilizing the family to accept help. The least common mechanisms for coping included maintaining family integration and understanding of the child's health condition (Smith, Jackson, & Sharpe, 2006).

3. Assessment
   a. Assess the level and sources of stress expressed by the client and family.
   b. Assess the client's ability to solve problems.
   c. Note changes in the client's and family's abilities to meet their needs.
   d. Note changes in communication patterns that reflect frustration (e.g., verbal manipulation, hostility).
   e. Note inappropriate behavior, activity, and responses that reflect frustration.
   f. Use the Assessment Instrument of Problem-Focused Coping, a self-report instrument that focuses on a person's own assessment of competence in coping with ADLs, personal problems, and level of satisfaction with ADLs (Tollen & Ahlstrom, 1998).

The Specialty Practice of Rehabilitation Nursing: A Core Curriculum, 5th Ed.

g. Use the Multidimensional Acceptance of Loss Scale, developed by Ferrin (2002), which evaluates ability to enlarge the scope of values, contain the disability, subordinate the physique, and change comparative status values to asset values.

h. Assess the continuing impact of chronic illness and exacerbation of symptoms (Stuifbergen, 2005).

i. Assess spirituality as a factor in QOL (Brillhart, 2005).

4. Nursing interventions

a. Provide rehabilitation and education and locate resources beyond personal care and independence, which can allow people with disability to expand their leisure and productive roles and promote socioeconomic integration (Pentland, Harvey, & Walker, 1998).

b. Explore the meaning of illness for the client and family, which can lead to understanding of their behaviors and responses.

1) The meaning the client or family associates with illness can have a profound effect on coping and adjustment and can influence relationships with the healthcare team.

2) The meaning of illness is influenced by cultural beliefs, religion, values, life philosophy, and past experiences (Howell, 1998).

c. Encourage purposeful and meaningful time expenditure, which contributes to a higher QOL, even more than the ability to be independent with ADLs (Cardol, Elvers, Oostendorp, Brandsma, & deGroot, 1996).

d. Understand the unique experience of the person with disability as influenced by his or her psychological, emotional, and spiritual needs and develop appropriate interventions to promote coping (Berman & Rose, 1998).

e. Encourage personal spirituality with the nuturing of friends, community, and family (Walton et al., 2004).

f. Educate the family about the impact of chronic illness on the roles and responsibilities of those with chronic illness (Walton et al., 2004).

H. Memory

1. Description

a. Memory is crucial to all aspects of cognition and learning.

1) Short-term memory: recall of immediate or recent events

2) Long-term memory: storage and retrieval of information

b. Memory disorders are very distressing to clients with head injuries and family caregivers.

2. Clinical examples

a. Ross (2000) reported that a 58-year-old woman who had a minor head injury presented with retrograde amnesia, anterograde memory loss, and mild impairment of executive thinking. This person had essentially normal computed tomography and electroencephalographic diagnostic tests; however, her magnetic resonance imaging scan indicated small vessel disease. Further assessment was needed to differentiate between memory loss caused by injury or psychological factors.

b. Those with mild cognitive impairment often have memory problems. Assessment for memory loss includes history of lost items, inability to repeat recent conversations, and difficulty with learning. Distinguishing memory loss from depression, hallucinations, and functional ability changes is important in planning care (Shah & Bennett, 2006).

3. Assessment

a. Assess the client's mental status early because it is an important element in planning and determining readiness for rehabilitation.

1) Mental changes affect functional abilities, family stress levels, rehabilitation success, social activities, and employment.

2) Early and continuing assessment is needed, and family input should be encouraged.

b. Use the Mini–Mental State Examination to assess memory and recall (Jarvis, 2004).

c. Assess the ability to learn new skills or facts.

d. Assess the client's ability to recall past experiences and ask family members to verify these descriptions.

e. Assess for differential physical diagnoses associated with memory loss (Shah & Bennett, 2005).

4. Nursing interventions for those with dementia and memory loss

a. Use memory aids and strategies such as family pictures, set schedules, calendars, familiar environments, and reminder notes (Remington et al., 2006).

b. Display pictures of self and family dated many years prior, a picture of self on the bedroom door and on a placemat at the dining room table, familiar furnishings, holiday decorations, and mementos.

c. Identify yourself and the relationship to the client with the initial and continuing contacts.

5. Nursing interventions for those with head injury and memory loss: Use the same interventions as are recommended for those with dementia. Additional interventions include personalized notebook day timers, white boards with daily schedules, and color coding to areas of the facility such as physical therapy. One effective intervention for medication reminders is to tape the medicines onto a large calendar posted to the refrigerator.

I. Self-Efficacy

1. Definition: a sense of control that consists of coping with, appraising, and managing one's life and leads to the conviction that the person can determine behaviors that lead to desired outcomes (Bandura, 1977)

2. Assessment

a. Investigate the client's and family's short- and long-term goals.

b. Identify fears of and barriers to self-efficacy.

c. Identify learning needs associated with self-efficacy.

d. Identify resources needed for self-efficacy.

e. Identify the client's ability to provide or direct self-care.

f. Identify the client's ability to manage the vocational and recreational aspects of life.

3. Nursing interventions

a. Individualize self-care education for the client and family.

b. Encourage the client to choose activities.

c. Encourage opportunities for self-responsibility.

d. Encourage behaviors and activities that lead to self-assurance.

e. Encourage alternative solutions for problem solving.

f. Provide opportunities to practice and direct self-care.

g. Provide resources for education and vocational development.

h. Provide opportunities for recreation and socialization.

i. Provide resources for goal achievement.

j. Encourage the client to evaluate the situation completely.

k. Plan with goal setting and identification of resources.

V. Behaviors That Affect Psychosocial Health

A. Denial

1. Definition: a defense mechanism in which a person is unable to admit reality or the presence of something that produces anxiety.

a. Initially, the client and family may experience shock and disbelief about the injury or illness and its effect on the client and family. Adjustment does not occur in even stages but may be characterized by many approaches and avoidance adjustment measures (Davidhizar, 1997).

b. Clients reported that denial is common until they were in formal rehabilitation programs and interacting with peers (Brillhart & Johnson, 1997).

2. Assessment

a. Note avoidance of discussion of the disability, injury, or illness.

b. Note unrealistic discussion of the permanence or severity of the disability.

c. Note unrealistic expectations about treatment or rehabilitation.

d. Note inappropriate mood for the situation (e.g., extreme cheerfulness).

e. Note disregard for the need for treatment or rehabilitation.

f. Note avoidance in rehabilitation program activities such as therapy and education sessions.

3. Nursing interventions

a. Encourage the client and family to express their feelings.

b. Use a nonjudgmental attitude toward the client.

c. Avoid making promises or giving false assurances.

d. Communicate empathy for the client's feelings.

e. Offer information about the disability, injury, illness, and available treatment and rehabilitation.

f. Encourage the client's peers to serve as role models and mentors.

g. Help the client build a support network.

h. Encourage vocational counseling and rehabilitation.

i. Encourage the client to have a realistic outlook on life (Davidhizar, 1997).

j. Suggest that the client participate in rehabilitation activities to meet current health needs even if he or she denies that disabilities are long term or lifelong.

4. Norris and Spelic (2002) reported that one of the initial reactions to body image disruption is denial. Denial is an attempt to minimize the awareness of change (e.g., a person with leg amputation falls in an attempt to walk; a person does not recognize her image after facial changes).

B. Depression

1. Definition: a state of sadness, seen as social withdrawal, crying, anxiety, irritability, or self-denigrating opinions

2. Research study findings

a. Harrison and Stuifbergen (2006) investigated the effect of functional decline and QOL among polio survivors. Depression symptoms were negatively correlated with QOL at the $p < .001$ level and negatively correlated with purpose of life at the $p < .001$ level. The findings of this study implied a need to address depression in these people.

b. A study by Livneh, Priebe, Wuermser, and Ottomanelli (2005) indicated that negative emotions such as depression and anxiety are related to disability denial and avoidance.

c. A study by Hughes, Swedlund, Petersen, and Nosek (2001) indicated that, among 64 women with spinal cord injury, depression was related primarily to stress. Other factors contributing to depression are pain, unemployment, abuse, poor vitality, and social isolation.

3. Assessment

a. Observe for overt signs of depression such as depressed mood, loss of interest, loss of pleasure, weight loss or gain, insomnia or excessive sleep, fatigue, agitation, worthlessness, guilt, and diminished concentration (Santos, Boyle, & Lyness, 2005).

b. Use the Geriatric Depression Scale for admission and ongoing assessment (Diamond, Holroyd, Macciocchi, & Felsenthal, 1995).

c. Use the Center for Epidemiological Studies Depression Scale, a 10-item assessment tool used to examine depression symptoms that have occurred in the last week. It is used as a screening instrument, not a diagnostic tool (Harrison & Stuifbergen, 2006; Nelson & Tucker, 2006).

d. Assess for contributing factors with depression (e.g., chronic illness, disease symptoms, lower socioeconomic status, lack of social support, and lower functioning level).

e. Assess for risk factors of depression and potential suicide, such as substance abuse, hopelessness, impulsiveness, negative thoughts, medication refusal, and impairment of executive processes (Carmine & Murphy, 2006).

4. Nursing interventions

a. Ensure the availability of psychological services during rehabilitation and after discharge (Scivoletto, Petrelli, Di-Lucente, & Castellano, 1997).

b. Establish a therapeutic relationship of trust.

c. Use therapeutic listening and reflection techniques.

d. Reinforce successful coping skills from past experiences.

e. Establish short-term realistic goals and build on successes.

f. Encourage family, friends, and others to provide personal support.

g. Encourage socialization and recreational activities because they increase the overall life satisfaction of those with disabilities (Johnson & Klaas, 2000; Reeves, 2006).

h. Encourage work modification and employment to increase purpose in life status, foster independence, and reduce depression (Harrison & Stuifbergen, 2006).

i. Refer clients to cognitive–behavioral therapy to help them identify and replace depressive thoughts with more realistic, positive thoughts (Crowe & Lutz, 2005).

j. Encourage volunteering, which has been shown to reduce depression (Yuen, Burik, & Krause, 2004).

C. Apathy

1. Definition: an attitude characterized by bland affect, lethargy, and decreased motivation. Apathetic clients may exhibit few goal-

directed behaviors, a lack of productivity, decreased goal-directed thinking, decreased interest, and decreased concern about health or personal problems.

2. Assessment
    a. Observe mood and activity level on an ongoing basis.
    b. Determine lack of goal formation and follow-up on established goals.
    c. Assess for poor self-regulated health maintenance.
    d. Note lack of motivation and initiation.
    e. Use the Apathy Evaluation Scale, an 18-item instrument that rates a person's thoughts, actions, and emotions during 1 month. This scale has been helpful in identifying clients whose apathy is associated with stroke, dementia, or depression (Resnick et al., 1998).

3. Nursing interventions
    a. Identify the client's short- and long-term life goals.
    b. Ensure the availability of vocational counseling.
    c. Introduce client to recreational activities and encourage active participation (Reeves, 2006; Thomas, 2006).
    d. Encourage family involvement and cohesiveness.
    e. Promote the benefits of peer counseling.
    f. Treatment of depression can also restore interest and involvement with friends and family and decrease apathy (Clancy, 2006).

4. Research study findings
    a. Leger's (2005) study of adolescents with spina bifida indicated that higher levels of life satisfaction resulted from success at school, participation in recreation or sports, and socialization.
    b. Brillhart (2005) investigated the relationship between spirituality and life satisfaction among those with SCI. Results of the study indicated that higher levels of life satisfaction were positively correlated with higher levels of spirituality. Interventions to promote spirituality include establishing trust, sharing feelings, and treating the client as a person of worth.
    c. Walton et al. (2004) investigated spirituality among those with chronic illnesses living in rural areas. Findings of this study indicated that spirituality was a source of strength, purpose, and direction.

d. Steffens, Maytan, Helms, and Plassman (2005) investigated behavioral symptoms and their association with preexisting medical conditions among those with dementia. Investigation involving 211 subjects indicated that those with prior head injury, alcohol abuse, and stroke commonly had neuropsychological problems. Common problems included apathy (39.3%), agitation (31.8%), and aberrant motor behaviors (31.1%).

VI. Pathological Behaviors That Affect Psychosocial Health

A. Confusion
    1. Definition: the inability to recall minute-to-minute, hour-to-hour, or day-to-day events
    2. Assessment
        a. Observe inaccuracies with name, date, location, and situation.
        b. Observe the client's ability to understand a situation as reflected by past events.
        c. Note the client's level of ability to follow directions.
        d. Note the client's lack of recall.
        e. Use the Mini–Mental State Examination (Jarvis, 2004), a two-part, accurate assessment instrument for baseline and ongoing mental status evaluation:
            1) Part 1 focuses on name, date, season, and location.
            2) Part 2 focuses on object recognition, sentence formation, the ability to follow commands, and conceptualization.
            3) The entire examination can be administered in 10 minutes.
            4) A score of 27–30 indicates no mental impairment, a score of 20–26 indicates mild impairment, a score of 16–19 indicates moderate impairment, and a score of 15 or less indicates severe mental deficits.
    3. Nursing interventions
        a. Help the client with reorientation. Name, date, and environment reminders can be useful for clients resolving memory deficits and clients with some types of traumatic brain injury (TBI).
        b. Use orientation cues (e.g., printed names, personal or family pictures, calendars, seasonal decorations, schedules, clocks), especially for clients with dementia or Alzheimer's disease.

c. Ensure consistency in the environment, schedules, and staff.

B. Impulsiveness

1. Definition: the tendency to act without considering the consequences.

2. Assessment: Use a behavior flowsheet to document impulsive behaviors (e.g., pacing, banging on doors, darting across the street, getting up from the wheelchair, going over siderails).

3. Nursing interventions

a. Ensure environmental safety.

b. Use door alarms.

c. Use alarm bracelets.

d. Establish a routine with meaningful activities.

e. Monitor clients closely to prevent injury.

f. Provide family education and guidance in dealing with impulsiveness.

g. Help clients avoid fatigue by developing a sleep–wake cycle.

h. Encourage the family's involvement with the client.

C. Perseveration

1. Definition: the reflexive repetition of behaviors, vocalizations, or activities

2. Assessment

a. Observe the client's reflexive responses.

b. Document the onset, duration, and situational factors that aggravate perseveration.

c. Document the factors that decrease perseveration.

3. Nursing interventions

a. Provide visual distractions.

b. Engage the client in simple activities (e.g., taking a walk).

c. Conduct a meaningful conversation with the client.

d. Use pet therapy.

e. Help the client avoid social isolation.

f. Use music therapy that involves the client (e.g., play music while exercising).

g. Gather family input about the cause and symptoms of perseveration.

h. Encourage family involvement and interaction with the client.

D. Confabulation

1. Description

a. Confabulation is the invention of detail or life experiences in an attempt to compensate for memory deficits.

b. The person substitutes imaginary experiences or confuses experiences with those he or she cannot recall.

c. Confabulation can be quite convincing even for healthcare professionals.

2. Assessment

a. Gather observations from family, relatives, or friends who know the client's life and history.

b. Assess and document incidents of confabulation at frequent intervals to determine an indication of disease progression.

3. Nursing interventions

a. For the family
1) Provide family education about the physiological causes of confabulation.
2) Assure the family that confabulation is a symptom of memory deficits.
3) Communicate frequently with the family to help them understand situations (e.g., the client's statements about a bruise, no breakfast, no one visits) and the true circumstances of the client's status and routine.
4) Maintain a logbook in the client's room in which staff members record their encounters with the client. Staff and family members can use the logbook to track the day's activities and interact appropriately with the client.

b. For the client
1) Provide distraction with meaningful conversation.
2) Engage in simple activities.
3) Avoid correcting or making negative comments to the client about confabulation.

E. Emotional Lability

1. Definition: uncontrollable, fluctuating emotional behaviors, usually alternating gaiety, somberness, and crying

2. Assessment

a. Observe and document emotional lability (e.g., duration, timing, cycles).

b. Observe and document factors that increase or diminish emotional lability.

3. Nursing interventions

a. Provide adequate rest and sleep–wake cycles.

b. Provide distraction in the early stages of emotional lability.

c. Play soothing music.

d. Ensure a calm atmosphere.

e. Reduce situations that promote frustration or anger.

f. Help staff or family members avoid overreacting to emotional episodes.

g. Use reminiscence therapy.

h. Encourage the client to sing familiar songs (e.g., "Row, Row, Row Your Boat").

i. Use physical activities (e.g., chair exercises).

j. Provide family education about emotional lability as a symptom of disease and tips on managing emotional lability.

k. Encourage the client to gain control of feelings of loss of control and frustration by simplifying normal daily events and preventing fatigue (Paterson & Stewart, 2002).

F. Disinhibition

1. Definition: uncontrolled behaviors or activities that are considered socially inappropriate. The person is unable to inhibit inappropriate behaviors, cannot foresee the consequences of inappropriate actions, and exhibits egocentric behaviors (Montgomery, Kitten, Niemiec, 1997).

2. Assessment

a. Observe inappropriate behavior (e.g., undressing in public, sexual overtures, physical or verbal abuse).

b. Evaluate the client's psychosocial status, focusing on impaired self-control and social withdrawal, on an ongoing basis (Spatt, Zebenholzer, & Oder, 1997).

3. Nursing interventions

a. Discourage behaviors involving sexual disinhibition.
1) Offer distractions that promote meaningful behavior.
2) Provide opportunities for adequate sleep and rest.
3) Encourage appropriate touch and contact by family, friends, and staff.

b. Discourage behaviors involving disrobing disinhibition.
1) Take the client to the bathroom or provide toileting routinely.
2) Maintain elimination hygiene if the client uses adult padding or incontinence briefs.

3) Provide appropriate clothing for the season and situation.
4) Provide special clothing that is difficult to remove.
5) Help the client redress himself or herself to regain dignity and privacy.

c. Discourage behaviors involving swearing.
1) Offer distractions that promote meaningful activities.
2) Avoid making the client feel shameful about swearing.
3) Help the family and staff avoid overreacting to client swearing.
4) Use music therapy with familiar tunes.
5) Provide family education and awareness of disease and injury processes related to swearing disinhibition.

G. Agitation

1. Definition: uncontrolled behaviors such as restlessness, irritability, anger, vocalization, and combativeness

2. Assessment

a. Assess for the triggers of agitation, which may include overstimulation, fatigue, forceful communication by others, pain, confusion, fear, and anxiety (Price, 2006).

b. Observe characteristic agitated behaviors (e.g., pacing, verbal aggression, physical aggression, frustration, confusion).

c. Assess for nonverbal cues such as facial expressions and body language that often precede agitation. Also assess for patterns of agitation and individualized triggers for agitation (Remington et al., 2006).

d. Document the type and duration of behaviors, time of day, preceding incidents, situational influences, and response to interventions.

e. Use the Agitation Behavior Scale (Riedel & Shaw, 1997), designed to evaluate people with TBI experiencing agitation.

3. Nursing interventions

a. To provide environmental control:
1) Avoid using physical restraints (e.g., Posey belts, arm restraints).
2) Reduce environmental noise, light, and activity.
3) Provide rest periods and quiet environment, ideally in a private room (Price, 2006).
4) Limit visitors.
5) Ensure the client's protection by using Craig beds.

6) Provide a consistent personal aide (Riedel & Shaw, 1997) and consistent routines.
7) Allow the client to pace in a safe environment with 1:1 supervision (Price, 2006).
8) Give instructions simply and one at a time (Price, 2006).

b. To take a specialized approach to an agitated client:
1) Provide staff education.
   a) Client and staff safety
   b) Staff morale issues
   c) Phases and causes of agitation
   d) Strategies for dealing with agitation
2) Prevent agitation by decreasing stressors such as fatigue, pain, change of routine, or confusing stimuli (Remington et al., 2006).
3) Defuse the situation before it reaches physical aggression.
4) Give simple instructions (e.g., "Don't kick," "Don't hit").
5) Avoid scolding or belittling the client.
6) Maintain a calm, controlled approach and vocalizations (Montgomery et al., 1997; Price, 2006).

c. To approach the client:
1) Continue to orient the client to the environment.
2) Explain all actions to the client.
3) Allow time away from required activities if agitation is heightened.
4) Use distraction to avoid cycles of agitation.
5) Avoid reasoning with the client during a period of agitation because he or she will have difficulty processing his or her thoughts.
6) Provide physical reassurance and comfort (Flannery, 1998).
7) Avoid arguing with the client during times of preagitation and during actual agitation (Price, 2006).

VII. Sensation and Perception Factors That Affect Psychosocial Health

A. Deficits in Hearing
1. Physiology of hearing: Hearing is a complex sensory perception that incorporates a stimulus, which activates the acoustic nerve (cranial nerve [CN] VIII) and then the cochlear nucleus, the nuclei, tracts of the lateral lemniscus, and the inferior colliculus.

The stimulus activates the structures along the brainstem's auditory pathways. Interpretation of the stimulus is based on conduction properties of various portions of the auditory tract.
2. Disruption in hearing: Disruptions of this complex system caused by injury or illness can lead to partial or total deafness (see Table 8-2).
3. Assessment
   a. Use the whisper test on both ears to assess gross hearing: The examiner stands behind the client and whispers a number. The client covers one ear at a time and repeats the whispered number (Jarvis, 2004).
   b. Inspect the external ear canal and tympanic membranes and use the Weber test (Jarvis, 2004) to assess conduction hearing loss.
   c. Use the Rinne and Weber tests (Jarvis, 2004) to assess neurogenic hearing loss.
   d. Evaluate the family's descriptions of the client's prior hearing status.
   e. Observe the appropriateness of the client's conversational flow.
   f. Observe whether the client can appropriately follow commands.
   g. Note unusual volume of the radio or television.
   h. Note the condition of the client's hearing aid.
4. Nursing interventions
   a. Reduce background noise.
   b. Keep sentences and messages short.
   c. Do not rush the client.
   d. Listen and seek feedback from the client.
   e. Encourage the use of bilateral hearing aids.
   f. Avoid shouting to the client.
   g. Use a low tone of voice.
   h. Face the client when speaking to him or her.
   i. Use alternative methods of communication (e.g., written notes, sign language).

B. Deficits in Vision
1. Pathophysiological factors in vision deficits involving the optic nerve: The major function of the optic nerve (CN II) is vision, which includes visual fields and visual acuity (see Table 8-3 and Figure 8-2).
   a. Assessment
      1) Test peripheral vision (i.e., visual field) using the technique of

Table 8-2. Pathophysiology of Hearing

Injury	Symptoms
Damage to lateral lemniscus	Partial deafness bilaterally, with more severe deafness on the side opposite the lesion
Destruction of cortex of one hemisphere of brain	Difficulty in judging direction and distance from the source of sound

Table 8-3. Pathophysiology of Vision: Part 1 (CN II)

Injury	Symptoms
Interruptions of optic pathways to calcarine cortex in occipital lobe	Visual field deficits
Retinal tears	Visual field deficits
Damage to one optical tract before unification of the left and right tract	Monocular vision loss in ipsilateral eye, associated with multiple sclerosis
Transient ischemic attacks affecting blood supply to optic nerve	Transient monocular vision loss
Pressure to optic chiasm	Permanent blindness, associated with brain tumors
Damage to optic pathway	Homonymous hemianopia, or vision loss in the same side of each eye, associated with cerebrovascular accidents

confrontation (e.g., the client gazes straight at the examiner and notes the examiner's fingers, which move into all visual fields).

    2) Use the Snellen chart tests (Jarvis, 2004) and reading material (e.g., newspaper) to assess visual acuity.

    3) Obtain information on prior visual status from the client and family.

    4) Note unilateral neglect.

    5) Note the client's ability to read materials at near and far distances.

  b. Nursing interventions

    1) Teach the client to scan the visual field.

    2) Provide environmental control for safety.

    3) Identify family, friends, and staff when interacting with the client.

    4) Ensure adequate lighting.

    5) Provide large-print reading materials.

    6) Provide current prescription for glasses and encourage client to wear the glasses.

2. Deficits in vision involving the oculomotor (CN III), trochlear (CN IV), and abducens (CN VI) nerves: These nerves unite to control the functions of the extraocular muscles, responsible for eye motion and binocular vision. The oculomotor nerve also controls the elevation of the upper eyelids and the constriction of the pupils (see Table 8-4).

  a. Assessment

    1) Inspect the eyelid for drooping (ptosis).

    2) Examine the size, shape, equality, position, and light reflexes of the pupils.

    3) Test the ocular movements of the eye for imbalance and conjugate deviation.

    4) Evaluate accommodation and convergence.

    5) Observe ocular movements.

  b. Nursing interventions

    1) Have the client use an eye patch to diminish double vision (diplopia).

    2) Address the cause of symptoms (e.g., elevated intracranial pressure).

C. Deficits in Touch

  1. Physiology of touch: The gray matter of the spinal cord has both motor and sensory components. The sensory (afferent) component consists of the dorsal (posterior) columns and the intermediate areas. Posterior horn cells remain within the central nervous system. Axons from these cells project to the anterior or ventral horn cells of the spinal cord, where they divide to become ascending and descending intersegmental tracts (see Table 8-5).

  2. Assessment

    a. Determine whether the client can differentiate between levels of temperature.

    b. Evaluate the client's pain.

    c. Evaluate the client's sense of light touch.

    d. Evaluate proprioception.

    e. Evaluate the client's sense of vibration.

    f. Evaluate the client's ability to identify familiar objects (use items such as a key or coin) just by touch (Jarvis, 2004).

    g. Evaluate the client's ability to identify a number drawn in the palms of the hand by touch only. The numbers 0, 1, and 8 are good to use because they are symmetrical (Jarvis, 2004).

    h. Evaluate the client's ability to distinguish between sharp and dull sensations of the extremities. Assess in a distal to proximal pattern (Jarvis, 2004).

  3. Nursing interventions

Figure 8-2. Visual Field Deficits Associated with Lesions of the Optic Pathway of Different Locations

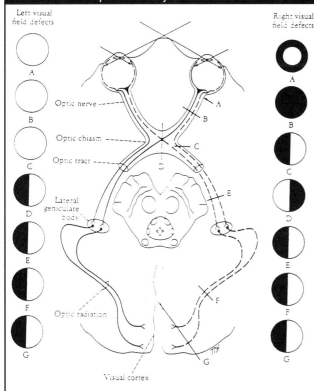

Left visual field defects — Right visual field defects

Optic nerve
Optic chiasm
Optic tract
Lateral geniculate body
Optic radiation
Visual cortex

A Right-sided circumferential blindness resulting from retrobulbar neuritis

B Total blindness of right eye resulting from division of the right optic nerve

C Right nasal hemianopia resulting from a partial lesion of the right side of the optic chiasm

D Bitemporal hemianopia resulting from a complete lesion of the optic chiasm

E Left temporal and right nasal hemianopia resulting from a lesion of the right optic radiation

G Left temporal and right nasal hemianopia resulting from a lesion of the right visual cortex

Reprinted with permission of Little, Brown and Company Inc. from Snell, R.S. (1980). *Clinical neuroanatomy for medical students* (p. 382). Boston: Little, Brown. Copyright 1980 by Little, Brown and Company Inc.

Table 8-4. Pathophysiology of Vision: Part 2 (CN III, IV, VI)

Injury	Symptoms
Injury to CN III, IV, or VI	Marked miosis, seen with brainstem strokes
	Dilation of pupils, seen with elevated intracranial pressure
	Ptosis of eyelid, associated with multiple sclerosis or elevated intracranial pressure
	Unequal pupil size, associated with ipsilateral hemisphere lesions
	Nystagmus with jerking movements of eyes
Disruptions of CN III or VI	Diplopia with disruption of conjugate movements of the eyes and impaired binocular vision

VIII. Communication: A Function of Sensory, Cognitive, and Physiological Status

A. Communication

  1. Is a complex process between sender and receiver

  2. Depends on the sensory, cognitive, emotional, and physical status of all components of the interaction

B. Assessment

  1. Characteristics of a person with cognitive communication deficits

    a. Does not speak

    b. Has problems finding words

    c. Uses inappropriate words

    d. Is unable to name familiar objects

    e. Appears confused or disoriented

    f. Displays attention deficits

    g. Is unable to speak a second language (e.g., the client initially spoke Spanish and was bilingual with English but now can speak only Spanish)

    h. Displays emotional lability

    i. Has decreased comprehension

  2. Characteristics of a person with sensory communication deficits

    a. Has diminished hearing or deafness

    b. Lacks or has diminished vision

    c. Lacks appropriate responses to touch because of sensory deficits

  3. Characteristics of a person with physiological communication deficits

    a. Slurs speech

    b. Speaks in a whisper

    c. Has difficulty with motor planning

    d. Has difficulty with articulation

C. Nursing Interventions

  1. For cognitive communication problems

    a. Ensure safety with extreme temperature exposures.

    b. Observe and control the sources of pain (e.g., pressure, burns, lesions).

a. Use short, simple sentences.
b. Use one-step commands.
c. Use nonverbal cues.
d. Use repetition and patterning when giving directions.
e. Communicate during times of peak energy and attentiveness.
f. Control the environment (e.g., eliminate background noise, light, activity, confusion).
g. Limit the time spent on communication sessions.
h. Use a communication board with symbols.
i. Teach the family strategies for effectively communicating with the client.

2. For sensory communication problems
a. Assess for intact, diminished, or absent sensation.
b. Provide sensory stimulation therapy (e.g., different textures and temperatures).
c. Focus family education on affectionate touch in areas of intact sensation.
d. Ensure that the client uses necessary hearing aids (especially bilateral aids).
e. Provide translators for clients who are deaf or use sign language.
f. Use nonverbal cues or gestures.
g. Ensure that the client uses necessary corrective lenses.
h. Use voice-operated computers.

3. For physiological communication problems
a. Ensure that the client receives speech therapy.
b. Provide computers with word processing programs.

Table 8-5. Physiology of Touch: Spinal Cord

Region of Spinal Cord	Function
Gray matter	
Afferent portion composed of dorsal (posterior) columns and intermediate areas	Modification of pain and temperature information
Substantia gelatinosa in dorsal horn of spinal cord	Conveys touch, pressure, and proprioception information to cerebellum
Nucleus dorsalis of the ventromedial portion of spinal cord	Serves as connections for spinal reflexes and transmission of sensory information to the brain
Nucleus proprius of the dorsal portion of the cord	Causes impairment of sensation on the side opposite the lesion
White matter	
Dorsal area	Carries impulses from extremities that involve proprioceptors, tactile endings, and end organs to the medulla, to pons, to midbrain, to general sensory nucleus of thalamus, to cerebral cortex
	Transmits location of stimuli, fine gradations of stimulus intensity; modulates tactile sensations of vibration, pressure, touch, and proprioception
Spinothalamic tract	
Anterior spinothalamic tract	Conducts impulses for light touch to sensory cortex
Lateral spinothalamic tract	Conducts pain and temperature stimuli from peripheral areas to thalamus and general sensory nucleus; responsible for crude awareness of pain and temperature, localization and quantitative assessment of pain and temperature
	Includes conditions such as tumors, trauma, infections, and degenerative processes

IX. Self-Perception and Self-Concept Issues Related to Psychosocial Health

A. Powerlessness
1. Definition: the inability to use personal energy to initiate and guide personal behavior.
a. The lack of personal power makes a person powerless, which is destructive to the self (Satir, 1988).
b. Powerlessness can be learned through negative reinforcement of dependency.
c. Powerlessness as a reaction to threats can lead to patterns of impotence, withdrawal, and passiveness.
2. Clinical example: Injury or illness leading to disability can destroy a person's normal level of life control and predictability. Relocation stress, experienced during the recovery and rehabilitation process, and powerlessness are influenced by a decrease in biopsychosocial status, anxiety, depression, apprehension, guilt, denial, and lowered self-esteem (Nypaver, Titus, & Brugler, 1996).
3. Assessment

a. Note lack of initiative in goal planning and achievement.

b. Note passivity.

c. Note withdrawal from family, social, and vocational decisions and interactions.

d. Assess apprehension and fear.

4. Nursing interventions

a. Encourage the client and family to maintain control in decision making and promote environmental predictability and emotional support (Nypaver et al., 1996).

b. Help the client realize that although the injury or illness that led to the disability cannot be changed, his or her response to the disability is a personal choice (Davidhizar, 1997).

c. Enable the client and family to recognize and mobilize their strengths and resources, feel confident, and use effective coping skills.

d. Encourage the client to achieve self-direction and self-determination.

e. Encourage the client and family to seek spiritual support.

f. Encourage and value the client's and family's involvement as participants in the interdisciplinary team.

g. Encourage the client's involvement with group and community support systems.

h. Provide follow-up rehabilitation care in the home setting if applicable.

B. Hopelessness

1. Definition: The feeling that a situation or condition is without solution. Associated feelings of hopelessness include powerlessness, despair, helplessness, and apathy.

2. Assessment

a. Observe for the characteristics of powerlessness, despair, and apathy.

b. Observe for the lack of initiative for self-help.

c. Observe for depression.

3. Nursing interventions

a. Enhance the client's sense of power, which precedes hopefulness.

b. Establish short- and long-term goals with the client and family.

c. Encourage family and social support.

d. Encourage spiritual empowerment and strength.

e. Encourage use of the word *hope*,

characterized by active responsibility, rather than *hopeful*, which is more passive (Kautz, 2006).

4. Research study findings: Lohne and Severinsson (2006) conducted a qualitative study to examine the experience of hope for those with SCI. The findings indicated that hope was important because it provided the energy and power to achieve progress and personal development after injury.

C. Helplessness

1. Definition: the belief that a person is dependent on others for support for a situation that seems to be impossible to alter. The person may perceive that events are beyond his or her control.

2. Assessment

a. Observe for inactivity and nonparticipation in rehabilitation.

b. Observe for self-isolation and withdrawal.

c. Observe for general behaviors (e.g., slow movements, low voice tones, sitting alone quietly).

d. Observe for disturbances in motivation, cognition, and emotion.

e. Observe for the absence of voluntary response to a situation.

f. Observe for learned dependence (i.e., the inability to act and make decisions).

g. Observe for fear and depression.

3. Nursing interventions

a. Foster voluntary responses and independence.

b. Encourage learning and reinforce successes.

c. Form the expectation of independence for the client and family.

d. Encourage the client to evaluate his or her personal assets and affirm his or her feelings or expressions of hope.

e. Encourage memory and increased coping abilities (Davidhizar, 1997).

D. Self-Perception

1. Problems with self-concept

a. Definition of self-concept: a person's perception of himself or herself as related to others and the environment. Self-concept addresses all aspects of the person.

b. Assessment

1) Observe for self-criticism (e.g., negative thinking, expectations of failure).

2) Observe for self-diminution (e.g., avoiding, neglecting, or refusing to recognize personal assets) (Stuart & Laraia, 1995).

c. Nursing interventions
1) Encourage activity in community-based social integration programs to develop social skills (Burleigh, Farber, & Gillard, 1998).
2) Encourage the client to approach life with open, realistic expectations.
3) Encourage and reinforce the client's evaluations of his or her personal assets.
4) Encourage the client to interact with family and friends.
5) Reinforce success, which can academically and vocationally increase self-concept (Brillhart & Johnson, 1997; Hayes, Balfanz-Vertiz, & Ostrander, 2005).
6) Participation in artistic activities can contribute to positive self-identification (Reynolds, 2003).

2. Problems with self-esteem
a. Definition of self-esteem: an attitude, feeling, and self-concept represented by behavior
1) Self-esteem is the person's sense of personal value and ability to consider himself or herself with dignity, love, and reality.
2) Self-esteem affects the inner person and the person's relationships with others.
3) Positive self-esteem is fostered by integrity, honesty, responsibility, compassion, and competence.
4) Self-esteem is based on personal evaluation of self-worth and competence (Norris & Speclic, 2002).
5) People with low self-worth have a "victim mentality" and expect deprecation.

b. Assessment
1) Observe for feelings of defeat, failure, and worthlessness (Satir, 1988), weakness, helplessness, hopelessness, fright, vulnerability, fragility, incompleteness, and inadequacy (Antle, 2004; Stuart & Laraia, 1995).
2) Assess the client to identify a personal situation in which mastery was achieved through positive coping

with disability effects (Norris & Spelic, 2002).

c. Nursing interventions
1) Allow time for relaxation.
2) Help the client realize what is occurring and his or her reaction to the situation.
3) Encourage the client to communicate with family members and share experiences.
4) Encourage the client to listen to others and try to reflect how both parties perceive the communication.
5) Foster relaxed, flexible family expectations.
6) Encourage the client to declare, "I am unique," "I can love myself," and "I am okay" (Satir, 1988).
7) Encourage family and friends to express that the client is a person of value (Norris & Spelic, 2002).
8) Prepare the client to perform to personally identified standards for life functions and roles (Norris & Spelic, 2002).
9) Encourage spirituality as a basis for self concept, which has been related to positive rehabilitation outcomes (Faull & Hills, 2006).

3. Poor body image
a. Definition of body image: a person's subjective picture of his or her own appearance that is based on observations, comparisons, and reactions by others
b. Assessment
1) Observe for grooming and hygiene status.
2) Observe for initiation of self-care activities.
3) Observe the functional abilities for self-care and ADLs.
4) Observe the effect of the client's appearance on family, friends, and the community.
c. Nursing interventions
1) Provide for independent or assisted grooming.
2) Ensure that the client has appropriate street clothing for activities.
3) Coordinate barber and hairdressing services.
4) Encourage the use of prosthetics.
5) Reinforce occupational therapy.
6) Provide recreational therapy and community reentry activities.
7) Encourage the client to recognize

successful people with disabilities (e.g., athletes who use wheelchairs).

8) Promote positive, public images of people with disabilities in business, politics, and the media.

9) Incorporate people with disabilities into play therapy (e.g., childhood books that include characters with disabilities, dolls in wheelchairs, cartoons with positive images of people with disabilities).

10) Encourage the client to attend support groups for people with disabilities.

E. Unresolved Grief Associated with Disability

1. Definition: prolonged grief and mourning that progresses beyond the initial grief associated with having an injury or illness and that incorporates the loss of function

2. Assessment

a. Observe for appetite loss, fatigue, apathy, lack of socialization, somatic complaints, and decreased activities.

b. Observe the client's emotions (e.g., feelings of emptiness and numbness, low self-esteem, sadness, guilt) (Stuart & Laraia, 1995).

c. Observe the client's level of willingness to participate in rehabilitation.

3. Nursing interventions

a. Encourage family and friends to reassure the client that he or she is loved for himself or herself, not for his or her appearance, physical abilities, or work capacity.

b. Foster peer modeling and mentoring (Davidhizar, 1997).

c. Encourage the client and family to seek psychological counseling.

d. Help the client build a social, cultural, and economic network of support (Davidhizar, 1997).

e. Help the client cultivate a positive and realistic outlook (Davidhizar, 1997).

f. Allow time for adjustment, because clients often do not internalize the entire impact of a disability until the rehabilitation phase of treatment (Brillhart & Johnson, 1997).

g. Refer the client for interpersonal psychotherapy, which focuses on grief, interpersonal role disputes, and role transitions (Crowe & Lutz, 2005).

F. Stress

1. Definition: the cognitive awareness of any external or internal unmet demands on a person that unbalances the equilibrium. Effects of stress are expressed physically, emotionally, intellectually, spiritually, and socially (Barry, 1996).

2. Assessment

a. Observe for physiological manifestations of stress (e.g., gastrointestinal distress, cardiac palpitations, anxious facial expressions, tremors).

b. Observe for emotional manifestations of stress (e.g., anxiety, emotional lability, restlessness, fright).

c. Observe for intellectual manifestations of stress (e.g., difficulty in concentration and memory, poor coping strategies).

d. Observe for spiritual manifestations of stress (e.g., value conflicts).

e. Observe for social manifestations of stress (e.g., role conflict, status incongruity, withdrawal, antagonism, role rigidity).

3. Nursing interventions

a. Examine the source of stress (e.g., fears of failure, lack of resources, lack of support system, role loss, ambiguity).

b. Examine and reinforce prior successful coping measures.

c. Provide crisis management.

d. Consult with the client's case managers and social workers.

e. Encourage the client to appraise stressors and his or her responses to stress and approaches to problem solving.

f. Encourage the client and family to be flexible with roles and problem solving.

g. Promote psychological hardiness by fostering control, commitment, and challenge for growth and development.

h. Encourage the client to seek spiritual counseling and support (Barry, 1996; Lazarus & Folkman, 1984).

i. Encourage prayer in times of stress, set limits on activities, and give rationale to others for relief of activities leading to stress (Walton et al., 2004).

j. Encourage guided imagery as a relaxation technique to decrease stress (Nathenson, 2006).

4. Research study findings: Rintala, Robinson-Whelen, and Matamoros (2005) reported that stressors among men with SCI were focused

on problems with physical abilities, health, and finances. Stress was positively related to depression and anxiety and negatively related to life satisfaction. Finally, those with low levels of social support were more vulnerable to negative effects of stress.

G. Stigma

1. Definition: The application of set attitudes about and stereotypes of people with disabilities. Stigma begins in the attitudes of others but may be internalized by the person with a disability and eventually influence that person's behaviors (Goffman, 1974).

2. Assessment

   a. Observe for statements of self-deprecation.

   b. Observe for self-isolating behaviors.

   c. Observe alienation and hostility by others.

   d. Note family's and friends' attitudes toward people with disabilities.

3. Nursing interventions

   a. Encourage the client to reevaluate the importance of physique.

   b. Encourage a realistic appraisal of the difficulties of dealing with disability.

   c. Encourage evaluation of personal assets and abilities.

   d. Encourage the client and family to focus on the total person, not just the disability.

   e. Provide counseling on dealing with stigma in the community.

   f. Encourage positive images of those with disabilities in the media, business, academia, athletics, and music.

   g. Ensure that children and adults with disabilities are mainstreamed into educational and recreational activities.

X. Roles and Relationships Related to Psychosocial Health

A. Family Roles

1. Description [Refer to Chapter 15 for additional information on family roles and theories.]

   a. The family unit is an active, operating system.

   b. The person with disability is not in isolation but is considered in the context of family.

   c. Family relationships are the living links that bind the family together.

   d. As a system, the family assigns roles and rules that are established for each member.

   e. Functions of the family include acquiring the means to provide for the necessities of daily life.

   f. The family is essential in dealing with internal change and external disruptions.

2. Nurturing families:

   a. Characteristics include a sense of aliveness, affection, genuineness, honesty, open communication, and love.

   b. These families make plans, adjust plans, problem solve without panic, and accept change as part of life.

3. Troubled families:

   a. Characteristics include coldness, rigidity, control, guarded communication, tolerance rather than love, and secrecy.

   b. Adjustment and problem solving are difficult as family members rigidly hold onto assigned roles and responsibilities (Satir, 1988).

4. The effect of disability on a family:

   a. Any family member's disability can cause permanent disruptions in family patterns.

   b. Established roles and responsibilities of the family change.

   c. Life patterns continue to change as children mature, siblings marry, individuals move away, parents grow older, health status changes within the family, and members die.

   d. Problem solving and adapting to change are necessary family skills for positive family life.

5. Assessment

   a. Observe the family members' communication patterns.

   b. Observe the family's cohesiveness during change.

   c. Examine the family's planning strategies.

   d. Examine the family's actions, behaviors, and roles.

6. Nursing interventions

   a. Encourage family therapy with a focus on the entire family, which should include information about the injury or illness, strategies for handling emotional distress, assistive services, opportunities to share concerns, and assistance with coping (Butcher, 1994).

   b. Provide training in communication skills (e.g., structured marriage enrichment programs, effective listening, self-awareness, conflict resolution) (Captain, 1995).

   c. Provide the means for lifetime planning for continued care (costs of long-term needs, costs of care and rehabilitation) (Deutsch, Allison, & Cimino-Ferguson, 2005).

   d. Help the client and family identify and cope with changes in roles and responsibilities caused by disability (Paterson & Stewart, 2002).

  7. Research study findings: People with TBI associated life satisfaction 1 year after injury with family satisfaction, employment, intact marriage, memory, and independence (Warren, Wrigley, Yoels, & Fine, 1996).

B. Social Support

  1. Definition: a multifaceted concept that includes instrumental support (e.g., equipment, services), affective support (e.g., concern, being loved, feeling important, support presence), and cognitive support (e.g., education, advice, information, role modeling, counseling) (Rintala, Young, Spencer, & Bates, 1996).

  2. Clinical examples

   a. Social support was seen as a strong predictor of life satisfaction among survivors of TBI who live in the community (Smith, Magill-Evans, & Brintnell, 1998).

   b. People with TBI or SCI and their partners indicated having low availability of social support and inadequate social integration in the years after injury. This social isolation led to high levels of depression (Hammell, 1994).

   c. People with multiple sclerosis and their partners had socialization difficulties because of their inability to keep up the pace of socialization, the inability of others to understand the limitations of multiple sclerosis, the need for mechanical or personal assistance, the uncertainty of daily energy levels, and inadequate finances (Stuifbergen, 1992).

  3. Research study findings

   a. Fairfax (2002) investigated QOL among stroke survivors. Analysis of data from 102 adults indicated a positive but nonsignificant relationship of QOL and social support. Level of disability contributed to 27% of prediction of QOL.

   b. Ferguson, Richie, and Gomez (2004) conducted a qualitative study to investigate the psychological factors contributing to the recovery for those with traumatic amputations. Results of the study indicated that acceptance of the loss and level of psychological recovery were greatly influenced by social support and societal attitudes toward the disabled.

  4. Assessment

   a. Observe for barriers in socialization (e.g., fatigue, multiple problems, isolation, lack of self-confidence, apathy) (Abjornsson, Orbaek, & Hagstadius, 1998).

   b. Observe the frequency of contact with family and friends and leisure and physical activities.

   c. Use the Life Satisfaction Index (Diener, 1984).

   d. Use the Sickness Impact Profile (Smith et al., 1998).

   e. Use the Community Integration Questionnaire (Smith et al., 1998).

   f. Use the Quality of Social Support instrument (Bethoux, Calmels, Gautheron, & Minaire, 1996).

   g. Observe the client's patterns of behaviors such as alcohol use after injury. Increased consumption of alcohol is associated with lower levels of social support (Boraz & Heinemann, 1996).

  5. Nursing interventions

   a. Encourage the client to use problem- and emotion-focused coping skills.

   b. Encourage social networking (Cormier-Daigle & Stewart, 1997).

   c. Involve the spouse with instrumental (task-oriented) and emotional support.

   d. Encourage the client to engage in meaningful, rewarding activities.

   e. Encourage social roles for identity, power, and family position (Nir, Wallhagen, Doolittle, & Galinsky, 1997).

   f. Encourage the client to attend support groups.

   g. Provide crisis therapy and stress management.

   h. Encourage cognitive activation and memory training (Abjornsson et al., 1998).

   i. Encourage the use of support groups using the computer-based systems. This is especially helpful for those in rural areas or those with fewer transportation resources (Hill, Schillo, & Weinert, 2004).

j. Provide access for social support to support participation in life situations (Lund, Nordlund, Nygard, Lexell, & Bernspang, 2005).

k. Encourage the peer mentoring experience as a complement to social support (Sherman, Sperling, & DeVinney, 2004).

l. Encourage emotion-focused coping as a major factor to promote social reintegration. Other pertinent factors for social reintegration include family support, information, and removal of social barriers (Song, 2005).

6. Research study findings: Isaksson, Skar, and Lexell (2005) conducted a qualitative study among women with SCI to investigate perceptions of social networking. Data analysis indicated that the subjects needed the social support to function in their occupations. The subjects also reported that they established new relationships with others having disabilities.

C. Independence and Dependence

1. Independence can be fostered when people with disabilities have responsibility for self-care and are expected to participate in family roles.

2. Assessment

a. Observe for initiation of ADLs.

b. Assess the client's level of functional abilities.

c. Assess the client's cognitive abilities.

d. Use the Functional Independence Measure™ instrument (Kelly-Hayes, 1996) to assess cognitive and functional abilities and the need for supervision, especially for clients with TBI (Smith & Schwirian, 1998).

e. Observe participation in academic and vocational activities.

f. Assess for initiation of recreational activities.

g. Assess for perceptions of poor health and emotional distress, which are often associated with increased dependency (Riegel, Dracup, & Glaser, 1998).

h. Use the FAMTOOL (a family health assessment tool) to evaluate communication, shared beliefs, shared work and play, value connectedness, and effort toward physical, emotional, social, and spiritual health (Weeks & O'Connor, 1997).

i. Assess role expectations from the different viewpoints of family members, especially those focusing on pressures, demands, personal resources, and family structure (Satir, 1988).

j. Use the Quality of Life Scale (Ferrans, 1996).

3. Nursing interventions

a. Encourage independence within the family unit.

b. Provide more intensive family support during transitional periods (e.g., moving from acute care to rehabilitation, rehabilitation to home, home to independence).

c. Eliminate environmental barriers.

d. Provide resources for adaptive housing, equipment, and attendant care (Brillhart & Johnson, 1997).

e. Encourage the thoughts such as "I have control of my life," "I can do things," "I feel close to others," and "Others understand me" to promote independence (Secrest, 2006).

f. Encourage family counseling:
   1) Appropriate support for the client
   2) Education about the client's discomfort with being a unilateral receiver and burden rather than a bidirectional receiver and giver
   3) The appropriate help needed by the client (Rintala et al., 1996)

g. Encourage the family to reestablish life trajectories, meet development needs, and reintegrate the survivor into the family (Brzuzy & Speziale, 1997).

4. Research study findings

a. Dependence was fostered by feelings of safety in a rehabilitation unit and reluctance to leave such security. Family attitudes that fostered dependency and the fear of risks associated with ADLs (e.g., falling during transfers) also led to dependency (Brillhart & Johnson, 1997).

b. Elfstrom, Ryden, Kreuter, Taft, and Sullivan (2005) investigated the relationship between coping strategies and QOL among 256 people with SCI. The findings of this study indicated that revaluation of life values (acceptance) and fewer dependency behaviors (social reliance) were positively related to QOL.

5. Clinical example: Effective coping styles and strategies by rehabilitation clients at discharge included confrontation, evasion, optimism, emotional expression, palliative

activities, support, and self-reliance. Generally, clients coped with discharge to home through positive thinking, humor, control of the situation and emotional control, prayer, taking problems step by step, and staying active (Easton, Zemen, & Kwiatkowski, 1995).

XI. Roles and Responsibilities of Advanced Practice Nurses in Rehabilitation Nursing

A. Background of Advanced Practice Nurses

1. Advanced degrees such as a master's in nursing, a doctorate in nursing science, or a PhD

2. Successful completion of national accreditation

3. Practice that establishes knowledge and skills as an advanced practice nurse

4. Advanced practice nurses, including clinical nurse specialists, are those with a registered nurse license and a master's degree in a clinical area of nursing from an accredited educational institution ("ANA hails Congress' support," 1997; "NP and CNS Medicare reimbursement," 1997).

B. Educator

1. Provide staff orientation and education for new employees and continuing education on the importance of assessment and provision of care for the psychosocial needs of the client with disability or chronic illness, including his or her support system.

2. Serve as mentor or preceptor for new nurses or students of nursing.

3. Develop and provide client education, including identification of psychosocial problems and care planning for those with disability and chronic illness. The advanced practice nurse can also identify important supportive resources for the client and family.

4. Prepare educational media such as textbooks, articles, handbooks, videos, and PowerPoint presentations focusing on the psychosocial impact of disability and chronic illnesses for the client and family.

5. The educator role in advanced practice nursing is seen in nursing homes (Mezey et al., 2005; Miller, 1995), acute care, rehabilitation units or facilities, subacute rehabilitation settings, outpatient rehabilitation facilities, and extended care facilities.

C. Clinician

1. Serve as a role model, mentor, or preceptor for the care of clients with psychosocial concerns such as stress, depression, denial, frustration, and grief.

2. Conduct advanced assessment for clients and family members experiencing psychosocial stress.

3. Develop care plans, practice guidelines, and critical pathways for clients with disability or chronic disease, focusing on acute or chronic psychosocial stress.

4. Participate in interdisciplinary groups to plan patient rehabilitation care and discharge planning. Collaboration with psychologists, social workers, counselors, vocational education counselors, and spiritual leaders is useful in addressing psychosocial stress for those with disability or chronic illness.

D. Researcher

1. Identify problems in patient care and delivery of care that warrant additional research. The advanced practice rehabilitation nurse has a unique opportunity to identify pertinent problems to stimulate research.

2. Serve on the human subjects review committee in a healthcare facility to ensure ethical practice in research.

3. Develop research proposals for studies in health care. Many CRRNs also have master's and doctoral degrees. These prepare the nurse to develop and conduct qualitative and quantitative studies for evidence-based practice. The studies often focus on the psychosocial needs of the client with disabilities or chronic illness and the client's family.

4. Disseminate research findings through presentations and publications. The Association of Rehabilitation Nurses provides opportunities for podium and poster presentations of research findings at the local, regional, and national level. The journal *Rehabilitation Nursing* provides an opportunity for the rehabilitation nurse to share important study results and suggestions for using the findings in practice.

5. Nurses can conduct research and evaluate the results of interventions in any setting with rehabilitation clients and their families.

6. Evidence-Based Practice as Applied to Rehabilitation Nursing

   a. Scope: Rehabilitation nurses care for the entire person as a social, psychological, physiological, and cognitive being. Past research and publications support the concept that the psychosocial aspects of disability can positively or negatively influence the outcome of rehabilitation. The plan of care should be based on the best research to enable evidence-based practice for the psychosocial needs of the client with disability.

   b. Clinical question: Can social support systems positively influence adaptation and rehabilitation for people with disability, as compared with other psychosocial interventions?

   c. Appraisal of Research Evidence Focused on the Clinical Question

E. Consultant or Leader

  1. Keep current on legislation focusing on those with disability and chronic disease.

  2. Remain active politically to protect the rights of those with disability and chronic illness. Advanced practice nurses are aware of many barriers clients with disabilities or chronic illnesses face. The barriers to positive QOL can be physical or more covert psychological barriers.

  3. Communicate with administrators and legislators about the needs of those with disability or chronic illness.

  4. Serve as a consultant regarding clients with rehabilitation needs. The advanced practice nurse can provide psychosocial care from the time of injury or illness diagnosis, through treatment and rehabilitation care, to tertiary care after discharge.

  5. Brunk (1992) wrote that the position of clinical nurse specialist often is eliminated when there are shortages of bedside nurses, budget constraints, and limited resources. To provide needed services, advanced practice nurses can act as external consultants on an as-needed basis.

F. Administrator

  1. Identify and support the role of advanced practicing nursing in rehabilitation settings. It is important that advanced practice nurses in an administrative role support the psychosocial and physical care of the client.

  2. Establish contracts with healthcare providers such as Medicare.

  3. Establish collaboration between facilities for services.

  4. Develop budgets and contracts to provide services that support both psychological care and physical rehabilitation care.

  5. Recruit and maintain a qualified staff to provide healthcare services.

  6. Supervise staff to provide high-quality health care. Criteria for excellence in health care should address all client and family needs, including psychosocial care and support.

G. Reimbursement as an Advanced Practice Nurse

  1. Advanced practice nurses, including nurse practitioners and clinical nurse specialists, deliver cost-effective, time-sensitive, high-quality health care to many populations in need, such as the poor and older adults. Pilot projects involving the care of the rural older adults since 1994 support these results of practice ("ANA hails Congress' support," 1997). Advanced practice nurses working with clients having disabilities or chronic illnesses can provide long-term psychosocial support in underserved areas.

  2. Documentation is essential to identify the roles and responsibilities of the advanced practice nurse, the contribution to health care, the cost effectiveness of the practice, client satisfaction, and the health outcomes of the practice.

  3. A study by Dellasega and Zerbe (2000) used both qualitative and quantitative research methods to identify the roles and cost effectiveness of advanced practice nursing. Findings of this study indicated that older adults receiving care involving advanced practice nurses had fewer emergency room visits and hospital readmissions. Caregivers reported significantly fewer work days missed. Clients reported that care by advanced practice nurses was more comprehensive for older adults and their caregivers.

    1) A qualitative study by Isaksson et al. (2005) found that women saw social networking as necessary to manage meaningful employment after injury. Level VI study with good evidence.

    2) A qualitative study by Smith, Jackson, et al. (2006) found that social support was less effective than spiritual support and client and family education for coping with disability. Level VI study with fair evidence because of its small sample size.

    3) Hill et al. (2004) compared coping among subjects who had social support via computers, those receiving written information, and a control group without intervention. Findings indicated that

online support groups had the most impact on coping, stress reduction, and QOL. Level I study with good evidence.

4) A study by Fairfax (2002) found that social support had an indirect relationship with QOL after a stroke. Level V study with fair evidence because of its nonrandomized sample.

5) In a survey conducted by Rintala, Robinson-Whelen, and Matamoros (2005), disabled veterans stated that lack of social support made them more vulnerable to the negative impact of stress. Level IV study with fair evidence because of its nonrandomized sample.

6) Elfstrom et al. (2005) found that social support improved QOL and coping among those with SCI. Level IV study with good evidence.

7) Song (2005) found that family support and client education were correlated with social reintegration for those with SCI. Level IV study with fair evidence because of its lack of randomized sample.

8) Antle (2004) found that the social support of close friends and family members were significantly correlated with self-worth among those with spina bifida. Level IV study with poor evidence because of the wide age range of subjects.

9) Hughes et al. (2001) found that high levels of stress were correlated with a lack of social support. Level IV study with fair evidence because of the lack of randomized sample.

4. Summary:
   1) One Level I study with good evidence
   2) One Level IV study with good evidence
   3) Three Level IV studies with fair evidence
   4) One Level V study with fair evidence
   5) One Level VI study with good evidence
   6) One Level VI study with fair evidence

5. Recommendation for best rehabilitation nursing practice: There is fair to good evidence that social support has a positive impact on the psychosocial rehabilitation of those with disability. There is a great need for Level I evidence based on controlled trials, randomized sampling with control and intervention groups of subjects, and adequate sample sizes for the studies. The current evidence did not compare the social support plan of care with other psychosocial interventions except for one study.

References

Abjornsson, G., Orbaek, P., & Hagstadius, S. (1998). Chronic toxic encephalopathy: Social consequences and experiences from a rehabilitation program. *Rehabilitation Nursing, 23*(1), 38–43.

ANA hails Congress' support for NP and CNS reimbursement. (1997). *Massachusetts Nurse, 67*(8), 1–2.

Anderson, K.H., & Tomlinson, P.S. (1992). The family health system as an emerging paradigmatic view for nursing. *Image: The Journal of Nursing Scholarship, 24*(1), 57–63.

Antle, B.J. (2004). Factors associated with self-worth in young people with disabilities. *Health and Social Work, 29*(3), 167–175.

Bandura, A. (1977). Self-efficacy: Toward a unifying theory of behavioral change. *Psychological Review, 84,* 191–215.

Barry, P.D. (1996). *Psychosocial nursing care of physically ill patients and their families* (3rd ed.). New York: Lippincott.

Berman, C., & Rose, L. (1998). Examination of a patient's adaptation to quadriplegia. *Physical Therapy Case Reports, 1*(3), 148–156.

Bethoux, F., Calmels, P., Gautheron, V., & Minaire, P. (1996). Quality of life of spouses of stroke patients: A preliminary study. *International Journal of Rehabilitation and Health, 2*(3), 189–198.

Boraz, M., & Heinemann, A. (1996). The relationship between social support and alcohol abuse in people with spinal cord injuries. *International Journal of Rehabilitation and Health, 2*(3), 189–199.

Brillhart, B. (2005). A study of spirituality and life satisfaction among persons with spinal cord injury. *Rehabilitation Nursing, 30*(1), 31–34.

Brillhart, B., & Johnson, K. (1997). Motivation and the coping process of adults with disabilities: A qualitative study. *Rehabilitation Nursing, 22*(5), 249–256.

Brunk, Q.A. (1992). The clinical nurse specialist as an external consultant: A framework for practice. *Clinical Nurse Specialist, 6*(1), 2–4.

Brzuzy, S., & Speziale, B. (1997). Persons with traumatic brain injuries and their families: Living arrangements and well-being post injury. *Social Work in Health Care, 26*(1), 77–88.

Burleigh, S.A., Farber, R.S., & Gillard, M. (1998). Community integration and life satisfaction after traumatic brain injury: Long-term findings. *American Journal of Occupational Therapy, 52*(1), 45–52.

Butcher, L.A. (1994). A family-focused perspective on chronic illness. *Rehabilitation Nursing, 19*(2), 70–74.

Captain, C. (1995). The effects of communication skills training on interaction and psychosocial adjustment among couples living with spinal cord injury. *Rehabilitation Nursing Research, 4*(4), 111–118.

Cardol, M., Elvers, J., Oostendorp, R., Brandsma, J., & deGroot, I. (1996). Quality of life in patients with amyotrophic lateral sclerosis. *Journal of Rehabilitation Sciences, 9*(4), 99–103.

Carmine, H.M., & Murphy, M.P. (2006, October). *Surviving suicide, a call to action: Essential risk assessment.* Paper presentation at the conference of the Association of Rehabilitation Nurses, Chicago, IL.

Clancy, F. (2006). Shortcutting darkness. *Neurology Now, 2*(4), 30–33.

Clark, M.S. (2000). Patient and spouse perceptions of stroke and its rehabilitation. *International Journal of Rehabilitation Research, 23*(1), 19–29.

Cormier-Daigle, M., & Stewart, M. (1997). Support and coping of male hemodialysis-dependent patients. *International Journal of Nursing Studies, 34*(6), 420–430.

Crowe, M., & Lutz, S. (2005). Nonpharmacological treatments for older adults with depression. *Geriatrics & Aging, 8*(8), 30–33.

Dacey, J., & Fiori, L. (2006). Psychological development: Challenges of adulthood. In K. Theis & J. Travers (Eds.), *Handbook of human development for health care professionals* (pp. 219–242). Boston: Jones and Bartlett.

Dacey, J., & Margolis, D. (2006). Psychological development: Adolescence and sexuality. In K. Thies & J. Travers (Eds.), *Handbook of human development for health care professionals* (pp. 191–218). Boston: Jones and Bartlett.

Davidhizar, R. (1997). Disability does not have to be the grief that never ends: Helping patients adjust. *Rehabilitation Nursing, 22*(1), 32–35.

Dellasega, C.A., & Zerbe, T.M. (2000). A multimethod study of advanced practice nurse postdischarge care. *Clinical Excellence for Nurse Practitioners, 4*(5), 286–293.

Deutsch, P.M., Allison, L., & Cimino-Ferguson, S. (2005). Life care planning assessments and their impact on life in spinal cord injury. *Topics in Spinal Cord Rehabilitation, 10*(4), 135–145.

Diamond, P., Holroyd, S., Macciocchi, S., & Felsenthal, G. (1995). Prevalence of depression and outcome of geriatric rehabilitation unit. *American Journal of Physical Medicine and Rehabilitation, 74*(3), 214–217.

Diener, E. (1984). Subjective well-being. *Psychological Bulletin, 95*(3), 542–575.

Easton, K., Zemen, D., & Kwiatkowski, S. (1995). The effects of nursing follow-up on the coping strategies used by rehabilitation patients after discharge. *Rehabilitation Nursing Research, 4*(4), 119–126.

Elfstrom, M.L., Ryden, A., Kreuter, M., Taft, C., & Sullivan, M. (2005). Relations between coping strategies and health-related quality of life in patients with spinal cord lesion. *Journal of Rehabilitation Medicine, 31*(1), 9–16.

Erikson, E. (1963). *Childhood and society.* New York: W.W. Norton.

Fairfax, J. (2002). *Theory of quality of life of stroke survivors.* Doctoral dissertation, Wayne State University, Detroit, MI.

Faull, K., & Hills, M. (2006). The role of the spiritual dimension of the self as the prime determinant of health. *Disability and Rehabilitation, 28*(11), 729–740.

Ferguson, A.D., Richie, B.S., & Gomez, M.J. (2004). Psychological factors after traumatic amputation in landmine survivors: The bridge between physical healing and full recovery. *Disability and Rehabilitation, 26*(14/15), 931–938.

Ferrans, C.E. (1996). Development of a conceptual model of quality of life. *Scholarly Inquiry for Nursing Practice: An International Journal, 10*(3), 293–304.

Ferrin, J.M. (2002). *Acceptance of loss after an adult-onset disability: Development and psychometric validation of the Multidimensional Acceptance of Loss Scale.* Doctoral dissertation, University of Wisconsin–Madison.

Flannery, J. (1998). Using the Levels of Cognitive Functioning Assessment Scale with patients with traumatic brain injury in an acute care setting. *Rehabilitation Nursing, 23*(3), 88–94.

Goffman, E. (1974). *Stigma.* New York: Jason Aronson.

Grzankowski, J.A. (1997). Altered thought processes related to traumatic brain injury and their nursing implications. *Rehabilitation Nursing, 22*(1), 24–28.

Hammell, K. (1994). Psychosocial outcome following severe closed head injury. *International Journal of Rehabilitation Research, 17*(4), 319–332.

Harrison, T.C., & Stuifbergen, A. (2006). Life purpose: Effect on functional decline and quality of life in polio survivors. *Rehabilitation Nursing, 31*(4), 149–154.

Hayes, E., Balfanz-Vertiz, K., & Ostrander, R.N. (2005). Building pathways to education and employment among individuals with spinal cord injury. *SCI Psychosocial Process, 18*(1), 17–26.

Hill, W., Schillo, L., & Weinert, C. (2004). Effect of a computer-based intervention on social support for chronically ill rural women. *Rehabilitation Nursing, 29*(5), 169–173.

Howell, D. (1998). Reaching to the depths of the soul: Understanding and exploring meaning in illness. *Canadian Oncology Nursing Journal, 8*(1), 22–23.

Hughes, R.B., Swedlund, N., Petersen, N., & Nosek, M.A. (2001). Depression and women with spinal cord injury. *Topics in Spinal Cord Injury Rehabilitation, 7*(1), 16–24.

Isaksson, G., Skar, L., & Lexell, J. (2005). Women's perceptions of changes in the social network after a spinal cord injury. *Disability and Rehabilitation, 27*(17), 1013–1021.

Jansen, D., & Keller, M. (1998). Identifying the attention demands perceived by elderly people. *Rehabilitation Nursing, 23*(1), 12–19.

Jarvis, C. (2004). *Physical examination and health assessment* (4th ed.). St. Louis: Saunders.

Johnson, K.A., & Klaas, S.J. (2000). Recreation involvement and play in a pediatric spinal cord injury population. *Topics in Spinal Cord Injury Rehabilitation, 6*(Suppl.), 105–109.

Johnston, T., Lauer, R.T., & Smith, B.T. (2006). Differences in scores between children with spinal cord injury and their parents using the Pediatric Quality of Life Inventory. *Pediatric Physical Therapy, 18*(1), 94–96.

Kautz, D.D. (2006, October). *Inspiring hope in our patients, their families, and ourselves.* Paper presented at the conference of the Association of Rehabilitation Nurses, Chicago, IL.

Kelly-Hayes, M. (1996). Functional evaluation. In S.P. Hoeman (Ed.), *Rehabilitation nursing: Process and application* (2nd ed., pp. 144–155). St. Louis: Mosby.

Knowles, M.S. (1984). *Andragogy in action.* San Francisco: Jossey-Bass.

Lazarus, R.S., & Folkman, S. (1984). *Stress, appraisal, and coping.* New York: Springer.

Leger, R.R. (2005). Severity of illness, functional status, and HRQOL in youth with spina bifida. *Rehabilitation Nursing, 30*(5), 180–187.

Livneh, M.E., Priebe, H., Wuermser, M., & Ottomanelli, L. (2005). Predictors of psychosocial adaptation among people with spinal cord injury or disorder. *Archives of Physical Medicine and Rehabilitation, 86*(6), 1182–1892.

Lohne, V., & Severinsson, E. (2006). The power of hope: Patients' experiences of hope a year after acute spinal cord injury. *Journal of Clinical Nursing, 15*(3), 315–523.

Lund, M.L., Nordlund, A., Nygard, L., Lexell, J., & Bernspang, B. (2005). Perceptions of participation and predictors of perceived problems with participation in persons with spinal cord injury. *Journal of Rehabilitation Medicine, 37*(1), 3–8.

Mezey, M., Greene, B.S., Bloom, H.G., Bourbonniere, M., Bowers, B., Burl, J.B., et al. (2005). Experts recommend strategies for strengthening the use of advanced practice nurses in nursing homes. *Journal of American Geriatric Society, 53*(10), 1790–1797.

Miller, S.E. (1995). The role of the clinical nurse specialist in home health care. *Journal of Home Health Care Practice, 7*(2), 62–72.

Montgomery, P., Kitten, M., & Niemiec, C. (1997). The agitated patient with brain injury and the rehabilitation staff: Bridging the gap of misunderstanding. *Rehabilitation Nursing, 22*(3), 20–23, 39.

Nathenson, N. (2006, October). *A new model in outpatient cardiac rehabilitation.* Paper presented at the conference of the Association of Rehabilitation Nurses, Chicago, IL.

Nelson, P.J., & Tucker, S. (2006). Developing an intervention to alter catastrophizing in persons with fibromyalgia. *Orthopaedic Nursing, 25*(3), 205–214.

Newton, M. (2006). Mental health disorders. In J. Rhoads (Ed.), *Advanced health assessment and diagnostic reasoning* (pp. 43–66). Philadelphia: Lippincott Williams & Wilkins.

Nir, Z., Wallhagen, M., Doolittle, N., & Galinsky, D. (1997). A study of the psychosocial characteristics of patients in a geriatric rehabilitation unit in Israel. *Rehabilitation Nursing, 22*(3), 143–151.

Norris, J., & Spelic, S.S. (2002). Supporting adaptation to body image disruption. *Rehabilitation Nursing, 27*(1), 8–10.

NP and CNS Medicare reimbursement. (1997, October). *Kansas Nurse, 72*(9), 10.

Nypaver, J., Titus, M., & Brugler, C. (1996). Patient transfer to rehabilitation: Just another move? *Rehabilitation Nursing, 21*(2), 94–97.

Pallett, P.J., & O'Brien, M.T. (1985). *Textbook of neurological nursing.* Boston: Little, Brown.

Paterson, J., & Stewart, J. (2002). Adults with acquired brain injury: Perceptions of their social world. *Rehabilitation Nursing, 27*(1), 13–18.

Pavlov, I. (1927). *Conditioned reflexes.* London: Oxford University Press.

Pentland, W., Harvey, A., & Walker, J. (1998). The relationships between time use and health and well-being in men with spinal cord injury. *Journal of Occupational Science, 5*(1), 14–25.

Piaget, J. (1952). *The origins of intelligence in children.* New York: Norton.

Ponsford, J., Willmott, C., Rothwell, A., Camerson, P., Ayton, G., Nelms, R., et al. (1999). Cognitive and behavioral outcome following mild traumatic head injury in children. *Journal of Head Trauma Rehabilitation, 14*(4), 360–372.

Price, T. (2006, October). *Behavioral strategies for management of disruptive behaviors associated with CHI.* Paper presented at the conference of the Association of Rehabilitation Nurses, Chicago, IL.

Reeves, J. (2006, October 9). Wounded warriors, *Tribune,* p. A8.

Remington, R., Abdallah, L., Melillo, K., & Flanagan, K. (2006). Managing problem behaviors associated with dementia. *Rehabilitation Nursing, 31*(5), 186–191.

Resnick, B., Zimmerman, S., Magaziner, J., & Adelman, A. (1998). Use of the Apathy Evaluation Scale as a measure of motivation in elderly people. *Rehabilitation Nursing, 23*(3), 141–147.

Reynolds, F. (2003). Reclaiming a positive identity in chronic illness through artistic occupation. *Occupation, Participation and Health, 23*(3), 118–127.

Riedel, D., & Shaw, V. (1997). Nursing management of patients with brain injury requiring one-on-one care. *Rehabilitation Nursing, 22*(1), 36–39.

Riegel, B., Dracup, K., & Glaser, D. (1998). A longitudinal model of cardiac invalidism following myocardial infarction. *Nursing Research, 47*(5), 285–292.

Rintala, D. H., Robinson-Whelen, S., & Matamoros, R. (2005). Subjective stress in male veterans with spinal cord injury. *Journal of Rehabilitation Research and Development, 42*(3), 291–304.

Rintala, D., Young, M., Spencer, J., & Bates, P. (1996). Family relationships and adaptation to spinal cord injury: A qualitative study. *Rehabilitation Nursing, 21*(2), 67–74.

Ross, S.M. (2000). Profound retrograde amnesia following mild head injury: Organic or functional? *Cortex, 36*(4), 521–537.

Santos, E., Boyle, L.L., & Lyness, J.M. (2005). *Geriatrics & Aging, 8*(8), 42–45.

Satir, V. (1988). *The new peoplemaker.* Mountain View, CA: Science and Behavior Books.

Scivoletto, G., Petrelli, A., Di-Lucente, L., & Castellano, V. (1997). Psychological investigation of spinal cord injury patients. *Spinal Cord, 35*(8), 516–520.

Secrest, J.A. (2006, October). *The relationship of continuity, functional ability, depression, quality of life over time in stroke survivors.* Paper presented at the conference of the Association of Rehabilitation Nurses, Chicago, IL.

Shah, R.C., & Bennett, D.A. (2006). Diagnosis and management of mild cognitive impairment. *Geriatrics & Aging, 8*(8), 53–56.

Sherman, J.E., Sperling, K.B., & DeVinney, D.J. (2004). Social support and adjustment after spinal cord injury: Influence of past peer-mentoring experiences and current live-in partner. *Rehabilitation Psychology, 49*(2), 140–149.

Skinner, B.F. (1974). *About behaviorism.* New York: Alfred Knopf.

Smith, A., & Schwirian, P. (1998). The relationship between caregiver burden and the TBI survivor's cognition and functional ability after discharge. *Rehabilitation Nursing, 23*(5), 252–257.

Smith, C.R., Cook, S., Frost, K., Jones, M., & Wright, P. (2006). A comparison of coping strategies of adolescents with and without physical disabilities. *Pediatric Physical Therapy, 18*(1), 105–106.

Smith, C.R., Jackson, L., & Sharpe, L. (2006). Coping behaviors of parents with school age/latency age children with disabilities. *Pediatric Physical Therapy, 18*(1), 106.

Smith, J., Magill-Evans, J., & Brintnell, S. (1998). Life satisfaction following traumatic brain injury. *Canadian Journal of Rehabilitation, 11*(3), 131–140.

Snell, R.S. (1980). *Clinical neuroanatomy for medical students.* Boston: Little, Brown.

Song, H. (2005). Modeling social reintegration in persons with spinal cord injury. *Disability and Rehabilitation, 27*(3), 131–141.

Spalding, J.A. (2005). Challenges of mentoring a brain-injured peer. *Rehabilitation Nursing, 30*(1), 3, 6.

Spatt, J., Zebenholzer, K., & Oder, W. (1997). Psychosocial long-term outcome of severe head injury as perceived by patients, relatives, and professionals. *Acta Neurologica Scandinavica, 95*(3), 173–179.

Steffens, D.C., Maytan, M., Helms, M.J., & Plassman, B.L. (2005). Prevalence and clinical correlates of neuropsychiatric symptoms in dementia. *American Journal of Alzheimer's Disease and Other Dementias, 20*(6), 367–373.

Stuart, G.W., & Laraia, M.T. (1995). *Principles and practice of psychiatric nursing.* St. Louis: Mosby.

Stuifbergen, A. (1992) Meeting the demands of illness: Types and sources of support for individuals with multiple sclerosis and their partners, *Rehabilitation Nursing, 1*(1), 14–23.

Stuifbergen, A. (2005). Secondary conditions and life satisfaction among polio survivors. *Rehabilitation Nursing, 30*(5), 173–178.

Thomas, J. (2006, October). *Wheeling into life: Wheelchair sports and rehabilitation.* Paper presented at the conference of the Association of Rehabilitation Nurses, Chicago, IL.

Tollen, A., & Ahlstrom, G. (1998). Assessment instrument for problem-focused coping: Reliability of APC, Part I. *Scandinavian Journal of Caring Sciences, 12*(1), 18–24.

Townsend, E., Lohr, J.L., & Nelson, C.A. (2006). Neurocognitive sequelae of repaired congenital heart disease. *Pediatric Physical Therapy, 18*(1), 107.

Travers, J. (2006). Cognitive development. In K. Theis & Travers, J. (Eds.), *Handbook of human development for health care professionals* (pp. 113–138). Boston: Jones and Bartlett.

Walton, J., Craig, C., Derwinski-Robinson, B., & Weinert, C. (2004). I am not alone: Spirituality of chronically ill rural dwellers. *Rehabilitation Nursing, 29*(5), 164–168.

Warren, L., Wrigley, J., Yoels, W., & Fine, P. (1996). Factors associated with life satisfaction among a sample of persons with neurotrauma. *Journal of Rehabilitation Research and Development, 33*(4), 404–408.

Weeks, S., & O'Connor, P. (1997). The FAMTOOL family assessment tool. *Rehabilitation Nursing, 22*(4), 188–191.

Wertheimer, M. (1959). *Productive thinking.* New York: Harper & Row.

Williams, A.M., & Dahl, C.W. (2002). Patient and caregiver perceptions of stroke survivor behavior: A comparison. *Rehabilitation Nursing, 27*(1), 19–24.

Yuen, H.K., Burik, J.K., & Krause, J.S. (2004). Physical and psychosocial well-being among adults with spinal cord injury. *Topics in Spinal Cord Injury Rehabilitation, 9*(4), 19–25.

Section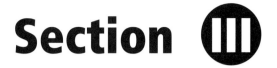

Nursing Management of Common Rehabilitation Disorders

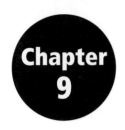

Chapter 9

Stroke

Carla J. Howard, MS RN CRRN • Kristen L. Mauk, PhD RN CRRN-A APRN BC

Stroke or "brain attack" (also called cerebrovascular accident [CVA]) affects hundreds of thousands of people each year. The effects of stroke may be slight or severe, temporary or permanent, and can be devastating to the person and the family. Patients who have had a stroke must cope with numerous sensorimotor, visual, perceptual, and language deficits. Rehabilitation should begin as soon after the stroke as possible. In patients who are stable, rehabilitation may begin within 2 days after the stroke has occurred and should be continued as necessary after the patient leaves the hospital. Rehabilitation is a team effort that focuses on regaining as much functional independence as possible. Rehabilitation also plays a major role in helping to prevent secondary complications and some long-term disabilities. To intervene effectively as a member of the rehabilitation team, nurses should have a good understanding of the physiological, perceptual, and psychological changes that occur after stroke.

I. Overview of Stroke

A. Description

1. A stroke is a sudden, nonconvulsive focal neurological deficit (Boss, 2002a).

2. A stroke, or brain attack, is an emergency; time is brain.

3. There are two major types of stroke: ischemic stroke and hemorrhagic stroke.

4. A stroke occurs when a blood clot blocks a blood vessel or artery (ischemic) or when a blood vessel breaks, interrupting blood flow to an area of the brain (hemorrhagic) (National Stroke Association [NSA], 2006d).

5. When a stroke occurs, blood flow to that part of the brain is disrupted, resulting in tissue anoxia and death of brain cells (infarction).

6. Neurons near the ischemic or infarcted areas undergo changes that disrupt plasma membranes, causing cellular edema and further compression of capillaries. Most people survive an initial hemispheric ischemic stroke unless there is massive cerebral edema (Boss, 2002a).

7. Massive brainstem infarcts from basilar thrombosis or embolism almost always are fatal. With hemorrhagic strokes, focal neurological deficits are found in 80% of people, and altered consciousness occurs in 50% of people (Boss, 2002a).

8. The economic cost is greater than $40 billion per year (Boss, 2002a).

B. Epidemiology (NSA, 2006b)

1. Stroke is the third leading cause of death in the United States, after heart disease and cancer.

2. 160,000 people per year die as a result of a stroke.

3. Stroke is the number one cause of adult disability.

4. Each year, 750,000 Americans have a stroke, and 1 out of every 5 will have another stroke within 5 years. In that 5-year period 24% of women and 42% of men have a second stroke.

5. Secondary strokes often have a higher rate of disability and death because parts of the brain that are already damaged by the original stroke may not be as able to withstand another insult.

6. Up to 35% of all people who experience a transient ischemic attack (TIA) go on to have a stroke.

7. Stroke occurs more often in people with risk factors that cannot be changed, such as being over the age of 55, being male or African American, having a family history of stroke, or having a history of diabetes. Others at risk include those who are of Hispanic or Asian/Pacific Islander origin.

8. The rate of first strokes in African Americans is almost twice the number of Caucasians, and African Americans are twice as likely to die from strokes as Caucasians.

9. The incidence of stroke in children is low, about 3 cases per 100,000 children per year. Strokes are slightly more common in children less than 2 years old.

C. Etiology (Buttaro, 2003; Graykoski, 2003; Sugerman, 2002)

1. Ischemic or hemorrhagic disruption of cerebral arteries is the major cause of stroke.

2. The arterial blood supply to the brain comes from the internal carotid arteries and the vertebral arteries. The internal carotid arteries supply the anterior portion of the brain with a greater amount of blood flow and originate from the common carotid arteries. They enter the cranium through the base of the skull, passing through the cavernous sinus and then branching off into the anterior and middle cerebral arteries. The vertebral arteries are posterior and originate as branches off the subclavian arteries. They pass through the foramen magnum and join at the junction of the pons and medulla oblongata to form the basilar artery. The basilar artery divides at the level of the midbrain to form the two posterior cerebral arteries (Sugerman, 2002).

3. The arterial circle (circle of Willis) is the structure in the brain with the ability to compensate for reduced blood flow from any of the major contributors (collateral blood flow). This circle is formed by the posterior cerebral arteries, posterior communicating arteries, internal carotid arteries, anterior cerebral arteries, and anterior communicating artery.

4. Ischemic stroke is the most prevalent, is occlusive in nature as the result of a cerebral embolism or cerebral thrombosis, and is categorized by vascular distribution or location.

5. Hemorrhagic stroke has a lower incidence than ischemic stroke but is associated with a higher mortality rate. A subarachnoid stroke is a rupture of a large vessel in the protective lining of the brain, and an intracerebral stroke is the rupture of a vessel in the brain itself.

6. TIAs are small ischemic events, often lasting only minutes, in which the neurological deficit resolves completely within a few hours and no longer than 24 hours (American Stroke Association [ASA], 2005).

7. There are several risk factors for stroke, many of which are preventable.
   a. Hypertension
   b. Obesity
   c. Smoking
   d. Diabetes
   e. Hypercholesteremia and hyperlipidemia
   f. Heavy ingestion of alcohol
   g. Sedentary lifestyle (lack of regular exercise)
   h. Cardiac disorders (e.g., atrial fibrillation)
   i. Carotid artery disease
   j. Family history of stroke
   k. Blood disorders (e.g., sickle cell anemia, polycythemia).
   l. TIA or previous stroke
   m. Older age: Approximately 72% of strokes occur in people who are at least 65 years of age or older (Hinkle, 2006).
   n. Gender: Stroke is most prevalent in men; however, women who use oral contraceptives, smoke, and have migraines are at a higher risk (Buttaro, 2003; Graykoski, 2003).
   o. Race: Stroke is more common in African Americans, Hispanics, and Pacific Islanders (NSA, 2006a).
   p. Substance abuse (e.g., cocaine, amphetamines, other illegal drugs) (Buttaro, 2003; Graykoski, 2003)

D. Signs and Symptoms of Stroke (NSA, 2006d)
   1. Sudden numbness or weakness of face, arm, or leg, especially unilaterally
   2. Sudden confusion, trouble speaking or understanding
   3. Sudden trouble seeing in one or both eyes
   4. Sudden ataxia, dizziness, loss of balance or coordination
   5. Sudden severe headache with no known cause

E. Pathophysiology
   1. Ischemic stroke (approximately 85%–88% of all strokes) (Buttaro, 2003; Sauerbeck, 2006)
      a. Process (Boss, 2002a; Buttaro, 2003)
         1) Begins as a result of atherosclerotic disease and progresses slowly as the affected artery becomes narrowed and eventually occluded. May also occur as a result of a rupture of an atherosclerotic plaque that travels as an embolus to the brain and blocks blood flow.
         2) Atherosclerotic plaques (stenotic lesions) form at branches and curves in the cerebral circulation. The stenotic area degenerates, which forms an ulcerated vessel wall. Platelets and fibrin adhere to the damaged wall and form clots, which eventually occlude the artery.
         3) The thrombus may enlarge in the vessel distally and proximally, or a portion of the clot may break off and travel up the vessel to a distant site, forming an embolus.

4) Focal areas of the brain and adjoining brain tissue are deprived of oxygen and glucose. When the deprivation is severe enough and lasts long enough, permanent damage occurs.

b. Types of ischemic strokes
  1) TIA (Keiser, 1999):
    a) Persists for several minutes or hours and then resolves.
    b) Usually lasts 5–15 minutes, followed by full recovery of neurological function within 24 hours; the majority last less than 1 hour.
    c) Resolution results in a negative neurological examination, and diagnosis may be based on history.
    d) People who experience TIA may have 9 times the risk of a stroke, and often this occurs within 30 days of the TIA. (A valid estimate of the incidence of TIA is not available because many go unreported because of the subtle nature of the symptoms.) After a stroke many patients or families report episodes that were likely to be TIAs preceding the stroke.
    e) Vertebrobasilar TIA is the result of inadequate blood flow from the vertebral arteries, usually secondary to a partially obstructed subclavian artery, which supplies this area (Keiser, 1999).
    f) Carotid TIA is the result of inadequate blood flow from the carotid artery, usually because of carotid stenosis.
  2) Reversible ischemic neurological deficit is a TIA or signs of a stroke that persist over 24 hours but eventually resolve completely, usually within 48 hours.
  3) Embolic stroke:
    a) A traveling clot, which typically originates from thrombi in the heart or from plaque in the aortic arch or carotid or vertebral arteries that becomes lodged and obstructs cerebral blood flow
    b) Commonly associated with history of cardiac disease, especially atrial fibrillation in older people
  4) Thrombotic stroke:
    a) Most common cause of stroke
    b) A stationary clot in a large blood vessel, usually caused by atherosclerotic plaque
      (1) Plaque forms when calcium and lipids collect and attach to the vessel wall, especially in bifurcations of a large artery. This produces narrowing that impedes or obstructs blood flow.
      (2) Atherosclerosis can produce degeneration of blood vessel walls. Can involve tearing or degeneration of a weakened vessel wall or plaque, which can trigger the normal clotting process, and this congestion further reduces circulation to the area.
      (3) Large vessel thrombosis: Thrombotic strokes occur most often in large arteries and usually are caused by a combination of long-term atherosclerosis followed by rapid blood clot formation. Thrombotic stroke patients are likely to have coronary artery disease, and heart attack is a common cause of death in patients who have had this type of stroke (NSA, 2006d).
  5) Lacunar infarcts (small vessel disease) (NSA, 2006d):
    a) Thrombotic strokes that affect the small arteries deep within the white matter of the brain (Buttaro, 2003; Graykoski, 2003)
    b) Are microinfarcts smaller than 1 cm in diameter and involve the small perforating arteries, predominantly in the basal ganglia, internal capsules, and pons (Boss, 2002b)
    c) Are caused by atherosclerosis
    d) Often result in pure motor or sensory deficits
    e) Are closely linked to hypertension or diabetes

c. Risk factors for ischemic strokes (Boss, 2002a)
  1) Arterial hypertension; elevated systolic and diastolic blood pressures are independent risk factors.
  2) Smoking increases the risk by 50%.
  3) Diabetes increases the risk by 2.5–3.5 times.

4) Insulin resistance is an independent risk factor.
5) Thrombocythemia and polycythemia increase the risk.
6) Impaired cardiac function and atrial fibrillation.
7) Elevated lipoprotein (a) is an independent risk factor.
8) Hyperhomocysteinemia is a strong and independent risk factor.
9) Estrogen deficiency in postmenopausal women increases the risk.

2. Hemorrhagic stroke (approximately 12%–15% of strokes) (Graykoski, 2003; Sauerbeck, 2006)
   a. Process (Boss, 2002a; Graykoski, 2003)
      1) Spontaneous rupture of a cerebral vessel occurs; blood enters the brain tissue or subarachnoid space.
      2) Most common causes of hemorrhagic stroke are hypertension (56% –81%), ruptured aneurysms, vascular malformations, bleeding into a tumor, hemorrhage from bleeding disorders or anticoagulation, head trauma, and illicit drug use (Boss, 2002a).
      3) The area around the injury dies within a few minutes from lack of oxygen and the failure of oxygen-dependent adenosine triphosphate metabolic pathway. The broader area of injury is called the penumbra, and this damage is more dynamic, taking 12–24 hours. The release of intracellular calcium initiates the programmed cell death or apoptosis (Graykoski, 2003).
   b. Types of hemorrhagic stroke
      1) Subarachnoid hemorrhage
         a) Spontaneous subarachnoid hemorrhage is primarily the result of a rupture of an intracranial saccular aneurysm or arteriovenous malformation on the surface of the brain (Graykoski, 2003).
         b) Presents clinically as abrupt onset of a severe headache ("the worst headache of my life"), nausea and vomiting, signs of meningeal irritation, and varying degrees of neurological dysfunction.
         c) Can result in elevated intracranial pressure, vasospasms, and ischemia, which reduces cerebral blood flow further.
      2) Intracerebral (intraparenchymal) hemorrhage
         a) Often caused by hypertension (blood pressure is elevated in almost all cases).
         b) Involves small, deep-penetrating blood vessels that rupture and release blood directly into the brain tissue.
         c) Usually invades deep white matter first.
         d) Neurological signs and symptoms vary with the site and size of the extravasation of blood (released blood puts pressure on surrounding tissue, which can cause small arterioles and capillaries to tear).
         e) May present clinically as an almost immediate lapse into stupor and coma, with hemiplegia and steady deterioration to death over several hours after initial presentation. More often presents with a headache, followed within a few minutes by unilateral neurological deficits involving face and limbs.
         f) Resulting hematoma acts as a space-occupying lesion that, if large enough, will cause brain shifting or herniation.
   c. Risk factors for hemorrhagic stroke
      1) High blood pressure is responsible for approximately 60% of intracerebral hemorrhages and is a controllable stroke risk factor.
      2) Excessive alcohol and drug use are associated with higher incidences of intracerebral hemorrhage and subarachnoid hemorrhage. Cocaine-related strokes are caused by an erosion of the vessel from the cocaine, which causes the vessel wall to become weaker and rupture (Keiser, 1999). Cocaine has been linked to aneurysm formation (Boss, 2002a). About 85%–90% of drug-associated intracerebral hemorrhages occur in people 20–30 years old.
      3) Anticoagulant medication may prevent ischemic stroke but may increase the risk of intracerebral hemorrhage if it is above the therapeutic range.
      4) Blood clotting disorders such as

hemophilia and sickle cell anemia can increase risk.

F. Clinical Manifestations of Stroke (Boss, 2002a; Buttaro, 2003)

1. Anterior cerebral artery supplies medial surfaces and upper areas of frontal and parietal lobes and medial surface of the hemisphere. Signs and symptoms of occlusion:
   a. Confusion
   b. Labile emotions, personality changes
   c. Weakness or numbness on affected side
   d. Paralysis of contralateral foot and leg
   e. Impaired mobility, sensation greater in lower extremities than upper extremities, impaired sensory function
   f. Urinary incontinence
   g. Loss of coordination

2. Middle cerebral artery (most commonly occluded vessel in stroke and the largest branch in the internal carotid artery) supplies part of the frontal lobe and lateral surface of the temporal and parietal lobes, including primary motor and sensory areas for the face, throat, hand, and arm and, in the dominant hemisphere, the areas for speech. Signs and symptoms of occlusion:
   a. Altered level of responsiveness
   b. Alterations in communication, including aphasia, dysphasia, reading difficulty (dyslexia), inability to write (dysgraphia)
   c. Visual field deficits
   d. Alterations in cognition, mobility, and sensation including contralateral sensory deficit and hemiparesis (more severe in the upper than lower)

3. Posterior cerebral artery supplies medial and inferior temporal lobes, medial occipital lobe, thalamus, posterior hypothalamus, and visual receptive area. Signs and symptoms of occlusion:
   a. Hemiplegia
   b. Receptive aphasia
   c. Sensory impairment
   d. Dyslexia
   e. Visual field deficits (cortical blindness from ischemia)
   f. Coma

4. Internal carotid artery supplies the cerebral hemispheres and diencephalon. Signs and symptoms of occlusion:
   a. Headaches
   b. Altered level of responsiveness
   c. Bruits over the carotid artery
   d. Profound aphasia
   e. Ptosis
   f. Unilateral blindness or retinal emboli
   g. Weakness, paralysis, numbness, sensory changes, and visual deficits on the affected side

5. Vertebral or basilar arteries supply the brainstem and cerebellum.
   a. Signs and symptoms of incomplete occlusion
      1) TIA
      2) Unilateral or bilateral weakness of extremities
      3) Visual deficits on affected side such as lack of depth perception, diplopia, or color blindness
      4) Nausea, vertigo, tinnitus
      5) Headache
      6) Dysarthria
      7) Numbness
      8) Dysphagia
      9) "Locked-in" syndrome: no movement except eyelids, sensation and consciousness preserved
   b. Signs and symptoms of complete occlusion
      1) Coma
      2) Decerebrate rigidity
      3) Respiratory and circulatory abnormalities

G. Residual Deficits of Stroke (see Table 9-1)

1. Significant alterations in many psychosocial areas
   a. Diminished affect
   b. Increased dependence in activities of daily living (ADLs)
   c. Decreased self-esteem
   d. Altered role performance
   e. Sexual dysfunction
   f. Change in leisure or social activity
   g. Decreased financial earning or vocational capability

2. General sequelae (all of which can influence safety)
   a. Hemiplegia: weakness or paralysis contralateral to the lesion
   b. Abnormal tone, including flaccidity initially and then hypertonicity on the affected side
   c. Sensorimotor problems, ataxia, imbalance

d. Language deficits if lesion is in the dominant hemisphere

e. Visuospatial perception impairments

f. Cognitive deficits

g. Memory changes

h. Emotional lability: inability to control emotions, especially crying and laughter (these may be expressed at inappropriate times)

i. Fatigue

j. Depression (may persist for months after the stroke)

k. Seizure activity

3. Left hemispheric stroke: common impairments and deficits

a. Right hemiparesis or hemiplegia

b. Impaired ability to think analytically

c. Inability to do mathematical computations or interpret symbols

d. Right homonymous hemianopsia

e. Behavioral changes (e.g., cautiousness, hesitancy)

f. Language difficulty, which includes not only the motor aspect of speech but also the ability to express and understand thoughts, ideas, and symbols in sequence

1) Expressive (Broca's dysphasia or nonfluent) (Boss, 2002a)

a) Occurs with lesions in the posterior part of the dominant frontal lobe (precentral gyrus) and usually is on the left hemisphere

b) Is responsible for the motor aspects of speech

Table 9-1. Residual Deficits of Stroke and Interventions

Manifestations	Left Hemispheric Damage	Interventions
Paresis or paralysis	Right side	Involve affected side during therapy or activities of daily living (ADLs).
Major deficits	Right homonymous hemianopsia; language deficits (e.g., aphasia, expression, comprehension, word finding); confuses left and right; has trouble gesturing, reading, writing	Incorporate techniques used by speech therapist when communicating with patient; use communication board and tools; incorporate affected side into ADLs and activities; use demonstration and positive feedback.
Thought processes	Has difficulty listening and understanding; cannot process incoming language normally	Be patient; work with patient in short timeframes to reduce frustration; offer encouragement; have same staff work with patient when possible; speak slowly.
Emotional style	Is easily frustrated or depressed; is aware of deficits	Be patient; offer encouragement; exhibit acceptance; educate family on realistic expectations for communication; have rehabilitation psychologist work with patient.
Attention span	Usually normal	Limit sessions, care, or treatments based on individual need.
Behavioral style	Is slow and cautious; needs encouragement	Allow plenty of time to work with patient; don't appear rushed; don't fragment care.

Manifestations	Right Hemispheric Damage	Interventions
Paresis or paralysis	Left side	Involve affected side during therapy or ADLs.
Major deficits	Left homonymous hemianopsia; displays visual, spatial, perceptual deficits (e.g., gets lost, cannot dress self correctly, misjudges distance and position in space, spills things, gets stuck in doorways); has distorted body image; may have agnosia	Use repetition and one-step commands; approach on left side and place objects in view past midline (e.g., affected arm on table while eating); orient patient in room so that all enter room on left side of patient.
Thought processes	Has poor judgment; may have unrealistic thoughts; has memory deficits; has difficulty with concrete thinking	Always be aware of safety for this patient (patient will take risks and will act impulsively); establish a routine and stick with it; use a memory book; mark patient's room so it can be easily found with cueing.
Emotional style	Is often cheerful or euphoric; will deny illness or deficits; is unaware of problems; neglects left side; exhibits socially inappropriate behavior	Cue to deficits; constant reminders to call for help; don't leave unattended in bathroom or shower; monitor for inappropriate behavior; educate family on expectations and deficits (patient will convince family that he or she is fine).
Attention span	Short; is highly distractible	Work with patient one to one in a quiet setting; minimize outside noise and distractions; keep sessions and treatments short.
Behavioral style	Is quick and impulsive; needs supervision to prevent injury	Do not leave unattended; may need to use bed and chair alarms or enclosure bed to prevent injury (patient will not call for help)

c) Damage in this area results in the inability to form or difficulty in forming or finding words, difficulty in writing (translating thoughts into symbols, not the physical act of writing), and impaired ability to read letters, numbers, or written material.
d) May have speech that is slow, effortful to produce, and punctuated by long pauses between words; verbal comprehension is largely intact
e) Altered comprehension of language
f) May have intact automatic speech (e.g., may express a word, phrase, profanity, or song unexpectedly in a clear manner)
g) May have anomia (difficulty finding words and naming objects), perseveration (unintentional repetition of a word or phrase), conductive aphasia (repeating words or phrases on command), and difficulty with sentence construction

2) Receptive (Wernicke's dysphasia or fluent) (Boss, 2002a)
a) Occurs with lesions in the posterior, superior temporal dominant lobe (superior temporal gyrus)
b) This area is responsible for reception and interpretation of speech.
c) Able to produce verbal language, but language content is meaningless; able to speak fluently, but words may be incorrect or inappropriate in context; unable to detect his or her own errors
d) Besides being impaired with verbal comprehension, is also impaired in naming, reading, and writing

3) Global dysphasia
a) Occurs with lesions in the frontal–temporal dominant lobes; anterior and posterior speech areas are extensively impaired.
b) Exhibits comprehension and speaking problems (produces very little speech, a few words or phrases)

c) Impaired reading, naming, and writing skills
d) May have intact automatic speech only for routines such as counting, singing a song, or stating the days of the week

4) Transcortical dysphasias (transcortical sensory dysphasia, mixed transcortical dysphasia, isolated speech center) (Boss, 2002a)
a) Occurs with lesions in anterior and posterior presylvian fissures
b) Have the ability to repeat (echolalia) and recite
c) Speech can be fluent but uses paraphrases
d) Inability to read and write
e) Comprehension is impaired.

5) Apraxia of speech
a) Occurs when there is damage to the motor centers in the cortex that controls speech
b) Inability to program the position of the speech muscles and the sequence of the muscle movements necessary to produce understandable speech.
c) Understanding of speech remains intact.
d) Speech may be clear at times and undecipherable the next.
e) Common for perseveration and inconsistency

6) Dysarthria
a) Occurs with damage to a central or peripheral motor nerve, brainstem, or cranial nerves
b) Exhibits poorly articulated speech, resulting from interference in the control and execution over the muscles of speech; muscle control of the palate and tongue may be abnormal.
c) May have abnormal voice quality (too soft or loud); speech is slow, may be slurred and hard to understand.

7) Anarthria
a) Total loss of articulation as a result of loss of control of the muscles of speech; inability to articulate words
b) Occurs with damage to a central or peripheral motor nerve or brainstem

4. Right hemispheric stroke: common impairments and deficits
   a. Left hemiplegia or hemiparesis
   b. Problems with depth perception and spatial relationships
   c. Visual disturbances (including left homonymous hemianopsia)
   d. Inability to distinguish directional concepts such as up–down, front–back, in–out
   e. Difficulty distinguishing foreground from background information (figure–ground, spatial–temporal perception)
   f. Decreased ability to distinguish between similar shapes and forms (form constancy, spatial–temporal perception)
   g. Anosognosia: lack of awareness or denial of a neurological deficit, especially paralysis, on one side of the body; reduced insight into the ramifications of the impairment
   h. Lack of awareness of others' nonverbal communication (e.g., facial expressions, tone of voice, territorial space, gestures); display of a flat affect
   i. Unilateral neglect: inability to integrate sensory and perceptual stimuli from one side of the body or environment
   j. Behavioral changes, including impulsiveness, egocentricity, quickness to try things, risk taking
   k. Social inappropriateness: sexual disinhibition and inappropriate self-disclosure
   l. Difficulty in finding locations, such as one's room, and understanding maps and objects (geographic–topographic memory)

5. Brainstem strokes
   a. Result from ischemic or hemorrhagic process in the midbrain, pons, or medulla
   b. Potential deficits: Many vital centers and nuclei of cranial nerves exist, so deficits can vary greatly, including dysarthria, dysphagia (chewing or swallowing difficulty), ataxia, quadriparesis or quadriplegia, poor balance or coordination, double or blurred vision, pinpoint pupils, horizontal gaze palsy (e.g., eye moves to the side, away from the cerebral lesion), vertigo with nausea, abnormal respiratory patterns, hyperthermia, coma or persistent vegetative state, locked-in syndrome

(quadriplegia and facial paralysis, except for eye or eyelid movement; intact cognition; stroke is in the pons).

H. Children and Stroke (NSA, 2004)
1. Etiology
   a. Incidence is low: about 3 cases in every 100,000.
   b. More common in children under the age of 2.
   c. On average it takes 48–72 hours for children to get to the hospital after recognizing the first symptom of stroke (related to widespread belief that strokes don't happen to children).
   d. Babies who have strokes in the womb or within the first month of life are at risk of cerebral palsy.
   e. Premature babies are at risk for stroke during or shortly after delivery if hypoxia occurs.
   f. Children have a greater ability to heal because of the greater plasticity or flexibility of their nervous system and brain. The brain is still developing, so it may be more likely to repair itself (children usually recover function with the help of physical and speech therapy).

2. Causes of childhood stroke
   a. Birth defects
   b. Infections such as meningitis or encephalitis
   c. Trauma
   d. Blood disorders such as sickle cell disease

3. Childhood stroke symptoms
   a. Severe headache (often the first complaint)
   b. Speech difficulties
   c. Problems with eye movement
   d. Numbness

4. Stroke-related disabilities
   a. Speech and communication from brain cell damage
   b. Paralysis or weakness unilaterally from brain cell damage
   c. Cerebral palsy (unique to children)
   d. Mental retardation (unique to children)
   e. Epilepsy (unique to children)

5. Stroke education for children
   a. NSA developed the Hip Hop Stroke Program in 2004.
   b. Program uses children to educate

families about stroke, primarily in urban elementary schools.

c. Program teaches children to develop lifelong healthy habits to prevent stroke and to recognize symptoms of stroke.

d. Program teaches children to identify stroke as an emergency and to call 911.

II. Primary Prevention of Stroke

A. Nonmodifiable Risk Factors

1. Age (greater than 65)

2. Gender (more common in men)

3. Race and ethnicity (more common in African Americans, Hispanics)

4. Family history (hereditary factors)

B. Modifiable or Treatable Risk Factors (Sauerbeck, 2006)

1. Hypertension (blood pressure 140/90 or higher for an extended period of time)

2. Heart disease (includes myocardial infarction, atrial fibrillation, heart failure)

3. Diabetes mellitus (1.8–6 times more likely to have a stroke; should have hemoglobin A1c less than 6)

4. Hyperlipidemia (low-density lipoprotein of 160 mg/dl or more; control with statins)

5. Carotid stenosis (carotid artery narrowed by 70% or more by atherosclerotic plaque doubles risk of stroke)

6. TIA (treat with aspirin or ticlopidine)

C. Lifestyle Risk Factors (Sauerbeck, 2006)

1. May be independent of or contribute to medical risk factors that could cause stroke.

2. Smoking: Toxic compounds contribute to atherosclerosis, increasing clustering of platelets and increasing clotting time and viscosity.

3. Physical inactivity: 30 minutes per day of moderate to vigorous exercise reduces risk of stroke; exercise controls obesity and diabetes, lowers blood pressure, and increases high-density lipoproteins, which also lowers risk.

4. Alcohol abuse increases triglycerides, can produce cardiac arrhythmias and cause heart failure.

5. Obesity: Body mass index greater than 30 increases risk; abdominal obesity (waist circumference greater than 40 inches in men, 35 inches in women) is an independent risk factor.

6. Stress reduction through lifestyle changes decreases release of stress hormones, which contribute to obesity.

7. Stroke Risk Scorecard can be used to rate or score personal risk (http://www.stroke.org).

III. Treatment of Stroke

A. Early Recognition of Stroke

1. A stroke is a "brain attack."

2. Time is brain.

3. Community education of emergency medical personnel and general public is key.

4. Any person experiencing signs and symptoms of a stroke should seek help immediately in a hospital setting.

5. Consultation with a neurosurgeon or neurologist is needed

B. Diagnostic Tests

1. Brain computed tomography scan (rule out hemorrhagic stroke in order to administer anticoagulants and recombinant tissue plasminogen activator [rt-PA])

2. Blood tests: complete blood cell count, electrolytes, liver and renal profiles, clotting studies, lipid panel

3. Angiogram (may be needed for patients with a subarachnoid hemorrhage to rule out an aneurysm or arteriovenous malformation [AVM])

4. Other tests that may be ordered are electrocardiogram, chest x-ray, echocardiogram, electroencephalogram, lumbar puncture, carotid studies, magnetic resonance angiography.

C. Medications

1. Thrombolytic therapy (ischemic strokes) (NSA, 2006d):

a. rt-PA

1) Must meet the inclusion criteria (arrival in emergency room [ER] within 3 hours of symptom onset, computed tomography rules out hemorrhage, exam consistent with symptoms of stroke)

2) Patient is assessed against exclusion criteria (e.g., current use of anticoagulants or prothrombin time more than 15 seconds, use of heparin in past 48 hours and prolonged partial thromboplastin time, recent previous stroke, major surgery within past 14 days, uncontrolled hypertension, seizure at onset of stroke, recent

myocardial infarction, blood glucose less than 50 mg/dl or more than 400 mg/dl, neurological signs that are improving rapidly) (Keiser, 1999).

   3) Patient is assessed using the National Institutes of Health Stroke Scale (the most widely accepted tool for neurological assessment of stroke) (http://www.strokecenter.org/trials/scales/nihss.html).

   4) The Cincinnati Stroke Scale often is used for initial screening of stroke by bedside clinicians (http://www.strokecenter.org/trials/scales/cincinnati.html).

   5) Only drug approved by U.S. Food and Drug Administration (in 1996) for ischemic stroke

   6) Intravenous dose rt-PA given as a bolus (10% of dose given over 1 minute) and followed by the remaining 90% of the dose as an infusion over 60 minutes

   7) Patient is monitored closely for bleeding complications during and after infusion.

  b. Antiplatelet and anticoagulation (Keiser, 1999; NSA, 2006d)

   1) Antiplatelet and anticoagulant drugs are the most common medications used to reduce risk of a secondary stroke.

   2) Aspirin is currently viewed as the gold standard because of its effectiveness and low cost.

   3) Antiplatelet drug dipyridamole (Aggrenox), in combination with aspirin, reduced risk of recurrent stroke by 37% in clinical trials (NSA, 2006d).

   4) Antiplatelet drug clopidogrel (Plavix) has also been compared with aspirin in clinical trials for prevention of secondary strokes.

   5) Antiplatelet drug ticlopidine (Ticlid) is prescribed for those allergic to aspirin.

   6) Heparin may be started as an anticoagulant (studies show no real benefit over aspirin for patients with atrial fibrillation who have an ischemic stroke), and then the person is placed on warfarin (Coumadin) for a maintenance dose that may last 90 days to a lifetime (warfarin is commonly prescribed for patients with atrial fibrillation).

  2. Anticonvulsants are controversial; some physicians may prescribe prophylactically if the stroke involves the temporal lobe; others use if seizures appear as a complication; medication is selected based on type of seizure (may use lorazepam initially and phenytoin in longer term).

  3. Vasopressors are used as needed to maintain cerebral perfusion pressure.

  4. Nimodipine (Nimotop) may be used to reduce the deficit produced by cerebral ischemia (vasospasm).

  5. Support and comfort: analgesics, antipyretics, sedation, pain medication (for central poststroke pain from damage to thalamus)

D. Surgery (Keiser, 1999)

  1. Ruptured aneurysms are repaired using a clip, or the aneurysm is treated from inside the vessel by embolization (a metal coil through the artery in the brain that reaches the aneurysm and allows a clot to form and prevent more bleeding).

  2. AVMs can be treated the same way using interventional neuroradiologic procedures and a coil to clot off the AVM or instillation of glue during an angiogram (keeps blood from flowing through the AVM).

  3. Aneurysms and AVMs may still warrant surgical excision.

  4. Evacuation of intracerebral hemorrhage

  5. Other procedures by interventional neuroradiologists are angioplasty, intraarterial thrombolysis, stenting, and mechanical retrieval devices (Bader & Palmer, 2006).

E. Intensive Care Management

  1. Management of elevated intracranial pressure through monitors and catheters (ventriculostomy)

  2. Respiratory support with mechanical ventilation if needed (supplemental oxygen and hyperventilation may be indicated for hypoxic patients)

  3. Cardiovascular support and management of blood pressure (labetalol, nicardipine, or nitroprusside is recommended if blood pressure exceeds recommended levels)

  4. Nutritional support (enteral or parenteral feeding) and management of serum glucose (hyperglycemia may increase neuronal damage, and hypoglycemia may extend infarct)

5. Management of body temperature (hypothermia may be neuroprotective after ischemia) and management of fluids (avoid aspiration, sustain cerebral perfusion, avoid cerebral edema or fluid overload). Normal saline is fluid of choice (dehydration and hypotension may exacerbate the infarction).

6. Early rehabilitation: physical, occupational, and speech therapy; rehabilitation psychologist; therapeutic recreation specialist

7. Most urban hospitals have special stroke units that provide patients with the complex interventions they need, including medical, nursing, and therapy professionals working as a team from the beginning toward stroke recovery. Early rehabilitation is the emphasis, and active participation by the patient and family is encouraged.

F. Stroke Centers

1. Primary stroke centers (Bader & Palmer, 2006)

   a. In 2000, a multidisciplinary group (Brain Attack Coalition [BAC]) conducted a literature search with objectives of improving the level of care and standardization of rapid diagnosis, treatment, and care for stroke patients.

   b. BAC focused hospitals on prioritizing care with 6 connecting elements: identification of stroke patient and rapid transport to a stroke-receiving hospital by emergency medical personnel; ER prioritization of stroke care with rapid triage, protocols for management, and procedures for rt-PA administration; organized acute stroke team for rapid response to the ER; written care protocols for the multidisciplinary team to follow using EB literature; designated stroke unit with highly skilled staff to deal with stroke patients; neurosurgeons available within 2 hours in case of need for neurosurgery.

   c. BAC recommended support services including a stroke center medical director, 24-hour neuroimaging and laboratory services, outcome and quality improvement tracking for patient outcomes, and educational programs for staff and the community.

   d. Goal of a primary stroke center is to provide the personnel and infrastructure to stabilize and treat the majority of stroke patients.

   e. Development of primary stroke centers led to further recommendations by BAC and the ASA to work with the Joint Commission (JC) on establishing criteria for certification of primary stroke center programs (American Heart Association [AHA], 2006).

   f. The ASA provides tools and resources to help hospitals become ready for certification (e.g., Acute Stroke Treatment Program toolkit, Get With the Guidelines/Stroke Quality Improvement program) and numerous professional education opportunities (online continuing medical education, International Stroke Conference) (AHA, 2006).

   g. For more information about JC Primary Stroke Center Certification, visit http://www.jointcommission.org (AHA, 2006).

   h. A state-by-state list of stroke centers is available from the National Stroke Association Web site or by calling 1-800-STROKE.

2. Comprehensive stroke centers (Bader & Palmer, 2006)

   a. BAC met in late 2004 and 2005 and used an evidence-based approach to establish criteria for comprehensive stroke centers (CSCs).

   b. A CSC would have the personnel and infrastructure to care for stroke patients needing high-intensity care with specialized tests or interventional therapies.

   c. A CSC would be capable of taking care of patients with strokes involving larger areas of the brain (large ischemic strokes, complex hemorrhagic strokes).

   d. A CSC would provide more advanced care and would serve as a resource for a primary stroke center.

G. Future Treatment for Strokes (Health News Digest, 2006; Seppa, 2003)

1. Vampire bat (*Desmodus rotundus*) saliva

   a. *Desmodus rotundus* salivary plasminogen activator (DSPA) or desmoteplase (recombinant form of potent bat saliva) has been trialed at Ohio State University Medical Center and approximately 80 centers around the world; studies include animals and humans.

   b. Vampire bat secretes an enzyme in the saliva that prevents the blood of its prey from clotting; in a study with mice DSPA targeted the protein fibrin without causing

collateral damage to the brain from
further bleeding.

    c. Has been used in studies with humans
9 hours after onset of stroke symptoms
without evidence of neurotoxicity or
bleeding into the brain

  2. Advantages over rt-PA

    a. Only about 3%–5% of stroke patients
arrive within the necessary 3-hour
timeframe for this drug because their
symptoms are too subtle.

    b. DSPA can be introduced into the circulatory
system in 1–2 minutes, compared to the 60-
minute infusion of rt-PA.

    c. Has been studied up to 9 hours after
onset of symptoms with good results
and without negative side effects such as
bleeding into the brain (occurs with rt-PA
in about 6% of patients)

    d. Disadvantage is that it is not approved by
the U.S. Food and Drug Administration
at this time but continues to be studied
throughout the world.

IV. Family and Caregiver Support

A. General Facts

  1. A stroke alters not only the life of the patient
but the entire family, more than any other
type of disability; however, most Americans
believe that home rather than a long-term
care facility is the best place for family
members who are disabled (Pierce, Steiner,
Hicks, & Holzaepfel, 2006).

  2. Caregivers must meet an enormous challenge
in caring for the physical and emotional
needs of the stroke survivor without
neglecting their own needs.

  3 Caregivers must suspend their own feelings
of grief, fear, and frustration to take care of
the stroke survivor.

B. Education

  1. Caregivers need information about stroke,
its impact, the expected prognosis, and the
rehabilitation process.

  2. Caregivers need to understand the physical
and psychological needs of the stroke
survivor.

  3. Caregivers need assistance in enhancing their
own caring and coping skills.

  4. Caregivers need to be aware of community
services and resources available to them
(used by less than 33% of stroke survivors
and caregivers) (King & Semik, 2006).

  5. Caregivers need support groups to share
ideas, information, and coping, including
peer counseling in which they can share
methods with others in the same situation.

  6. Caregivers need to understand the
changes that occur in their partner, such as
depression, fatigue, frustration, egocentricity,
loss of companionship, and lack of support.

  7. Caregivers need to understand their own role
changes (may become the shopper, cook,
nurse, financier, handyman).

C. Considerations by Medical Professionals

  1. Age and health of caregiver and stroke survivor

  2. Gender (men not generally socialized to
provide care)

  3. Financial status (may have limited resources)

  4. Safety concerns (e.g., handling emergencies
such as falls)

  5. Level of caregiver stress (can lead to neglect
or abuse of stroke survivor)

D. Problems Identified by Caregivers (Pierce et al.,
2006)

  1. Independence (not enough personal time or
ability to maintain own role in society)

  2. Emotions (anger, frustration, isolation)

  3. Balancing duties (e.g., caregiver role,
personal role, taking care of house and
finances)

  4. Having a partner with physical limitations
(change in relationship, need to be a physical
therapist as well as spouse)

  5. Sleep and rest (sleep patterns altered because
of caregiving role or worry)

E. Resources for Caregivers and Families

  1. Family Caregiver Alliance: 76% of family
caregivers need respite (transportation,
errands, meal preparation, time away for
personal needs, visits by others to decrease
isolation) (National Family Caregivers
Association [NFCA], 2002).

  2. NFCA Web site (http://www.nfcacares.org).

  3. NSA partnered with Lotsa Helping Hands,
a free, personalized online tool through
the NSA Web site that helps organize a
community of family and friends (can
create a Web calendar) (http://stroke.
lotsahelpinghands.com) (NSA, 2004).

  4. Stroke Links (an NSA pilot program) is an
online tool to help organize and develop
local teams of family, friends, and coworkers
and provides them education in caring for
and supporting the stroke survivor.

5. Stroke Recovery Scorecard is available from the NSA Web site (can be filled out by stroke survivor and discussed with physician or healthcare provider).

6. Support and counseling may be needed for stroke survivors, family, and caregivers (both caregivers and the stroke survivor may experience depression).

V. Nursing Process

A. Assessment by Nurses and the Interdisciplinary Rehabilitation Team (see Figures 9-1, 9-2, and 9-3)

1. Medical management: assessed by the nurse and physicians (e.g., rehabilitation physiatrist, primary physician, and consulting physicians)

   a. Patient's medical stability: the initial primary focus in rehabilitation

   b. Assessment of medical needs that can impede rehabilitation progress if left unmanaged (e.g., hypotension, hypertension, hyperglycemia, oxygen saturation, cardiac irregularities, other chronic illnesses affecting medical stability)

2. Communication: assessed by speech–language pathologist (SLP), nurse, and registered occupational therapist (OTR)

   a. Presence of aphasia; expressive or receptive communication

   b. Other methods of communication (e.g., nodding, pointing, gesturing, using symbols)

   c. Premorbid communication pattern: history from family or significant other

   d. Vocalization problems from motor inability; tracheostomy

   e. Agnosia, apraxia, dysarthria

   f. Hearing aid or glasses

3. Memory: assessed by SLP, OTR, nurse, and physical therapist (PT)

   a. Premorbid ability

   b. Short-term memory

   c. Long-term memory

   d. Memory problems involving auditory or visual information

4. Problem-solving ability: assessed by nurse, SLP, OTR, PT

   a. Premorbid ability

   b. Ability to make appropriate choices

   c. Ability to find solutions

   d. Presence of planning or organizational skills

5. Sensory and visual perception: assessed by nurse, OTR, PT

   a. Premorbid use of hearing aid or glasses

   b. Perceptual responses; acuity of senses (e.g., vision, hearing, touch, taste, smell)

   c. Medications that may alter sensation or perception

Figure 9-1. Assessment of a New Patient with Stroke

- Obtain verbal report from a nurse on the unit that sent the patient.
- Make appropriate room assignment based on deficits (e.g., turn affected side toward door for stimulation, place close to nursing station if at high risk for falls).
- When patient arrives, assist with the patient's transfer to bed. The nursing assessment begins now as the nurse observes how much the patient can do during the transfer.
- Determine whether the patient can answer questions and is cognitively aware. This can be determined in a short time with conversation while welcoming the patient to the unit. If the patient is unable to provide his or her own history, ask a family member to attend the assessment.
- Assess general data (e.g., allergies, medications, identification band on).
- Obtain complete medical history and complete a head-to-toe assessment, including neurological checks (e.g., for strength, orientation). During this time, also assess communication and cognition skills.
- Assess bowel and bladder function, using information obtained from the report of other nurses, combined with information from the patient and family. This assessment may not be complete until the nurse actually toilets the patient during the first 24 hours.
- Obtain histories for sleep, nutrition, safety, and sex.
- Assess psychosocial history and educational wants, needs, and preferences for learning style.
- Assess leisure interests, community reentry needs, and discharge planning needs.
- Provide the patient and family with verbal and written orientation information about the unit and the staff.
- Communicate pertinent information to team members as soon as possible.
- Provide the patient with necessary safety equipment (e.g., bed alarm, wheelchair alarm) as soon as the assessment is complete.
- Follow the assessment pattern of the unit but keep in mind that the patient may get tired or frustrated if several team members assess the same things at different times.

Figure 9-2. Modified Rankin Scale

Grade	Description
0	No symptoms at all.
1	No significant disability despite symptoms. Able to carry out all usual duties and activities.
2	Slight disability: Unable to carry out all previous activities but able to look after own affairs without assistance.
3	Moderate disability: Needs some help but able to walk without assistance.
4	Moderately severe disability: Unable to walk without assistance and unable to attend to own bodily needs without assistance.
5	Severe disability: Bedridden, incontinent, and needing constant nursing care and attention.

Source consulted

Stroke, 1988, Vol. 19, pp. 604–607.

Figure 9-3. Barthel Index

1. Feeding

Unable	- totally dependent	☐ 0
Needs help	- cutting, spreading butter but feeds self	☐ 5
Independent	- can eat normal food (not only soft food) provided by others but not cut up	☐ 10

2. Bathing

Dependent		☐ 0
Independent	- can get in and out unsupervised and wash self. In shower, independent if unsupervised/unaided	☐ 5

3. Grooming (personal care)

Needs help		☐ 0
Independent	- washes face, does hair, brushes teeth, shaves (implements can be provided by helper)	☐ 5

4. Dressing

Dependent		☐ 0
Needs help	- e.g. with buttons, zips etc. but can do about half task unaided	☐ 5
Independent	- can select and put on all clothes (including buttons, zips, laces, etc)	☐ 10

5. Bowel control (preceding week)

Incontinent		☐ 0
Occasional accident	- once a week or less often	☐ 5
Continent		☐ 10

6. Bladder Control

Incontinent	- or catheterized and unable to manage catheter	☐ 0
Occasional accident	- less than once a day (24 h)	☐ 5
Continent	- for over 7 days. If catheterized, can manage catheter alone	☐ 10

7. Toilet Use

Dependent		☐ 0
Needs some help	- can wipe self plus can do some of other tasks required of independent person	☐ 5
Independent	- can reach toilet/commode, undress, sufficiently, wipe self, dress and leave	☐ 10

8. Chair/Bed transfer

Unable	- no sitting balance, cannot sit, requires two people to lift	☐ 0
Major help	- can sit, requires one strong/skilled or two normal people to lift	☐ 5
Minor help	- one person can lift easily or needs any supervision for safety	☐ 10
Independent		☐ 15

9. Mobility

Immobile		☐ 0
Wheel chair independent	- can negotiate corners/doors unaided	☐ 5
Walks with help	- one untrained person providing physical help, supervision or moral support	☐ 10
Independent	- can walk 50 m or around house. May use any aid e.g. stick, except rolling walker	☐ 15

10. Stairs

Unable		☐ 0
Needs help	- verbal or physical help or carrying aid	☐ 5
Independent	- up and down, carrying any walking aid	☐ 10

Source

Mahoney, F.J., & Barthel, D.W. (1965). Functional evaluation: The Barthel Index. *Maryland State Medical Journal, 14,* 61– 65.

6. ADLs and self-care: assessed by RN, OTR
   a. Ability to bathe, dress, or toilet self
   b. Premorbid abilities
   c. How much help is needed
   d. Ability to gather needed equipment, supplies, clothing
   e. Mobility to carry out activities
   f. Adaptive equipment needed (e.g., bath sponge, reacher, shoe horn)

7. Dysphagia and swallowing: assessed by nurse, SLP, OTR
   a. Ability to feed self; amount of assistance needed
   b. Ability to chew, drink, swallow without difficulty
   c. Correct diet and consistency ordered
   d. Adequate caloric and fluid intake
   e. Use of correct position for eating, alertness
   f. Presence of drooling and pocketing, not swallowing
   g. Presence of cough and gag reflex
   h. Voice quality (e.g., wet, gurgly, nasal while eating)
   i. Use and fit of dentures
   j. Use of upper extremities (e.g., grip, able to lift utensils, able to cut and prepare food)
   k. Ability to see food (e.g., hemianopsia)

8. Bowel management: assessed by nurse
   a. Neurogenic bowel (sudden, involuntary defecation)
   b. Continence history before stroke; bowel history (e.g., when, how often)
   c. Awareness of need to defecate
   d. Medication use, digital stimulation
   e. Bowel sounds, abdominal tenderness or distention
   f. Ability to get to bathroom, ability to don and doff clothing
   g. Hygiene needs, assistance needed
   h. Positioning, privacy

9. Bladder management: assessed by nurse
   a. Neurogenic bladder: decreased capacity and involuntary voiding as soon as urge is perceived
   b. Continence history before stroke
   c. Premorbid history (e.g., nocturia, stress incontinence)
   d. Recent history (e.g., urgency, frequency, urinary tract infection)
   e. Awareness of need to urinate, cognition

   f. Ability to perform toileting and to get to the bathroom
   g. Hygiene needs, assistance, privacy
   h. Catheter (e.g., intermittent, indwelling)
   i. Fluid intake
   j. Medication use

10. Mobility: assessed by nurse, PT, OTR
    a. Bed mobility: moving up, down, side to side; bridging; sitting up; amount of assistance needed
    b. Transfers: bed to chair, wheelchair to toilet, to bath bench or shower chair, to car; amount of assistance needed (see Figure 9-4)
    c. Wheelchair mobility: type of wheelchair, ability to self-propel, amount of assistance needed
    d. Gait, sitting, standing; need for devices (e.g., walker, cane, crutches)
    e. Endurance, strength, balance, tone, and proprioception
    f. Environment (e.g., lighting, open space)

11. Sexual functioning: assessed by nurse, physician, psychologist
    a. Premorbid sexual history (e.g., preferences, frequency, initiation [partner or self])
    b. Sensory deficits
    c. Mobility
    d. Ability to communicate, visual or perceptual deficits
    e. Emotional status, fear
    f. Fatigue
    g. Knowledge
    h. Libido
    i. Need for birth control
    j. Bowel and bladder management before sex

12. Skin integrity: assessed by nurse, PT, OTR
    a. Immobility
    b. Loss of sensation
    c. Incontinence and hygiene
    d. Presence of pressure, friction, shearing
    e. Poor circulation
    f. Hydration and nutrition

13. Equipment: assessed by OTR, PT, nurse, social worker (SW), discharge planner
    a. Need for assistance with mobility
    b. Need for assistance with ADLs
    c. Financial resources available

14. Psychosocial needs: assessed by nurse, SW, psychologist
    a. Role changes

Figure 9-4. Transfer Techniques for Patients Who Have Had a Stroke

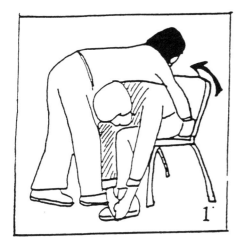
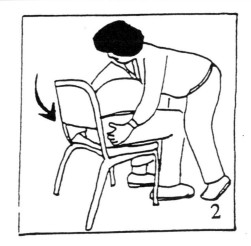
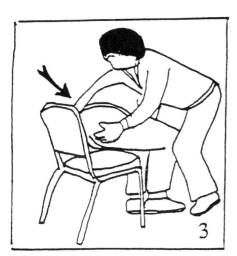
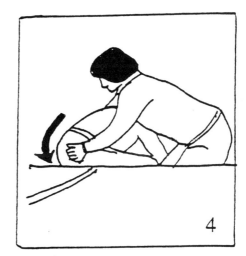

Maximal Assist

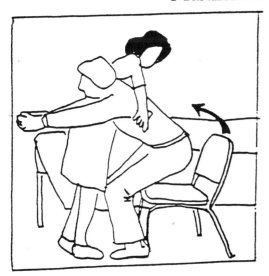

Position feet flat on floor, heels behind knees.
Bring trunk well forward prior to standing.
Encourage bilateral weight bearing.
Approximate knees through hips.
Assist by using leverage, not by lifting.

Modified Stand-Pivot Transfer: Moderate Assist

b. Relationships with family members

c. Family and community support

d. Coping skills and stressors

15. Leisure: assessed by nurse and certified therapeutic recreation specialist

    a. Premorbid leisure history

    b. Current physical ability and endurance related to leisure interest

    c. Cognitive status

16. Education: assessed by each rehabilitation team member

    a. Cognitive status, intellectual capacity

    b. Attention span

    c. Premorbid learning needs (e.g., visual, auditory, kinesthetic, combination)

    d. Level of formal education

    e. Ability to read or write

    f. Language and cultural barriers

    g. Motivation and readiness to learn

    h. Environmental barriers

    i. Knowledge of disability and self-care needs

    j. Support and presence of caregivers

17. Safety: assessed by each rehabilitation team member

    a. Cognition and awareness

    b. Risk for and history of falls

    c. Environment (e.g., hospital, home)

    d. Medication that alters level of consciousness

    e. Sensory impairments

18. Comfort and pain level: assessed by nurse

    a. Subluxation and shoulder pain: Subluxation is painless; however, manipulation and improper positioning of a subluxed shoulder cause pain.

    b. Shoulder–hand syndrome

    c. Pain and its location, frequency; use different pain scale for nonverbal aphasic patients. [Refer to Chapter 13 for pain scales.]

    d. Pain related to activity or randomly occurring

    e. What relieves pain

    f. Effectiveness of medicine

    g. Changes in sleep pattern; may have reversal of sleep–wake cycle

    h. Sleep history (e.g., normal bedtime, need for white noise, lights)

    i. Sleep problems: onset, frequent awakenings, nocturia

j. Environmental (e.g., hot, cold, comfortable bed)

19. Spiritual: assessed by nurse and chaplain

    a. Sources of hope and strength

    b. Religious practices

    c. Scheduled time for privacy

20. Discharge planning: assessed by discharge planner in conjunction with rehabilitation team

    a. Physical deficits and need for adaptive equipment

    b. Caregiver knowledge and support

    c. Financial resources available

    d. Need for community resources

    e. Adaptations needed for home environment with rehabilitation team input

B. Nursing Diagnoses

    1. Impaired physical mobility

    2. Self-care deficits (specify level)

    3. Sensory–perceptual alteration

    4. Impaired verbal communication

    5. Altered elimination (bowel and bladder)

    6. High risk of aspiration or impaired swallowing

    7. Potential for injury

    8. Impaired home maintenance management and discharge planning

    9. Impaired thought processes

    10. Disturbance in body image

    11. Altered sexuality pattern

    12. Caregiver distress

    13. Spiritual distress

    14. Alteration in skin integrity

    15. Knowledge deficit

    16. Alteration in comfort

C. Planning and Patient Goals

    1. Demonstrate maximal independence in mobility.

    2. Perform ADLs at optimal level of independence with or without the use of assistive devices.

    3. Be free from injury.

    4. Identify diversional activities to decrease stress (by caregivers).

    5. Verbalize satisfaction with sexuality.

    6. Identify negative feelings related to self-image.

    7. Verbalize understanding of the diagnosis and treatment of stroke (CVA).

D. Interventions

1. Medical management:

    a. Monitor vital signs (more frequently during early rehabilitation); medication for hypertension as needed; intravenous fluids for hypotension (if the patient is hypotensive, hemoconcentration can occur and cerebral perfusion decreases, potentially worsening the infarct).

    b. Monitor blood glucose and regulate with insulin as needed.

    c. Use intravenous solutions of normal saline.

    d. Provide oxygen as ordered and titrate to 90% or more.

    e. Use telemetry monitoring or electrocardiogram for cardiac abnormalities.

    f. Check lung sounds and risk of aspiration.

    g. Check for fever (e.g., urinary tract infection, pneumonia).

    h. Check lab values (e.g., activated partial thromboplastin time, hemoglobin and hematocrit, electrolytes).

    i. Measure legs daily for swelling; assess for deep vein thrombosis.

2. Communication: "Language is the most human of mental skills" (Mace & Rabins, 1981, p. 29). Without language, the person with a stroke is lonely, depends on others, and loses self-confidence.

    a. Determine communication method: All disciplines should use consistent methods.

    b. Ensure that hearing aids and glasses are available if needed.

    c. Use symbols and communication boards.

    d. Provide a supportive environment; be patient and calm.

    e. Include the family when possible.

    f. Use music therapy: The person may be unable to speak but able to sing.

    g. Speak slowly and distinctly; use short, simple sentences; maintain eye contact.

    h. Establish yes–no reliability.

    i. Try cueing; prompt if the direction of verbalization is understood.

    j. Provide opportunities for success; offer praise.

3. Memory:

    a. Use memory books.

    b. Use cueing and repetition.

    c. Use memory games and allow the patient to reminisce.

    d. Work from simple to complex concepts and promote success.

    e. Present material in different ways (e.g., written, verbal, pictures, demonstration)

4. Problem-solving ability:

    a. Allow the patient to make choices, beginning with safe and simple options.

    b. Help with planning.

    c. Organize and prioritize information.

    d. Break problems into steps and cue the patient through the steps.

5. Sensory and visual perception:

    a. Provide adaptive equipment (e.g., glasses, hearing aid).

    b. Ensure appropriate lighting and color contrast.

    c. Make large-print books and materials available.

    d. Place items to allow for visual cuts (homonymous hemianopsia) and teach the patient to visually scan the environment.

    e. Reduce environmental noise (e.g., radio, television).

    f. Adapt environment to accommodate hearing loss (e.g., flashing light for phone).

    g. Use aromatherapy.

    h. Provide various textures and temperatures.

    i. Ensure safety (e.g., hot or cold, especially with decreased sensation).

    j. Serve foods of various colors, tastes, and smells.

    k. Review medications (e.g., sedatives).

    l. Set up room to stimulate the neglected side.

    m. Eliminate spatial difficulties (e.g., use colored food on white plate).

6. ADLs and self-care:

    a. Ensure privacy and a safe environment (e.g., grab bars, tub bench).

    b. Establish a bathing and toileting routine and provide adaptive equipment for bathing, dressing, and toileting.

    c. Involve caregivers in ADL training.

    d. Incorporate crossover neurodevelopmental techniques (NDTs) (i.e., the patient's uninvolved side helps the involved side during activity).

    e. Provide ongoing comprehensive history and assessment for ADL training and for determining the patient's home care assistance needs (documentation of this may be required by the patient's insurance company).

f. Adapt the home environment for wheelchair, equipment, and accessibility.

g. Allow the patient to choose his or her clothing; encourage use of clothing that is loose or easy to put on.

h. Allow time for activity and rest between self-care activities and promote energy-saving techniques, beginning in bed and progressing throughout the day.

i. Dress the patient's affected side first.

7. Dysphagia and swallowing:

a. Evaluate swallowing (via bedside or radiology) as identified by videofluoroscopic swallow study.

b. Position the patient upright for feeding and administering medication.

c. Ensure the correct level of dysphagia diet and consistency (e.g., thicken if needed); ensure that dentures fit properly; obtain a dental consult.

d. Observe during meals for pocketing, drooling, swallowing.

e. Provide adaptive equipment (e.g., divided plate, cutout cup).

f. Crush medications into applesauce; turn the patient's head to the affected side if he or she has difficulty swallowing medications.

g. Monitor weight changes and lab values.

h. Consult with dietitian about the patient's food preferences.

i. Monitor hydration: Patients on oral dysphagia diets need adequate fluids to avoid dehydration.

j. Use supplemental tube feedings: Check for residual and placement of tube and position the patient upright for feedings.

k. Use supplemental parental nutrition: Maintain tube site and monitor labs.

8. Bowel management:

a. Verify premorbid bowel evacuation routine and adapt bowel program to accommodate previous routine.

b. Increase fluid intake, bulk, fiber; monitor intake and output.

c. Monitor bowel sounds and abdominal distention; avoid gas-forming foods.

d. Position the patient upright; use toilet or commode rather than bedpan; allow time for complete evacuation.

e. Provide appropriate medications (e.g., stool softeners, enemas, suppositories).

f. Teach digital stimulation as needed.

g. Encourage the patient to wear loose clothing and use good hygiene after each stool.

9. Bladder management:

a. Determine continence history, provide adequate lighting if the patient has a history of nocturia.

b. Set up bladder program to decrease or avoid incontinence.

c. Assess medications that contribute to incontinence (e.g., diuretics, sedatives, anticholinergics, antihypertensives).

d. Provide adequate hydration (i.e., fluid intake of 2,000–3,000 cc/day if tolerated) and monitor intake and output.

e. Use bladder scan and catheterize for postvoid residuals greater than 150 cc generally or greater than 300 cc if the patient is unable to void.

f. Provide time, privacy, and adaptive equipment for hygiene.

g. Provide medication to facilitate bladder tone and emptying.

10. Mobility:

a. Work with patient on bed mobility, bridging, sitting up, moving up and down, and increasing endurance.

b. Use general concepts of NDTs (e.g., normalizing muscle tone, integration vs. compensation, meaningful activities vs. simulated activities) to help with proprioception.

c. Consider possible use of NDTs for transfers.

d. Provide safe environment for mobility practice (space and lighting).

e. Encourage the patient to wear sturdy shoes to prevent foot drop.

f. Ensure safety when the patient attempts to sit or stand: According to clinical experience, more than one-third of falls in patients who have had a stroke occur while rising or sitting down.

11. Sexual functioning:

a. Encourage the use of times of day when the patient is most rested.

b. Provide education and support with significant other.

c. Teach positioning (e.g., supine or on affected side, use pillows for support).

d. Discuss fear of another stroke.

e. Instruct partner on the emotional lability of the patient.

f. Encourage tactile stimulation to enhance communication, especially if the patient is aphasic.

g. Discuss birth control methods.

h. Encourage the patient to evacuate the bowel and bladder before sex.

12. Skin integrity:

a. Inspect skin regularly for friction, shearing, pressure.

b. Teach weight-shifting techniques.

c. Use pressure-relieving devices.

d. Keep patient clean and dry.

e. Consult with dietitian for nutritional needs to promote healing.

f. If the patient has sensory loss, guard for contact with extreme hot and cold temperatures (e.g., bath water).

g. Assess for medications that may alter level of consciousness, sensation, or awareness.

13. Equipment:

a. Provide adaptive equipment as needed; attempt to increase the patient's functional ability without equipment if possible.

b. Verify insurance payment for durable medical equipment.

c. Reinforce the use of equipment that therapists have obtained.

14. Psychosocial needs:

a. Provide time for verbalization and counseling for patient and family with psychologist.

b. Facilitate team and family conferences as needed.

c. Provide socialization opportunities (e.g., eating meals in dining room, group therapy, stroke support groups).

d. Role changes occur and should be discussed with patient and family.

e. Allow the patient and family to grieve their losses (e.g., function, role, relationships).

f. Reduce stress when possible and allow the patient and family to have as much control over care as possible.

15. Leisure:

a. Incorporate the patient's leisure interests into therapy (e.g., card games).

b. Promote community reentry using adaptive equipment (e.g., outing to a wheelchair-accessible fishing dock using a mounted fishing rod holder).

c. Use memory games to work on cognition in group therapy.

d. Use NDTs during games (e.g., incorporate hemiplegic side using strong side hand over hand to hit balloon or reach for cards).

e. Try to adapt the patient's leisure interests that use equipment (e.g., fasten an embroidery hoop to a wheelchair).

f. Encourage pet therapy.

16. Education:

a. Determine readiness and motivation to learn.

b. Provide information at the patient's ability and intellectual level.

c. Use a variety of teaching methods.

d. Use an interpreter if language barriers exist.

e. Plan family teaching sessions.

f. Reduce distraction and noise when teaching.

g. Make use of the time when the patient is most alert, attentive, and rested.

h. Test cognition and use return demonstration or verbalization.

i. Check awareness of current status and build knowledge base.

17. Safety:

a. Ensure that the environment is free of hazards.

b. Use bed alarms, electronic wristband monitors, vest restraints as necessary.

c. Assess medications that may alter awareness.

d. Evaluate the patient's home (e.g., handrails, throw rugs, wheelchair ramp).

e. Ensure kitchen and bathroom safety for patients with sensory impairments (e.g., stove, hot and cold water).

f. Teach postmorbid impulse control and fall prevention techniques.

18. Comfort and pain level:

a. Position the patient comfortably, be aware of shoulder pain (subluxation possible), and position in bed so the patient's shoulder is protracted (see Figure 9-5).

b. Do not use the patient's arms or shoulders to move the patient up in bed.

Figure 9-5. Bed Positioning for Patients Who Have Had a Stroke

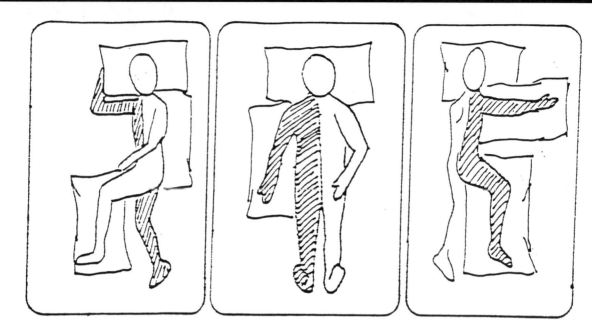

On Involved Side   Supine   On Non-Involved Side

Reprinted with permission of International Clinical Educators, Inc., from Davis, J. (1997). *NDT course for nursing.* Port Townsend, WA: International Clinical Educators, Inc. Available: International Clinical Educators, Inc., PO Box 1990, Port Townsend, WA 98368, 888/665-6556, www.strokehelp.com.

c. Assess the intensity and location of pain and medicate as appropriate.

d. Watch for shoulder–hand syndrome: Reduce edema; maintain range of motion of metacarpal phalangeal, proximal interphalangeal, and distal interphalangeal joints; maintain wrist in slight extension; encourage movement of the involved shoulder; and maintain correct bed positioning.

e. Allow rest periods but decrease frequency if patient cannot sleep at night.

f. Provide night lighting and white noise if needed.

g. Monitor the room with cameras if the patient is impulsive at night.

19. Spiritual

a. Notify the chaplain if requested.

b. Make spiritual readings available (e.g., scriptures, daily devotions).

c. Arrange for the patient to attend chapel services if requested.

d. Schedule time for meditation and prayer.

20. Discharge planning

a. Discuss discharge goals with patient and family at conferences.

b. Set up follow-up appointments.

c. Arrange home health care, outpatient therapy, or long-term care placement.

d. Obtain durable medical equipment.

e. Arrange for prescriptions.

f. Provide discharge instructions and explain medications (e.g., side effects, administration).

g. Assist with financial and community resource information.

E. Evaluation and Expected Outcomes

1. Evaluate the patient's optimal level of functioning.

2. Individualize each patient's outcomes based on goals related to nursing diagnoses.

F. Posthospitalization Follow-Up

1. Education about stroke prevention is essential because stroke can be a recurring disorder.

2. Research suggests that stroke survivors who adapt well use positive coping strategies

such as hoping that things will improve, prayer, and humor and that nursing follow-up may have a positive impact on coping after stroke (Easton, Rawl, Zemen, Kwiatkowski, & Burczyk, 1995; Rawl, Easton, Zemen, Kwiatkowski, & Burzcyk, 1998).

3. Stroke survivors may go through a predictable recovery process (Easton, 1999; 2001). If so, nursing interventions may be targeted to the patient's unique needs throughout the rehabilitation process and after discharge to the home setting (Mauk, 2006).

4. Stroke recovery may be facilitated by several controllable and uncontrollable factors such as age, life experience, knowledge of the cause of stroke, expectations, social support, and faith (Mauk, 2006) (see Figure 9-6).

5. Rehabilitation nurses can gain insight into the concerns and challenges facing stroke survivors who have returned to the community by assessing their learning needs and making referrals for follow-up care.

6. Many patients who have had a stroke suffer from depression, lack of concentration, anxiety, fatigue that continues even years after stroke, and memory loss (Easton, 2001; Sisson, 1998).

7. Quality of life is also affected by stroke (Secrest, 2002).

8. It is important to refer the patient and family for counseling if needed.

G. Future Reimbursement

1. In this time of chronic disease management, rehabilitation plays an important role in the clinical management of patients.

2. According to the AHA (2006), the estimated direct and indirect cost of stroke for 2006 is nearly $58 billion.

3. Reimbursement changes affect the length of stay in rehabilitation units.

4. Rehabilitation nurses will be challenged to meet the needs of patients who have had a stroke more rapidly and with fewer resources available.

VI. Advanced Practice

Advanced practice nurses (APNs), whether clinical nurse specialists or nurse practitioners, can play a significant role in the care of stroke survivors. In many situations, APNs may engage in several role components of advanced practice simultaneously. Whether as direct care providers, educators, consultants, researchers, theorists, or leaders, APNs should be at the forefront in improving the quality of life for stroke survivors.

A. Clinician: The APN as clinician possesses advanced assessment skills. APNs should be knowledgeable about current best practices for care of stroke patients. Specifically, the APN specializing in stroke could reasonably be expected to have mastered knowledge related to the content of this chapter but with greater depth and expertise.

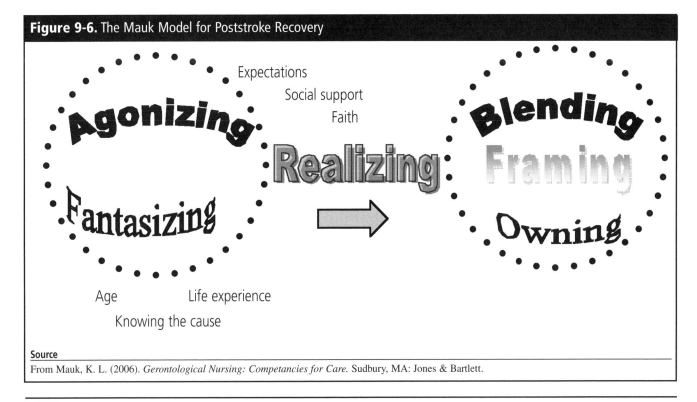

Figure 9-6. The Mauk Model for Poststroke Recovery

Agonizing
Fantasizing

Expectations
Social support
Faith

Realizing

Blending
Framing
Owning

Age   Life experience
Knowing the cause

Source

From Mauk, K. L. (2006). *Gerontological Nursing: Competencies for Care.* Sudbury, MA: Jones & Bartlett.

1. Practice settings
   a. Emergency room
   b. Acute care hospital
   c. Acute rehabilitation
   d. Transitional care
   e. Skilled care
   f. Long-term care facility
      1) Intermediate or skilled care
      2) Independent living
      3) Assisted living
   g. Home care
   h. Community–living in the home or residential setting after stroke
2. Additional skills as direct care provider (clinical nurse specialist or nurse practitioner)
   a. Comprehensive physical exam
   b. Thorough history
   c. Screening for dysphagia, risk for skin breakdown, deep vein thrombosis risk
   d. Identification of risk factors for stroke
   e. Assessment of stroke severity using standardized scales
   f. Assessment of cranial nerve function
   g. Clinical management of acute stroke
   h. Knowledge of stroke rehabilitation principles and concepts
   i. Making appropriate referrals to stroke service and initiation of rehabilitation
   j. Outpatient follow-up visits with survivor and family
   k. Coordination of stroke support groups
   l. Staff, patient, and family education about treatment plan and discharge plans, including ordering of appropriate adaptive equipment
   m. Care management or coordination
   n. Home care supervision
   o. Management of potential common complications
      1) Skin breakdown
      2) Dysphagia
      3) Deep vein thrombosis
      4) Aphasia
      5) Ongoing functional limitations including gait disorders, hemiplegia
      6) Depression and anxiety
      7) Sleep disorders
      8) Shoulder subluxation
      9) Altered nutrition/dehydration
   p. Prescribing and managing medications
B. Educator: The APN as educator focuses on identifying areas of need; providing essential knowledge of stroke prevention, treatment, and rehabilitation to the target audience; and fostering a positive learning environment.
   1. Educates various populations in all levels of stroke prevention
      a. Nursing staff
      b. Patients and families
      c. Interdisciplinary team members
      d. Communities
      e. Students
   2. Educates in various settings
      a. Hospitals
      b. Acute rehabilitation units
      c. Transitional care
      d. Long-term care facilities
      e. Academia, universities and colleges of nursing
      f. Communities
   3. Uses evidence-based practice to develop teaching strategies in areas of need to improve the quality of care
      a. Promotes use of evidence-based practice in the clinical setting.
      b. Nursing follow-up after patient discharge shows positive results (Easton et al., 1995; Rawl et al., 1998).
      c. Nursing interventions related to education have both short- and long-term effects on a variety of variables (Nir, Zolotogorsky, & Sugarman, 2004).
      d. Web-based teaching interventions have shown positive outcomes with stroke survivors and caregivers (Pierce, Steiner, & Govoni, 2002; Pierce et al., 2004).
      e. Female stroke survivors may have unique needs related to body image and self-perception that are infrequently addressed by rehabilitation nurses (Kvigne, Kirkevold, & Gjengedal, 2005).
      f. Stroke survivors and their caregivers do not report perceiving therapeutic assistance from nurses (Secrest, 2002).
C. Leader: The APN as leader is active in organizations at the local, regional, state, national, and international levels. The APN may also demonstrate leadership through civic and professional involvement, presentations at conferences, publications, consulting work, and research programs.
   1. Tasks as leader
      a. Advocate for social reform.
      b. Act as a change agent by holding office in

professional organizations.

    c. Assist with development of clinical practice guidelines.

    d. Participate on committees within professional organizations and interdisciplinary national organizations of interest.

    e. Hold positions of influence or lobby within appropriate political arenas to support the rights of those with disabilities.

    f. Write grants for funding of stroke research.

    g. Become a fellow in a national organization such as the AHA.

  2. Organizations for involvement (Table 9-2)

    a. American Heart Association (AHA) and American Stroke Association (ASA)

    b. National Stroke Association (NSA)

    c. Association of Rehabilitation Nurses (ARN)

    d. American Geriatrics Society (AGS)

    e. American Association of Neuroscience Nurses (AANN)

D. Consultant: As consultant, the APN may engage in a variety of activities. The role of consultant is continually redefined as nurses increase their expertise in areas related to rehabilitation.

  1. Legal consulting

    a. Expert opinion

    b. Expert testimony, written and in court

    c. Clinical expert in law practice

    d. For attorneys, insurance companies, private clients, companies

  2. Educational consulting

    a. For academic institutions, on site

    b. For private clients needing one-on-one teaching

    c. For rehabilitation units providing educational seminars related to stroke

    d. For rehabilitation facilities or private

companies that provide outreach in different parts of the country

  3. Clinical consulting

    a. Expert clinician on research team

    b. Expert consultant for grant applications and funding

    c. Expert on complex cases (in a variety of settings)

    d. Share expertise with other team members

    e. Author or reviewer of publications (books, articles, case studies)

  4. Guardianship: generally court appointed; often complex cases that do not have appropriate family involvement or that require involvement of a healthcare expert

  5. Advocacy: care planning and mediation for those in care settings; interacting with the interdisciplinary team to ensure quality of care and continuity

  6. Life care planning

    a. "A life care plan is a comprehensive document designed to help meet the long-term financial and health needs of a person who has experienced a catastrophic injury" (Mauk & Mauk, 2006, p. 818).

    b. "A Life Care Plan is a dynamic document based upon published standards of practice, comprehensive assessment, data analysis and research, which provides an organized, concise plan for current and future needs with associated costs, for individuals who have experienced catastrophic injury or have chronic health care needs" (Weed, 1999, p. iii).

    c. Advanced practice status is not needed, but APNs generally have more credibility when involved in legal matters where credentialing and advanced education are important; a background in case management is helpful.

    d. Life care planning for stroke survivors could involve:

      1) Estimating lifetime cost of care and other needs related to medical malpractice in a lawsuit (e.g., in which the injured party suffered a stroke)

      2) Predicting lifetime care costs in relation to care coordination or management over time

E. Researcher: The APN as researcher will discover and facilitate the use of evidence-based practice for stroke survivors. Some APNs may hold

Table 9-2. Stroke Resources

American Heart Association: www.americanheart.org

American Stroke Association: www.strokeassociation.org

National Stroke Association: www.stroke.org

National Institute of Neurological Disorders and Stroke: www.ninds.nih.gov

Association of Rehabilitation Nurses: www.rehabnurse.org

American Association of Neuroscience Nurses: www.aann.org

positions whose major emphasis is research related to stroke.

1. Examples of APN involvement in stroke research
   a. Stroke program coordinator
      1) In acute care hospital (including those with primary or comprehensive stroke centers)
      2) In acute rehabilitation
      3) In freestanding rehabilitation facilities
   b. Researcher in research institutions or academic settings
   c. Research scientist in large rehabilitation institutes
   d. Writer of grants to seek funding for stroke research
2. Examples of current areas of stroke research by rehabilitation APNs
   a. Continuity and Discontinuity of Self Scale (Secrest & Thomas, 1999; Secrest & Zeller, 2003, 2006), which relates to quality of life after stroke
   b. Mauk model for poststroke recovery (Easton, 1999; Mauk, 2006), a grounded theory that suggests targeting of nursing interventions to each phase of stroke recovery
   c. Adaptation to stroke (King, Shade-Zeldow, Carlson, Feldman, & Philip, 2002)
   d. Caregivers of stroke survivors
      1) Web-based nursing interventions for caregivers of stroke survivors (Pierce et al., 2004; Steiner & Pierce, 2002)
      2) New caregivers of people with stroke (Pierce et al., 2006)
      3) Problems of stroke caregivers (Hartke & King, 2002)
3. Evidence-based practice example
   a. Background on evidence-based practice related to dysphagia screening for stroke patients:
      1) More than 700,000 strokes occur per year in America, with more than 2/3 of patients surviving.
      2) Prevalence of dysphagia after stroke is 40%–70% (Nishiwaki et al., 2005), although more than 80% of patients recover the ability to swallow 2–4 weeks after stroke (Ramsey, Smithard, & Kalra, 2003).
      3) Dysphagia is one of the most serious complications resulting from stroke and can lead to dehydration, aspiration, pneumonia, and death.
      4) The most reliable screening tool has

been radiography (videofluoroscopy [VFS]), but researchers have been working on developing a reliable bedside screening tool that is safe and efficient in predicting dysphagia.
   b. The clinical question: What is the best screening tool for dysphagia in patient with stroke?
   c. Appraisal of evidence: Eight relevant sources provide good evidence to address the question but with conflicting results. No qualitative studies have been found. The review is limited to patients with stroke and excludes dysphagic patients with other diagnoses.
      1) One level 1 source with good evidence (Scottish Intercollegiate Guidelines Network, 2004)
      2) One level 1 source with fair and poor evidence (Veterans Health Administration, 2003)
      3) Three level 3 articles with good evidence (Hinds & Wiles, 1998; McCullough, 1997; Smith, Lee, O'Neill, & Connolly, 2000)
      4) One level 4 article with good evidence (Nishiwaki et al., 2005)
      5) One level 4 article with good evidence (DePippo, Holas, & Reding, 1994)
      6) One level 5 article with good evidence (Ramsey et al., 2003)
   d. Recommendations for best rehabilitation nursing practice:
      1) The evidence cited here provides conflicting results about recommendations for best practice.
      2) All studies agree that early screening tools for dysphagia in stroke survivors are important and that VFS, though the standard, is not practical in all situations.
      3) Most researchers agree that a reliable bedside tool with which to screen those at risk for dysphagia and its complications would be useful. The Veterans Administration (2003) recommended that the speech–language pathologist perform a simple bedside screening on all stroke patients and that those with abnormal findings receive a comprehensive bedside exam. Those assessed to have swallowing problems would then undergo VFS. However, these recommendations are

supported by only fair evidence.

4) The major methods studied for screening of dysphagia include:

   a) VFS, the gold standard and reliable.

   b) Clinical observation of wet voice and spontaneous cough during swallow or dysarthria and poor speech intelligibility (McCollough, 1997).

   c) 30 ml water swallowing tests were found to be highly accurate in one study (DePippo et al., 1994) but had variable sensitivity and were poor at detecting silent aspiration (Ramsey et al., 2003).

   d) Oxygen saturation was found to detect 86% of aspirators and was most accurate in combination with bedside swallowing assessment with a 10-ml water swallow screening (Smith et al., 2000).

5) The practice guidelines examined recommend that water swallow test be used as part of the screening for aspiration risk in stroke patients.

6) VFS is still the most reliable and accurate screening tool for dysphagia, but the water test, clinical observation for signs and symptoms of dysphagia, and oxygen saturation all show promise as screening tools for stroke survivors.

7) More Level I evidence is needed to determine other evidence-based practice for screening for dysphagia in stroke survivors.

References

American Heart Association. (2006). *Primary stroke center certification program.* Retrieved October 23, 2006, from http://www.strokeassociation.org

American Stroke Association. (2005). *Warning signs.* Retrieved February 6, 2005, from http://www.strokeassociation.org

Bader, M., & Palmer, S. (2006, April–June). What's the "hyper" in hyperacute stroke? *AACN Advanced Critical Care, 17*(2), 194–214.

Boss, B.J. (2002a). Alterations of neurologic function. In K.L. McCance & S.E. Huether (Eds.), *Pathophysiology: The biologic basis for disease in adults & children* (4th ed., pp. 487–549). St. Louis: Mosby.

Boss, B.J. (2002b). Concepts of neurologic dysfunction. In K.L. McCance & S.E. Huether (Eds.), *Pathophysiology: The biologic basis for disease in adults & children* (4th ed., pp. 438–486). St. Louis: Mosby.

Buttaro, T.M. (2003). Cerebrovascular accident. In T.M. Buttaro, J. Trybulski, P.P. Bailey, & J. Sandberg-Cook (Eds.), *Primary care: A collaborative practice* (2nd ed., pp. 150–153). St. Louis: Mosby.

Davis, J. (1997). *NDT course for nursing.* Port Townsend, WA: International Clinical Educators.

DePippo, K.L., Holas, M.A., & Reding, M.J. (1994). The Burke dysphagia screening test: Validation of its use in patients with stroke. *Archives of Physical Medicine & Rehabilitation, 75*(12), 1284–1286.

Easton, K.L. (1999). The post-stroke journey: From agonizing to owning. *Geriatric Nursing, 20*(2), 70–75.

Easton, K.L. (2001). The post-stroke journey: From agonzing to owning. Doctoral dissertation. Wayne State University.

Easton, K.L., Rawl, S., Zemen, D.M., Kwiatkowski, S., & Burczyk, B. (1995). The effects of nursing follow-up on the coping strategies used by rehabilitation patients after discharge. *Rehabilitation Nursing, 4*(4), 119–126.

Graykoski, J.J. (2003). Cerebrovascular events. In T.M. Buttaro, J. Trybulski, P.P. Bailey, & J. Sandberg-Cook (Eds.), *Primary care: A collaborative practice* (2nd ed., pp. 929–934). St. Louis: Mosby.

Hartke, R.J., & King, R.B. (2002). Analysis of problem types and difficulty among older stroke caregivers. *Topics in Stroke Rehabilitation, 9*(1), 16–33.

Health News Digest. (2006, October 9). Vampire bats help battle strokes. Retrieved October 24, 2006, from http://healthnewsdigest.com

Hinds, N.P., & Wiles, C.M. (1998). Assessment of swallowing and referral to speech and language therapists in acute stroke. *QJM: An International Journal of Medicine, 91,* 829–835.

Hinkle, J.L. (2006, February). Variables explaining functional recovery following motor stroke. *Journal of Neuroscience Nursing, 38*(1), 6–12.

Keiser, M.M. (1999). Neurologic disorders. In A. Gawlinski & D. Hamwi (Eds.), *Acute care nurse practitioner: Clinical curriculum and certification review* (pp. 295–384). Philadelphia: W.B. Saunders.

King, R.B., & Semik, P.E. (2006, April). Stroke caregiving: Difficult times, resource use, and needs during the first 2 years. *Journal of Gerontological Nursing,* pp. 37–44.

King, R.B., Shade-Zeldow, Y., Carlson, C.E., Feldman, J.L., & Philip, M. (2002). Adaptation to stroke: A longitudinal study of depressive symptoms, physical health, and coping process. *Topics in Stroke Rehabilitation, 9*(1), 46–66.

Kvigne, K., Kirkevold, M. & Gjengedal, E. (2005). The nature of nursing care and rehabilitation of female stroke survivors: The perspective of hospital nurses. *Journal of Clinical Nursing, 14*(7), 897–905.

Love, R.J., & Webb, W.G. (1996). *Neurology for the speech–language pathologist* (3rd ed.). Newton, MA: Butterworth-Heinemann.

Mace, N.L., & Rabins, P.V. (1981). *The 36-hour day.* Baltimore, MD: Johns Hopkins University Press.

Mahoney, F.J., & Barthel, D.W. (1965). Functional evaluation: The Barthel Index. *Maryland State Medical Journal, 14,* 61–65.

Mauk, K.L. (2006). Nursing interventions within the Mauk model of poststroke recovery. *Rehabilitation Nursing, 31*(6), 267–263.

Mauk, KL., & Mauk, J.M. (2006). Future trends in gerontological nursing. In K. Mauk (Ed.), *Gerontological nursing: Competencies for care* (pp. 815–828). Sudbury, MA: Jones and Bartlett.

McCullough, G.H. (1997). *Sensitivity and specificity of a clinical/bedside examination of swallowing for detecting dysphagia in adults subsequent to stroke.* Doctoral dissertation, Vanderbilt University, Nashville, TN.

National Family Caregivers Association. (2002). *About NFCA.* Retrieved December 28, 2006, from http://www.nfcacares.org

National Stroke Association. (2004). *"What can I do to help?"* Retrieved December 28, 2006, from http://stroke.lotsahelpinghands.com

National Stroke Association. (2006a). *African Americans and stroke.* Retrieved December 28, 2006, from http://www.stroke.org

National Stroke Association. (2006b). *Kids and stroke.* Retrieved December 28, 2006, from http://www.stroke.org

National Stroke Association. (2006c). *Managing the demands of caregiving.* Retrieved December 28, 2006, from http://www.stroke.org

National Stroke Association. (2006d). *What is stroke?* Retrieved December 28, 2006, from http://www.stroke.org

Nir, Z., Zolotogorsky, Z., & Sugarman, H. (2004). Structured nursing intervention versus routine rehabilitation after stroke. *American Journal of Physical Medicine & Rehabilitation, 83,* 522–529.

Nishiwaki, K., Tsuji, T., Liu, M., Hase, K., Tanaka, N., & Fujiwara, T. (2005). Identification of a simple screening tool for dysphagia in patients with stroke using factor analysis of multiple dysphagia variables. *Journal of Rehabilitation Medicine, 37,* 247–251.

Pierce, L., Steiner, V., Govoni, A.L. (2002). In-home online support for caregivers of survivors of stoke. *CIN & Computers Information Nursing, 20*(4), 154–164.

Pierce, L., Steiner, V., Govoni, A., Hicks, B., Thompson, T., & Friedemann, M. (2004). Caring-Web: Internet-based support for rural caregivers of persons with stroke show promise. *Rehabilitation Nursing, 29*(3), 95–99, 103.

Pierce, L.L., Steiner, V., Hicks, B., & Holzaepfel, A.L. (2006). Problems of new caregivers of persons with stroke. *Rehabilitation Nursing, 31*(4), 166–172.

Ramsey, D.J.C., Smithard, D.G., & Kalra, L. (2003). Early assessments of dysphagia and aspiration risk in acute stroke patients. *Stroke, 34,* 1252–1257.

Rawl, S.M., Easton, K.L., Zemen, D., Kwiatkowski, S., & Burczyk, B. (1998). Effectiveness of a nurse-managed follow-up program for rehabilitation patients after discharge. *Rehabilitation Nursing, 23*(4), 204–209.

Sauerbeck, L.R. (2006, November). Primary stroke prevention. *AJN, 106*(11), 40–50.

Scottish Intercollegiate Guidelines Network (SIGN). (2004). *Management of patients with stroke: Identification and management of dysphagia. A national clinical guideline.* Edinburgh: Author.

Secrest, J.S. (2002). How stroke survivors and primary support persons experience nurses in rehabilitation. *Rehabilitation Nursing, 27*(5), 176–181.

Secrest, J., & Thomas, S.P. (1999). Continuity and discontinuity: The quality of life following stroke. *Rehabilitation Nursing, 24*(6), 240–246.

Secrest, J., & Zeller, R. (2003). Measuring continuity and discontinuity following stroke. *Journal of Nursing Scholarship, 35*(3), 243–249.

Secrest, J., & Zeller, R. (2006). Replication and extension of the Continuity and Discontinuity of Self Scale (CDSS). *Journal of Nursing Scholarship, 38*(2), 154–159.

Seppa, N. (2003, January 18). *Nifty spittle: Compound in bat saliva may aid stroke patients.* Retrieved October 24, 2006, from http://www.sciencenews.org

Sisson, R.A. (1998). Life after a stroke: Coping with change. *Rehabilitation Nursing, 23*(4), 198–203.

Smith, H.A., Lee, S.H., O'Neill, P.A., & Connolly, M.J. (2000). The combination of bedside swallowing assessment and oxygen saturation monitoring of swallowing in acute stroke: A safe and humane screening tool. *Age and Ageing, 29,* 495–499.

Steiner, V., & Pierce, L. (2002). Building a web of support for caregivers of persons with stroke. *Topics in Stroke Rehabilitation, 9*(3), 102–111.

Stroke. (1988). *Stroke, 19,* 604–607.

Sugerman, R.A. (2002). Structure and function of the neurologic system. In K.L. McCance & S.E. Huether (Eds.), *Pathophysiology: The biologic basis for disease in adults & children* (4th ed., pp. 363–396). St. Louis: Mosby.

Veterans Health Administration, Department of Defense. (2003). *VA/DoD clinical practice guideline for the management of stroke rehabilitation in the primary care setting.* Washington, DC: Author.

Weed, R.O. (1999). *Life care planning and case management handbook.* Boca Raton, FL: CRC Press.

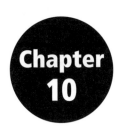

Chapter 10

Traumatic Injuries: TBI and SCI

Linda Dufour, MSN RN CRRN • Joan Williams, MSN RN CRRN ARNP-C
Tiffany Lecroy, RN CMSN CCRC • Rachel Emery, BA • Kristen L. Mauk, PhD RN CRRN-A APRN BC

Catastrophic injuries of the brain and spinal cord affect millions of people each year. Falls, motor vehicle accidents, violence, and sporting and recreational injuries are the major causes. Annually, about 11,000 new spinal cord injuries (SCIs) occur (CDC, unpublished data), and an estimated 1.4 million people sustain a traumatic brain injury (TBI) (National Center for Injury Prevention and Control [NCIPC], 2007). Both injuries largely affect the younger population and tend to occur more often in men. Both types of injuries produce alterations that vary according to the specific location and severity of injury.

Rehabilitation nurses play an important role in enhancing patient outcomes through astute assessment, timely interventions, and thorough evaluation. The rehabilitation process is interdisciplinary and works to improve all aspects of the individual's life.

I. Traumatic Brain Injury (TBI)

A. Overview
1. Definitions
   a. Refers to a blow or a jolt to the head or a penetrating injury to head that disrupts the function of the brain (Brain Injury Association, 2005)
   b. May produce altered levels of consciousness, changes in cognition and behavior, and physical limitations (Brain Injury Association, 2005)
   c. The severity of brain injury may range from mild to moderate or severe (Brain Injury Association, 2005)
2. Impact
   a. Affects roles and relationships for individual and family (Baggerly & Le, 2001)
   b. Often affects employment, finances, and leisure activities (Baggerly & Le, 2001)
3. General symptoms (Table 10-1)

B. Types of Injuries
1. Concussion
   a. Definition: an immediate, temporary loss of consciousness resulting from a mechanical force to the brain (Hickey, 2003b)
   b. Symptoms: may or may not report unconsciousness (Evans, 2003), momentary loss of reflexes or memory, headache, confusion, dizziness, irritability, visual and gait disturbances (Hickey, 2003b)

2. Contusion: bruising to the brain cortex; may be moderate or severe; associated with a loss of consciousness, stupor, and confusion; outcomes vary according to location and severity of injury (Blank-Reid & Barker, 2002)

3. Hemorrhagic injuries
   a. Subdural hematoma
      1) Results from bleeding between the dura and arachnoid interface
      2) May be acute, subacute, or chronic.
      3) Occurs in 5%–22% of patients with intracranial injuries and is more common in older adults
      4) Changes in level of consciousness, elevated intracranial pressure and associated symptoms, seizure, paresis
      5) Surgical evacuation may be needed for larger sizes (more than 1 cm in adult); smaller sizes may benefit from medical management (Chanda & Nanda, 2003).
   b. Epidural hematoma
      1) Develops as a rapid arterial or venous bleed often associated with skull fracture or a lacerated meningeal artery (most common cause)
      2) More common in young adults and adults over age 60
      3) Accounts for about 2% of traumatic intracranial insults
      4) Changes in level of consciousness, elevated intracranial pressure and associated symptoms, seizure, paresis
      5) Usually warrants surgical management (Chanda & Nanda, 2003)

c. Intracerebral hemorrhage
   1) Develops from bleeding into the cerebral tissue and is associated with contusions
   2) May act as a space-occupying lesion compressing brain tissue; poor prognosis
   3) Headache, deteriorating consciousness, coma, contralateral paresis, ipsilateral dilated pupil, signs of herniation (Hickey, 2003b)
d. Subarachnoid hemorrhage
   1) Develops from bleeding into the subarachnoid space
   2) Is associated with severe head injury and aneurysmal ruptures
   3) Symptoms related to elevated intracranial pressure and meningeal irritation (Hickey, 2003b)

4. Penetrating injuries
   a. Missile injuries (high-velocity trauma)
      1) Caused by gunshots, nail guns, or other types of missiles. The location, path of injury, and depth of penetration directly affect the severity of the injury.
      2) May be associated with infection caused by bone fragments, hair, and skin entering the brain with the missile (Blank-Reid & Barker, 2002).
   b. Stab wounds
      1) Refers to the piercing of the scalp, skull, or brain by a foreign object (e.g., knife, ice pick, pencil, scissors)
      2) May cause severe neurologic impairment depending on the location of the insult (Vinas et al., 2006)

C. Epidemiology
   1. It is estimated that at least 5.3 million people have a need for extended or permanent assistance in activities of daily living (ADLs) because of a TBI. Annually 80,000–90,000 people experience the onset of long-term or permanent disability caused by TBI.
   2. Based on 1995–2001 data about emergency department (ED) visits, hospitalizations, and deaths, the NCIPC (2006) reported that each year:

Table 10-1. General Symptoms of Traumatic Brain Injury

Physical	Cognitive and Behavioral
Paresis	Poor initiation
Dysphagia	Disinhibition
Dysarthria	Agitation
Cerebrospinal fluid leaks	Restlessness
Balance and coordination impairments	Impulsivity
Visual impairments	Aphasias
Loss of bowel control	Memory and thinking deficits
Loss of bladder control	Sequencing difficulties
Spasticity and loss of tone	Attention and concentration deficits
Seizures	Problem solving and reasoning deficits
Dysautonomia ("storming")	Anxiety
Sleep–wake disturbance	Depression
Pain	Emotional lability
Metabolic effects (higher nutritional needs)	Loss of social competence

Sources consulted

Baggerly, J., & Le, N. (2001). Nursing management of the patient with head trauma. In J.B. Derstine & S.D. Hargrove (Eds.), *Comprehensive rehabilitation nursing* (pp. 331–367). Philadelphia: W.B. Saunders.

Hickey, J. (2003b).Craniocerebral trauma. In J. Hickey (Ed.), *Clinical practice of neurological and neurosurgical nursing* (5th ed., pp. 373–406). Philadelphia: Lippincott.

Hickey, J. (2003c). Overview of neuroanatomy and neurophysiology. In J. Hickey (Ed.), *Clinical practice of neurological and neurosurgical nursing* (5th ed., pp. 45–92). Philadelphia: Lippincott.

---

   a. 1.1 million people are treated and released for TBI from hospital EDs.
   b. 235,000 people are hospitalized and survive TBI, and 50,000 do not survive.
   3. The NCIPC (2006) also reported the following 1995–2001 data:
   a. Adults age 75 and older have the highest rate of TBI-related hospitalizations and deaths, whereas very young children ages 0–4 and adolescents ages 15–19 have the highest rates of ED visits.
   b. Men are approximately 1.5 times more likely to sustain a TBI than women.
   c. Boys age 0–4 have the highest rate of TBI-related deaths, hospitalizations, and ED visits combined, followed by girls ages 0–4, adolescents ages 15–19, and adults 75 and older.

D. Etiology and Causes of TBI
   1. Falls (28%); leading cause of TBI. Rate is highest among children ages 0–4 and adults ages 75 and over (NCIPC, 2006).
   2. Motor vehicle accidents (20%); highest rate is among adolescents ages 15–19 (NCIPC, 2006).
   3. Struck by or against events (19%): includes sports-related injuries. An estimated 300,000

sports-related mild to moderate brain injuries occur annually (Sosin, Sniezek, & Thurman, 1996).

4. Assaults (11%); highest rate is among adolescents ages 15–19 (NCIPC, 2006).

5. Other (13%) (NCIPC, 2006).

6. Unknown (9%) (NCIPC, 2006).

E. Pathophysiology

1. Primary injuries

   a. Primary injury: damage to the brain that occurs at the moment of impact (Gennarelli & Graham, 2005).

   b. Acceleration and deceleration injuries: caused by changes in velocity when the head has a rapid forward movement and then stops abruptly; causes strain on the brain tissue in the form of compression, tension, or shearing (Hickey, 2003b); associated with motor vehicle crashes, falls, and objects striking the head (Blank-Reid & Barker, 2002).

   c. Diffuse axonal injuries (DAI):

     1) DAIs are caused by microscopic damage to neuronal axons; microscopic lesions are not seen on traditional computed tomography (CT) scan; they may appear as small areas of hemorrhage (Meythaler, Peduzzi, Eleftheriou, & Novack, 2001; Wasserman & Koenigsberg, 2004).

     2) Destruction occurs in the cerebral hemispheres, corpus callosum, and brainstem; often seen in areas where brain densities differ, such as the junctions of gray and white matter.

     3) Severity depends on the magnitude of the acceleration forces involved in the traumatic event and usually is worse than what is noted on imaging studies (Wasserman & Koenigsberg, 2004).

     4) Classified as mild, moderate, or severe; about 45% of patients fall into the moderate category, with incomplete recovery in those that survive (Hickey, 2003b).

   d. Focal injuries: areas damaged by a localized trauma, involving consolidated areas of tissue destruction such as contusions, lacerations, hematomas, and intracranial hemorrhages; symptoms vary according to type, extent, and location of injury (Hickey, 2003b).

2. Secondary injuries

   a. Complications after a primary event

(Gennarelli & Graham, 2005)

   b. Causes (Blank-Reid & Barker, 2002; Povlishock & Katz, 2005)

     1) Cerebral edema

     2) Elevated intracranial pressure

     3) Hypoxia and ischemia

     4) Infection and inflammatory response

     5) Hypotension

     6) Electrolyte imbalance, hypocapnia

     7) Hyperthermia

     8) Vasospasm

F. Assessment

1. Classification

   a. Mild brain injury

     1) Description:

       a) May result in a loss of consciousness for 30 minutes or less (NCIPC, 2003)

       b) Glasgow Coma Scale (GCS) scores of 13–15 (NCIPC, 2003) and negative neuroimaging (see Table 10-2)

       c) A complicated mild brain injury has the same GCS score but with positive CT findings (Kennedy et al., 2006).

       d) About 75% of TBIs are classified as mild (NCIPC, 2006).

     2) Symptoms may include dizziness, headache, insomnia, fatigue, decreased memory, and irritability (NCIPC, 2006).

   b. Moderate brain injury

     1) Description:

       a) GCS scores ranging from 9 to 12 (van Baalen et al., 2003)

       b) Abnormal CT findings

     2) Physical, cognitive, and behavioral symptoms last several months or are permanent (DOD, 1999).

     3) May have a good recovery or learn to compensate for neurological deficits with proper treatment (Department of Defense [DOD], 1999)

   c. Severe brain injury

     1) Description

       a) Loss of consciousness lasting hours, days, months, or years (DOD, 1999).

       b) GCS scores less than 8 (van Baalen et al., 2003).

       c) May make significant improvements but often are left with permanent residual neurological deficits (DOD, 1999)

     2) Severe disorders of consciousness

Table 10-2. Glasgow Coma Scale Categories

Category	Response	Score
Eye opening	Spontaneous: Eyes open spontaneously without verbal or noxious stimulation.	4
	To speech: Eyes open with verbal stimuli but not necessarily to command.	3
	To pain: Eyes open with various forms of noxious stimuli.	2
	None: No eye opening with any type of stimulation.	1
Verbal response	Oriented: Aware of person, place, time, reason for hospitalization, and personal data.	5
	Confused: Answers not appropriate to question but correct use of language.	4
	Inappropriate words: Disorganized, random speech, no sustained conversation.	3
	Incomprehensible sounds: Moans, groans, and mumbles incomprehensibly.	2
	None: No verbalization, even to noxious stimuli.	1
Best motor response	Obeys commands: Performs simple tasks on command and able to repeat task on command.	6
	Localizes to pain: Organized attempt to localize and remove painful stimuli.	5
	Withdraws from pain: Withdraws extremity from source of painful stimuli.	4
	Abnormal flexion: Decorticate posturing that occurs spontaneously or in response to noxious stimuli.	3
	Extension: Decerebrate posturing that occurs spontaneously or in response to noxious stimuli.	2
	None: No response to noxious stimuli; flaccid.	1

Source consulted

Hickey, J. (1997). *Clinical practice of neurological and neurosurgical nursing* (4th ed.). Philadelphia: Lippencott. Reprinted with permission of Elsevier.

(subcategories of severe brain injury) (Giacino & Whyte, 2005; Giacino et al., 2002)

a) Coma: complete absence of arousal or responsiveness.
   (1) Eyes do not open spontaneously or in response to stimulation
   (2) Absent sleep–wake cycle
   (3) No purposeful motor activity, distinct defensive movements, or localization to noxious stimuli
   (4) No ability to follow commands or intelligible verbalization
   (5) No conscious awareness of self or environment

b) Vegetative state: no distinct evidence of conscious awareness of self or environment.
   (1) Eyes open spontaneously.
   (2) Sleep–wake cycle resumes; arousal is sluggish, poorly sustained.
   (3) No signs of intentional, purposeful, or reproducible behavioral responses to stimuli
   (4) No signs of language perception or communication

c) Minimally conscious state: distinct behavioral signs of conscious awareness as evidenced by at least one of the following:
   (1) Basic command following
   (2) Intelligible verbalization
   (3) Yes–no responses, whether verbal or by gesture
   (4) Nonreflexive emotional or motor behavior that occurs in response to related environmental stimuli (e.g., affective responses to emotional content, object manipulation, pursuit eye movements)

d) Locked-in syndrome
   (1) Eye opening is present; eye movement is the primary mode of communication.
   (2) Basic cognitive function evident on exam
   (3) Clinical evidence of quadriplegia
   (4) Often occurs as a result of a lesion in the pons

e) Akinetic mutism: condition characterized by diminished neurologic drive or inattention; movement and speech are extremely deficient.
   (1) Eye opening and spontaneous visual tracking are present.
   (2) Can be considered a

subcategory of minimally conscious state because purposeful responses often are inconsistent but can be elicited after application of stimulation

2. Assessment instruments and tools

a. Agitated Behavior Scale

1) Used for ongoing assessment of presence and intensity of agitation during the acute phase of recovery (Bogner, Corrigan, Bode, & Heinemann, 2000)

2) Composed of 14 items that are each rated from 1 (*absent*) to 4 (*present to an extreme degree*)

3) Best overall indicator for agitation is the total score, although subscales for disinhibition, aggression, and lability can be calculated (Corrigan & Bogner, 1994)

b. Coma/Near Coma (Rappaport, 2000, 2005)

1) Designed to expand the upper range of the Disability Rating Scale

2) Measures clinical changes in vegetative and persistent vegetative state

3) Has 8 items grouped into 5 categories ranging from *extreme coma* to *no coma*

c. Coma Recovery Scale Revised (Kalmar & Giacino 2005; Giacino, Kalmar, & Whyte, 2004)

1) Designed to assess subtle changes in cognitive status and to predict outcome in patients with severe disorders of consciousness

2) Differentiates between vegetative and minimally conscious state

d. Disability Rating Scale

1) Designed to quantitatively assess moderate to severe brain injury along a wide continuum of recovery, from severe vegetative state to no disability (Wright, 2000)

2) Composed of 8 items that are divided into 4 categories: arousability, cognitive ability for self-care, degree of dependence, and employability (Rappaport, 2005; van Baalen et al., 2003)

e. Functional Independence Measure (Grosswasser, Schwab, & Salazar, 1997; van Baalen et al., 2003)

1) Constructed to provide a uniform measure of function across rehabilitation settings

2) Measures items of self-care, sphincter control, mobility, locomotion, communication, and social cognition

f. Galveston Orientation and Amnesia Test: used to measure the duration of posttraumatic amnesia after a brain injury (Levin, O'Donald, & Grossman, 1975; van Baalen et al., 2003)

g. GCS (see Table 10-2)

1) Used to assess the level of consciousness after a brain injury

2) Categorized into three main assessment areas: motor, verbal, and eye-opening responses

3) Is very useful in the acute care setting (Rosebrough, 1998)

h. Glasgow Outcome Scale: developed to assess general outcome after brain injury; categories include *good recovery, moderate disability, severe disability, persistent vegetative state,* and *death* (van Baalen et al., 2003)

i. Neurobehavioral Functioning Inventory (Kreutzer, Seel, & Marwitz, 1999; Marwitz, 2000)

1) Used to assess the frequency of a variety of behaviors and symptoms that may occur after brain injury

2) Composed of 76 items divided into 6 categories: depression, somatic, memory and attention, communication, aggression, and motor

j. Neuropsychological testing

1) Refers to a variety of tests and test batteries that are used to measure cognitive function

2) May includes measures of attention, memory, concentration, reasoning, processing speed, and executive function (Girard et al., 1996)

k. Rancho Levels of Cognitive Function Scale: used to interpret the cognitive recovery process after a brain injury (Rancho Los Amigos National Rehabilitation Center, 2006) (see Table 10-3)

1) Levels range from 1 to 10. Lower scores indicate a more severe impairment of consciousness.

2) Hagen (personal communication, October 25, 2006) states that the Rancho Levels of Cognitive Function Scale was created as a team treatment scale.

Table 10-3. Rancho Los Amigos Levels of Cognitive Functioning Scale—Revised

Cognitive Level	Expected Behavior
Level I No response: Total assistance	Complete absence of observable change in behavior when presented visual, auditory, tactile, proprioceptive, vestibular or painful stimuli.
Level II Generalized response: Total assistance	Demonstrates generalized reflex response to painful stimuli. Responds to repeated auditory stimuli with increased or decreased activity. Responds to external stimuli with physiological changes generalized, gross body movement and/or not purposeful vocalization. Responses noted above may be same regardless of type and location of stimulation. Responses may be significantly delayed.
Level III Localized response: Total assistance	Demonstrates withdrawal or vocalization to painful stimuli. Turns toward or away from auditory stimuli. Blinks when strong light crosses visual field. Follows moving object passed within visual field. Responds to discomfort by pulling tubes or restraints. Responds inconsistently to simple commands. Responses directly related to type of stimulus. May respond to some persons (especially family and friends) but not to others.
Level IV Confused/agitated: Maximal assistance	Alert and in heightened state of activity. Purposeful attempts to remove restraints or tubes or crawl out of bed. May perform motor activities such as sitting, reaching and walking but without any apparent purpose or upon another's request. Very brief and usually non-purposeful moments of sustained alternatives and divided attention. Absent short-term memory. May cry out or scream out of proportion to stimulus even after its removal. May exhibit aggressive or flight behavior. Mood may swing from euphoric to hostile with no apparent relationship to environmental events. Unable to cooperate with treatment efforts. Verbalizations are frequently incoherent and/or inappropriate to activity or environment.
Level V Confused, inappropriate non-agitated: Maximal assistance	Alert, not agitated but may wander randomly or with a vague intention of going home. May become agitated in response to external stimulation and/or lack of environmental structure. Not oriented to person, place or time. Frequent brief periods, non-purposeful sustained attention. Severely impaired recent memory, with confusion of past and present in reaction to ongoing activity. Absent goal directed, problem solving, self-monitoring behavior. Often demonstrates inappropriate use of objects without external direction. May be able to perform previously learned tasks when structured and cues provided. Unable to learn new information. Able to respond appropriately to simple commands fairly consistently with external structures and cues. Responses to simple commands without external structure are random and non-purposeful in relation to command. Able to converse on a social, automatic level for brief periods of time when provided external structure and cues. Verbalizations about present events become inappropriate and confabulatory when external structure and cues are not provided. *Continued*

Table 10-3. Rancho Los Amigos Levels of Cognitive Functioning Scale—Revised *(Continued)*

Cognitive Level	Expected Behavior
Level VI Confused, appropriate: Moderate assistance	Inconsistently oriented to person, time, and place.
	Able to attend to highly familiar tasks in non-distracting environment for 30 minutes with moderate redirection.
	Remote memory has more depth and detail than recent memory.
	Vague recognition of some staff.
	Able to use assistive memory aid with maximum assistance.
	Emerging awareness of appropriate response to self, family, and basic needs.
	Moderate assist to problem solve barriers to task completion.
	Supervised for old learning (e.g., self care).
	Shows carry over for relearned familiar tasks (e.g., self care).
	Maximum assistance for new learning with little or no carry over.
	Unaware of impairments, disabilities and safety risks.
	Consistently follows simple directions.
	Verbal expressions are appropriate in highly familiar and structured situations.
Level VII Automatic, appropriate: Minimal assistance for daily living skills	Consistently oriented to person and place, within highly familiar environments. Moderate assistance for orientation to time.
	Able to attend to highly familiar tasks in a non-distraction environment for at least 30 minutes with minimal assist to complete tasks.
	Minimal supervision for new learning.
	Demonstrates carry over of new learning.
	Initiates and carries out steps to complete familiar personal and household routine but has shallow recall of what he/she has been doing.
	Able to monitor accuracy and completeness of each step in routine personal and household ADLs and modify plan with minimal assistance.
	Superficial awareness of his/her condition but unaware of specific impairments and disabilities and the limits they place on his/her ability to safely, accurately, and completely carry out his/her household, community, work, and leisure ADLs.
	Minimal supervision for safety in routine home and community activities.
	Unrealistic planning for the future.
	Unable to think about consequences of a decision or action.
	Overestimates abilities.
	Unaware of others' needs and feelings.
	Oppositional/uncooperative.
	Unable to recognize inappropriate social interaction behavior.
Level VIII Purposeful, appropriate: Stand-by assistance	Consistently oriented to person, place, and time.
	Independently attends to and completes familiar tasks for 1 hour in distracting environments.
	Able to recall and integrate past and recent events.
	Uses assistive memory devices to recall daily schedule, "to do" lists and record critical information for later use with stand-by assistance.
	Initiates and carries out steps to complete familiar personal, household, community, work and leisure routines with stand-by assistance and can modify the plan when needed with minimal assistance.
	Requires no assistance once new tasks/activities are learned.
	Aware of and acknowledges impairments and disabilities when they interfere with task completion but requires stand-by assistance to take appropriate corrective action.
	Thinks about consequences of a decision or action with minimal assistance.
	Overestimates or underestimates abilities.
	Acknowledges others' needs and feelings and responds appropriately with minimal assistance.
	Depressed.
	Irritable.
	Low frustration tolerance/easily angered.
	Argumentative.
	Self-centered.
	Uncharacteristically dependent/independent.
	Able to recognize and acknowledge inappropriate social interaction behavior while it is occurring and takes corrective action with minimal assistance. <div align="right">*Continued*</div>

Table 10-3. Rancho Los Amigos Levels of Cognitive Functioning Scale—Revised *(Continued)*

Cognitive Level	Expected Behavior
Level IX Purposeful, appropriate: Stand-by assistance on request	Independently shifts back and forth between tasks and completes them accurately for at least two consecutive hours.
	Uses assistive memory devices to recall daily schedule, "to do" lists and record critical information for later use with assistance when requested.
	Initiates and carries out steps to complete familiar personal, household, work and leisure tasks independently and unfamiliar personal, household, work and leisure tasks with assistance when requested.
	Aware of and acknowledges impairments and disabilities when they interfere with task completion and takes appropriate corrective action but requires stand-by assist to anticipate a problem before it occurs and take action to avoid it.
	Able to think about consequences of decisions or actions with assistance when requested.
	Accurately estimates abilities but requires stand-by assistance to adjust to task demands.
	Acknowledges others' needs and feelings and responds appropriately with stand-by assistance.
	Depression may continue.
	May be easily irritable.
	May have low frustration tolerance.
	Able to self monitor appropriateness of social interaction with stand-by assistance.
Level X Purposeful, appropriate: Modified independent	Able to handle multiple tasks simultaneously in all environments but may require periodic breaks.
	Able to independently procure, create, and maintain own assistive memory devices.
	Independently initiates and carries out steps to complete familiar and unfamiliar personal, household, community, work and leisure tasks but may require more than usual amount of time and/or compensatory strategies to complete them.
	Anticipates impact of impairments and disabilities on ability to complete daily living tasks and takes action to avoid problems before they occur but may require more than usual amount of time and/or compensatory strategies.
	Able to independently think about consequences of decisions or actions but may require more than usual amount of time and/or compensatory strategies to select the appropriate decision or action.
	Accurately estimates abilities and independently adjusts to task demands.
	Able to recognize the needs and feelings of others and automatically respond in appropriate manner.
	Periodic periods of depression may occur.
	Irritability and low frustration tolerance when sick, fatigued and/or under emotional stress.
	Social interaction behavior is consistently appropriate.

Sources consulted

Rancho Los Amigos Levels of Cognitive Functioning Scale—Revised. Reprinted with permission. Original scale co-authored by Hagen, C., Malkmus D., Durham P., (2006).

Communication Disorders Service, Rancho Los Amigos Hospital, 1972. Revised 1974 by Hagen, C., Malkmus, D. & Stenderup, K. Revised scale 1997 by Hagen, C.

3) After level I patients may fluctuate between three levels, with the mid-level being the most common.

4) All members of the team determine what factors help the patient remain at his or her most common level of cognitive functioning, what factors facilitate movement to higher levels, and what factors cause regression.

l. Sensory Stimulation Assessment Measure: designed to expand the GCS and used to standardize sensory presentation (Duff & Wells, 1997; O'Dell & Riggs, 1996; Rader, Alston, & Ellis, 1989)

m. Western Neuro Sensory Stimulation Profile

1) Used to assess auditory and visual comprehension, tracking, object manipulation, attention, arousal, tactile, and olfactory function

2) Contains 33 items in 6 areas (Ansell & Keenan, 1989)

3. Physical assessment

a. General: Determine location of brain injury and corresponding symptoms (see Tables 10-4 and 10-5).

b. Neurologic:

1) Assess cognitive, motor, and sensory status, reflexes, and cranial nerves.

2) Monitor anticonvulsant levels.

3) Monitor for signs and symptoms of elevated intracranial pressure.

4) Monitor changes in behavior (excesses and deficits).

5) Monitor changes in level of consciousness.

6) Monitor effects of medications prescribed for cognition and behavior (at present most of these are often used off label).

c. Respiratory: Assess airway patency, oxygen saturation, nature of sputum, lung fields, and potential for aspiration.

Table 10-4. Location of Injury and Associated Symptoms

Region of Brain	Symptoms
Frontal lobe	Impaired judgment, reasoning, concentration, abstraction, executive functions, behavior, and impulse control; expressive aphasia in dominant hemisphere (usually the left hemisphere); impaired voluntary motor function
Temporal lobe	Impaired somatic, auditory, olfactory, and visual association; receptive aphasia in dominant hemisphere (usually the left hemisphere); impaired learning and detailed memories such as past experiences, conversations, art, music, and taste
Parietal lobes	Impaired sensory association; impaired ability to recognize size, shape, texture, presence of touch, pressure, and body position; impaired recognition of own body parts (often called neglect)
Occipital lobe	Impaired visual perception and visual reflexes
Cerebellum	Impaired fine motor movement, balance, coordination
Brainstem	Abnormalities of cranial nerve function depending on location in brainstem; impaired cardiac, respiratory, and vasomotor function; wakefulness

Sources consulted

Barker, E. (2002). Neuroanatomy and physiology of the nervous system. In E. Barker (Ed.), *Neuroscience nursing: A spectrum of care* (pp. 3–50). St. Louis: Mosby.

Hickey, J. (2003c). Overview of neuroanatomy and neurophysiology. In J. Hickey (Ed.), *Clinical practice of neurological and neurosurgical nursing* (5th ed., pp. 45–92). Philadelphia: Lippincott.

Table 10-5. Cerebral Hemispheres and Symptoms

Right Hemisphere	Left Hemisphere
Motor impairment on left side of body	Motor impairments on right side of body
Impulsivity	Impaired speech and language; aphasias
Impaired judgment	Impaired comprehension
Impaired insight into condition (may not realize that deficits exist)	Cautious, slow to perform
Left-sided neglect	Aware of deficits, depression, anxiety
Spatial–perceptual deficits	Impaired right–left discrimination

Source consulted

Barker, E. (2002). Neuroanatomy and physiology of the nervous system. In E. Barker (Ed.), *Neuroscience nursing: A spectrum of care* (pp. 3–50). St. Louis: Mosby.

d. Cardiovascular: Assess blood pressure, pulse, heart rate, rhythm, risk for or existence of deep vein thrombosis, and risk factors for emboli (atrial fibrillation); presence of dysautonomia.

e. Nutritional: Assess weekly weights, intake and output, daily hydration status, and dietary intake; anticipate that the patient will have increased metabolic demands; modify diet if dysphagia is present (e.g., use of thickener).

f. Sensory and perceptual: Assess responses to various types of stimuli, sleep–wake cycles, level of consciousness, presence of neglect.

g. Elimination:
1) Assess bowel sounds and premorbid bowel patterns.
2) Assess premorbid elimination history, urinary output, and bowel movements.
3) Assess bowel and bladder continence and effectiveness of bowel and bladder programs (e.g., scheduled toileting programs, medications).
4) Monitor for potential alterations in elimination (e.g., constipation, diarrhea, urinary tract infection, and retention).

h. Musculoskeletal:
1) Assess for heterotropic ossification, orthopedic injuries, premorbid history of joint disease, contractures, tone, spasticity, range of motion (ROM), need for adaptive equipment.
2) Observe safety with transfers, gait, and mobility as appropriate.
3) Assess handedness.
4) Assess padding and positioning needs to maintain ROM.

i. Integumentary: Assess skin condition (turgor, color, wounds, and high-risk places under pressure such as areas with orthotic devices).

j. Communication: Assess for expressive, receptive, and global aphasias, dysarthria, and alternative communication strategies (e.g., augmentative communication devices).

k. Behavior: Assess for behavior excesses (e.g., agitation, disinhibition, impulsivity, poor judgment, motor restlessness, perseveration, emotional lability) and deficits (e.g., apathy, poor initiation).

l. Safety:
1) Assess for risk of falls, wandering, impulsivity, balance, strength, judgment, and insight.
2) Assess need for least restrictive restraint or 1:1 sitter if necessary.

m. Psychosocial: Assess family support, coping mechanisms, and potential response to fear and anxiety.

n. Sexual: Assess function issues and related physical, cognitive, and behavioral alterations:
   1) Last menstrual period
   2) Pregnancy at time of admission
   3) Premorbid sexual problems
   4) Developmental stage

o. Educational needs of patient and caregiver:
   1) Physical, psychosocial, safety care
   2) Preferred learning style
   3) Barriers to learning
   4) Readiness to learn

p. Vocational: Assess potential for returning to work, school, or other purposeful activity (e.g., volunteering).

G. Planning: Patient and Family Goals
   1. Set individualized goals upon admission:
      a. Bowel and bladder continence or established elimination schedules depending on cognition and level of consciousness
      b. Improved cognition
      c. Improved mobility
      d. Improved functional independence
      e. Improved safety (see Table 10-6)
      f. Improved judgment
      g. Manageable behavior

h. Increased knowledge to care for self or patient

i. Resolution of medical problems

j. Adequate nutritional status or plan to achieve such

   2. Meet at regular intervals to evaluate status of goal achievement.

   3. Add or delete goals based on patient's progress and condition.

H. Nursing Plan of Care and Interventions for Cognitive Rehabilitation (see Table 10-7)

I. Evaluation
   1. Evaluate progress toward patient and family goals listed in Section G.
   2. Use instruments described in Section F.2.

J. Discharge Planning and Community Resources
   1. Discharge planning should begin before admission to the rehabilitation facility.
   2. Discharge planning should incorporate extensive exploration of community resources for a lifetime of disability management.
      a. Financial resources
         1) Private insurance
         2) Auto insurance
         3) Medicare and Medicaid
         4) Social Security Disability Insurance
         5) Litigation awards
         6) Donations
      b. Continuum of care options

Table 10-6. Safety Tips

Don't	Do
Leave sharp objects in reach.	Provide the recommended supervision levels at home (as suggested by the rehabilitation team).
Leave poisons, chemicals, and household cleaners within reach.	Communicate with patient as an adult.
Leave car keys or keys to heavy equipment within reach.	Speak to patient in a regular tone of voice.
Leave patient alone near fire or heat sources (stove, barbecue, matches, lighters, cigarettes).	Praise small accomplishments and do so at the time of occurrence.
Assume that the patient has the same preinjury abilities or can resume his or her previous roles at home, at work, or in society.	Provide brain injury awareness information to the patient's neighbors and fire and police departments.
Leave patient alone near bodies of water (ocean, lakes, swimming pools).	Provide structure and consistency of schedules.
Leave patient unattended and at risk for wandering, falls, or other injuries.	Provide a balance of stimulation and quiet time; recognize signs of impending escalation or fatigue.
Leave patient alone with heavy machinery.	Provide information on positive coping strategies regarding changes in family, work, and social roles.
Leave patient alone or in charge of small children until level of supervision or assistance is known.	Maintain a safe physical environment related to cognitive, behavioral, and physical changes.
Provide meal types or diet textures that are outside the prescribed plan of care.	Reintegrate the patient into community activities as appropriate for the patient's cognitive and behavioral level.
Overstimulate the patient with a multitude of schedule changes, activities, or visitors.	Maintain diet type and texture to prevent aspiration.

Teaching Topics

Source consulted

Dufour, L., Williams, J., & Coleman, K. (2000). Traumatic injuries: TBI and SCI. In P.A. Edwards (Ed.), *The specialty practice of rehabilitation nursing: A core curriculum* (4th ed., p. 194). Glenview, IL: Association of Rehabilitation Nurses.

Table 10-7. Plan of Care for Cognitive Rehabilitation

Cognitive Level	Description	Nursing Management for Levels I, II, and III
I: No response	Unresponsive to touch, pain, or auditory or verbal stimuli	Orient patient.
		Encourage family to bring in favorite music, pictures, blankets.
		Begin to talk to the patient about family members and friends.
II: Generalized response	Displays inconsistent, nonpurposeful, reflexic responses to stimuli or pain	Talk in a normal tone of voice and use short simple phrases, explaining all nursing tasks.
		Be careful what you say in front of the patient.
		Guide patient to follow simple commands (wink, wiggle fingers).
III: Localized response	Responds in a more focused manner to certain types of stimuli (e.g., turns to sound, withdraws from pain, tracks); may follow simple commands inconsistently	Allow extra time for a response.
		Introduce smells, tactile, auditory, and visual stimulation.
		Engage in familiar activities.
		Nursing assessments and physical care.
		Monitor cardiovascular effects of pharmacological management (neurostimulants).
		Offer emotional support to family members.
		Talk to the patient about familiar topics of interest, family and close friends.
		Schedule nursing tasks to promote sleep/wake cycles.
		Begin family education; provide materials related to injury.
		Show family how to interact with patient – model behaviors; teach them not to overstimulate.
		Provide emotional support.

Nursing Management for Level IV

IV: Confused agitated	Alert and in heightened state of activity; possibly aggressive; may display inappropriate behavior in response to internal confusion; short attention span	Limit the number of visitors to 2 or 3.
		Provide a quiet, calm, environment; eliminate "noise clutter" from the environment.
		Reorient frequently.
		Reassure the patient that s/he is safe.
		Monitor sleep/wake cycles.
		Provide familiar objects or photos from home.
		Allow as much freedom of movement as is safe.
		Do nursing care in short blocks; take a break, the start the next task giving the patient a break.
		Have a helper for safety.
		Low stim during care; explain care in simple terms, avoiding "chatter."
		Consider 1:1 supervision v. restraints during certain times of day.
		Use quiet, low traffic areas for activities that require attention (eating for example).
		Remove items that might be frightening to the patient (TV/news).
		Use close circuit cameras for additional monitoring.
		Consider an enclosure bed.
		Do not force him to do things. Instead, listen to what he wants to do and follow his lead, within safety limits.
		Give breaks to prevent agitation or restlessness. Look for patterns. Work with team on this.
		Change activities frequently; redirect as needed.
		Consider that patient has no short-term memory so behavior plans with "consequences" typically don't work.
		Preventing agitation through controlling the external environment and therapeutic use of self are KEY.
		Monitor pharmacological management which may include anti-anxiety agents.
		Use structure; same staff, same routing, same way of doing things.
		Prevention is better than intervention.

Continued

Table 10-7. Plan of Care for Cognitive Rehabilitation *(Continued)*

Cognitive Level	Description	Nursing Management for Levels V and VI
V: Confused inappropriate (nonagitated)	Alert, easily distracted, responsive to commands; pays gross attention to environment; displays absent carryover from one situation to another	Use repetition. Reorient frequently to person, place and time. Use short and simple comments and questions. Assist with activity initiation; set-up. Show patient pictures and objects that were of interest pre-injury.
VI: Confused appropriate	Follows commands consistently but is inconsistently oriented to time and place; has short-term memory deficits; begins to participate in self-care	Provide frequent rest periods; collaborate with therapy team on schedule. Limit the number of visitors. Monitor nutrition with increased activity. Establish bowel and bladder continence; start toileting programs. Provide tasks appropriate to level (e.g. hygiene, simple meal preparation – cold cereal). Identify areas of motivation for self-care tasks. Schedule rest and quiet time; fatigue or stress is common. Introduce memory aids (i.e. calendars, schedules); help with schedule. Discuss events of the day to help improve memory. Monitor medication regimen; report sleep/wake, lethargy, agitation patterns to MD. Begin to incorporate the patient in the education process with family. Provide education to patient regarding injury and outcomes. Monitor for safety – still an important concern. Structure activities; staff should use a lot of cueing; the goal is for the patient to "figure it out" with your help. Provide daily structure. Encourage participation in all therapies. Give immediate positive feedback. May start to use behavior plans with simple rewards.

Cognitive Level	Description	Nursing Management for Levels VII and VIII
VII: Automatic–appropriate	May perform tasks in familiar environment but in a robot-like manner; begins to have insight into deficits; continues to have poor judgment and problem-solving skills	The main goal is to promote reintegration into the community. Ask the patient to remember more difficult things from day to day. Reduce environmental structure as necessary. Ask the patient to solve problems s/he might encounter at home (i.e. what would you do if you lost your keys to the house). Treat the individual as an adult.
VIII: Purposeful–appropriate	Consistently oriented; has correct responses; intact memory; needs supervision; has realistic planning skills	Provide guidance and assistance in decision-making. Encourage and allow the patient to use his/her judgment, reasoning and problem-solving skills within the home and safe community settings. Provide community outing to integrate patient back into social environment. Refer the patient to community-based programs that support his/her condition. Encourage the use of memory aids such as note taking, calendars and schedules. Encourage independent functioning. Help the patient to set reasonable goals for the future regarding education and employment. Discourage the use of alcohol and drugs. Help the patient with conversations relating to social interaction and sexuality. Identify situations that make the individual frustrated and discuss strategies for handling these situations. Help the patient identify new roles within the family. Decrease barriers that contribute to isolation; transportation and esthetics.

Continued

Table 10-7. Plan of Care for Cognitive Rehabilitation *(Continued)*

Cognitive Level	Description	Nursing Management for Levels IX and X
IX: Purposeful–appropriate (standby assistance)	Patient is aware and acknowledges impairments and disabilities when they interfere with tasks; initiates and carries out steps to complete familiar personal, household, work, and leisure tasks independently and unfamiliar personal, household, work, and leisure tasks with assistance when requested	Provide breaks with multiple tasks. Continue to provide memory aids with "to do" lists for use with assistance on request. Standby assistance is needed to anticipate a problem before it occurs and to take action to avoid it. Stand-by assistance to adjust to task demands. Monitor for depression, irritability and frustration; counsel as needed; may recommend a neuropsychologist. Stand-by assist to monitor for appropriateness of social interaction. Discuss consequences of decision-making; patient may take more time than usual or use compensatory strategies to select the appropriate decision. Discuss feelings and needs of others and how to respond to them appropriately. Discourage drugs and alcohol. Discuss difficulties of living with brain injury, provide counseling, resources and information about support organizations.
X: Purposeful–appropriate (modified independent)	Independently initiates and carries out steps to complete familiar and unfamiliar personal, household, community, work, and leisure tasks but may need more than usual amount of time or compensatory strategies to complete them	Patient is independent. Monitor for depression. Monitor for irritability and low frustration tolerance when sick, fatigued and/or under emotional stress. Encourage/support patient and family. Encourage participation in support group. Encourage counseling as needed. Follow up with MD as needed (medications, out-patient therapy).

Sources consulted

Brain Injury Association of America. (2006). *Scales and measurements of function*. Retrieved June 11, 2006, from http://www.biausa.org/Pages/what_is_the_rehab_process.html#ways

Rancho Los Amigos National Rehabilitation Center. (2006). *Family guide to the levels of cognitive functioning*. Retrieved June 11, 2006, from http://www.rancho.org/patient_education/bi_cognition.pdf-88k-2006-01-06

Brain injury.com. (2006a). *Recovery and rehabilitation*. Retrieved September 9, 2006, from http://www.braininjury.com/recovery.html

Brain injury.com. (2006b). *Symptoms of brain injury*. Retrieved September 9, 2006, from http://www.braininjury.com/symptoms.html

Gatens, C., & Hebert, A.R. (2001). Cognition and behavior. In S. Hoeman (Ed.), *Rehabilitation nursing: Process, application and outcomes* (pp. 599–630). St. Louis: Mosby.

Dufour, L., Williams, J., & Coleman, K. (2000). Traumatic injuries: TBI and SCI. In P.A. Edwards (Ed.), *The specialty practice of rehabilitation nursing: A core curriculum* (4th ed., pp. 196–198). Glenview, IL: Association of Rehabilitation Nurses.

Rosebrough, A. (1998). Traumatic brain injury. In P.A. Chin, D. Finocchiaro, & A. Rosebrough (Eds.), *Rehabilitation nursing practice, major neurological deficits and common rehabilitation disorders* (pp. 223–244). New York: McGraw-Hill.

1) Skilled nursing facilities
2) Long-term care facilities
3) Residential programs
4) Day therapy programs
5) Assisted living facilities
6) Clubhouse programs
7) Cognitive-based centers and neurobehavioral units
8) Home

c. Healthcare resources
1) Home health services
2) Outpatient programs
3) Local hospital network
4) Primary care provider
5) Durable medical equipment (DME) supplier

6) Telehealth programs

d. Community resources (for information)
1) Brain Injury Association
2) American Heart Association
3) National Stroke Association
4) Epilepsy Foundation of America
5) Local library
6) State-level brain and spinal cord injury trust funds (as available)
7) Centers for Disease Control and Prevention
8) Defense and Veterans Brain Injury Center
9) National Association of State Head Injury Administrators
10) National Center for Medical

Rehabilitation Research, National Institute of Child Health and Human Development, National Institutes of Health

    11) National Institute on Disability and Rehabilitation Research

    12) North American Brain Injury Society

    13) Social Security Administration

    14) State Department of Rehabilitation Services

II. Spinal Cord Injury (SCI)

A. Definitions

  1. SCI: traumatic insult to the spinal cord resulting in alterations or complete disruption of normal motor, sensory, and autonomic function

  2. Tetraplegia (replaced the term *quadriplegia*)

    a. Injury to one of the eight cervical segments of the spinal cord

    b. Impairment or loss of motor or sensory function in cervical segments causing loss of function in all four extremities

  3. Paraplegia

    a. Impairment or loss of motor or sensory function in the thoracic, lumbar, or sacral segments causing impairment in trunk, legs, and pelvic organs

    b. Usually occurs as a result of injuries at T2 or below

B. The Vertebral Segments [Refer to Chapter 5 for discussion of neuroanatomy.]

  1. Cervical vertebrae (7)

  2. Thoracic vertebrae (12)

  3. Lumbar vertebrae (5)

  4. Sacral vertebrae (5)

  5. Spinal cord segments correspond to muscles and associated movements.

C. Epidemiology (National Spinal Cord Injury Statistical Center [NSCISC], 2006)

  1. Incidence of SCI

    a. Approximately 40 cases per million in the United States, or approximately 11,000 new cases per year.

    b. No new overall incidence studies in America since the 1970s.

    c. In the 1970s SCI occurred primarily in young adults 16–30 years of age.

    d. Since 2000, median age of people with SCI in the United States has increased.

    e. Median age is 31.8 years (Dawodu, 2007).

    f. 11.5% of injuries are in those over age 60.

    g. 77.8% of those with SCI are male.

    h. More than 60% of SCI injuries are among Caucasians.

  2. Prognosis

    a. Life expectancy after SCI is slightly less than normal with paraplegia, and for those with tetraplegia, life expectancy is less than people with paraplegia.

    b. Mortality rates are significantly higher in the first year after injury and among those who are older at the time of injury.

    c. 10%–20% of patients with SCI do not survive.

    d. The higher the injury, the more negative the effect on life expectancy.

    e. Leading causes of death are pneumonia, pulmonary emboli, heart disease, and septicemia.

    f. Poor functional outcomes are associated with cervical cord injuries in people over 50 years of age (Alander, Parker, Stauffer, & Shannon, 1997).

D. Etiology (Dawodu, 2007)

  1. Motor vehicle accidents (44.5%)

  2. Falls (18.1%); more common in those over age 45

  3. Violence (16.6%)

  4. Sports and recreational injuries (12.7%); diving is the most common sport associated with SCI.

  5. Other:

    a. Tumors

    b. Infection

    c. Injuries after procedures such as spinal injections or epidural catheter placement

    d. Vertebral fractures

E. Mechanisms of Injury and Associated Common Abnormalities

  1. Direct trauma

    a. Flexion

      1) Occurs when head is thrown violently forward

      2) Occurs when head is struck from behind

      3) Occurs commonly in motor vehicle accidents and falls

    b. Flexion with rotation: occurs when the combination of forces causes severe twisting, resulting in ruptured ligaments and dislocation

c. Hyperextension: occurs in forward falls in which the face or chin is struck

d. Penetration: injuries that directly pierce the cord (e.g., gunshot wound, knife wound)

2. Compression

a. Flexion: axial

1) Occurs when vertebral bodies are wedged and compressed

2) Occurs in the thoracic and lumbar region

3) Caused by a fall onto the buttocks

b. Vertical

1) Occurs when vertebral bodies are shattered and burst into the spinal cord

2) Typically occurs in the cervical region

3) Caused by a high-velocity blow to the top of the head (e.g., diving)

3. Ischemia: injury as a result of damage or blockage, such as clots, in spinal arteries (Dawodu, 2007)

F. Pathophysiology

1. Varying degrees of damage associated with SCI

a. Severity of bony injury does not always correspond to the extent of neurological impairment.

b. Common sites of injury—the cervical and thoracolumbar junctures—are the most mobile parts of the spine.

c. The spinal cord itself may sustain contusion without vertebral fractures or dislocations.

d. The most common levels of injury are C4 and C5 (Dawodu, 2007).

e. Progressive tissue destruction occurs in the cord within hours and may involve several responses:

1) Decrease of microperfusion at site of injury

2) Hemorrhage in the gray matter

3) Development of hematoma and edema

4) Release of biochemicals at site of injury

5) Ischemia and necrosis in the cord, causing neurological damage

f. Clinical presentations related to edema and tissue damage:

1) Spinal shock

a) Temporary state of reflex depression of cord function occurring after injury

b) Initial increase in blood pressure

c) Flaccid paralysis, including bowel and bladder

d) Lasts several hours to days

2) Neurogenic shock

a) Characterized by hypotension, bradycardia, hypothermia

b) More common in injuries above T6

c) Need to differentiate between spinal and hypovolemic shock

3) Autonomic dysreflexia or hyperreflexia (Campagnolo, 2006)

a) A medical emergency

b) Occurs in 48%–90% of those with injuries at or above T6, especially cervical injuries; rare occurrences in as low as T10 injuries

c) More common in males than females (4:1)

d) Caused by stimulation below the level of injury, often in the area of the sacral segments or lower, such as overdistended bladder, fecal impaction, decubitus ulcers, urological procedures, pregnancy and delivery, gynecological procedures, ingrown toenails, fractures, restrictive shoes or clothing, deep vein thrombosis

e) Characterized by hypertension, bradycardia, flushing and perspiration above the level of the lesion, gooseflesh above the level of the lesion, nasal congestion

f) Blood pressure 20–40 mm Hg above patient's normal baseline may indicate autonomic dysreflexia.

g) Treatment is to reduce the causing stimulus (e.g., empty the bladder) and to lower blood pressure by raising head of the bed and administer appropriate medications.

h) Untreated, can result in stroke, coma, death

i) Many episodes can be prevented with good bowel and bladder care.

2. Levels of SCI

a. Upper motor neuron (UMN) injury

1) Is evident in lesions above T12–L1 vertebrae

2) Causes loss of cerebral control over all reflex activity below the level of lesion.

3) Causes spastic paralysis
4) UMNs lie within the spinal cord.
   b. Lower motor neuron (LMN) injury
1) Is evident in lesions below T12–L1 level (i.e., conus medullaris, cauda equina)
2) Causes destruction of the reflex arc
3) Causes flaccid paralysis
4) LMNs branch off from the spinal cord.
3. Clinical syndromes
   a. Central cord syndrome
1) Caused by damage to the central part of the cord
2) Usually is in the cervical region
3) Produces loss of motor power and sensation that affects upper limbs more than lower limbs
   b. Brown–Sequard syndrome
1) Caused by damage to one side (hemisection) of the cord
2) Produces loss of motor function and position sense on the same side as the damage and a loss of pain, temperature sensation, and light touch on the opposite side
   c. Anterior cord syndrome
1) Caused by damage to the anterior artery, affecting the anterior two-thirds of the cord
2) Produces paralysis and loss of pain and temperature sensation below the lesion with preservation of position sense
   d. Conus medullaris syndrome
1) Caused by damage to the conus and lumbar nerve roots
2) May produce areflexia (flaccidity) in bladder, bowel, and lower limbs
   e. Cauda equina syndrome
1) Caused by damage below conus to lumbar–sacral nerve roots
2) May produce areflexia in bladder, bowel, and lower limbs

G. Assessment
1. Classification
   a. Skeletal level of injury: the level at which, by radiographic examination, the greatest vertebral damage is found
1) Stable injury: occurs when the bone or ligaments support the injured cord area, preventing progression of neurological deficit
2) Unstable injury: occurs when the bone and ligaments are disrupted and unable to support and protect the injured cord area, possibly causing

further neurological deficit
   b. Neurological level of injury: the most caudal segment of the spinal cord with normal sensory and motor function on each side of the body (American Spinal Injury Association [ASIA], 1996)
1) Sensory level
   a) Refers to the most caudal segment of the spinal cord with normal sensory function on each side of the body
   b) Evaluated at a key sensory point within each of 28 dermatomes on the right and 28 dermatomes on the left side of the body
2) Motor level (see Table 10-8)
   a) Best predictor of a person's functional abilities (McKinley & Silver, 2006)
   b) Refers to the most caudal segment of the spinal cord with normal motor function on each side of the body
   c) Evaluated at a key muscle within each of 10 myotomes on the right and 10 myotomes on the left side of the body
   c. Complete injury: an absence of motor and sensory function in the lowest sacral segment
   d. Incomplete injury
1) Results in partial preservation of sensory or motor function below the neurological level and includes the lowest sacral segment
2) Includes sacral sensation at the anal mucocutaneous junction and deep anal sensation
3) Includes motor function of voluntary contraction of the external anal sphincter upon digital examination
   e. Zone of partial preservation (ASIA, 1996)
1) Consists of the dermatomes and myotomes that are caudal to the neurological level and remain partially innervated
2) Term used only with complete injuries (e.g., a person with a complete C5 injury may have patchy sensation at C6 or C7 but not have any anal reflexes, such as sacral sparing, and thus still be classified as a complete C5 injury)
2. Assessment instruments and tools
   a. Assessing impairment: ASIA Impairment Scale (1996):

Table 10-8. Neurological Levels and Functional Potential

Level	Activity
C1–C4	Dependent in feeding, grooming, dressing, bathing, bowel and bladder routines, bed mobility, transfers, and transportation
	Independent wheelchair propulsion with pneumatic or chin control and with electronically adapted communication and environmental control devices
C1–C3	Dependent on ventilation support
C5	Independent feeding and grooming with adapted equipment
	Dependent in dressing, bathing, bowel and bladder routines, and transportation
	Needs assistance for bed mobility and transfers
	Independent wheelchair propulsion in motorized chair and with electronically adapted communication and environmental control devices
C6	Independent feeding, grooming, upper extremity dressing, bathing, bowel routine, and bed mobility—all with adapted equipment
	Needs assistance for lower extremity dressing and bladder routine
	Potentially independent transfers with transfer board
	Independent manual wheelchair propulsion with plastic rims and lugs indoors
	Independent driving with adapted van
	Independent phone operation and page turning with equipment
C7	Independent feeding, grooming, and bathing with equipment
	Potentially independent in upper and lower extremity dressing and bowel and bladder routines
	Independent in bed mobility, transfers with and without board, manual wheelchair propulsion, driving with adapted car or van and communication activities
C8–T1	Independent in all personal care activities, bed mobility, transfers, wheelchair propulsion, driving with adapted car or van, and communication activities
T2–T10	Independent in all activities
	Ambulation with long leg braces and crutches or walker for exercise only (nonfunctional)
T11–L2	Independent in all activities
	Potentially independent functional ambulation indoors with long leg braces and crutches
L2–S3	Independent in all activities
	Independent ambulation indoors and outdoors with short leg braces and crutches or canes

Reprinted with permission of Springer Publishing Co., from Hanak, M. (1993). *Spinal cord injury: An illustrated guide for health care professionals* (2nd ed., p. 92). New York: Springer Publishing.

1) Frequently used scale that reflects severity of impairment
2) Modified version of Frankel Grading System for SCI
3) Levels of ASIA scale
    a) A—Complete: No sensory or motor function preserved in S4–S5
    b) B—Incomplete: Sensory function (but not motor function) preserved below the neurological level and extends through S4–S5
    c) C—Incomplete: Motor function preserved below the neurological level; the majority of muscles below the level are grade 3 or lower.
    d) D—Incomplete: Motor function preserved below the neurological level; the majority of muscles below the level are grade 3 or higher.
    e) E—Normal: Normal sensory and motor function
  b. Motor grading scale
  c. Sensory impairment scale scores: 0 = absent, 1 = impaired, 2 = normal, NT = not tested
  d. Other: Spinal Cord Independence Measure assesses 16 categories of self-care, mobility, and respiratory and sphincteric function; Quadriplegic Index of Function detects slight changes in ADLs among those with tetraplegia; Modified Barthel Index is a 15-item measure of self-care and mobility (McKinley & Silver, 2006).
3. Physical assessment
  a. Neurologic:
    1) Assess cognitive, motor, and sensory status, reflexes, and cranial nerves.
    2) Monitor for signs and symptoms of increase or decrease in function, pain, and abnormal sensations.

b. Respiratory: Assess breath sounds, airway patency, oxygen saturation, diaphragm movement, nature of sputum and potential for aspiration, and potential for pulmonary emboli.

c. Cardiovascular: Assess blood pressure, pulse, heart rate, rhythm, edema, deep vein thrombosis, and signs and symptoms of orthostatic hypotension.

d. Nutritional:
   1) Assess weekly weight, daily hydration status, and dietary intake.
   2) Monitor complete blood cell count, electrolytes, albumin and prealbumin levels for anemia, electrolyte imbalance, and nutritional status.

e. Elimination:
   1) Assess abdomen for tenderness, distention, masses, and bowel sounds, premorbid and current bowel patterns, current bladder program; assess urine for color, odor, clarity, and amount.
   2) Review effectiveness of bowel and bladder programs.

f. Musculoskeletal: Assess for swelling, spasticity, ROM, tone, contractures, orthopedic injuries, and heterotopic ossification.

g. Integumentary:
   1) Assess entire body for skin breakdown, especially bony prominences for redness, warmth, and blanching.
   2) Assess and record size, appearance, and location of any skin breakdown.
   3) Assess knowledge and practices to prevent skin breakdown.

h. Psychosocial: Assess family support, coping mechanisms, adjustment to disability, and potential response to fear and anxiety; monitor for suicidal ideation.

i. Sexual:
   1) Assess level of injury in relation to physical capabilities, emotional state, behavior consistent with denial, anger, or depression.
   2) Assess current home situation: presence of significant other or spouse, children, history of birth control practices (if applicable).

H. Planning
   1. Setting goals (Hoeman, 2002)
      a. Goals should be developed with the patient's strengths and limitations in mind.
      b. Rehabilitation goals should be directed toward helping the patient achieve and maintain maximum independence and safe performance of self-care activities.
      c. Goals should focus on the person, not the disability.
      d. Family involvement with goals from the beginning can influence the success of the patient's rehabilitation.
      e. Support and instructions from rehabilitation team members can help the family assist the patient in achieving maximum independence throughout life.
   2. Functional outcomes of SCI (see Table 10-8)

I. Interventions (Hoeman, 2002; Mahoney, 2001)
   1. In the acute phase, interventions emphasize spinal stability, preservation of life, and prevention of complications.
      a. Spinal stability
         1) Use log rolling; avoid twisting.
         2) Surgery may be needed to stabilize the spine (i.e., spinal fusion).
         3) Various orthotics are used depending on level of injury; the name of the brace indicates the part of the spine it immobilizes (Kulkarni & Sam, 2005).
            a) Halo brace or cervical tongs immobilize cervical spine; the halo brace is skeletal traction that provides maximal restriction of movement for those with cervical or high thoracic injuries (to T3).
            b) Sternal occipital mandibular immobilizer brace is used in minimally unstable fractures; allows greater movement than the halo brace but must be fitted correctly; ideal for bedridden patients.
            c) Thoracic lumbar sacral orthosis
            d) Thoracolumbar orthosis is used to treat T10–L2 fractures.
            e) Lumbar sacral orthosis stabilizes L1–L4.
         4) Instruct patient that immobilizer is to remain on at all times.
         5) Immobilizers often are worn for about 3 months to allow the spine to heal.
         6) Emphasize importance of immobilization to allow time for healing and prevent further injury that could result in more damage to the spinal cord.

b. Prevention of secondary complications, especially common in older adults (Krassioukov, Furlan, & Fehlings, 2003)
   1) Infections
   2) Psychiatric disorders
   3) Pressure sores
   4) Cardiovascular problems

2. Interventions are determined with the patient's and family's input to promote maximum health, independence, and safety.

3. Interventions may involve teaching the patient and family about the problem-solving process, providing adaptive devices as necessary, and educating the patient and family about safe and effective performance of skills.

4. Rehabilitation nurses must encourage the patient and family to work toward achieving goals and to continue to perform goals that have already been accomplished.

5. Little research has been done on the unique needs of women experiencing spinal cord injury, and women have specific needs to be addressed (Newman, 2006).

6. Additional suggestions for patient care (Hickey, 2003a):
  a. Establish a therapeutic nurse–patient relationship.
  b. Cultivate a climate of trust.
  c. Allow the patient to verbalize feelings.
  d. Accept the patient's behavior without being judgmental.
  e. Let the patient know that it will take time to adjust to the disability.
  f. Answer questions, referring those that you are unable to answer to the appropriate source.
  g. Include written reports of the patient's emotional and psychological reactions in the chart.
  h. Incorporate steps for meeting the emotional and psychological needs of the patient into the care plan.
  i. Promote a good self-concept and body image by encouraging the patient to use good grooming habits.
  j. Use team conferences to discuss the patient's emotional and psychological status.
  k. Involve the patient in the decision-making process related to his or her care so as to foster a feeling of self-control.
  l. Address common concerns expressed by people with SCI (Lindsey, 1998):

   1) Wanting to walk again
   2) Sexual dysfunction
   3) Pain
   4) Impaired bowel and bladder function
   5) Financial difficulties
   6) Loss of independence
   7) Anxiety

  m. Adapt strategies for older patients with SCI that optimize the length of stay and provide resources after discharge (Scivoletto, Morganti, Ditunno, Ditunno, & Molinari, 2003).

  n. Address the needs of the family caregiver, particularly in the following areas (Lindsey, 1998):
   1) Negative attitudes toward the person with SCI
   2) Feelings of guilt
   3) Frustration at lack of appreciation from the patient
   4) Loss of alone time
   5) Feeling overwhelmed
   6) Setting boundaries in the relationship of caregiving

7. Nursing plan of care (see Table 10-9).

J. Evaluation
1. ASIA Impairment Scale
2. Functional Independence Measure™ instrument
3. Residual deficits and systemic dysfunction that may occur after SCI (Mahoney, 2001; National Institute of Neurological Disorders and Stroke [NINDS], 2007)
  a. Neurological manifestations
   1) Loss or decrease of voluntary motor function below level of injury
   2) Loss or decrease of sensation
   3) Loss of normal reflex activity
   4) Autonomic dysfunction caused by loss of normal sympathetic nervous system functioning
    a) Autonomic dysreflexia
    b) Hypotension
    c) Loss of thermoregulation
    d) Loss of vasomotor tone or control
  b. Cardiovascular manifestations
   1) Hypotension and vasodilation, causing decreased cardiac output
    a) Orthostatic hypotension: Rapid drop in blood pressure when the erect position is assumed; patients with cervical or high thoracic injury have poor vasomotor control, so there is

Table 10-9. Plan of Care for Patients with SCI

System-Specific Considerations	Nursing Diagnosis and Collaborative Problems	Nursing Management	Level of Injury
Respiratory system			
If possible, wean the patient from the ventilator. If weaning is not possible, plan for long-term ventilation management options (discharge home on ventilator, diaphragmatic pacer, or other options). Patients with cervical injuries usually have decreased volumes of air exchange in tidal volumes, movement of the chest with each respiration, forced expiration volume, and responsiveness to chemical stimuli for respirations, resulting in chronic alveolar hypoventilation.	Ineffective airway clearance High risk for aspiration Ineffective breathing pattern High risk for respiratory infection Impaired gas exchange Risk of altered respiratory function Hypoxemia Atelectasis, pneumonia	Continue with the pulmonary program initiated in the acute phase (e.g., chest physical therapy, deep breathing and assistive coughing, use of incentive spirometer). Begin a patient and family teaching program (e.g., respiratory care, breathing exercises, assisted coughing, suction technique, oxygen, intermittent positive pressure breathing and other therapy treatments).	Cervical injuries
Cardiovascular system			
Bradycardia and orthostatic hypotension may occur. Orthostatic hypotension may be a problem when the head of the bed is raised or when the patient is in a wheelchair.	Risk of peripheral neurovascular dysfunction Impaired gas exchange Dysrhythmias Deep vein thrombosis Pulmonary embolus Hypovolemia Orthostatic hypotension	Apply abdominal binder and thigh-high elastic stockings. Continue with air boots. Slowly position patient from supine to sitting (e.g., first sit patient upright in bed, then sit patient on edge of bed with support; if patient becomes hypotensive in wheelchair, tilt wheelchair into recline position and elevate legs).	Cervical injuries High-thoracic injuries May occur in low-thoracic injuries
Nervous system			
Autonomic hyperreflexia can occur with injuries at the level of T6 or above. Initially, pain may be experienced at the level of injury. Some sensation (ranging from mild tingling to severe pain) may return if the lesion is incomplete. Pain may be caused by scar tissue or posttraumatic sympathetic dystrophy. Parathesias and hyperthesias may be noted.	Dysreflexia Pain Knowledge deficit Impaired physical mobility Self-care deficit Sensory and perceptual alterations Sexual dysfunction Sleep pattern disturbance Risk of injury	Manage autonomic hyperreflexia. Assess pain and use pain control strategies. Provide information to patient and family. Provide for total care needs of patient. Begin patient and family teaching related to prevention and treatment of dysreflexia, comfort measures, and prevention of injury to tissue.	Autonomic dysreflexia (T6 and above) Pain (all levels of injury) Parathesias and hyperthesias (all levels of injury)
Integumentary system			
Skin pressure problems are a concern, although there is decreased sensation below the level of injury.	Impaired skin integrity Risk of peripheral neurovascular dysfunction Impaired tissue integrity Altered tissue perfusion peripheral Pressure ulcers Osteomyelitis	Provide skin care and turn the patient every 2 hours. Inspect skin, especially bony prominences, twice a day. Provide for weight shifts in wheelchair every 15–30 minutes. Provide for range-of-motion exercises once daily. Begin patient and family education about the potential and prevention of skin breakdown.	Skin breakdown (all levels of injury)

Continued

Table 10-9. Plan of Care for Patients with SCI *(Continued)*

System-Specific Considerations	Nursing Diagnosis and Collaborative Problems	Nursing Management	Level of Injury
Musculoskeletal system			
Prolonged immobility and paralysis have significant effects on bone, joints, and muscles. Spasticity may be present.	Impaired physical mobility Disuse syndrome Contractures Ankylosis Muscle atrophy Osteoporosis Spasticity		
Gastrointestinal (GI) system			
Neurogenic bowel may be present. Peristalsis returns but is sluggish. Other GI reflexes are sluggish. The development of gastric ulcers or hemorrhage remains a concern.	Altered bowel elimination Paralytic ileus GI bleeding Constipation	Implement aggressive physical therapy program. Provide for range-of-motion exercises once daily. Position the patient's extremities in proper body alignment. Monitor spasticity.	Bones, joints, and muscles (all levels of injuries can have significant effects) Spasticity (T12 and above)
Genitourinary system			
Neurogenic bladder may be present. Altered sexual function may be present.	Altered urinary elimination High risk for infection Sexual dysfunction Renal calculi Kidney disease	Initiate a bowel program.	Neurogenic bowel (potentially all levels of injury)
Metabolic system			
A high-fluid, high-carbohydrate, and high-protein diet is still needed for energy and tissue repair.	Fluid volume deficit Altered nutrition, less than body needs Electrolyte imbalances	Initiate a bladder program.	Neurogenic bladder (potentially all levels of injury)
Psychological and emotional responses			
The effect of the injury on the patient's previous functional level and lifestyle begins to be realized.	Impaired adjustment Body image disturbance Ineffective denial Grieving	Provide adequate fluid and nutritional intake.	Altered nutrition (all levels of injury)
System-Specific Considerations			
The patient begins the loss, grief, and bereavement process. The effect of the injury on the family and significant others begins to be realized.	Anxiety Fear Depression Altered family processes Hopelessness Powerlessness Impaired social interaction Social isolation Spiritual distress High risk for self-directed violence	Communicate with the patient and the family. Be supportive. Set realistic goals.	Altered psychological and emotional response (all levels of injury)

Source consulted

Hickey, J. (1997). *Clinical practice of neurological and neurosurgical nursing* (5th ed.). Philadelphia: Lippincott.

difficulty getting blood out of the lower extremities and back to the heart.

  b) Vasodilation: Results from loss of sympathetically induced vasoconstriction, which triggers pooling of blood in abdomen and lower extremities.

  2) Bradycardia caused by unopposed vagal tone (10th cranial nerve)

  3) Impaired temperature regulation manifested by poikilothermia, a condition in which the body assumes the environmental temperature because of the inability to sweat or shiver below the injury

  4) Cardiac dysrhythmias, which usually appear in the first few weeks and are more common in severe injuries

  5) Blood clots (risk is three times higher than in the non-SCI person)

c. Respiratory manifestations
  1) Injury above C4: Results in paralysis of respiratory muscles, including the diaphragm; patient is dependent on a ventilator.

  2) Injury between C4 to T6: Results in paralysis of the intercostal and abdominal muscles; patient usually is weaned from the ventilator but needs aggressive pulmonary management.

  3) Injury between T6 and T12: Results in paralysis of some abdominal muscles; patient does not need a daily respiratory program unless an upper respiratory infection is present.

  4) Pneumonia is a common complication; intubation increases the risk of ventilator-acquired pneumonia, which accounts for about 25% of deaths (NINDS, 2007).

d. Metabolic and musculoskeletal manifestations
  1) Negative nitrogen balance
  2) Decreased basal metabolic rate and expenditure of energy
  3) Hypercalcemia or hypercalciuria
  4) Altered secretion of pituitary-derived hormones
  5) Heterotopic ossification
  6) Contractures
  7) Muscle spasms

e. Gastrointestinal manifestations
  1) Peristaltic slowing, causing paralytic ileus
  2) Increased acidity, causing

gastrointestinal bleeding
  3) Pancreatitis after injury (Sugarman, 1985)
  4) Abnormal liver function caused by trauma
  5) Neurogenic bowel [Refer to Chapter 7.]
  6) Constipation and hemorrhoids

f. Genitourinary manifestations
  1) Neurogenic bladder [Refer to Chapter 7.]
    a) Reflexic (UMN dysfunction)
    b) Areflexic (LMN dysfunction)
  2) Urinary outlet sphincter dysfunction
  3) Autonomic dysreflexia

g. Sexual manifestations [Refer to Chapter 7.]
  1) Males
    a) Reflexogenic erection
    b) Psychogenic erection
    c) Variability in sperm production, penile erection, fertility, or ejaculation, depending on level of injury
  2) Females
    a) Menses cease and then resume within 6 months to a year.
    b) May still conceive and bear children but should be under the care of a physician specializing in women with SCI.
    c) Autonomic dysreflexia may be a problem during delivery.
    d) Discuss contraception practices.

h. Psychosocial manifestations
  1) Stressors and losses
    a) Stressors
      (1) Survival
      (2) Quality of life
      (3) Lifestyle alterations
      (4) Occupational changes
      (5) Participation in recreational activities
      (6) Change in relationships and roles
      (7) Possibly neurogenic pain
    b) Losses
      (1) Sensation
      (2) Mobility
      (3) Bowel and bladder control
      (4) Sexual function
      (5) Control and independence
      (6) Former roles
      (7) Self-esteem
  2) Emotions and behaviors
    a) Anxiety
    b) Frustration

c) Anger

d) Hostility

e) Fear

f) Sarcasm

g) Regression

h) Denial

i) Guilt

j) Depression

k) Sensory overload

K. Discharge Planning

1. Begins before admission to rehabilitation.

2. Is a collaborative effort between the patient, family, and interdisciplinary team.

3. Includes the following considerations:

a. Identify key family members who will be learning or performing care.

b. Provide education using return demonstration by the patient and family throughout the rehabilitation stay; teach patient and family members about prevention of complications, including bladder infections, pressure sores, respiratory problems, fatigue, and constipation (Blackwell, Krause, Winkler, & Stiens, 2001).

c. Identify the location or setting to which the patient is being discharged.

d. Perform a home evaluation.

e. Identify and order necessary DME.

f. Identify funding sources.

4. Ensure that the patient is discharged to a safe environment.

5. Make referrals to a life care planner if needed.

L. Research on Aging with SCI (Charlifue, 2007a, 2007b, 2007c; Charlifue & Gerhart, 2004; Charlifue, Lammertse, & Adkins, 2004; Gerhart, Charlifue, Menter, Weitzenkamp, & Whiteneck, 1999; Gerhart, Weitzenkamp, Kennedy, Glass, & Charlifue, 1999; McColl, Arnold, & Gerhart, 2001; Winkler, 2007)

1. Longitudinal study began in 1990 in Great Britain to track more than 800 people with SCI (Gerhart, Charlifue et al., 1999).

a. Three phases: 1990, 1993, and 1996.

b. Results of this study published beginning in the late 1990s

2. Death rates and causes of death:

a. SCI survivors have a higher death rate than the general population.

b. Causes of death include cardiovascular disease, pneumonia, septicemia, cancer, and suicide.

c. Rate of cardiovascular disease is more than 200% higher in people with SCI than people the same age without spinal injury (Winkler, 2007).

3. Morbidity (illnesses and complications):

a. Urinary tract infections

b. Pressure sores

c. Problems with chest infections, spasticity, perceived abdominal pain, and general malaise (more likely in people with tetraplegia)

d. Musculoskeletal problems such as joint pain, stiffness, pressure sores, diarrhea, and constipation (especially in people with paraplegia)

e. Increased fractures, cystitis, and motor and sensory changes (especially in people with incomplete injuries)

f. Functional decline or decreasing physical independence

g. Gastrointestinal problems are common and worsen with age, including hemorrhoids and difficulty with bowel evacuation (Winkler, 2007).

4. General health, life satisfaction, stress:

a. More than 75% reported feeling generally healthy.

b. 74% were generally satisfied with their lives.

c. Stress and depression seemed to decrease as more years passed since the injury.

d. Stress was related to adaptation and coping but unrelated to injury severity or physician independence.

5. Risk factors:

a. Pressure sores:

1) More likely in people with paraplegia.

2) More likely in people who had already developed one pressure sore.

3) Increased risk for those with abnormal pulses in feet and lower extremities.

4) Increased risk with unemployment.

5) Number of pressure ulcers increased with time according to data from the National Spinal Cord Injury Database in one study of those 5–25 years postinjury (Charlifue et al., 2004).

b. Upper extremity pain:

1) Decreased psychosocial well-being coincided with an increase in upper extremity pain.

2) Limitations in ROM increased the risk of upper extremity pain.
c. Life satisfaction:
   1) Younger participants who had increased psychosocial well-being and increased finances reported a higher life satisfaction.
   2) Participants who reported social involvement had less fatigue and were less likely to be overweight.
   3) Declined over time (Charlifue & Gerhart, 2004)
   4) Decreased life satisfaction was associated with decreased community reintegration.
d. Factors related to decreased physical independence:
   1) Increased age, especially among people with paraplegia
   2) Changes in DME
   3) Changes in bladder management program
   4) Increased fatigue over time
e. Fatigue: Those with a poor self-perception of health had more fatigue.
f. Community integration and social support (Charlifue & Gerhart, 2004):
   1) General decline in community integration over time related to decreased physical independence, decreased mobility, and lack of social integration.
   2) Life satisfaction was related to community reintegration.
   3) In a study of 132 Canadians and 158 Britons with SCI (mean age of 57 and length of time since injury averaged 33 years) (McColl et al., 2001):
      a) Informational support was less available than emotional support.
      b) Age had a negative effect on satisfaction with social support.
g. Spirituality and depression (Charlifue, 2007a):
   1) No significant relationship between spiritual well-being and age
   2) No significant relationship between spiritual well-being and length of time post-injury
   3) Individuals reporting better spiritual well-being were less depressed and reported better quality of life

6. Conclusions:
   a. Pressure sores and respiratory problems appear to be more common with age.
   b. Musculoskeletal problems are associated more with longer durations of injury.
   c. Life satisfaction and quality of life are vital concepts, neither of which is totally dependent on the level or severity of the disability or on the number of medical complications; however, each seems to be very important as a predictor of future outcomes.
   d. Fatigue appears to be an important predictor of future problems.
   e. Fatigue, depression, and decreased life satisfaction should not go unaddressed because they may lead to costly and compromising complications.
   f. There is a general decline in community integration based on a variety of factors.

M. Other Research
   1. Clinical and rehabilitative research focusing on understanding the nature of SCI and defining the nervous system's response to injury (The Miami Project, 1999a, 1999b; NINDS, 2007)
      a. Study of the pathology of human SCI: A detailed analysis of postmortem human spinal cords is under way to compare actual spinal cord anatomy with diagnostic radiography (e.g., magnetic resonance images) and define the nature of the cellular damage that results from SCI.
      b. Electrophysiology of the spinal cord: Researchers have identified the appearance of a newly formed reflex, which demonstrates that nerve circuits may be altered and new connections formed after injury in humans.
      c. Spasticity and fatigue in paralyzed muscle: These factors provide essential information for designing exercise programs that optimize function in muscles that have lost some or all of their nerve supply.
      d. Central pattern generator: This group of nerve cells synchronizes muscle activity during alternating stepping of the legs.
      e. Pain research group: This group is evaluating the effect of SCI pain on quality of life.
      f. Neural prostheses: Bioengineers are trying to restore functional connections through computers and functional electrical stimulation systems to control the muscles of the arms and legs, especially to stimulate walking, reaching, and gripping.

g. Surgery to relieve pressure: Some research has shown improvement with early decompression surgery in animals but has not been replicated reliably in humans.

h. Pain treatment: Chronic pain syndromes are thought to continually trigger functional changes in neurons; drugs that interfere with neurotransmitters related to pain syndromes are being investigated.

i. Spasticity: Drug interventions, surgery, and electrical stimulation below the injury may decrease spasms.

j. Bladder control: Electrical stimulation, surgical procedures, and root stimulator implants (or combinations thereof) may be helpful for those with reflex incontinence.

2. Basic science research (NINDS, 2007) concentrating on techniques that hold the promise of repairing different types of spinal cord damage

a. Stopping excitotoxicity: When nerve cells are damaged, they release the neurotransmitter glutamate, which can cause secondary damage. Researchers are examining receptor antagonists that may block a specific type of glutamate receptor.

b. Controlling inflammation:
1) Cooling the body immediately after injury protects tissue and nerve cells.
2) Boosting T-cell response may reduce secondary damage.

c. Preventing apoptosis:
1) Research is aimed at understanding cellular mechanisms that cause damage after SCI.
2) Research is exploring how to promote axonal regrowth and repair.

d. Promoting regeneration:
1) Cell grafts show some promise.
2) Fetal spinal cord tissue implants have had some success in animal trials.
3) Stem cells are still under investigation, and more research must be done.

e. Axonal regrowth research is focusing on
1) Encouraging growth
2) Clearing away debris
3) Examining axon connections to reconnect to the spinal cord

3. General notes
a. No one theory or approach will encompass all the effects of SCI.

b. Many scientists believe that significant new treatments will not be found in a single approach but rather in a combination of techniques.

III. Advanced Practice Considerations: Role of the Advanced Practice Nurse in TBI Rehabilitation

A. Educator
1. Design patient and family caregiver education curriculum to be used by rehabilitation nurses in inpatient and outpatient settings (e.g., behavior, safety, cognition and memory, seizures, medications, bowel and bladder, community reentry).

2. Present professional papers and posters at national and international brain injury meetings.

3. Coordinate or teach certification review material to facility staff in order to increase the numbers of certified rehabilitation nurses.

4. Collaborate with academic institutions to place nursing students in brain injury rehabilitation practicums.

5. Collaborate with community agencies and academic institutions to teach rehabilitation nursing care for the patient with TBI.

B. Leader
1. Collaborate with local and national legislators to advocate for people with TBI regarding rehabilitation benefit coverage, accessibility, community resources, and other funding issues.

2. Participate on local and state committees such as TBI trust funds (check your local state).

3. Participate in your local chapter of the Association of Rehabilitation Nurses.

4. Participate in national Association of Rehabilitation Nurses committees; run for office.

C. Consultant
1. Serve as a resource to clinical staff in inpatient and outpatient settings for complex patient care problems (assist with treating a complex wound, assess a patient's bowel problems, assist with strategies to facilitate cognitive and behavioral function, assist the case manager with discharge planning supplies related to nursing and medical care).

2. Attend team conferences and offer information; collaborate with the rehabilitation team.

3. Collaborate with external case managers regarding funding issues for brain injury rehabilitation stays.

4. Collaborate with community service agencies serving people with TBI (and their caregivers) for the purpose of providing information and additional resources.

5. Consult with community-based physicians about the care of their patients with TBI (for questions related to behavior, cognition, spasticity, nutrition).

D. Researcher

1. Research question: What is the standard of practice for pharmacological management of agitation after TBI?

2. There have been many clinical studies evaluating pharmacology in TBI.

3. Many of the studies have been found to lack a rigorous method, thus limiting evidence for the prescribing clinician (Levy et al., 2005).

4. Case study reports usually are not generalizable (Pachet, Friesen, Winkelaar, & Gray, 2003; Sugden, Kile, Farrimond, Hilty, & Bourgeois, 2006; Wroblewski, Kupfer, & Kalliel, 1997) even though the researchers achieved favorable or interesting results.

5. Several true experiments were reviewed, with varied results, ranging from inconclusive evidence to "general support," but most suggest further study with larger samples. See Levy et al. (2005) and Deb and Crownshaw (2004) for comprehensive analyses of the relevant literature.

6. Based on a critical review of the scientific literature, there is no established practice standard for the management of agitation after TBI. Many new studies are in progress, and it is important for the advanced practice nurse to design well-controlled randomized clinical trials or to continually appraise the literature in this particular area for new and efficacious evidenced-based practices.

References

Alander, D., Parker, J., Stauffer, E., & Shannon, M.D. (1997). Intermediate-term outcome of cervical spinal cord-injured patients older than 50 years of age. *Spine, 22*(11), 1189–1192.

American Spinal Injury Association (ASIA). (1996). *International standards for neurological and functional classification of spinal injury patients* (Rev. ed.). Atlanta: Author.

Ansell, B., & Keenan, J. (1989). The Western Neuro Sensory Stimulation Profile: A tool for assessing slow-to-recover head injured patients. *Archives of Physical Medicine and Rehabilitation, 70,* 104–108.

Baggerly, J., & Le, N. (2001). Nursing management of the patient with head trauma. In J.B. Derstine & S.D. Hargrove (Eds.), *Comprehensive rehabilitation nursing* (pp. 331–367). Philadelphia: W.B. Saunders.

Barker, E. (2002). Neuroanatomy and physiology of the nervous system. In E. Barker (Ed.), *Neuroscience nursing: A spectrum of care* (pp. 3–50). Saint Louis: Mosby.

Blackwell, T.L., Karuse, J.S., Winkler, T., & Stiens, S.A. (2001). *Spinal cord injury desk reference.* New York: Demos Medical Publishing.

Blank-Reid, C., & Barker, E. (2002). Neurotrauma: Traumatic brain injury. In E. Barker (Ed.), *Neuroscience nursing: A spectrum of care* (pp. 409–437). St. Louis: Mosby.

Bogner, J.A., Corrigan, J.D., Bode R.K., & Heinemann A.W. (2000). Rating scale analysis of the Agitated Behavior Scale. *The Journal of Head Trauma Rehabilitation, 15*(1), 656–669.

Brain Injury Association of America. (2005). *Facts about traumatic brain injury.* Retrieved October 18, 2006, from http://www.biausa.org/elements/aboutbi/factsheets/factsaboutBI.8.29.05.pdf

Brain Injury Association of America. (2006). *Scales and measurements of function.* Retrieved June 11, 2006, from http://www.biausa.org/Pages/what_is_the_rehab_process.html#ways

Brain injury.com. (2006a). *Recovery and rehabilitation.* Retrieved September 9, 2006, from http://www.braininjury.com/recovery.html

Brain injury.com. (2006b). *Symptoms of brain injury.* Retrieved September 9, 2006, from http://www.braininjury.com/symptoms.html

Campagnolo, D.I. (2006). *Autonomic dysreflexia in spinal cord injury.* Retrieved May 1, 2007, from http://www.emedicine.com/pmr/topic217.htm

Chanda, A., & Nanda, A. (2003). Subdural and epidural hematomas. In R.W. Evans (Ed.), *Saunders manual of neurologic practice* (pp. 500–506). Philadelphia: Saunders.

Charlifue, S. (2007a). A collaborative longitudinal study of aging with spinal cord injury: Overview of the background and methodology. *Topics in Spinal Cord Injury Rehabilitation, 12*(3), 1–14.

Charlifue, S. (2007b). Effects of aging on individuals with chronic SCI. *Topics in Spinal Cord Injury Rehabilitation, 12*(3), 1–96.

Charlifue, S. (2007c). Living well: Aging and SCI: Some good news. *PN/Paraplegia News, 61*(1), 12–13.

Charlifue, S., & Gerhart, K. (2004). Community integration in spinal cord injury of long duration. *NeuroRehabilitation, 19*(2), 91–101.

Charlifue, S., Lammertse, D.P., & Adkins, R.J. (2004). Aging with spinal cord injury: Changes in selected health indices and life satisfaction. *Archives of Physical Medicine and Rehabilitation, 85*(11), 1848–1853.

Corrigan, J.D., & Bogner, J.A. (1994). Factor structure of the Agitated Behavior Scale. *Journal of Clinical and Experimental Neuropsychology, 16*(3), 386–392.

Dawodu, S. T. (2007). *Spinal cord injury: Definition, epidemiology, pathophysiology.* Retrieved April 30, 2007, from http://www.emedicine.com/pmr/topic185.htm

Deb, S., & Crownshaw, T. (2004). The role of pharmacotherapy in the management of behavior disorders in traumatic brain injury. *Brain Injury, 18*(1), 1–31.

Department of Defense (DOD) and Veteran's Head Injury Program & Brain Injury Association of America. (1999). *Brain injury and you.*

Duff, D., & Wells, D. (1997). Postcomatose unawareness/ vegetative state following severe brain injury: A content methodology. *Journal of Neuroscience Nursing. 29*(5), 305–317.

Dufour, L., Williams, J., & Coleman, K. (2000). Traumatic injuries: TBI and SCI. In P.A. Edwards (Ed.), *The specialty practice of rehabilitation nursing: A core curriculum* (4th ed., pp. 223–244). Glenview, IL: Association of Rehabilitation Nurses.

Evans, R.W. (2003). Mild head injury and postconcussion syndrome. In R.W. Evans (Ed.), *Saunders manual of neurologic practice* (pp. 488–493). Philadelphia: Saunders.

Gatens, C., & Hebert, A.R. (2001). Cognition and behavior. In S. Hoeman (Ed.), *Rehabilitation nursing: Process, application and outcomes* (pp. 599–630). St. Louis: Mosby.

Gennarelli, T.A., & Graham, D.I. (2005). Neuropathology. In J.M. Silver, T.W. McAllister, & S.C. Yudofsky (Eds.), *Textbook of traumatic brain injury* (pp. 27–50). Washington, DC: American Psychiatric Publishing.

Gerhart, K., Charlifue, S., Menter, R., Weitzenkamp, D., & Whiteneck, G. (1999, August 10). *Aging with spinal cord injury.* Retrieved July 1, 2007 from http://www.ed.gov/pubs/ AmericanRehab/spring97/sp9706.html

Gerhart, K.A., Weitzenkamp, D.A., Kennedy, P., Glass, C.A., & Charlifue, S. (1999). Correlates of stress in long-term spinal cord injury. *Spinal Cord, 37*(3), 183–190.

Giacino, J., Kalmar, K., & Whyte, J. (2004). The JFK Coma Recovery Scale—Revised: Measurement characteristics and diagnostic utility. *Archives of Physical Medicine and Rehabilitation, 85*(12), 2020–2029.

Giacino, J. & White, J. (2005). The vegetative and minimally conscious states. *Journal of Head Trauma Rehab.* (20) 1, 30–50.

Giacino, J.T., Ashwal, S., Childs, N., Cranford, R., Jennett, B., Katz, D.I., et al. (2002). The minimally conscious state: definition and diagnostic criteria. *Neurology, 58,* (3), 1–11.

Girard, D., Brown, J., Burnett-Stolnack, M., Hashimoto, N., Hier-Wellmer, S., Perlman, O.Z., et al. (1996). The relationship of neuropsychological status and productive outcomes following traumatic brain injury. *Brain Injury, 10,* 663–676.

Grosswasser, Z., Schwab, K., & Salazar, A. (1997). Assessment of outcome following traumatic brain injury in adults. In R. Herndon (Ed.), *Handbook of neurologic rating scales* (pp. 187–208). New York: Demos Vermande.

Hanak, M. (1993). *Spinal cord injury: An illustrated guide for health care professionals* (2nd ed.). New York: Springer.

Hickey, J. (2003a). *Clinical practice of neurological and neurosurgical nursing* (5th ed.). Philadelphia: Lippincott.

Hickey, J. (2003b).Craniocerebral trauma. In J. Hickey (Ed.), *Clinical practice of neurological and neurosurgical nursing* (5th ed., pp. 373–406). Philadelphia: Lippincott.

Hickey, J. (2003c). Overview of neuroanatomy and neurophysiology. In J. Hickey (Ed.), *Clinical practice of neurological and neurosurgical nursing* (5th ed., pp. 45–92). Philadelphia: Lippincott.

Hoeman, S.P. (2002). *Rehabilitation nursing: Process, applications, and outcomes.* Philadelphia: Mosby.

Kalmar, K., & Giacino J.T. (2005). The JFK Coma Recovery Scale—Revised. *Neuropsychological Rehabilitation, 15*(3–4), 454–460.

Kennedy, R.E., Livingston, L., Marwitz, J.H., Gueck, S., Kreutzer, J.S., & Sander, A.M. (2006). Complicated mild traumatic brain injury on the inpatient rehabilitation unit: A multicenter analysis. *Journal of Head Trauma Rehabilitation, 21*(3), 260–271.

Krassioukov, A.V., Furlan, J.C., & Fehlings, M.G. (2003). Medical co-morbidities, secondary complications, and mortality in elderly with acute spinal cord injury. *Journal of Neurotrauma, 29*(4), 391–399.

Kreutzer, J.S., Seel, R.T., & Marwitz, J.H. (1999). *Neurobehavioral Functioning Inventory (NFI).* San Antonio, TX: The Psychological Corporation, Harcourt Brace & Company.

Kulkarni, S. & Sam, H. (2005). Spinal orthotic. Retrieved July 17, 2007 from http://www.emedicine.com/pmr/topic173.htm.

Levin, H., O'Donald, V., & Grossman, R. (1975). The Galveston orientation and amnesia test: A practical scale to assess cognition after head injury. *Journal of Nervous and Mental Disease, 167,* 675–686.

Levy, M., Berson, A., Cook, T., Bollegala, N., Seto, E., Turanski, S., et al. (2005). Treatment of agitation following traumatic brain injury: A review of the literature. *Neurorehabilitation, 20,* 279–306.

Lindsey, L. (1998). *Caregivers for SCI: SCI infosheet #17.* Spinal Cord Injury Information Network. Retrieved May 21, 2007, from http://www.spinalcord.uab.edu/show.asp?durki=22479

Mahoney, D. (2001). Nursing management of the patient with spinal cord injury. In J.B. Derstine & S.D. Hargrove (Eds.), *Comprehensive rehabilitation nursing* (pp. 368–423). Philadelphia: W.B. Saunders.

Marwitz, J. (2000). *NFI background.* The Center for Outcome Measurement in Brain Injury. Retrieved October 23, 2006, from http://www.tbims.org/combi/nfibg.html

McColl, M.A., Arnold, R., Charlifue, S., & Gerhart, K. (2001). Social support and aging with a spinal cord injury: Canadian and British experiences. *Topics in Spinal Cord Injury Rehabilitation, 6*(3), 83–101.

McKinley, W., & Silver, T.M. (2006). Functional outcomes per level of spinal injury. Retrieved May 8, 2007, from http:// www.emedicine.com/pmr/topic183.htm

Meythaler, J.M., Peduzzi, J.D., Eleftheriou, E., & Novack, T.A. (2001). Current concepts: Diffuse axonal injury–associated traumatic brain injury. *Archives of Physical Medicine and Rehabilitation, 82*(10), 1461–1471.

The Miami Project. (1999a). *Basic science research* [Brochure]. Miami, FL: Author.

The Miami Project. (1999b). *Clinical and rehabilitative research* [Brochure]. Miami, FL: Author.

National Center for Injury Prevention and Control (NCIPC). (2003). *Report to Congress on mild traumatic brain injury in the United States: Steps to prevent a serious health problem.* Atlanta, GA: Centers for Disease Control and Prevention.

National Center for Injury Prevention and Control (NCIPC). (2006). *Heads up: Brain injury in your practice tool kit.* Retrieved September 7, 2006, from http://www.cdc.gov/ncipc/ pub-res/tbi_toolkit/toolkit.htm

National Center for Injury Prevention and Control. (2007). What is traumatic brain injury? Retrieved July 18, 2007 for http:// www.cdc.gov/ncipc/tbi/TBI.htm

National Institute of Neurological Disorders and Stroke (NINDS). (2007). *Spinal cord injury: Hope through research.* Retrieved May 21, 2007, from http://www.ninds.nih.gov/disorders/sci/ detail_sci.htm

National Spinal Cord Injury Statistical Center (NSCISC). (2006). *Facts and figures at a glance*. Retrieved April 27, 2007, from http://www.spinalcord.uab/show.asp?durk?=21446

Newman, S.D. (2006). Community integration of women with spinal cord injury: A case for participatory research. *SCI Nursing*. Retrieved May 21, 2007, from http://www.unitedspinal.org/publications/nursing/2006/08/27/community-integration-of-women-with-spinal-cord-injury-a-case-for-participatory-research/

O'Dell, M., & Riggs, R. (1996). Management of the minimally responsive patient. In L. Horn & N. Zasler (Eds.), *Medical rehabilitation of traumatic brain injury* (pp. 103–132). Philadelphia: Hanley & Belfus.

Pachet, A., Friesen, S., Winkelaar, D., & Gray, S. (2003). Beneficial behavioral effects of lamotrigine in traumatic brain injury. *Brain Injury, 17*(8), 715–722.

Povlishock, J.T., & Katz, D.I. (2005). Update of neuropathology and neurological recovery after traumatic brain injury. *Journal of Head Trauma Rehabilitation, 20*(1), 76–94.

Rader, M., Alston, J., & Ellis, D. (1989). Sensory stimulation of severely brain injured patients. *Brain Injury, 3*, 141–147.

Rancho Los Amigos National Rehabilitation Center. (2006). *Family guide to the levels of cognitive functioning*. Retrieved June 11, 2006, from http://www.rancho.org/patient_education/bi_cognition.pdf-88k-2006-01-06

Rappaport, M. (2000). *The Coma/Near Coma Scale*. The Center for Outcome Measurement in Brain Injury. Retrieved October 22, 2006 from http://www.tbims.org/combi/cnc

Rappaport, M. (2005). The Disability Rating and Coma/Near-Coma scales in evaluating severe head injury. *Neuropsychological Rehabilitation, 15*(3–4), 442–453.

Rosebrough, A. (1998). Traumatic brain injury. In P.A. Chin, D. Finocchiaro, & A. Rosebrough (Eds.), *Rehabilitation nursing practice, major neurological deficits and common rehabilitation disorders* (pp. 223–244). New York: McGraw-Hill.

Scivoletto, G., Morganti, B., Ditunno, P., Ditunno, J.F., & Molinari, M. (2003). Effects on age on spinal cord lesion patients' rehabilitation. *Spinal Cord, 41*(8), 457–464.

Sosin, D.M., Sniezek, J.E., & Thurman, D.J. (1996). Incidence of mild and moderate brain injury in the United States, 1991. *Brain Injury, 10*, 47–54.

Sugarman, B. (1985). Medical complications of spinal cord injury. *Quarterly Journal of Medicine, 54*(213), 3–18.

Sugden, S.G., Kile, S.J., Farrimond, D.D., Hilty, D.M., & Bourgeois, J.A. (2006). Pharmacological intervention for cognitive deficits and aggression in frontal lobe injury. *Neurorehabilitation, 21*, 3–7.

Thurman D, Alverson C, Dunn K, Guerrero J, & Sniezek J. (1999). Traumatic brain injury in the United States: a public health perspective. *Journal of Head Trauma Rehabilitation, 14*(6), 602–15.

van Baalen, B., Odding, E., Maas, A.I.R., Ribbers, G.M., Bergen, M.P., & Stam, H.J. (2003). Traumatic brain injury: Classification of initial severity and determination of functional outcome. *Disability and Rehabilitation, 25*(1), 9–18.

Vinas, F.C., Pilitsis, J., Nosko, M.G., Talavera, F., Pluta, R.M., Zamboni, P., et al. (2006). *Penetrating head trauma*. Retrieved October 18, 2006, from http://www.emedicine.com/med/topic2888.htm

Wasserman, J.R., & Koenigsberg, R.A. (2004). *Diffuse axonal injury*. Retrieved October 18, 2006, from http://www.emedicine.com/radio/topic216.htm

Winkler, T. (2007). *Spinal cord injury and aging*. Retrieved on May 18, 2007, from http://www.emedicine.com/pmr/topic185.htm

Wright, J. (2000). *The Disability Rating Scale*. The Center for Outcome Measurement in Brain Injury. Retrieved October 17, 2006, from http://www.tbims.org/combi/drs

Wroblewski, B.A., Joseph, A.B., Kupfer, J., & Kalliel, K. (1997). Effectiveness of Valproic acid on destructive and aggressive behaviors in patients with acquired brain injury. *Brain Injury, 11*(1), 37–47. ForwardSourceID:NT00030FAA

Suggested Reading

Azouvi, P., Jokic, C., Attals, N., Denys, P., Markabi, S., & Bussel, B. (1999). Carbamazepine in agitation and aggressive behavior following severe closed-head injury: Results of an open trial. *Brain Injury, 13*(10), 797–804.

Baguley, I.J., Cameron, I.D., Gree, A.M., Slewayounan, S., Marosszeky, J.E., & Gurka, J.A. (2004). Pharmacological management of dysautonomia following traumatic brain injury. *Brain Injury, 18*(5), 409–417.

Bell, K.R., & Williams, F. (2003). Use of botulinum toxin type A and type B for spasticity in upper and lower limbs. *Physical Medicine and Rehabilitation Clinics of North America, 14*, 821–835.

Brooke, M.M., Patterson, D.R., Questad, K.A., Cardenas, D., & Farrel-Roberts, L. (1992). The treatment of agitation during initial hospitalization after traumatic brain injury. *Archives of Physical Medicine and Rehabilitation, 73*, 917–921.

Brooke, M.M., Questad, K.A., Patterson, D.R., & Bashak, K.J. (1992). Agitation and restlessness after closed head injury: A prospective study of 100 consecutive admissions. *Archives of Physical Medicine and Rehabilitation, 73*, 320–323.

Burnett, M.D., Kennedy, R.E., Cifu, D.X., & Levenson, J, (2003). Using atypical neuroleptic drugs to treat agitation in patients with a brain injury: A review. *Neurorehabilitation, 13*, 165–172.

Cicerone, K.D., Dahlberg, C., Malec, J.F., Langenbahn, D.M., Felicetti, T., Kneipp, S.S., et al. (2005). Evidence-based cognitive rehabilitation: Updated review of the literature from 1998 through 2002. *Archives of Physical Medicine and Rehabilitation, 86*, 1681–1692.

Demark, J., & Gemeinhardt, M. (2002). Anger and its management for survivors of acquired brain injury. *Brain Injury, 16*(2), 91–108.

Francisco, G.E., Hu, M.M., Boake, C., & Ivanhoe, C.B. (2005). Efficacy of early use of intrathecal baclofen therapy for treating spastic hypertonia due to acquired brain injury. *Brain Injury, 19*(5), 359–364.

Giacino, J.T., Ashwal, S., Childs, N., Cranford, R., Jennett, B., Katz, D.I., et al. (2002). The minimally conscious state: Definition and diagnostic criteria. *Neurology, 58*(3), 1–11.

Giacino, J., & Whyte, J., (2005). The vegetative and minimally conscious states: Current knowledge and remaining questions. *Journal of Head Trauma Rehabilitation, 20*, 30–50.

Glen, M.B. (1998). Methylphenidate for cognitive and behavioral dysfunction after traumatic brain injury. *Journal of Head Trauma Rehabilitation, 13*(5), 87–90.

Harvey, C.V. (2005). Spinal surgery patient care. *Orthopaedic Nursing, 24*(6), 426–440.

Hughes, S., Colantonio, A., Santaguida, P.L., & Paton, T. (2005). Amantadine to enhance readiness for rehabilitation following severe traumatic brain injury. *Brain Injury, 19*(14), 1197–1206.

Kajs-Wyllie, M. (2002). Ritalin revisited: Does it really help in neurological injury? *Journal of Neuroscience Nursing, 43*(6), 303–313.

Kraus, M.F., Smith, G.S., Butters, M., Donnell, A.J., Dixon, E., Yilong, C., et al. (2005). Effects of dopaminergic agent and NMDA receptor antagonist amantadine on cognitive function, cerebral glucose metabolism and D2 receptor availability in chronic traumatic brain injury: A study using positron emission tomography. *Brain Injury, 19*(7), 471–479.

Leone, H., & Polsonetti, B.W. (2005). Amantadine for traumatic brain injury: Does it improve cognition and reduce agitation? *Journal of Clinical Pharmacy and Therapeutics, 30*, 101–104.

Llemke, D.M. (2004). Riding out the storm: Sympathetic storming after traumatic brain injury. *Journal of Neuroscience Nursing, 36*(1), 4–7.

Maryniak, O., Manchanda, R., & Velani, A. (2001). Methotrimeprazine in the treatment of agitation in acquired brain injury patients. *Brain Injury, 15*(2), 167–174.

Meythaler, J., Brunner, R., Johnson, A., & Novack, T. (2002). Amantadine to improve neurorecovery in traumatic brain injury–associated diffuse axonal injury: A pilot double-blind randomized trial. *Journal of Head Trauma Rehabilitation, 17*(4), 300–313.

Meythaler, J.M., Clayton, W., Davis, L.K., Guin-Renfroe, S., & Brunner, R.C. (2004). Orally delivered baclofen to control spastic hypertonia in acquired brain injury. *Journal of Head Trauma Rehabilitation, 19*(2), 101–108.

Meythaler, J.M., Depalma, L., Devivo, M.J., Guin-Renfroe, S., & Novack, T.A. (2001). Sertraline to improve arousal and alertness in severe traumatic brain injury secondary to motor vehicle crashes. *Brain Injury, 15*(4), 321–331.

Mooney, G.F., & Haas, L.J. (1993). Effect of methylphenidate on brain injury-related anger. *Archives of Physical Medicine and Rehabilitation, 74*, 153–160.

Pachet, A., Friesen, S., Winkelaar, D., & Gray, S. (2003). Beneficial behavioral effects of lamotrigine in traumatic brain injury. *Brain Injury, 17*(8), 715–722.

Pena, C.G. (2003). Seizure emergency. *American Journal of Nursing, 103*, 73–81.

Port, A., Willmott, C., & Charlton, J. (2002). Self-awareness following traumatic brain injury and implications for rehabilitation. *Brain Injury, 16*(4), 277–289.

Povlishock, J.T., & Katz, D.J. (2005). Update on neuropathology and neuronal recovery after traumatic brain injury. *Journal of Head Trauma Rehabilitation, 20*(1), 76–94.

Rao, V., & Lyketsos, C.G. (2002). Psychiatric aspects of traumatic brain injury. *Psychiatric Clinics of North America, 25*(1), 1–24.

Rhijn, J.V., Molenaers, G., & Ceulemans, B. (2005). Botulinum toxin type A in the treatment of children and adolescents with an acquired brain injury. *Brain Injury, 19*(5), 331–335.

Schiff, N.D., Rodriguez-Moreno, D., Kamal, A., Kim, K.H.S., Giacino, J.T., Plum, F., et al. (2005). fMRI reveals large-scale network activation in minimally conscious patients. *Neurology, 64*, 514–523.

Schneider, W.N., Drew-Cates, J., Wong, T.M., & Dombovy, M.L. (1999). Cognitive and behavioral efficacy of amantadine in acute traumatic brain injury: An initial double-blind placebo-controlled study. *Brain Injury, 13*(11), 863–872.

Shoumitro, D., & Crownshaw, T. (2004). The role of pharmacotherapy in the management of behavior disorders in traumatic brain injury patients. *Brain Injury, 18*(1), 1–31.

Silver, J.M., Kourmara, B., Chen, M., Mirski, D., Potkin, S.G., Reyes, P., et al. (2006). Effects of rivastigmine on cognitive function in patients with traumatic brain injury. *Neurology, 67*, 748–755.

Stanislav, S.W., & Childs, A. (2000). Evaluating the usage of droperidol in acutely agitated persons with brain injury. *Brain Injury, 14*(3), 261–265.

Sugden, S.G., Kile, S.J., Farrimond, D.D., Hilty, D.M., & Bourgeois, J.A. (2006). Pharmacological intervention for cognitive deficits and aggression in frontal lobe injury. *Neurorehabilitation, 21*, 3–7.

Thorley, R.R., Wertsch, J.J., & Klingbeil, G.E. (2001). Acute hypothalamic instability in traumatic brain injury: A case report. *Archives of Physical Medicine and Rehabilitation, 82*, 246–249.

Whiteneck, G. (Ed.). (1993). *Aging with spinal cord injury.* New York: Demos.

Wiercisiewski, D.R. (2001). Pharmacologic management of behavior in traumatic brain injury. *Physical Medicine and Rehabilitation: State of the Art Review, 15*(2), 267–281.

Wroblewski, B.A., Joseph, A.B., Kupfer, J., & Kalliel, K. (1997). Effectiveness of valproic acid on destructive and aggressive behaviors in patients with acquired brain injury. *Brain Injury, 11*(1), 37–47.

Zafonte, R.D., Lexell, J., & Cullen, N. (2001). Possible applications for dopaminergic agents following traumatic brain injury: Part 1. *Journal of Head Trauma Rehabilitation, 16*(1), 1179–1182.

Zafonte, R.D., Lexell, J., & Cullen, N. (2001). Possible applications for dopaminergic agents following traumatic brain injury: Part 2. *Journal of Head Trauma Rehabilitation, 16*(1), 112–116.

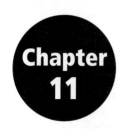

Chapter 11

Musculoskeletal and Orthopedic Disorders

Sue Pugh, MSN RN CRRN CNRN • Elizabeth Yetzer, MSN RN CRRN
Barbara Naden-Blucher, MSN RN CRRN GNP

Rehabilitation nurses often come in contact with clients who have musculoskeletal disorders. Whether the client has a chronic condition (e.g., rheumatoid arthritis) or a fracture related to a fall, rehabilitation nurses are members of an interdisciplinary team that treats the whole person. Rehabilitation nurses take on the essential roles of care provider, educator, and counselor to achieve a well-rounded plan of care for these clients.

By the year 2020, it is expected that the number of people older than age 65 in the United States will be 51 million. With age can come chronic illness. Chronic illnesses can take several forms and can occur suddenly or very slowly. Chronic illnesses can involve periodic flare-ups or remain in remission with an absence of symptoms for many years.

Osteoporosis is a chronic illness that comes on slowly and often is not diagnosed until after a sudden acute event, such as a fracture. Osteoporosis has only recently become an international issue, in part because of the growth and aging of the world's population and the recent improvements in diagnostic testing capacity. Financial considerations related to osteoporosis also have become a concern.

One of the objectives of the Healthy People 2010 initiative is to decrease the incidence of osteoporotic fractures. One way of achieving this is by taking a comprehensive, interdisciplinary approach in which prevention is of primary concern. Preventive programs should target infants, children, adolescents, and young adults because they are still building up calcium stores. For adults older than 30, the focus should be to prevent further loss of calcium and build existing stores of calcium. Preventable safety programs should be stressed, especially with people older than 65 years.

According to the Healthy People 2010 Report, arthritis resulted in 44 million visits to a healthcare provider, over 700,000 hospitalizations per year with $15 billion in medical costs related to arthritis (www.healthypeople.gov, 2007).

In recent years, preventive health care has taken a much larger role. In fact, statistics show that people are already living longer, healthier, and more productive lives. However, health workers are still seeing chronic illnesses in older Americans. This is due in part to a lifetime of unhealthy habits. Advances in medical science and technology have shown us that once-unknown disease processes are amenable to preventive treatments and that complications can be decreased with good medical management and preventive care.

By performing accurate, thorough assessments, rehabilitation nurses can monitor chronic illnesses such as arthritis over time and adjust treatments to meet each client's needs. Client and family education are essential elements of care, especially with musculoskeletal disorders. The client must understand the diagnosis (e.g., what it is, how it affects the body, what the natural progression is) to make informed decisions about treatment plans. Client buy-in is needed because the treatment plan often is long and requires a great deal of effort to achieve functional outcomes. This chapter discusses rehabilitation nursing care of patients with osteoporosis, fractures, arthritis, and amputation. Rehabilitation nurses play many roles in the treatment plan, which is designed to return the client to functional independence.

I. Osteoporosis

A. Overview

1. A degenerative disease that causes bones to become fragile and break with little or no trauma

2. Affects more than 10 million people in the United States (8 million women and 2 million men)

3. About 34 million Americans are at risk for osteoporosis because of low bone mass (National Osteoporosis Foundation, 2006).

4. A major health problem for more than half of Americans over age 50

5. Leads to 1.5 million fractures at an annual cost of $18 billion per year to the U.S. healthcare system (National Osteoporosis Foundation, 2006)

6. A leading cause of disability in the aging population

7. Affects not only the ability to perform activities of daily living (ADLs) but also social and psychological functioning

8. Leads to a decrease in quality of life

9. Osteoporosis, or porous bone, is a disease characterized by low bone mass and structural deterioration of bone tissue, leading to bone fragility and greater susceptibility to fractures, especially of the hip, spine, and wrist, although any bone can be affected (National Osteoporosis Foundation, 2006).

10. Is associated with elevated risk of fractures of the hip, wrist, spine, ribs, and pelvis

11. Occurs when bone reabsorption is greater than bone formation

12. Often is not diagnosed until a fracture is sustained

B. Etiology

1. Cause remains unknown

2. Contributing risk factors (National Osteoporosis Foundation, 2006):

   a. Genetic factors
      1) Female
      2) Asian or Caucasian, especially northern European ancestry
      3) Family history of hip fracture, kyphosis (dowager's hump), osteoporosis
      4) Red or blond hair
      5) Fair skin
      6) Scoliosis
      7) Rheumatoid arthritis
      8) Small-framed body

   b. Nutritional problems
      1) Limited calcium and vitamin D intake
      2) High-protein diet
      3) Poor gastrointestinal absorption
      4) Eating disorders (e.g., anorexia, bulimia)
      5) Heavy alcohol use
      6) High caffeine intake

   c. Lifestyle factors
      1) Low level of activity
      2) Immobilization
      3) Previous falls
      4) Heavy cigarette smoking

   d. Endocrine disorders
      1) Hyperthyroidism
      2) Diabetes mellitus
      3) Gonadal dysfunction in men, low testosterone levels in men
      4) Early or surgically induced menopause
      5) Exercise-induced amenorrhea
      6) Nulliparity
      7) Abnormally low weight or leanness
      8) Low bone density

   e. Pharmacological factors
      1) Antacids containing aluminum. cause calcium loss in stool.
      2) Antiseizure medications (e.g., phenytoin, phenobarbital, primidone) interfere with vitamin D metabolism and decrease calcium absorption.
      3) Tetracycline, isoniazid, and furosemide cause increased calcium loss in urine.
      4) Vitamin A: More than 5,000 IU/day increases calcium loss in the urine.
      5) Corticosteroids (e.g., prednisone, dexamethasone): Long-term use results in severe osteoporosis.
      6) Thyroid hormones in excessive dosages
      7) Heparin
      8) Lithium

   f. Other risk factors
      1) Hyperparathyroidism
      2) Neoplasm
      3) Renal dysfunction
      4) High vitamin D intake
      5) High calcium carbonate intake
      6) Previous fracture
      7) Selected chemotherapy agents
      8) Osteomalacia

3. Incidence (National Osteoporosis Foundation, 2006):

a. Osteoporotic fractures most often involve the hip, vertebra, or wrist.
b. One in 2 women and 1 in 4 men over age 50 will sustain a related fracture sometime before end of life.
c. About 24% of patients age 50 and older die in the year after a hip fracture.
d. Only 15% of patients at 6 months after hip fracture can walk any distance without assistance.
e. Hip fracture accounts for a significant number of nursing home admissions.

4. Types of osteoporosis (NYU Hospital, 2005):
   a. Type I (postmenopausal)
      1) Related to rapid drop in estrogen production around the time of menopause. Estrogen is essential for normal calcium absorption.
      2) Diet low in calcium and vitamin D
   b. Type II (senile or age-related)
      1) Occurs in men and women older than age 70
      2) Is the result of the normal aging process and chronic lack of calcium
      3) May be caused by renal dysfunction, which affects the conversion of vitamin D to a form usable for calcium absorption
   c. Disuse osteoporosis (National Institutes of Health [NIH] Consensus Development Panel on Optimal Calcium Intake, 1994)
      1) Seen with paraplegia, quadriplegia, and other disorders that limit mobility
      2) Involves an initial rapid decrease in bone mass caused by increased bone reabsorption and decreased bone formation
      3) Associated with high calcium intake, which must be monitored carefully because of potential risks (NIH Consensus Development Panel, 1994)
         a) Hypercalcemia
         b) Ectopic ossification
         c) Ectopic calcification
         d) Nephrolithiasis

C. Pathophysiology
   1. Skeletal system influence
      a. The normal bone remodeling cycle is constant and is governed by reabsorption activities of osteoclasts and bone-forming osteoblasts (Kessenich, 1997).
         1) There are two basic types of bone.
            a) Cortical bone: dense and less metabolically active; forms the outer shell of the bone
            b) Trabecular bone: metabolically active; is concentrated in the flat bones of the pelvis, vertebrae, forearms, and ribs
         2) All bones are made of both types, but the proportions differ.
      b. Normally, 10% of bone is undergoing a remodeling cycle at a given time (Kessenich, 1997).
      c. The cycle is balanced until approximately age 30, when bone loss outweighs bone growth at a rate of 3%–5% per decade (Kessenich, 1997).

   2. Endocrine system involvement
      a. Bone reabsorption is affected by parathyroid hormone, 1,25-dihydroxyvitamin D, and calcitonin.
      b. Each affects the regulation of serum calcium (see Figure 11-1).
      c. Parathyroid hormone increases the reabsorption of bone by increasing osteoclast activity and, ultimately, bone breakdown.
      d. Release of parathyroid hormone activates vitamin D to 1,25-dihydroxyvitamin D3 and allows calcium to be absorbed in the gastrointestinal tract.
      e. Release of calcitonin inhibits osteoclasts, thus decreasing bone resorption and causing a decrease in serum calcium levels.
      f. Estrogen may affect these hormones and has been noted to increase the osteoblastic cells available for new bone growth (Crowley, 2004).

   3. Menopausal influence
      a. Menopause begins a marked acceleration in bone loss—as much as 15% during the perimenopausal period.
         1) Bone loss begins approximately 1.5 years before the last menstrual period.
         2) Continued rapid bone loss continues until about 1.5 years after the last menstrual period.
      b. Bone loss is caused by a decrease in natural estrogen.
      c. Estrogen replacement decreases the effects of menopause on bone loss.

D. Diagnosis
   1. Thorough history (Yurkow & Yudin, 2002)
      a. Family history
      b. Excessive height loss (more than 2 in.)

c. Fractures from minimal trauma before age 40

d. Complaints of bone pain, particularly in the back

e. Onset of menopause and estrogen deficiency, the single most common cause of osteoporosis (Yurkow & Yudin, 2002)

f. Low intake of calcium, lactose intolerance

g. Steroid use

h. Northern European heritage

i. Gum disease or tooth decay

j. Excessive caffeine use

k. Cigarette use

l. High alcohol intake

m. Sedentary lifestyle or long-term immobilization

n. History of specific conditions
   1) Thyroid problems
   2) Liver problems
   3) Diabetes mellitus
   4) Renal failure
   5) Malignancies (Watts, 1997)
   6) Other endocrine disorders

o. Medication history
   1) Corticosteroids
   2) Isoniazid
   3) Heparin
   4) Tetracycline
   5) Anticonvulsants
   6) Thyroid supplements

2. Physical examination (Yurkow & Yudin, 2002)

a. Fracture of wrist or femur, vertebral compression fractures

b. Marked kyphosis, dowager's hump

c. Shortened status

d. Muscle atrophy

e. Muscle spasms in back

f. Difficulty bending forward

g. Impaired breathing

h. Poor dentition

3. Laboratory tests (Yurkow & Yudin, 2002)

a. 24-hour urine calcium level

b. Serum calcium, phosphorus, alkaline phosphatase levels

c. Serum osteocalin

d. Thyroid tests

e. Fasting urine sample for calcium and hydroxyproline, corrected for creatinine (Woodhead & Moss, 1998)

4. Bone mineral density (BMD) evaluation ("AACE clinical practice guidelines," 2003)

Figure 11-1. Hypocalcemia and Hypercalcemia

Hypocalcemia

⇓ Calcium blood level
⇓
Release of parathyroid hormone from parathyroid gland
⇓
⇑ Release of calcium from bones
⇑ Calcium reabsorption from kidneys
⇑ Calcium absorption from the gut (requires presence of vitamin D)
⇓
⇑ Blood calcium levels normal

Signs and symptoms
• Nerve excitability
• Paresthesias
• Muscle cramping
• Muscle spasm
• Tetany
• Death

Hypercalcemia

⇑ Calcium blood levels
⇓
Release of calcitonin from thyroid gland
⇓
⇓ Release of calcium from bones
⇓ Calcium reabsorption from kidneys and gut
⇓
⇓ Blood calcium levels normal

Signs and symptoms
• Muscle weakness
• Ataxia, coma
• Arrhythmia, cardiac arrest
• Fractures
• Extreme polyuria

a. Results are measured against two standard norms:
   1) Age- and sex-matched readings (the z-score): Compare a patient's results (the t-score) with what is expected in someone of the same age and sex.
   2) BMD t-scores: This represents a patient's BMD, expressed as the number of standard deviations (SD) above or below the mean BMD value for a normal young adult.

b. WHO has established diagnostic criteria for women who have not experienced fractures, based on the BMD t-scores:
   1) Normal: BMD within 1 SD of the young adult mean
   2) Osteopenia or low bone mass: BMD between 1.5 and 2.5 SD below the young adult mean

3) Osteoporosis: BMD at least 2.5 *SD* below the young adult mean

5. Radiographic studies
   a. Quantitative computed tomography
   b. Quantitative ultrasound
   c. Radiographic absorptiometry
   d. Single-energy x-ray absorptiometry

E. Resulting Disabilities
   1. Hip fracture (National Osteoporosis Foundation, 2006)
      a. In 2001, more than 300,000 Americans over age 45 sustained hip fracture necessitating hospitalization, with an underlying cause of osteoporosis.
      b. Caucasian women over age 65 are twice as likely to sustain a hip fracture as African American women.
      c. The incidence of hip fracture in women is more than twice that of men worldwide, but men with hip fracture are twice as likely to die in the first year as women.
      d. The incidence of hip fracture is greater in older adults who are institutionalized.
      e. A woman's risk for hip fracture is greater than her risk of breast, uterine, or ovarian cancer.
      f. Prompt surgical fixation allows earlier ambulation, which helps to decrease the complications of immobility.
      g. The cause of the hip fracture must be investigated; it may be a sign of an underlying medical problem (e.g., cardiac, neurological, oncological).
   2. Vertebral compression fracture (VCF) (Tanner, 2003–2004)
      a. Most common complication of osteoporosis
      b. 750,000 VCFs occur per year in the United States. One-third of these are painful, and the rest are subclinical.
      c. After first fracture, there is a 5-fold higher risk of another VCF.
      d. Treatment options include:
         1) Restore mineral bone density with adequate calcium and vitamin D supplementation
         2) Medications to treat underlying osteoporosis
         3) Bracing, bed rest, and analgesics; will take 8–10 weeks to recover
      e. Surgical interventions:
         1) Vertebroplasty
            a) Started in 1997 in North America

      b) Transpedicle approach to the vertebral body with the patient in the prone position
      c) Small incision with an injection of polymethylmethacrylate, a low-viscosity bone cement, under radiographic guidance
      d) Restoration of vertebral height occurs in 30% of patients.
         2) Kyphoplasty
            a) Similar to vertebroplasty except that a balloon is inserted into vertebral body to reestablish height of vertebral body.
            b) Cement is then injected when the balloon is withdrawn.
            c) Multiple levels can be done, but usually only 1–2 vertebral bodies are done at one time.
            d) Restoration of vertebral height occurs in 97% of patients.
      f. Complications after surgery:
         1) The complication rate after kyphoplasty is 0.4% per patient versus 1.2% per patient for vertebroplasty.
         2) Major concern is cement leakage onto nerve root or into spinal canal.
         3) Some patients have fever and pain related to a reaction to the cement.
         4) These patients are at high risk for future fracture because of the hardness of the cemented vertebrae compared with the surrounding osteoporotic vertebrae. A 6-month follow-up x-ray is recommended to check for additional fractures.
   3. Wrist fracture, usually seen in younger postmenopausal women
   4. Balance disturbances as a result of kyphosis and scoliosis
   5. Falls resulting from balance disturbances

F. Client Education
   1. Ensure a balanced diet with calcium-rich foods and vitamin D and calcium supplements when indicated.
   2. Promote a regular weight-bearing exercise program.
   3. Decrease or eliminate risk factors (e.g., smoking, consuming caffeine or alcohol).
   4. Instruct in home and community safety measures.
   5. Evaluate BMD.
   6. Maintain a record of client's height.

7. Discuss with physician hormone replacement therapy or other osteoporosis medication.

8. Manage medications.

G. Interventions After Diagnosis

  1. Pharmacological management:

    a. Calcium

      1) Adequate calcium intake is essential to achieving optimal peak bone mass (NIH Consensus Development Panel, 1994).

      2) Most Americans do not get the recommended daily allowance (RDA) of calcium based on their age and physiological need.

      3) Optimal recommended calcium intakes are as follows (NIH Consensus Development Panel, 1994):

        a) Children: 800–1,200 mg/day

        b) Adolescents: 1,200–1,500 mg/day

        c) Premenopausal adult women: 1,000–1,500 mg/day

        d) Postmenopausal women not taking hormone replacement: 1,500 mg/day

        e) Postmenopausal women taking hormone replacement: 1,200–1,500 mg/day

        f) Men aged 60 and older: 1,300 mg/day

        g) Older adults: 1,000–1,500 mg/day

        h) Average RDA: 1,400–1,500 mg/day

      4) There are many sources of calcium:

        a) Milk, yogurt, cheese, cottage cheese, ice cream, tofu, salmon, broccoli, spinach, kale, eggs, beans, sardines, clams, oysters

        b) Calcium-fortified foods (e.g., cereal)

        c) Supplements

          (1) Calcium carbonate (e.g., Tums), inexpensive and efficient

          (2) Tricalcium phosphate or calcium citrate (e.g., Os-Cal): effective alternatives if gastrointestinal symptoms occur (McClung, 1999)

          (3) Alkali antacids

    b. Estrogen replacement therapy

      1) Slows the rate of bone loss.

      2) Is surrounded by controversy: The decision to supplement must be explored carefully.

    c. Vitamin D, needed for adequate calcium absorption

      1) Deficiency occurs when there is inadequate exposure to the sun, inadequate dietary intake, and acquired resistance to vitamin D (NIH Consensus Development Panel, 1994).

      2) Deficiency can be corrected by eating foods that are fortified with vitamin D and supplementing the diet with 600–800 IU/day of vitamin D (NIH Consensus Development Panel, 1994).

    d. Alendronate (Fosamax)

      1) Proven to prevent bone resorption, reduce the risk of fractures, and slow the course of disease (Spratto & Woods, 1998)

      2) Necessitates special precautions for ingestion (see Figure 11-2)

    e. Calcitonin (Miacalcin) nasal spray

      1) Indicated for women who are 5 or more years postmenopausal

      2) Has been shown to increase spinal bone mass

      3) Must be taken with 1,200–1,500 mg calcium and 400 IU of vitamin D (Heaney, 1998; Solomon, 1998)

    f. Raloxifene (Evista, http://www.evista.com; Eli Lilly, 1998)

      1) A selective estrogen receptor modulator that imitates some of estrogen's positive effects.

      2) Prevents bone loss through the body.

      3) Special precaution: Avoid use in sedentary patients because of blood clot formation risk.

    g. Ibandronate sodium (Boniva, http://www.boniva.com), first and only once-monthly medication

---

Figure 11-2. Client Education: Precautions for Fosamax Therapy

Instruct the client to take the medication correctly

- Take on an empty stomach, first thing in the morning.
- Take with a full 8 oz. of tap water (not bottled water, coffee, or juice).
- Take with 1,200–1,500 mg of calcium and 400 IU of vitamin D.
- Wait at least 30 minutes before eating or drinking anything, including taking any other medication.
- If possible, wait 60 minutes before eating or drinking to ensure an enhanced absorption of the medication.
- Do not lie down after taking the medication.

Provide information about therapeutic side effects of the medication.

Explain the safety issues for proper storage of the medication.

Teaching Topics

---

h. Teriparatide (Forteo, http://www.
   forteo.com/control/pen_user_manual;
   http://www.fda.gov/bbs/topics/
   ANSWERS/2002/ANSO1176.html)
   1) Synthetic form of parathyroid
      hormone
   2) Recommended daily dose: 20 mcg

2. Exercise and weight bearing:
   a. Walk, jog, use a stationary bike, do
      theraband or aerobic exercise on a regular
      basis to promote bone remodeling and
      increase bone density.
   b. Limit, as much as possible, any event that
      may cause prolonged immobilization.

3. Pain management: Manage pain resulting
   from changes in the musculoskeletal system
   and compression fractures to allow early and
   progressive activity.

4. Safety issues: Conduct a fall prevention
   safety assessment, asking the following
   questions (Mosby Great Performance, 1995,
   pp. 6–7):
   a. Is there adequate lighting in each room?
   b. Are nightlights placed throughout the
      house where they're needed?
   c. Are stairways adequately lighted?
   d. Are light switches within reach and easy
      to use?
   e. If the person uses a wheelchair, can he or
      she still reach the light switches?
   f. Are you using lights that may produce
      glare?
   g. Have you removed throw rugs that might
      cause falls?
   h. Do carpets have worn areas or places that
      have come loose or untacked?
   i. Are floors free of phone and extension
      cords?
   j. Are walkways clear of clutter, boxes, or
      low furniture that might cause a fall?
   k. Are there nonskid strips in potentially
      dangerous areas such as on stairs, on
      bathroom floors, in front of the toilet, and
      in the bath or shower?
   l. Are the stairs free of cracks and sagging
      carpeting?
   m. Are there sturdy railings on both sides of
      the stairway?
   n. Are carpets low-pile monotone rather
      than shag?
   o. Does the bathroom have grab bars around
      the toilet and in the tub or shower,
      capable of supporting a 250-lb load?
   p. Does the house have heat sources such as
      radiators and space heaters that may be
      obstacles for a person using a cane?
   q. Is there a possibility that the person's
      medications may affect his or her
      movement, balance, or consciousness?

H. Prevention Strategies
   1. Set a goal to have the optimal level of bone
      mass by the time menopause begins.
   2. Manage diet to take in the RDA of calcium
      and vitamin D throughout the lifespan.
   3. Exercise and continue an active, healthy
      lifestyle throughout life.
   4. Decrease or eliminate risk factors:
      a. Stop smoking.
      b. Decrease caffeine intake.
      c. Decrease alcohol intake.
      d. Maintain a balanced diet.
      e. Limit medications that reduce bone mass.
      f. Maintain an ideal weight.
      g. Prevent falling episodes.

I. Research Topics (University of Minnesota
   Research, 2006; Canadian Association of
   Radiologists, 2005)
   1. The role of hip protectors in decreasing the
      risk of hip fracture
   2. Risk factors associated with fractures in
      postmenopausal women
   3. Recommendations for BMD reporting
   4. Study of osteoporotic fractures
   5. Outcomes of various drug studies, including
      alendronate, parathyroid hormone, raloxifene
   6. Estrogen replacement therapy
   7. Osteoporotic fractures in men

II. Arthritis

A. Overview
   1. The inflammation of a joint
   2. Affects connective tissues (e.g., muscle,
      tendons, bursa, fibrous tissue)
   3. A term that the public uses to describe pain
      and stiffness of the musculoskeletal system
      (sometimes called rheumatism)
   4. A medical term that is restricted to
      rheumatic diseases that involve inflammatory
      conditions affecting the joints
   5. Has more than 100 different Arthritis
      Foundation classifications
   6. The second leading cause of limitation of
      movement (after heart disease)

7. The leading cause of absenteeism in the workplace and the second leading reason for disability payments (after mental illness)

8. Involves more than $8.6 billion annually in lost wages and medical bills

9. An increasing problem for the growing older population in the United States that is putting an increased strain on Medicare

B. Classification

    1. Inflammatory

    2. Degenerative

    3. Metabolic

C. Rheumatoid Arthritis (RA)

    1. Definition:

        a. A chronic inflammatory systemic condition that affects primarily joints but can also damage muscles, lungs, skin, blood vessels, nerves, and eyes

        b. Associated with a symmetrical involvement of the peripheral joints

        c. Common symptoms: fatigue and weight loss

    2. Etiology:

        a. Cause remains unknown.

        b. Theories:

            1) A genetically controlled host immune response to an unknown stimulus (Thalgott, LaRocca, & Gardner, 1993)

           2) An infectious microorganism (which has not been isolated yet)

           3) Genetic predisposition

               a) Affects more women than men by a 3:1 ratio

               b) Tends to be seen in families with a history of RA

           4) Trauma

           5) Alteration of the normal peripheral vascular bed by an autonomic influence (Schoen, 2001)

           6) Increased stress (emotional and physical), known to cause acute exacerbations

    3. Pathophysiology:

        a. Process (Thalgott et al., 1993)

           1) Involves synovial proliferation, joint effusion, and edema in the small joints

           2) Causes cartilage to erode and be destroyed

           3) Forms pannus in the articular cartilage and destroys the joint. Pannus is the membrane of inflammatory cells and granulation tissue that covers and erodes the articular cartilage (Schoen, 2001)

           4) Affects ligaments and the joint capsule, making it impossible to maintain proper alignment and position, which causes deformity

           5) Results in a generalized osteoporosis that develops in these areas and makes surgical stabilization difficult

           6) Produces fibrous adhesions, bony ankylosis, and uniting of opposing joint surfaces, which occur in the later stages of RA

           7) Involves irreversible effects

        b. Effects of RA on the joint

           1) Joint destruction

           2) Joint inflammation and effusion, particularly in the feet, hands, fingers, wrists, and elbows

           3) Redness, swelling, and pain with motion

        c. Effects of RA on the body (Arthritis Foundation, 2006)

           1) General: fatigue, anorexia, weight loss, aching, and stiffness

           2) Lymph: enlarged glands

           3) Pulmonary:

               a) Caplan's syndrome (i.e., rheumatic nodules with cavitation)

               b) Pleuritis

               c) Interstitial fibrosis

               d) Pleural effusion

               e) Interstitial pneumonia

           4) Neurologic: localized neuropathy:

               a) Foot drop as a result of nerve injury secondary to ischemia, compression, or obstruction of the nerves going to the ankle

               b) Entrapment neuropathy

               c) Spinal cord compression

           5) Ocular: uveitis, Sjögren's syndrome

           6) Cardiovascular:

               a) Fibrous pericarditis in 10% of cases

               b) Cardiomyopathy

               c) Vasculitis

           7) Skin: thinning

           8) Rheumatic: Nodules may occur.

               a) Present in 20% of cases

               b) Presence is associated with a poor prognosis.

               c) Firm, nontender, oval mass up to 2 cm in diameter

               d) Found in subcutaneous tissue over pressure points (e.g., elbows, sacrum, dorsal surface of the hand)

e) Found in other areas (e.g., lungs, heart valves, vocal cords, eyes)
4. Incidence (Arthritis Foundation, 2006):
   a. About 46 million adults have some form of arthritis, and this is projected to increase to 64.9 million by the year 2030. About 2.1 million or 1% of the population has RA.
   b. 85%–90% of RA clients have a positive rheumatoid factor (RF).
   c. Affects women more frequently than men.
   d. Affects people of all races
   e. Is not affected by climate
   f. Onset usually occurs between 20 and 50 years. Most cases are diagnosed when people are in their 40s.
   g. Can affect older adults: 25% of older adults develop RA with sudden onset when they are affected by another severe disease. In these patients RA is best managed aggressively with disease-modifying antirheumatic drugs.
5. Types of RA:
   a. Juvenile arthritis (JA)
      1) A chronic inflammatory condition that has an onset before age 16 years.
      2) Includes three types of onset, which are classified during the first 6 months of the illness (Youngblood & Edwards, 1999):
         a) Systemic onset
         b) Pauciarticular arthritis
         c) Polyarticular onset
            (1) RF negative
            (2) RF positive
      3) Clinical aspects vary with onset type (see Table 11-1).
      4) Affects approximately 1 in 1,000 children
      5) Affects slightly more girls than boys
      6) Is generally mild
   b. Adult RA
6. Classification, based on four or more criteria (Arnett et al., 1988):
   1) Morning stiffness for at least 1 hour, present for at least 6 weeks
   2) Arthritis of 3 or more joints:
      a) Soft tissue swelling or fluid
      b) Affects joints such as right and left proximal interphalangeal (PIP) joint, metacarpophalangeal (MCP) joint, metatarsophalangeal (MTP) joint, wrist, elbow, knee, or ankle
      c) Present for at least 6 weeks
   3) Arthritis of hand joints:
      a) Soft tissue swelling or fluid
      b) Affects at least one area in a wrist, PIP, or MCP
      c) Present for at least 6 weeks
   4) Symmetrical arthritis:
      a) Bilateral involvement of the same joint
      b) Affects PIPs, MCPs, or MTPs but may not be absolutely symmetrical
      c) Present for at least 6 weeks
   5) Rheumatoid nodules: Subcutaneous, over bony prominences, extensor surfaces, or juxta-articular regions
   6) Serum RF: Determined by a method that is positive in fewer than 5% of normal control subjects

Table 11-1. Juvenile Arthritis: Onset Types and Clinical Aspects

Systemic onset	Any age; female = male; about 20% of cases
	Recurrent, intermittent fever greater than 103° F, usually high once or twice each day
	Rheumatoid rash—pale red, nonpruritic, macular on trunk and extremities
	Joint manifestations vary and lag behind systemic symptoms
	Internal organ involvement—liver, spleen, heart
Polyarticular onset RF negative	Females 4:1, any age but peaks 1–3 years and 8–10 years
	Involves four joints or more—wrists, knees, ankles, elbows, feet
	Insidious or precipitated by infection—progression early, tends to get worse over time
	Morning sickness—systemic distribution
Polyarticular onset RF positive	Female, younger than 10 years of age
	Family history
	Clinical features as adult form—more likely to develop severe chronic arthritis
	Fever usually less than 103° F, rash, anemia, fatigue, anorexia, failure to gain weight
Pauciarticular arthritis	Most common type, females younger than 4 years of age
	Four or less joints; knee most common, also ankles and hips
	Painless swelling, child is walking "funny"
	Few systemic signs—irritable, tired, poor weight gain, chronic eye inflammation

Reprinted with permission of W.B. Saunders from Youngblood, N.M., & Edwards, P.A. (1999). Autoimmune and endocrine conditions. In P.A. Edwards, D.L. Hertzberg, S.R. Hays, & N.M. Youngblood (Eds.), *Pediatric rehabilitation nursing* (p. 414). Philadelphia: W.B. Saunders.

7) Radiologic changes: Posterior and anterior hand and wrist roentgenograms show erosions or unequivocal bony decalcifications.

7. Diagnosis (Yurkow & Yudin, 2002):
    a. Thorough history and physical assessment
        1) Assess for fatigue, malaise, and weakness.
        2) Note reports of vague arthralgias, myalgias, joint pain and stiffness, decreased range of motion (ROM).
        3) Note joint size, shape, color, symmetry.
        4) Assess for presence and history of joint swelling, redness, cyanosis, warmth, tenderness, family history of arthritis.
        5) Note shiny, taut skin over joint.
        6) Assess for muscle atrophy and flexion contractures.
        7) Note subluxation in metacarpal and metatarsal joints and ulnar deviation of fingers.
        8) Assess for deformities or fibrous or bony ankylosis:
            a) Spindle-shaped fingers
            b) "Swan neck," "boutonniere," "cock-up toes"
            c) Broadening of the forefoot, clawing of the toes, plantar calluses
        9) Assess for side effects of steroid therapy:
            a) Buffalo hump, moon face
            b) Abdominal distention
            c) Ecchymosis after minimal trauma
            d) Impotence
            e) Amenorrhea
            f) Hypertension
            g) Generalized weakness
            h) Muscle atrophy
        10) Cutaneous nodules over bony prominences
        11) Assess for vascular deficits.
        12) Assess muscle strength and presence of muscle spasm and sensation.
        13) Note joint mobility, crepitus, function, and sensation.
        14) In children, look for longer, shorter, or larger bones than normal. Inflammation can affect the growth plates in the bones.
        15) In children, behavioral and physical changes (Youngblood & Edwards, 1999):
            a) Irritability
            b) Morning stiffness
            c) Pain
            d) Limping or walking funny
            e) Heat and swelling in a joint
            f) Intermittent rash
            g) Altered posture
        16) Recent trauma or infection
        17) In children, changes in facial appearance and dental problems
    b. Laboratory studies
        1) Anemia
        2) Elevated white blood cell count
        3) Erythrocyte sedimentation rate
        4) Protein electrophoresis
        5) RF
        6) Antinuclear antibodies
        7) C-reactive protein
        8) Urinalysis
    c. Radiologic studies
        1) Early signs
            a) Soft tissue swelling
            b) Periarticular osteoporosis
            c) New bone formation
            d) Subchondral cyst formation
        2) Late signs
            a) Subchondral erosions
            b) Narrowing of joint spaces
            c) Diffuse osteoporosis
    d. Other
        1) Arthroscopy
        2) Thermograph and bone scan
        3) Joint aspirations

8. Resulting disabilities (JA is the primary cause of disability in children):
    a. Deforming contractures of joints
    b. Joint instability
    c. Spinal cord compression, usually cervical
    d. Depression and anxiety
    e. Deficits in ADLs and instrumental activities of daily living (IADLs)
    f. Mobility deficits
    g. Chronic pain

9. Client education:
    a. What does RA or JA mean?
    b. How will it affect the body?
    c. Why me?
    d. How is it diagnosed?
    e. What causes RA or JA?

10. Interventions after diagnosis for early arrest of the disease process:
    a. Goal: to maintain joint function and prevent deformities

b. Pharmacologic management (Table 11-2):
1) Anti-inflammatory agents
a) Salicylates
b) Nonsteroidal anti-inflammatory drugs (NSAIDs)
c) Phenylbutazone
d) Cyclooxygenase-2 inhibitors (e.g., celecoxib)
2) Glucocorticoids: infrequently used in JA, because of their effects on growth
3) Intraarticular steroids
4) Remission-inducing agents
a) Gold salts
b) Hydroxychloroquine
c) D-penicillamine
5) Disease-modifying antirheumatic drugs, which are immunosuppressants
a) Azathioprine (Imuran)
b) Cyclophosphamide (Cytoxan)
c) Chlorambucil (Leukeran)
d) Levamisole
e) Sulfasalazine (Azulfidine)
f) Methotrexate (Mexate)
g) Leflunomide (Arava)
6) Antitumor, necrotizing factor agents
a) Etanercept (Enbrel)
b) Infliximab (Remicade)
c) Adalimumab (Humira, http://www.humira.com)
7) Baseline urine and blood studies before initiating these medications
c. Physical therapy: Encourage participation in an exercise program and use of assistive devices to keep mobile and remain flexible (e.g., hydrotherapy).
d. Occupational therapy: Help make ADLs and IADLs easier by using adaptive aids.
e. Splints: Use to give joints rest, correct deformity, and provide physical support to unstable joints.
f. Psychological support:
1) Antidepressants
2) Support groups
g. Vitamins, minerals, and herbs (e.g., echinacea, ginkgo, St. John's wort).
h. Cartilage matrix enhancers (e.g., glucosamine and chondroitin sulfate).
i. Client education:
1) Choose a treatment regimen.
2) Teach how to incorporate treatment regimen into life.
3) Manage medication.
4) Teach how to prevent complications.

Table 11-2. Commonly Used Medications to Treat Arthritis Pain

Medication	Brand name	Nursing implication
Traditional NSAIDs	**Prescription:** Anaprox (naproxen sodium) Clinoril (sulindac) Indocin (indomethicin) Lodine (etodolac) Relafen (nabumetone) Voltaren (diclofenac sodium) **OTC:** Advil, Motrin IB, Nuprin (ibuprofen) Aleve (naproxyn sodium) Actron (ketoprofen)	**Side effects:** GI upset, stomach ulcers; CV complications; blood counts and liver enzymes; do not take with alcohol or blood thinners; take with food or antacids to reduce GI upset or heartburn
COX2 inhibitors	Celebrex (celecoxib)	**Most common side effects:** stomach pain, diarrhea, indigestion, headache; less risk of GI bleeding than with other NSAIDs; do not take with other NSAIDs; may be taken with low dose aspirin; does not interfere with blood clotting; primary treatment option for patients at risk of GI complications; careful monitoring needed when taken with warfarin, fluconazole, and lithium; risk of stomach ulcers may be increased in those drinking more than 3 alcoholic beverages per day
OTC Salicylates		
Aspirin	Bayer, Ecotrin, Ascriptin, Exedrin	Take with food; do not take with other NSAIDs; Confusion, dizziness, tinnitus are signs of toxicity; with high doses, monitor blood levels; may increase risk of bleeding and stomach ulcers

OTC=over the counter; nonprescription
Source
Mauk, K.L. (2006, Oct/Nov). Medications to treat arthritis. *ARN Network, 23*(5), 7–8.

5) Explain the importance of physical and occupational therapy.
6) Explain how to use assistive devices.
7) Teach joint conservation techniques.
8) Teach energy conservation techniques.
9) Explain what happens if techniques do not work.

11. Surgical interventions after diagnosis:
    a. Goals: to relieve pain, stabilize the joint, and correct deformity of the joint
    b. Total joint replacement
        1) Areas include hips, knees, ankles, shoulders, elbows, phalanges.
        2) Aggressive rehabilitation in acute care, rehabilitation facilities, or subacute care settings is essential to successful outcomes.
        3) For children, joint replacement is delayed as long as possible until bone growth has finished.
    c. Arthrodesis or fusion of the bony joint
    d. Laminectomy and spinal fusion for cord compressions
    e. Tendon repair (if done within 2 days of rupture)
    f. Tenosynovectomies and synovectomies

12. Research topics (Arthritis Foundation, 2007):
    a. Identification of genetic links to RA
    b. The effects of biologics in arthritis
    c. Anticyclic citrullinated proteins in RA
    d. Use of glucosamine and chondroitin treatment
    e. Causes of relapse in JA
    f. Immune cell involvement
    g. Treatment options for systemic sclerosis
    h. Anakinra use in JA

D. Degenerative Joint Disease (DJD) or Osteoarthritis (OA)
    1. Definition
        a. A progressive, noninflammatory process that affects weight-bearing joints in particular
        b. Characterized by degeneration of the articular cartilage at the joint
    2. Etiology
        a. Cause remains unknown.
        b. Contributing risk factors:
            1) Age
                a) Strongest risk factor but not solely responsible for causing OA.
                b) Changes related to aging in cells and tissues may induce development of the disease.
            2) Trauma
                a) Injury to articular cartilage, leaving fragments in the joint
                b) Recurrent dislocation of the patella
                c) Congenital dislocation of the hip
            3) Obesity: increases the load on the joints that causes changes in posture and gait
            4) Lifestyle
                a) Athlete's knee
                b) Dancer's ankle
                c) Tennis elbow
            5) Intraarticular sepsis
            6) Primary diagnoses affecting joints
                a) Hemophilia
                b) Paget's disease
                c) Diabetes mellitus
                d) Charcot–Marie–Tooth disease
            7) Menopause
            8) Immune response
            9) Preexisting joint abnormalities
                a) RA
                b) Legg–Calvé–Perthes disease
                c) Avascular necrosis

    3. Pathophysiology (Schoen, 2001)
        a. Articular cartilage pits, softens, and frays, losing elasticity and becoming more susceptible to stress damage.
        b. Gradually, full-thickness loss of the articular cartilage occurs, leaving exposed subchondral bone that then goes through a remodeling process.
        c. This bone hypertrophies and forms spurs at the joint margins and at ligaments, tendons, and the joint capsule.
        d. Spurs or osteophytes break off into the joint.
        e. A secondary synovitis occurs later in the process, further affecting the joint's function.
        f. With advanced disease, all the cartilage may be destroyed.

    4. Incidence (National Council on Aging, 2005)
        a. DJD or OA is the most common form of arthritis.
        b. The disease may begin when the person is in his or her 20s, but it peaks when the person is in his or her 50s or 60s.
        c. 20 million Americans suffer with OA
        d. Incidence is higher in Caucasians.
        e. The disease affects women twice as often as men who are older than 55.
        f. Hip, knee, cervical, and lumbosacral joints are most frequently involved.

g. Women's hands are affected most after menopause.

h. Lifestyle and occupation may be factors.

i. Weight gain, lower self-esteem, and loss of sleep may result.

5. Diagnosis

a. History

1) Early stages: joint stiffness, relieved with activity

2) Later: pain on movement, relieved with rest

3) Advanced stages

a) Night pain and pain at rest

b) Limping

c) Paresthesias

b. Physical

1) Localized symptoms

2) Enlarged joints

3) Decreased ROM

4) Crepitus

5) Joint instability

6) Changes in alignment with flexion deformity

7) Pain on movement

c. Diagnostic tests

1) Radiologic tests

a) An X-ray of involved joint will not necessarily reflect the severity of clinical symptoms.

b) X-rays taken during weight bearing may show deformity.

2) Laboratory tests

a) Sedimentation rate: may be minimally elevated

b) Analysis of synovial fluid after aspiration of the involved joint

6. Resulting disabilities

a. Pain with rest and movement

b. Joint contractures

c. Loss of joint function

d. Loss of independence

e. Depression and anxiety

7. Client education

a. What does DJD mean?

b. How will it affect my body?

c. Why me?

d. How is it diagnosed?

e. What causes it?

f. How can it be prevented?

8. Interventions

a. Goals of treatment

1) Reduce pain

2) Regain joint ROM

3) Regain independence with mobility and ADLs

b. Pharmacological management

1) Administer early in the morning and before activity.

2) Aspirin

3) NSAIDs: used when aspirin is no longer effective

4) Adrenocorticoids: local intraarticular injection for severely symptomatic joints

5) Analgesics

6) Vitamins, minerals, and herbal remedies

c. Interdisciplinary approaches

1) Physical therapy to establish an exercise program

a) Pool therapy

b) Home exercise program

2) Heat and cold applications

3) Splinting or bracing

4) Use of assistive devices

5) Use of transcutaneous electrical nerve stimulation for pain reduction

6) Weight loss

7) Nontraditional remedies

a) Meditation

b) Relaxation exercises

c) Massage

d) Biofeedback

d. Surgical interventions

1) Arthroscopy of joint to remove osteophytes and loose bodies (e.g., particles and fragments of cartilage and bone floating freely in the synovial fluid of the joint)

2) Total joint replacement: relieves pain, restores motion, and increases joint stability

a) Contraindications to elective surgery

(1) Acute or chronic infection

(2) Major bone loss

(3) Poor muscle function

(4) History of noncompliance

(5) Age

(6) Malnutrition

(7) Bone marrow disease

b) Possible complications

(1) Wound or joint infection with possible prosthesis removal, with extensive intravenous antibiotic therapy and lengthy time before new prosthesis could be used (Anderson & Dale, 1998)

(2) Dehiscence of incision line

(3) Hematoma

(4) Deep vein thrombosis (DVT) or pulmonary embolism

(5) Neurovascular compromise

(6) Dislocation

(7) Loosening or fracture of components

(8) Wear on components

3) Laminectomy and spinal fusion

4) Arthrodesis: surgical fusion of the joint

e. Psychological support

9. Trends in total joint replacement

a. Use of critical pathways, which begin 3–4 weeks before surgery and include the following components:

1) Total joint classes to educate the client and coach about what to expect

2) Preoperative therapy session to teach total joint exercises

3) Home evaluation, if necessary, before surgery

4) Preadmission coordination of all equipment and follow-up services

b. Decreased length of stay; on average, 3 days of acute care

c. Discharge with home therapy or outpatient therapy or transfer to a rehabilitation facility or subacute care unit for the remainder of rehabilitation (usually less than 1 week)

10. Client education

a. Choice of treatment regimen

b. How to incorporate it into lifestyle

c. Medication management

d. The importance of physical and occupational therapy and assistive devices

e. Other treatment options

1) Arthroscopy

2) Arthroplasty

3) Arthrodesis

f. Complications and risks of surgery

g. Precautions after surgery

h. Life with an artificial joint

11. Future research

a. Outcome studies on the use of critical pathways

b. Improvements in the components used in total joint arthroplasty

c. Debates about which protocol best prevents DVT (Hyers, Hull, & Weg, 1995)

E. Metabolic Arthritis (Gout)

1. Definition: disturbance in uric acid metabolism in which urate salts are deposited into joints and subcutaneous tissues

2. Etiology

a. Cause remains unknown.

b. Primary gout results from a genetic defect in purine metabolism and leads to elevated uric acid production or retention of uric acid.

c. Secondary gout:

1) Hydrochlorothiazide and pyrazinamide, which affect urate excretion

2) Malignant disease, myeloproliferation psoriasis, and sickle-cell anemia may lead to gout because of the increased cell turnover, breakdown, or renal dysfunction

3) Caused by overindulgence in foods high in protein (e.g., organ meat, shellfish) or alcohol

3. Pathophysiology

a. Four stages of gout (Schoen, 2001)

1) Asymptomatic: Urate levels increase, but no signs or symptoms are present.

2) Acute attack: First attack is sudden.

a) Involves extreme pain in one or more joints, usually the great toe

b) Characterized by tissue damage and inflammation

3) Intercritical period: between attacks, symptom free

4) Chronic gout: persistent pain and renal dysfunction

a) Tophi: Uric acid crystal lumps found in joints and cartilage (usually the earlobe, fingers, hands, knees, and feet) that lead to the erosion of surrounding tissues, as in RA

b) Renal tubules: Affected by kidney stone formation

b. Uric acid crystal deposits surrounded by an inflammatory process that leads to fibrous tissue, giant cells, and local necrosis

4. Incidence

a. Affects about 5.1 million Americans

b. Affects men in 95% of all cases, with the first attack happening after age 30

c. Affects the foot and great toe in 90% of diagnosed cases

5. Diagnosis
   a. History
      1) Frequency of attacks and severity and location of symptoms
      2) Pain history
      3) Dietary history (e.g., high protein intake)
   b. Physical assessment of specific signs and symptoms
      1) Red, swollen, deformed, tender, dusty cyanotic joints, especially in the great toe, ankles, fingers, and wrists
      2) Fever
      3) Tachycardia, hypertension
      4) Headache
      5) Joint effusion
      6) Severe pain in the joint
      7) Decreased ROM
      8) Severe back pain
   c. Diagnostic tests
      1) Laboratory tests
         a) Serum uric acid levels: elevated
         b) Urinary uric acid levels: elevated in secondary gout
         c) Urinalysis: albuminuria
         d) Complete blood count: leukocytosis
         e) Sedimentation rate: elevated
      2) Radiological examination of the affected joint
         a) Initially, the joint looks normal.
         b) Later, the joint looks punched out as urate crystals replace bony structures (Crowley, 2004).
         c) Eventually, a narrowing of the joint space is apparent, degenerative arthritic changes occur, and cartilage is destroyed.
      3) Aspiration of synovial fluid
      4) Renal studies to determine whether kidneys are affected
6. Resulting disabilities
   a. Deformation of the involved joint
   b. Renal dysfunction
   c. Cardiovascular lesions
   d. Tophi deposits, leading to infection
   e. Thrombosis
   f. Hypertension
   g. Chronic pain
7. Interventions
   a. Goals of treatment: to control symptoms and decrease the frequency of acute attacks

   b. Pharmacological management
      1) Aspirin and acetaminophen for pain management of mild attacks
      2) Colchicine
         a) Prevents or relieves acute attacks
         b) Does not affect uric acid synthesis
         c) Is a prophylactic agent
         d) Is taken at the first sign of an acute attack
         e) Involves side effects (e.g., B12 deficiency, diarrhea)
      3) Uricosurics: probenecid, sulfinpyrazone
         a) Inhibits reabsorption of uric acid
         b) Is not effective in an acute attack
      4) Allopurinol
         a) Reduces synthesis of uric acid
         b) Is not effective in acute attack
         c) Increases activity of anticoagulants and hypoglycemics
      5) Corticosteroids: used for inflammation resistant to colchicine therapy
      6) Sodium bicarbonate, citrate solutions: used to increase urine pH, which increases uric acid excretion by the kidney
   c. Nutrition
      1) Protein-limited diet
      2) Alcohol and purine restriction
      3) Weight loss encouraged
   d. Joint protection
   e. Pain and symptom management
      1) Acute attack
         a) Bed rest during episode and until 24 hours after
         b) Immobilization of affected joint
         c) Joint protection
         d) Pain management
      2) Chronic attack
         a) Treat with uricosurics
         b) Increase fluids
   f. Surgical
      1) Inject corticosteroids into the joint
      2) Aspirate joints
      3) Excise and drain joint to remove crystals
      4) Use surgery to improve function and decrease deformity
   g. Psychological support
8. Client education
   a. What is gout?
   b. What are the stages of gout?

c. What are the symptoms and signs of gout?

d. What do you do when you see the signs of gout?

e. How do you decrease the chances of an attack?
1) Medication management
2) Diet education
3) Weight loss

f. What are joint conservation techniques?

g. How do you manage the pain of an attack?

9. Future research: clinical drug trials

III. Amputation

A. Overview

1. Clients with amputations account for a significant part of the population in most rehabilitation facilities.

2. Loss of a body part is permanent, leaving the person with alterations in mobility and body image and self-care deficits.

3. Rehabilitation interventions are critical for successful adaptation and reintegration into the community.

4. A national health objective for 2010 is to decrease diabetes-related amputations by 40%, from 8.2 per 1,000 people to 4.9 per 1,000 people with diabetes (U.S. DHHS, 2000). To achieve this goal, regular foot assessments and client education on proper foot care must be stressed long before any problem is noted.

B. Prevention of Amputations

1. Get regular foot assessments by a medical practitioner or podiatrist.

2. Check daily for cracks, sores, and blisters, with prompt medical attention if anything is noted.

3. Cleanse with a mild soap and water daily and dry well.

4. Get special care if the person is diabetic.

5. Keep diabetes controlled.

C. Types of Amputation

1. Congenital: absence of part or all of an extremity at birth

2. Acquired: loss of part or all of an extremity as a direct result of disease, trauma, or surgery

D. Incidence

1. Age:
a. Rate of amputation increases with age.
b. Peak incidence occurs between 41 and 71 years of age; 75% of all amputations occur in people age 65 or older.

2. Sex: Incidence of amputations is higher in men.

3. Race: African Americans with diabetes have 1.5:1 to 3.5:1 and Hispanic Americans 3.6:1 amputation rates compared with Caucasians with diabetes (Limb Loss Research & Statistics Program, 2006).

4. Type: Lower extremity amputations usually are related to disease, and upper extremity amputations are usually related to trauma.

E. Etiology

1. Disease-related amputations (American Academy of Physical Medicine and Rehabilitation, 2005):

a. Diabetes mellitus [Refer to Chapter 14 for more information about diabetes.]
1) Diabetes is the leading cause of nontraumatic amputation in the United States, accounting for a majority of all nontraumatic amputations.
2) 50% of these clients are older than age 65 and have vascular, peripheral nerve, cardiac, respiratory, visual, and kidney problems.

b. Peripheral vascular disease (PVD)
1) In the past, 80% of clients with amputations had PVD, and 75% had diabetes (ACA Fact Sheet, 2007).
2) PVD is 2.5 to 3 times more common in diabetic clients.
3) PVD advances more rapidly in diabetic clients.
4) A diabetic client with PVD is unable to form collateral circulation (Spollett, 1998).

c. Osteomyelitis
1) Inflammation of the bone (localized or generalized) caused by a pyrogenic infection
2) Causes bone destruction, acute pain, and fever
3) Can be aggravated by diabetes and PVD

d. Gangrene
1) The death of body tissue, usually associated with a loss of vascular supply and followed by bacterial invasion

2) Dry gangrene: common because of the gradual reduction in blood flow to the area

    e. Thrombosis: results from an atherosclerotic event

2. Trauma-related amputations:

    a. Account for 75% of upper extremity amputations and 30% of all amputations

    b. Result from motor vehicle accidents, gunshot wounds, falls, frostbite, explosions, war injuries, burns, and industrial and farm accidents

    c. Occur more often in men 17–55 years of age

3. Tumor-related amputations: 5% are caused by sarcomas and are most common in people 10 to 20 years of age.

F. Presurgical Interventions

1. Preamputation treatments

    a. Local treatment of wounds

    b. Intravenous antibiotics

    c. Debridement procedures:
       1) Appropriate dressings
       2) Whirlpool treatment
       3) Surgical debridement

    d. Revascularization procedures

    e. Hyperbaric oxygen treatments

    f. Pain management: Pain must be managed aggressively before the amputation to decrease phantom limb pain after surgery (Beer, 2005).

2. Client and family education

    a. What to expect from the preamputation interventions

    b. What happens when conservative treatment fails

    c. What to expect after the amputation

    d. What causes phantom pain

    e. The rehabilitation process

    f. Therapy before surgery (Yetzer, 1996)
       1) Transfer training
       2) Strengthening exercises
       3) Use of assistive devices

    g. The normal grieving process

G. Surgery

1. Types of surgery:

    a. Closed procedure
       1) A full-thickness flap of skin covers the distal end of bone.
       2) Accounts for most amputations.

    b. Open procedure (or guillotine procedure)
       1) Performed when infection is present or likely to develop

       2) Leaves the end of the residual limb open

2. Level of amputation:

    a. Based on the level of viable tissue, the amputation usually is done as distally as possible.

    b. Preservation of the knee joint is preferred for optimal mobility and function.

    c. Energy expenditure is an issue (Walters, 1992).
       1) Using a unilateral below-knee prosthesis uses 10%–40% more energy than normal.
       2) Using an above-knee prosthesis uses 60%–100% more energy than normal.
       3) Energy needs are compounded if the client is a bilateral amputee. A person with a bilateral below-knee amputation uses less energy for walking than a person with a unilateral above-knee amputation.

3. Presence of comorbidities that affect outcomes:

    a. Cardiopulmonary deconditioning
       1) Occurs as a result of presurgical treatments (e.g., bed rest)
       2) Increases if the client also has a severe cardiac or pulmonary history
       3) Can be limited with presurgical therapy interventions that are continued after surgery

    b. Peripheral vascular disease: determines level of amputation needed

    c. Diabetes: affects wound healing

4. Replantation, which has high success rates with upper extremities and digits and is considered in the following cases (O'Hare & LineaWeaver, 1990):

    a. Amputation of thumbs or multiple digits

    b. Amputations in children

    c. Clean amputations at the palm, wrist, or forearm

    d. Complex injuries that might benefit from acute microsurgical reconstruction (e.g., revascularization, free flap coverage)

5. Tumor-related surgery (Piasecki, 1991):

    a. An alternative treatment done less often because of advances in limb salvage surgical procedures

    b. Indicated when tumor margins are not microscopically clean or local resection is not possible

H. Postoperative Interventions

1. Complications after amputation surgery (see Figure 11-3)
2. Pain management
   a. Acute postoperative pain: Early intervention has been shown to decrease phantom pain the most; the use of epidural analgesia both preoperatively and postoperatively has shown promise (Williams & Deaton, 1997).
   b. Phantom limb pain:
      1) Painful sensations perceived in the missing limb
      2) Often described as knifelike, burning, or squeezing sensations
      3) Often described as similar to presurgical pain
      4) Occurs to some extent in all amputees
      5) Has no known cure but many theories as to why it occurs
3. Contracture prevention
   a. Goal: to keep the joint above the site of the amputation in full extension to allow a more functional gait
   b. Lying in prone position
      1) Stretches the hip muscles into full extension
      2) Usually done 3 or 4 times a day for 20 minutes each time
      3) Counteracts decreased mobility and increased chair dependency
   c. Knee extension
      1) Prevents contracture of the knee joint and allows a more functional gait:

      a) Some surgeons cast the extremity immediately after surgery to decrease the chance of a flexion contracture. A disadvantage of this method is that the surgical incision cannot be examined.
      b) Removable rigid dressing can be used to prevent contractures and can be removed for limb inspection and care.
      c) Some surgeons place a knee immobilizer over the top of the surgical dressing. A benefit of this method is that wound checks can be done.
      2) Splints, boards, and wheelchair extensions attempt to keep the limb in extension and allow for wound checks.
   d. Elbow extension: usually done with a splint made specifically for the client
4. Psychological support
   a. Allow the client to grieve at his or her own pace.
   b. Watch for signs of disturbance. Along with the physical discomfort, psychological distress has been cited as a major reason for nonuse of the prosthesis (Butler, Turkal, & Seidl, 1992).
      1) Refusal to look at or touch residual limb
      2) Unwillingness to discuss predicted limitations or use of prosthesis
      3) Refusal to participate in self-care
      4) Social withdrawal
   c. Make referrals to psychologist and to support groups for amputees.
5. Therapy
   a. Transfer training
      1) Standing pivot transfers
      2) Sliding board transfers
   b. Ambulation training
      1) Begin with parallel bars and progress to a walker.
      2) Balance training (sitting and standing)
   c. Preprosthetic training
      1) Teach client to be functional at the wheelchair level.
      2) Condition the residual limb.
      3) Practice ROM exercises.
   d. Deconditioning and strengthening exercises for the entire body
   e. Functional activity training
   f. Prosthetic evaluation and recommendation

Figure 11-3. Potential Complications After Amputation Surgery

Pressure ulcers and skin breakdown (e.g., buttocks, heels)

Nonhealing surgical incisions necessitating revision surgery healing by secondary intention

Infection

Osteomyelitis

Gangrene

Falls without injury

Falls with injuries (e.g., fractures, dehiscence of incision)

Postoperative confusion related to anesthesia, medication, sepsis

Altered mental status, which can worsen dementia, Alzheimer's disease

Depression, anxiety, fear, and adjustment disorders

Embolism (e.g., pulmonary embolism, deep vein thrombosis)

Heart attack or stroke

Diabetic reactions

Flexion contracture

Deconditioning secondary to decreased mobility before surgery

6. Wound management
   a. For clients with immediate postoperative casting, monitor for the following:
      1) Signs of increased edema, drainage, and odor
      2) Lack of pulse in the next joint proximally
   b. For clients without casting, monitor for the following:
      1) Dehiscence
      2) Nonhealing
      3) Infection
      4) Progressive gangrene
      5) Lack of pulse in the next joint proximally
   c. For clients with residual limb edema:
      1) Decrease pain and prepare limb for prosthetic fitting.
      2) Use appropriate methods of shrinkage and bandaging (see Figure 11-4):
         a) Ace wrap: Rewrap limb every 3–4 hours.
         b) Residual limb (stump) shrinker: Remove every 3–4 hours to assess incision line. Shrinkers should be washed daily, so 2 are needed.
         c) Jobst compression boot: Use for 20 minutes, 3 or 4 times a day, along with an ace wrap or shrinker.
         d) Elevation: Do not allow limb to hang down for extended periods of time.
7. Desensitization to decrease pain
   a. Tap the distal aspect
   b. Rub the distal aspect
   c. Stroke the distal aspect
   d. Massage the residual limb

I. Prosthetic Management
1. Remember that prostheses can be functional or cosmetic.
2. Develop a wearing schedule:
   a. Usually start with 2 hours on, 2 hours off, 1 or 2 times a day when sitting.
   b. Perform prewearing and postwearing skin check, looking for areas of redness, irritation, or skin breakdown, which means the adjustment is needed.
   c. If open area on limb, should not wear prosthesis until healed.
3. Build up wearing times as tolerated.
4. May need to use numerous prostheses over the long term for specific needs related to work, school, home, sports, and leisure activities and growth of child.

5. Provide prosthetic care before donning the prosthesis:
   a. Check prosthesis for mechanical stability.
   b. Wipe off with damp cloth daily.
   c. Wipe out socket daily and allow to dry before donning the prosthesis.
   d. Apply clean, dry socks to the residual limb:
      1) Sock thickness depends on amount of shrinkage of limb.
      2) Need several socks of different thicknesses so worn socks can be washed daily.
      3) Weight loss or gain of as little as 5 lb can affect prosthesis fit and function.
6. Proper foot care of remaining foot to prevent amputation.

J. Geriatric Considerations
1. Many amputees are older than 65, and the effects of aging can affect their rehabilitation.
2. Dual diagnoses and rehabilitation problems are common in this population (Edelstein, 1992).
   a. Cardiopulmonary capacity
   b. Poor neuromuscular coordination
   c. Visual impairments
   d. Weakened musculature
   e. Limited ROM

K. Research Topics
1. The causes of phantom limb pain and phantom sensations (Davis, 1993)
2. Preoperative education and pain management's effects on outcomes after surgery (Jahangiri, Jayatunga, Bradley, & Dark, 1994)
3. Client outcome studies: inpatient rehabilitation, home care, and outpatient rehabilitation, which helps the client become more functional faster

IV. Nursing Diagnoses Associated with Musculoskeletal and Orthopedic Disorders

A. Overview
1. Rehabilitation nurses work in many settings: acute care hospitals, rehabilitation hospitals, home care, schools, long-term care facilities, ambulatory care centers, and insurance companies.
2. Nearly every rehabilitation nurse will someday care for a person with musculoskeletal and orthopedic disorders,

Figure 11-4. Wrapping a Residual Limb

WRAPPING ABOVE KNEE — always wrap in a "figure 8" pattern

If the elastic bandage slips or was not wrapped well the first time, unwrap it and wrap it again.

The elastic bandage needs to be changed every 4 to 6 hours, or more often if it becomes loose.

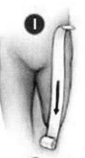 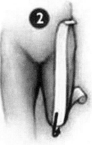 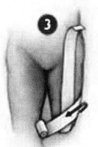 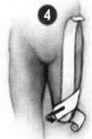 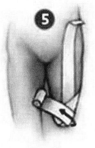

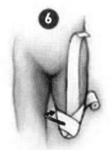 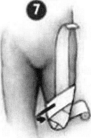 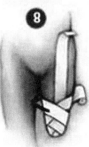

Continue wrapping in this pattern until the entire residual limb is covered and you can fasten the bandage in place.

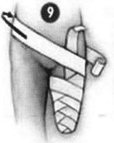 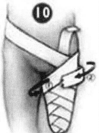

WRAPPING BELOW KNEE — always wrap in a "figure 8" pattern

If the elastic bandage slips or was not wrapped well the first time, unwrap it and wrap it again.

The elastic bandage needs to be changed every 4 to 6 hours, or more often if it becomes loose.

 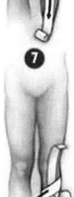 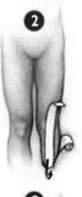 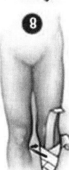 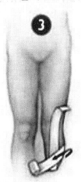 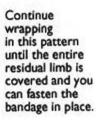 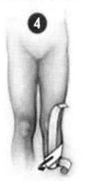 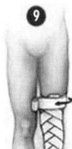

Continue wrapping in this pattern until the entire residual limb is covered and you can fasten the bandage in place.

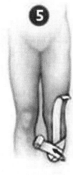 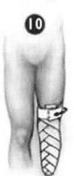

no matter what practice setting he or she works in.

3. As the population ages, nurses will see more clients with these chronic illnesses in everyday practice.

B. Assessment

1. Thorough health history

2. Thorough physical examination

3. Functional assessment, focusing on the musculoskeletal and neuromuscular systems

4. Psychological assessment

C. Nursing Diagnoses and Plans of Care

1. Impaired physical mobility (see Table 11-3): Adjust for client's age, physical ability, and support systems available for assistance.

2. Knowledge deficit (see Table 11-4):

   a. Adjust based on the following factors:
      1) Client's diagnosis
      2) Prior knowledge about the disease
      3) Age of the client
      4) Educational level

   b. Provide information in several forms (e.g., verbal, written) at numerous times.

3. Self-care deficit (see Table 11-5): Tailor to the client's abilities and disabilities, but do not encourage dependency on others.

D. Other Potential Nursing Diagnoses

1. Ineffective individual coping: denial

   a. Lack of comprehension of the seriousness of the diagnosis

   b. Denial used as a defense mechanism

2. Alterations in comfort: pain

   a. Surgical procedures

   b. Joint destruction

   c. Pathology of the injury or disease

   d. Therapy procedures and exercises

   e. Medical treatment plan

   f. Activity restrictions

3. Alteration in family processes

   a. Role changes necessitated by the disability

   b. Diagnosis of a chronic illness with disabling features

4. Potential for injury

   a. Activity restrictions

   b. Balance changes created by weight-bearing restrictions

   c. Use of assistive devices

Table 11-3. Nursing Plan of Care: Impaired Physical Mobility

Related to the following:
- Limited movement ability.
- Activity restrictions.
- Need to use assistive devices.
- Need for assistance for ambulation and transfers.
- Intolerance to activity.
- Pain and discomfort.
- Limited strength.

Goals	Interventions
Demonstrate optimal independence in mobility skills and ADLs.	Teach safe use of assistive devices (e.g., walkers, canes).
	Encourage participation in self-care tasks with or without assistive devices.
	Consult physical therapist (PT) and occupational therapist (OT) for a prescribed exercise program.
	Encourage participation in recreational activities and community outings.
	Teach home safety and fall prevention.
Help client and family with activity restrictions.	Determine prescribed activity education restrictions and length of the restrictions.
	Educate client and family about why restrictions are needed.
	Teach client and family how to maintain restrictions in real-life situations.
	Educate client and family on what to do if restrictions are broken (e.g., notify physician).
Improve tolerance to activity.	Encourage the use of assistive devices.
	Provide adequate rest periods between activities.
	Teach ways to combine activities.
	Teach client to pace activities to allow for rest periods.
	Encourage compliance with exercise program created by PT and OT.
	Educate about the need to adapt environment to maximize independence.
Manage pain.	Teach about prescribed pain medications and the best times to take them.
	Provide nonpharmacological options for pain management (e.g., heat, ice).
	Provide comfort measures.
	Educate about the need to stay active to avoid further complications of deconditioning.

Expected Outcomes

Maintain a level of independence with mobility and ADLs.

Understand and adhere to activity restrictions as prescribed.

Report improved tolerance to activity.

Report effective pain management program.

Maintain safety precautions with all activities.

---

d. Rushing to get things done and not thinking about safety

e. Unsafe environment

5. Noncompliance: medical

   a. Medication regimen

   b. Diet restrictions

   c. Failure to comply with exercise program

   d. Failure to obtain preventive medical care

6. Alteration in skin integrity

   a. Surgical procedures

   b. Immobility

   c. Pressure sores

   d. Nutritional deficits

   e. Nodule development in RA

   f. Crystal development in gout

   g. Use of splints, casts, braces, orthotics, and prosthetics

7. Social isolation

   a. Prescribed activity restrictions

   b. Lack of transportation

   c. Lack of social support network

   d. Self-imposed isolation

   e. Self-esteem issues

   f. Lack of motivation

   g. Chronic pain issues

8. Disturbance in body image

9. Altered sexuality pattern

E. Diagnoses Specifically Relevant for Children

1. Alteration in self-esteem

2. Alteration in body image

3. Alteration in growth and development

4. Ineffective family coping

5. Knowledge deficit related to community resources

Table 11-4. Nursing Plan of Care: Knowledge Deficit

Related to the following:
• Chronic illness diagnosis.
• Prescribed treatment regimen.
• Possible complications.

Goals	Interventions
Verbalize understanding about diagnosis and prescribed treatment plan.	Teach client and family about the diagnosis. • What does the diagnosis mean? • How will it affect the body? • Why me? • How is it diagnosed? • What causes the disease? • What does the future look like? Explain the treatment options presented by the physician. Teach the specifics of the treatment plan. • Medication management • Nutritional management • Activity restrictions, use of assistive devices, need for regular exercise • Consult PT or OT for exercise program • Encourage proper health maintenance (e.g., eye exams, foot assessments) • Community resources available • The importance of complying with the treatment plan Tailor information to the client's and family's educational level. Integrate cultural and religious differences. Be creative when presenting information. Use age-appropriate education principles. Progress from simple to complex topics. Repeat information to reinforce learning. Provide written information if possible.
Verbalize understanding of possible complications and what to do about them.	Offer information frequently about complications associated with the diagnosis. Teach the client and family what to do if signs and symptoms develop. Teach the consequences of complications that are not addressed in a timely manner.
Verbalize understanding of the disease process and what the future may hold	Explain the natural progression of the disease. Describe treatment changes that may occur as the result of the disease progression (e.g., more aggressive medications, surgical procedures, need for more assistance with mobility and ADLs). Describe possible comorbidities that may occur as a result of the disease.

Expected Outcomes

Actively participate in the prescribed treatment plan.

Understand the disease condition and possible complications and comorbidities.

Know what to do if signs and symptoms of complications arise.

V. **Advanced Practice**

A. Clinician

1. Coordination of the multidisciplinary team

   a. Communicating rehabilitation therapy interventions to the beside nurse

   b. Coordinating patient's physical needs to discharge personnel to ensure continuity of care and a safe transition.

2. Medical and nursing care

   a. Monitoring of relevant lab values and

Table 11-5. Nursing Plan of Care: Self-Care Deficit

Related to the following:
- Decreased activity tolerance.
- Pain and discomfort.
- Fear, anxiety, and depression.
- Lack of motivation.
- Inability to perform or complete bathing.
- Inability to perform or complete dressing and grooming self-care activities.
- Inability to perform toileting self-care activities.

Goals	Interventions
Demonstrate the ability to use adaptive equipment.	Teach or reinforce the use of assistive devices provided by therapy (e.g., plate guards, swivel utensils, universal cuffs, reachers, long-handled sponges, wash mitts, grab bars, tub or shower seats, walkers, crutches, canes).
	Educate the family about what the client can do and what he or she may need help with.
Perform toileting, bathing, and dressing activities at optimal level of independence.	Set up the environment so the client has easy access to all equipment, hygiene products, and clothing.
	Allow extra time to complete tasks.
	Encourage the use of safety measures.
	Provide privacy based on the client's safety level.
Maintain safe bathing practices.	Teach and reinforce safety measures often (e.g., adequate lighting, no-slip strips on floors and tub or shower floors, electric appliances placed away from water sources, need for rails and grab bars).
	Provide a means of calling for help as needed (e.g., call bells, panic buttons).
	Teach how to test water temperature to prevent burns if the client has neurological problems.
Improve tolerance in performing self-care activities.	Teach the client how to pace himself or herself during ADLs.
	Provide rest periods between activities as necessary.
	Educate the client and family about energy conservation techniques.
	Provide assistance to the client to prevent exhaustion.
	Encourage the client to choose loose-fitting clothes that are easy to put on.
Show an interest in hygiene and wear own clothes.	Encourage the client to see himself or herself as becoming healthier.
	Encourage the client to wear his or her own clothes as much as possible.
	Adapt clothing for easier application as necessary (e.g., Velcro closures, adjustments to clothing to fit over bulky appliances).
	Provide assistance with hair, makeup, or shaving as needed.
	Foster an atmosphere that promotes wellness.
	Provide psychological counseling as necessary (e.g., for adjustment disorders, depression, anxiety).

Expected Outcomes

Use assistive devices for eating, grooming, dressing, and toileting in a correct, safe, and efficient manner.

Maintain an independent level of functioning for toileting, bathing, grooming, and dressing activities.

Maintain a safe environment.

Demonstrate improved tolerance to performing ADLs.

Demonstrate improved motivation to perform ADLs.

---

follow-up interventions related to lab values (e.g., hemoglobin and hematocrit levels after joint replacement)

b. Monitoring and intervening to prevent complications (e.g., DVT prophylaxis, activity)

c. Troubleshooting problem-prone and high-risk patient care

d. Creating protocols to make care seamless and reduce chance of error (e.g., develop bowel regimen to prevent constipation in patient taking a lot of pain medication)

B. Educator

1. Nursing personnel

a. Importance of mobility to prevent complications

b. Universal precautions to minimize spread of infection

c. Identification of high-risk patients for falls, complications, development of medical problems

d. Instruct on pain management techniques and interventions to prevent oversedation complications

2. Multidisciplinary personnel
   a. Outline role of nursing in the multidisciplinary team.
   b. Learn rehabilitation techniques that can be carried over to the bedside nursing personnel.
   c. Coordinate new staff orientation to rehabilitation department and the treatments offered to patients.
3. Community
   a. Health promotion
      1) Early identification of musculoskeletal diseases
      2) Dietary intake needs of preteens and teenagers in osteoporosis prevention
      3) Safety awareness for injury prevention in sports and leisure activities
   b. Illness avoidance
      1) Community methicillin-resistant *Staphylococcus aureus* epidemic
      2) Fall prevention
      3) Circulatory and diabetes care to prevent the need for amputations

C. Leader
1. Facilitate the incorporation of clinical practice guidelines into the patient care setting.
2. Participate in relevant hospital committees:
   a. Safety committee
   b. Pharmacy and therapeutics
   c. Specialty program development, evaluation, and treatment
   d. Quality improvement initiatives
3. Interact with relevant community and national organizations to assist in disease prevention and implement evidenced-based practice:
   a. National Osteoporosis Foundation
   b. National Institutes of Health
   c. Arthritis Foundation
   d. Society of Vascular Surgery
   e. American Academy of Orthopedic Surgeons
   f. National Association of Orthopedic Nurses
4. Contact local and state representatives related to health promotion and safety:
   a. Dietary intake in the school settings
   b. Helmet and seatbelt laws
   c. Funding for catastrophic care

D. Consultant
1. Identify key areas of care related to specific diagnosis (e.g., joint replacement: vital signs, lab values, blood loss, activity level, pain management, and incision care).
2. Develop effective mechanisms to communicate this information to the physician and other healthcare providers.
3. Communicate with internal and external financial resources to ensure optimum billing and reimbursement.
4. Product adoption (e.g., assist in medical equipment purchasing to facilitate patient recovery and mobility).

E. Researcher
1. Evidence-based practice related to pain management in orthopedic surgery:
   a. Pain management is a fundamental component of nursing care in the orthopedic patient.
   b. Multiple routes of administration of pain relief are available for use: epidural and intrathecal opioid analgesia, patient-controlled analgesia with systemic opioids, and regional techniques.
   c. Many factors affect how a patient experiences pain, such as age, race, sex, and culture.
   d. Pain management treatment continues to be driven by practitioner preference and familiarity of treatment options.
2. Clinical question: Are around-the-clock scheduled pain medications more effective in pain management than patient-controlled analgesia or as-needed pain management practices?
3. Appraisal of evidence:
   a. Two national guidelines with good evidence: "Practice Guidelines for Acute Pain Management in the Perioperative Setting: An Updated Report by the American Society of Anesthesiologists Task Force on Acute Pain Management" (2004) and *Acute Pain Management: Operative or Medical Procedures and Trauma. Clinical Practice Guideline* (AHCPR, 1992).
   b. Two level II articles with good evidence (Gimbel, Brugger, Zhao, Verburg, & Geis, 2001; Moizo, Marchetti, Albertin, Muzzolon, & Antonino, 2004; Sinatra et al., 2005).
   c. Two level VI articles with good evidence (Pellino, Willens, Polomano, & Heve, 2003; Titler & Herr, 2004).

4. Recommendations for best rehabilitation nursing practice:
   a. There is good support for around-the-clock use of certain analgesic medications such as NSAIDs, coxibs, and acetaminophen.
   b. Patients' perceptions of the staff's ability to care for them influences their satisfaction with pain relief.
   c. Multimodal pain management treatments can and should be used for effective pain relief.

References

AACE clinical practice guidelines for the prevention and treatment of postmenopausal osteoporosis. (2003). Retrieved April 20, 2007, from http://www.aace.com/pub/pdf/guidelines/osteoporosis2001revised.pdf

AHCPR. (1992). *Acute pain management: Operative or medical procedures and trauma. Clinical practice guideline.* Rockville, MD: AHCPR.

American Academy of Physical Medicine and Rehabilitation. (2005). *Amputations/prosthetics.* Retrieved October 15, 2005, from http://www.aapmr.org/condtreat/rehab/amputations.htm

Amputee Coalition of America (ACA). (2007). Fact sheet. Retrieved July 19, 2007 from www.amputee-coalition.org/fact-sheet/dysvascular.html

Anderson, L.P., & Dale, K.G. (1998, January–February). Infections in total joint replacements. *Orthopaedic Nursing, 17*(1), 117–119.

Arnett, F.C. et al (1987). The American Rheumatism Association 1987 revised criteria for the classification of rheumatoid arthritis. *Arthritis, 31,* 315–323.

Arthritis Foundation. (2006). http://www.arthritis.com

Arthritis Foundation. (2007, January). *Research update.* Atlanta: Author.

Beare, P.G., & Myers, J.L. (1990). *Principles and practice of adult health nursing.* St. Louis: Mosby.

Beer, M.H. (2005). *Merck manual of geriatrics.* Whitehouse Station, NJ: Merck Research Laboratories.

Butler, D., Turkal, N., & Seidl, J. (1992). Amputation: Preoperative psychological preparation. *Journal of American Board of Family Practice, 5*(1), 69–73.

Canadian Association of Radiologists. (2005). *Osteoporosis Research News, 26.*

Crowley, L.V. (2004). *An introduction to human disease: Pathology and pathophysiology correlations.* Sudbury, MA: Jones and Bartlett.

Davis, R.W. (1993). Phantom sensation, phantom pain, and stump pain. *Archives of Physical Medicine and Rehabilitation, 74,* 243–256.

Edelstein, J. (1992). Preprosthetic and nonprosthetic management of older patients. *Topics in Geriatric Rehabilitation, 8*(1), 22–29.

Eli Lilly. (1998). *Evista (raloxifene hydrochloride).* Indianapolis: Author.

Gimbel, J., Brugger, A., Zhao, W., Verburg, K., & Geis, G. (2001). *Clinical Therapeutics, 23*(2), 228–241.

Healthy People 2010. (2007). Retrieved on July 19, 2007 from www.healthypeople.gov.

Heaney, R.P. (1998). Recommended calcium intakes revisited: Round table. In P. Burckhardt, B. Dawson-Hughes, & R.P. Heaney (Eds.), *Nutritional aspects of osteoporosis* (pp. 317–325). New York: Springer-Verlag.

Hyers, T.M., Hull, R.D., & Weg., J.G. (1995). Anti-thrombotic therapy for venous thrombo-embolic disease. *Chest, 108*(4), 335S–351S.

Jahangiri, M., Jayatunga, A.P., Bradley, J.W., & Dark, C.H. (1994). Prevention of phantom pain after major lower limb amputation by epidural infusion of diamorphine, clonidinell and bupivacaine. *Annals of the Royal College of Surgeons of England, 76,* 324–326.

Kessenich, C.R. (1997). The pathophysiology of osteoporotic vertebral fractures. *Rehabilitation Nursing, 22*(4), 192–195.

Limb Loss Research & Statistics Program. (2006). *People with amputations speak out.* http://www.amputee-coalition.org/people-speak-out/background.html

McClung, B.L. (1999). Using osteoporosis management to reduce fractures in elderly women. *The Nurse Practitioner, 24*(3), 26–42.

Moizo, E., Marchetti, C., Albertin, A., Muzzolon, F., & Antonino, S. (2004). *Minerva Anesthesiology, 70*(11), 779–787.

Mosby Great Performance. (1995). *Helping at home, preventing falls* [Pamphlet]. (Available from 14964 NW Greenbrier Parkway, Beaverton, OR 97006).

National Council on Aging. (2005). New survey uncovers impact of osteoarthritis on sufferer's everyday lives. Rerieved July 19, 2007 from www.ncoa.org.

National Institutes of Health (NIH) Consensus Development Panel on Optimal Calcium Intake. (1994). Optimal calcium intake. *Journal of the American Medical Association, 272,* 1942–1948.

National Osteoporosis Foundation. (2006). *Fast facts.* Retrieved April 6, 2006, from http://www.nof.org/osteoporosis/diseasefacts.htm

NYU Hospital for Joint Diseases Spine Center. (2005). *Types of osteoporosis.* Retrieved April 11, 2007, from http://www.med.nyu.edu/hjd/hjdspine/education/problems/osteoporosis/types.html

O'Hare, M., & LineaWeaver, W.C. (1990). Microsurgical replantation: Development and current status. *Critical Care Nursing Quarterly, 13*(1), 1–11.

Pellino, T., Willens, J., Polomano, R., & Heve, R. (2003). *Orthopedic Nursing, 22*(4), 289–297.

Piasecki, P. (1991). Limb salvage procedures for osteosarcoma. *Nursing Clinics of North America, 26,* 33–41.

Practice guidelines for acute pain management in the perioperative setting: An updated report by the American Society of Anesthesiologists Task Force on Acute Pain Management. (2004). *Anesthesiology, 100*(6), 1573–1581.

Schoen, D.C. (2001). *NAON core curriculum for orthopaedic nursing* (4th ed.). Pitman, NJ: Anthony J. Jannetti.

Sinatra, R., Jahr, J., Reynolds, L., Viscusi, E., Groudine, S., & Paen-Champenois, C. (2005). Efficacy and safety of single and repeated administration of 1 gram intravenous acetaminophen injection (paracetamol) for pain management after major orthopedic surgery. *Anesthesiology, 102*(4), 822–831.

Solomon, J. (1998). Osteoporosis: When supports weaken. *RN, 61*(5), 37–40.

Spollett, G.R. (1998). Preventing amputations in the diabetic population. *Nursing Clinics of North America, 33*(4), 629–637.

Spratto, G.R., & Woods, A.L. (1998). *PDR nurses' handbook* (3rd ed.). Montvale, NJ: Medical Economics.

Tanner, S. (2003–2004). Back pain, vertebroplasty, and kyphoplasty: Treatment of osteoporotic vertebral compression fractures. *Bulletin on the Rheumatic Diseases, 52*(2), 1–7.

Thalgott, J., LaRocca, H., & Gardner, V.O. (1993). Arthritides affecting the spinal column. In S.H. Hochschuler, H.B. Cotler, & R.D. Guyer (Eds.), *Rehabilitation of the spine.* St. Louis: Mosby.

Titler, M., & Herr, K. (2004). *Clinical Journal of Pain, 20*(5), 331–340.

University of Minnesota Research. (2006). *Osteoporosis research.* Retrieved April 11, 2007, from http://www.epi.umn.edu/research/osteop.shtm

U.S. Department of Health and Human Services (DHHS). (2000, August 14). Diabetes-related amputations of lower extremities in the Medicare population: Minnesota, 1993–1995. *Morbidity and Mortality Weekly Report (MMWR), 47*(31), 649–652.

Walters, R. (1992). Energy expenditure. In J. Perry (Ed.), *Gait analysis: Normal and pathological function* (pp. 475–479). New York: McGraw-Hill.

Watts, N.B. (1997, September). Osteoporosis: Prevention, detection and treatment. *Journal of the Medical Association of Georgia*, pp. 224–226.

Williams, A.M., & Deaton, S.B. (1997). Phantom limb pain: Elusive, yet real. *Rehabilitation Nursing, 22*(2), 73–77.

Woodhead, G.A., & Moss, M.M. (1998). Osteoporosis: Diagnosis and prevention. *The Nurse Practitioner, 23*(11), 18–35.

Yetzer, E.A. (1996). Helping the patient through the experience of an amputation. *Orthopaedic Nursing, 15*(6), 45–49.

Youngblood, N.M., & Edwards, P.A. (1999). Autoimmune and endocrine conditions. In P.A. Edwards, D.L. Hertzberg, S.R. Hays, & N.M. Youngblood (Eds.), *Pediatric rehabilitation nursing* (pp. 412–419). Philadelphia: W.B. Saunders.

Yurkow, J., & Yudin, J. (2002). Musculoskeletal problems. In V.T. Cotter & N.E. Strumpf (Eds.), *Advanced practice nursing with older adults: Clinical guidelines* (pp. 229–242). New York: McGraw-Hill.

Suggested Resources

Actonel, for HealthCare Professionals: http://www.fight-fracture.com

Amputee Coalition of America: http://www.amputee-coalition.org

Arthritis Health Professions Association. (1989). *A core curriculum in rheumatology for health professionals.* Atlanta, GA: Professional Education Department, Arthritis Foundation.

Bellantoni, M.F. (1996). Osteoporosis prevention and treatment. *American Family Physician, 54*(30), 986–991.

Bichler, L. (1999). Foot ulcers in diabetes. *Advance for Nurse Practitioners, 7*(1), 49–52.

Cannon, M. (2006). *Gold preparations.* Atlanta, GA: American College of Rheumatology. Retrieved August 27, 2006, from http://www.rheumatology.org/public/factsheets/gold.asp

Centers for Disease Control and Prevention. (2006). *Quick stats on arthritis.* Retrieved August 27, 2006, from http://www.cdc.gov/arthritis/pressroom/index.htm

Cosman, F., Nieves, J., Horton, J., Shen, V., & Lindsay, R. (1994). Effects of estrogen on response to edetic acid infusion in postmenopausal osteoporotic women. *Journal of Clinical Endocrinology and Metabolism, 78,* 939–943.

Darovic, G. (1997). Caring for patients with osteoporosis. *Nursing '97, 27*(5), 50–51.

Edwards, P.A., Hertzberg, D.L., Hays, S.R., & Youngblood, N.M. (Eds.). (1999). *Pediatric rehabilitation nursing.* Philadelphia: W.B. Saunders.

Heaney, R.P. (1987). Prevention of osteoporotic fracture in women. In L.V. Avioli (Ed.), *The osteoporotic syndrome: Detection, prevention, and treatment* (pp. 67–90). Orlando, FL: Grune & Stratton.

Levin, M. (1993). Diabetic foot ulcers: Pathogenesis and management. *Journal of ET Nursing, 20,* 191–198.

Matheson, A.J., & Figgitt, D.P. (2001). Rofecoxib: A review of its use in the management of osteoarthritis, acute pain and rheumatoid arthritis. *Drugs, 61*(6), 833–865.

Medline Plus® medical encyclopedia: Compression fractures of the back. http://www.nlm.nih.gov/medlineplus/print/ency/article/000443.htm

National Institutes of Health. (2006). Celecoxib. Retrieved August 27, 2006, from http://www.nlm.nih.gov/medlineplus/druginfo/medmaster/a699022.html

The Osteoporosis Center: http://endocrineweb.com/osteoporosis/

Silverstein, F.E., Faich, G., Goldstein, J.L, Simon, L.S., Pincus, T., Whelton, A., et al. (2000). Gastrointestinal toxicity with celecoxib vs nonsteroidal anti-inflammatory drugs for osteoarthritis and rheumatoid arthritis: The CLASS study: A randomized controlled trial. Celecoxib Long-Term Arthritis Safety Study. *Journal of the American Medical Association, 284,* 1247–1255.

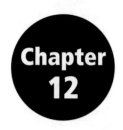

Chapter 12

Cardiovascular and Pulmonary Rehabilitation: Acute and Long-Term Management

Lynn Carbone, RN CRRN

Cardiovascular disease (CVD) affects 79.4 million Americans according to the American Heart Association (AHA, 2007g), and 35 million Americans experience some form of chronic lung disease according to the American Lung Association (ALA, 2006a). Heart disease is the leading cause of death, and chronic obstructive lung disease is the fourth leading cause of death in the United States (AHA, 2007g; ALA, 2006a). Complications of CVD and pulmonary disease greatly affect quality of life and the economy. Pulmonary disease is the leading cause of disability in the United States according to the ALA. Rehabilitation specialists need to be aware of the differences between men and women and how they cope with chronic obstructive pulmonary disease (COPD) as the incidence rises among women (Ninot et al., 2006). COPD is the third ranking condition after congestive heart failure and stroke in necessitating home care services (Connors & Hilling, 1998).

Early detection and rehabilitation can prevent the progression of cardiac and lung diseases to a disabling state. Cardiac and pulmonary rehabilitation programs use a comprehensive interdisciplinary approach to achieve positive patient outcomes. These programs have a comprehensive approach focused on individualized preventive and therapeutic interventions. Rehabilitation programs help patients make lifestyle adjustments, decrease risky health behaviors, optimize physical status without endangering life, and reduce the rate of morbidity and mortality. Rehabilitation is a continuous process that begins in the critical care period and extends to a lifelong program of lifestyle adaptation (Scottish Intercollegiate Guidelines Network [SIGN], 2002). Acute care and home health rehabilitation nurses can adapt the information in this chapter for their patients' health promotion and disease prevention needs. Assessments, interventions, and goals should be individualized according to the patient and the practice setting.

Cardiac rehabilitation programs serve patients with manifestations of congenital or acquired heart disease (e.g., myocardial infarction [MI], chronic stable angina, cardiomyopathy, postsurgical or post–procedural intervention) and those who have multiple uncontrolled risk factors or have had cardiac surgery. Cardiac rehabilitation enhances recovery, and secondary prevention measures prevent further complications from disease. Ades (2001) stated that only 10%–20% of eligible people participate in cardiac rehabilitation programs. This low rate may be attributed to low referral rates by physicians, low reimbursement rates by insurance companies, lack of availability of programs, and unwillingness of patients to alter their lifestyles. Some health reasons that may limit participation in a program include unstable angina, elevated resting blood pressure, uncontrolled arrhythmias, uncontrolled diabetes, and other high-risk heart conditions. Physical deconditioning that follows a cardiac event can promote a decline in cardiovascular health. Exercise and knowledge of the disease process help protect patients from further decline. Rehabilitation should begin when the patient is medically stable and under the care of medical professional (SIGN, 2002). There are four phases of cardiac rehabilitation programs (Aldana et al., 2003; SIGN, 2002):

- Phase I: Usually during the inpatient hospital stay
- Phase II: Early after discharge
- Phase III: Structured exercise program in the hospital
- Phase IV: Maintenance of physical activity and lifestyle change

Pulmonary rehabilitation programs serve patients with manifestations of COPD, nonobstructive lung disease, and other lung disorders. Assessment, patient training, exercise, psychosocial intervention, and follow-up are essential components of a pulmonary rehabilitation program (American Association for Respiratory Care [AARC], 2002).

Both cardiac and pulmonary rehabilitation improve physical functioning, leading to a potential decrease in morbidity and mortality by enhancing the life of the person with the disease (AARC, 2002; Krau, Ward, & Parsons, 2001). Risk factor interventions vary significantly between cardiac rehabilitation programs, with much focus on the exercise component. Although exercise is an important part of the reconditioning of the myocardium and other organs, a multifaceted program improves clinical outcomes. The incorporation of multiple intervention applications is inconsistent across medical care settings. Scientific evidence demonstrates that comprehensive risk factor interventions extend overall survival, improve quality of life, decrease the need for interventional procedures, and reduce the incidence of subsequent MI (Adams et al., 2007; American Association of Cardiovascular and Pulmonary Rehabilitation [AACVPR], 2005; Aldana et al., 2003).

I. Cardiovascular Disease (CVD)

A. Types of CVD

1. Coronary artery disease (CAD): disorder of the coronary arteries that leads to disruption of the blood flow that supplies oxygen and nutrients to the myocardium

2. Congestive heart failure (CHF) or heart failure: complex syndrome that results from the heart's inability to increase cardiac output sufficiently to meet the body's metabolic demands

3. Cardiomyopathy: disease that diffusely affects the myocardium, resulting in enlargement or restriction, and leads to ventricular dysfunction

4. Congenital heart defects (CHDs): structural or functional abnormalities of the heart or great vessels existing from birth that obstruct blood flow in and to the heart and cause the blood to flow abnormally through the heart (AHA, 2007a)

   a. Aortic stenosis

   b. Atrial septal defect

   c. Atrioventricular canal defect

   d. Bicuspid aortic valve

   e. Coarctation of the aorta

   f. Ebstein's anomaly

   g. Eisenmenger's complex

   h. Hypoplastic left heart syndrome

   i. Patent ductus arteriosus

   j. Pulmonary atresia

   k. Subaortic stenosis

   l. Tetralogy of Fallot

   m. Total anomalous pulmonary venous connection

   n. Transposition of the great arteries

   o. Tricuspid atresia

   p. Truncus arteriosus

   q. Ventricular septal defect

B. Epidemiology and Incidence

1. CVD (AHA, 2007g)

   a. Leading cause of morbidity and mortality in United States: 871,517 deaths in 2004.

   b. 79,400,000 American adults have 1 or more types of CVD. Accounts for 476,124 deaths per year, or 1 of every 4.9 deaths.

   c. 37,500,000 Americans are 65 years of age or older.

   d. The decrease in mortality rates suggests that primary and secondary interventions have contributed to the decline in CVD mortality in the United States.

   e. Heart disease is the most costly healthcare expenditure, estimated at $431.8 billion for 2007.

2. CHF (AHA, 2007h) or heart failure

   a. Affects 5.2 million Americans: 2.2 million men and 2.3 million women

   b. Involves 550,000 new cases annually

3. CHD (AHA, 2007e)

   a. Affects approximately 8 infants of every 1,000 births, or 35,000 births yearly

   b. Affects 1 million Americans

   c. Costs of inpatient surgery are estimated at $2.2 billion.

   d. Mortality rates have dropped from 30% in 1960–1970 to 20% today.

C. Etiology

1. Causes

   a. CAD: atherosclerosis (WebMD, 2006b)

   b. CHF (AHA, 2007h; WebMD, 2007)

      1) Decreased myocardial contractility

         a) CAD

         b) Myocarditis

         c) Cardiomyopathy

         d) Infiltrative diseases (e.g., amyloidosis, tumors, sarcoidosis)

         e) Collagen-vascular diseases (e.g., systemic lupus erythematosus, scleroderma)

         f) Drugs (e.g., beta-adrenergic blocking agents, calcium antagonists)

      2) Increased myocardial workload

         a) Hypertension

         b) Pulmonary hypertension

         c) Vascular disease

         d) Cardiomyopathy

         e) Intra-aortic shunting

         f) Hyperthyroidism

      3) Congenital heart disease

      4) Other

         a) Smoking

         b) Elevated cholesterol

         c) Diabetes

         d) Obesity

   c. Cardiomyopathy

      1) Dilated (AHA, 2007c; WebMD, 2004a)

         a) Excessive alcohol use

         b) Third trimester of pregnancy

         c) Infections (myocarditis)

         d) Immunological abnormalities (e.g., thiamine deficiency,

thyrotoxicosis, diabetes mellitus)
- e) Ischemia
- f) Noninfectious conditions (e.g., rheumatic heart disease, scleroderma, systemic lupus erythematosus, polyarteritis)
- 2) Hypertrophic (idiopathic): genetic
- 3) Restrictive (AHA, 2007c; WebMD, 2004b)
  - a) Infiltrative or fibrotic processes in the myocardium
  - b) Amyloidosis: abnormal buildup of protein in the heart muscle
  - c) Hemochromatosis: abnormal buildup of iron in the heart muscle
  - d) Glycogen storage disease
  - e) Sarcoidosis: abnormal inflammatory nodules
  - f) Neoplasm and its treatment
  - g) Genetics
  - h) Loeffler's syndrome and endomyocardial fibrosis: buildup of white blood cells, causing scarring
- 4) Others
  - a) Toxic metals
  - b) Illegal drugs
  - c) Chemotherapy
  - d) CAD
- d. CHDs (AHA, 2007a, 2007e)
  - 1) Unknown causes
  - 2) Genetics
  - 3) Teratogens
- 2. Risk factors for CVD (AHA, 1996)
  - a. Nonmodifiable
    - 1) Heredity
    - 2) Race
    - 3) Gender
    - 4) Age
  - b. Modifiable
    - 1) Smoking
    - 2) Hypertension
    - 3) Elevated serum cholesterol
    - 4) Diabetes mellitus
    - 5) Sedentary lifestyle
    - 6) Stress
    - 7) Oral contraceptives
    - 8) Alcohol
    - 9) Obesity
- D. Pathophysiology
  - 1. CAD: Involves formation of plaque inside a vessel, impeding the flow of blood (see Figure 12-1):
    - a. Theories (AHA, 1996)

- 1) Plaque formation
  - a) Endothelium is damaged by a variety of factors.
    - (1) Elevated serum cholesterol and triglycerides
    - (2) Hypertension
    - (3) Cigarette smoke
  - b) Fats, cholesterol, fibrin, platelets, cellular debris, and calcium deposit in arterial wall.
  - c) Thickened endothelium narrows arterial lumen, impeding blood flow and decreasing oxygen supply to myocardium.
  - d) Formation of thrombus or hemorrhage around plaque blocks blood flow.
- 2) Abnormal growth of smooth muscle cells
  - a) Platelets form prostaglandins that may destroy the walls of arteries.
  - b) Platelets also contain platelet growth factor, which stimulates the growth of smooth muscle cells.
  - c) Abnormal growth of smooth muscle cells may be one of the earliest events in the atherosclerotic process.
- 3) Deposition of connective tissue cells
  - a) Lipoproteins from the blood that are trapped in the arterial wall accumulate and become oxidized.
  - b) Lipoproteins become modified and are absorbed by smooth muscle cells.
  - c) Foam cells are formed, causing connective tissue cells to become deposited.

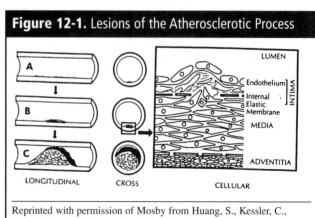

Figure 12-1. Lesions of the Atherosclerotic Process

Reprinted with permission of Mosby from Huang, S., Kessler, C., McCulloch, C., & Dasher, L. (1989). Cardiac rehabilitation of the myocardial patient. In *Coronary care nursing* (2nd ed., p. 133). Philadelphia: W.B. Saunders.

b. Severity of disease
    1) Measured by degree of obstruction in each coronary artery and the number of arteries involved
    2) Involves an increased risk of death with arterial lumen obstructions exceeding 70% of one or more coronary arteries
2. CHF (functional defects): impaired cardiac output (AHA, 2007d):
    a. Left-sided heart failure
        1) Left ventricle works harder to circulate blood out of the heart.
        2) Increasing fluid pressure in pulmonary vessels makes it hard to breathe.
    b. Right-sided heart failure
        1) Damaged right ventricle increases venous congestion and swelling in the hands, legs, and abdomen.
        2) Tricuspid valve regurgitation
        3) Right ventricular infarct
        4) Pulmonary disease
    c. Decreased ability of kidneys to remove sodium and water
3. Cardiomyopathy (AHA, 2007c) (structural defects) (see Figure 12-2):
    a. Dilated
        1) Enlarged (dilated) and stretched heart chambers with normal to low myocardium wall thickness
        2) Decreased ejection fraction
        3) Decreases blood flow, causing blood to clot
        4) Risk for dysrhythmias
    b. Restrictive
        1) Endocardium and myocardium become rigid.
        2) Impairs relaxation of the heart muscle, causing fatigue
    c. Hypertrophic

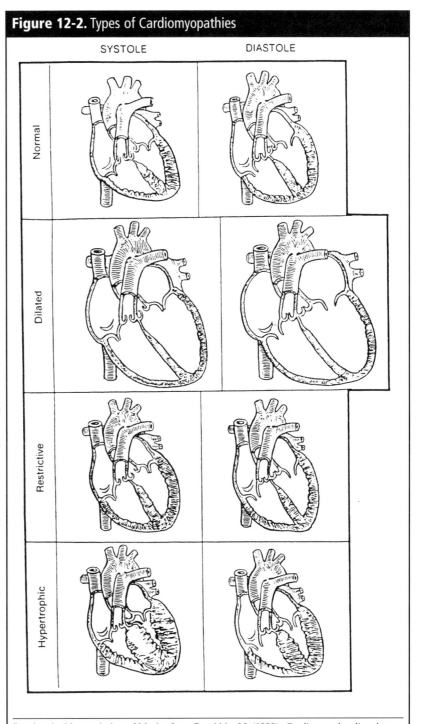

Figure 12-2. Types of Cardiomyopathies

Reprinted with permission of Mosby from Canobbio, M. (1990). *Cardiovascular disorders* (p. 93). St. Louis: Mosby.

        1) Heart muscle walls thicken, obstructing blood flow.
        2) Causes mitral valve to leak
4. CHDs: Severity of symptoms depends on the type of defect.

E. Residual Deficits (AHA 1996; WebMD, 2004b)
    1. Dysrhythmias:
        a. Cardiac arrest

b. Sudden death

c. Atrial fibrillation

2. Ischemia, manifested as chest pain (i.e., angina pectoris) (Tierney, McPhee, & Papadakis, 1994):

   a. Stable angina (precordial chest pain)

      1) Precipitated by hypertension, tachycardia, other dysrhythmia, strenuous activity, cold temperature, emotional stress, or a large meal.

      2) Has a short duration that subsides completely when the aggravating factor is removed (e.g., rest after exertion). If attack is precipitated by anger or a large meal, it may last as long as 20 minutes.

      3) Involves substernal sensation (chest pain), often characterized as aching, sharp, tingling, burning, or pressure radiating to the left arm and shoulder, neck, jaw, or scapular inner aspects of both arms.

   b. Unstable angina

      1) Occurs with minimal activity or at rest

      2) Involves chest pain lasting longer than 30 minutes

      3) Is less responsive to medications and may progress to infarction

      4) Involves sensations similar to stable angina but may be more severe

   c. Variant (Prinzmetal's) angina

      1) Characteristically occurs in early morning and awakens patient

      2) Involves chest pain that intensifies quickly and lasts longer than stable angina

      3) Involves sensations similar to stable angina

3. MI: death of myocardial tissue from inadequate coronary perfusion; blood supply to heart is severely reduced or stopped (AHA, 2007f; Tierney et al., 1994):

   a. May occur at rest or with exertion

   b. May last longer than 30 minutes, is continuous, and is unrelieved by rest, position change, or nitroglycerin tablets

   c. Involves chest pain characterized as crushing, squeezing, stabbing, or heavy pressure that radiates down the left arm and to neck, jaws, teeth, epigastric area, and back

   d. Is associated with other symptoms (e.g., diaphoresis, weakness, apprehension, lightheadedness, syncope, dyspnea, orthopnea, nausea, vomiting)

4. Embolus formation from diminished blood flow:

   a. Stroke

   b. Pulmonary embolus

5. Psychosocial effects:

   a. Sense of helplessness

   b. Fear of dying

   c. Anxiety

   d. Apathy

   e. Depression

   f. Social withdrawal

   g. Guilt

6. Poor tissue perfusion:

   a. Renal failure from diminished blood flow

      1) Fluid retention

      2) CHF

      3) Edema (e.g., peripheral, sacral, genitalia, abdominal)

      4) Electrolyte imbalance

   b. Malnutrition

      1) Decreased nutrient absorption

      2) Decreased gastrointestinal motility

      3) Nausea, vomiting, fatigue

   c. Hypoxic encephalopathy from diminished cerebral blood flow

   d. Hypoxemia

F. Management Measures (AHA, 2007p; Krau et al., 2001; SIGN, 2002)

   1. Risk factor modification

      a. Stop smoking.

      b. Control blood pressure.

      c. Control cholesterol:

         1) AHA-recommended cholesterol levels

            a) Lower low-density lipoproteins (LDLs) to <100 mg/dl

            b) Raise high-density lipoproteins (HDLs) to >60 mg/dl

            c) Maintain total cholesterol level of <200 mg/dl

            d) Fasting triglyceride levels <150 mg/dl

         2) Ways to lower elevated cholesterol levels (see Figure 12-3)

            a) Diet

            b) Exercise

            c) Weight control

            d) Medications

            e) Smoking cessation

      d. Control diabetes:

         1) Control weight.

         2) Modify diet.

         3) Administer medication properly.

Figure 12-3. Ways to Lower Cholesterol Levels

Less than 7% of total calories from saturated fat.

No more than 25% of total calories from fat.

Less than 300 mg of cholesterol per day; if low-density lipoprotein (LDL) levels are high, then less than 200 mg daily.

Less than 2,000 mg of sodium daily (1 teaspoon of salt).

14 grams of fiber per 1,000 calories.

25–30 grams of dietary fiber daily.

Limit total calories to achieve and maintain a healthy weight.

Food Options

Poultry, fish, and lean cuts of meat (remove skin from chicken and trim fat).

Fat-free, nonfat, or low-fat milk products.

Salt-free seasonings.

Drain and rinse canned foods to remove some of the sodium.

Eat fresh vegetables and fruit.

For desserts choose fresh fruit, sherbet, gelatin, or angel food cake.

Bake, broil, roast, boil, or microwave foods rather than frying.

Substitute polyunsaturated margarine or oil for a tablespoon of butter; substitute one egg white with unsaturated oil for one egg.

Ask for more healthful substitutes when eating out.

Benefits of Physical Activity

Lowers LDL levels.

Raises high-density lipoprotein (HDL) levels.

Lowers blood pressure.

Lowers triglyceride levels.

Reduces weight.

Improves fitness of the heart and lungs.

Controls diabetes.

Medications

If LDL and triglyceride levels remain high after dietary changes and physical activity, the physician may introduce medications.

Clofibrate (Atromid-S): raises HDL and lowers triglyceride levels.

Gemfibrozil (Lopid): raises HDL levels.

Nicotinic acid (works in liver): lowers triglyceride and LDL and raises HDL levels.

Resins (bile acid binding in intestines): increase the excretion of cholesterol.

Cholestyramine (Questran, Prevalite, Lo-Cholest).

Colestipol (Colestid).

Colesevelam (WelChol).

Statins (interrupt the formation of cholesterol in the blood): lower LDL levels.

Atorvastatin (Lipitor).

Fluvastatin (Lescol).

Lovastatin (Mevacor).

Pravastatin (Pravachol).

Rosuvastatin calcium (Crestor).

Simvastatin (Zocor).

Niacin (nicotinic acid): not regulated by the Food and Drug Administration; may have varying amount of niacin and must not be used as a substitute for prescription niacin.

Smoking Cessation

Smoking lowers HDL.

Source consulted

American Heart Association (AHA). (2007p). *What your cholesterol levels mean.* Retrieved June 23, 2007 from http://www.americanheart.org/presenter. jhtml?identifier=183

e. Perform physical activity (AHA, 2007i, 2007k) (see Figure 12-4):
   1) Consult with physician before beginning an exercise program.
   2) Exercise regularly.
   3) Monitor target heart rate.
   4) Follow walking program.
   5) Take appropriate precautions.
f. Manage stress:
   1) Identify stressors.
   2) Use relaxation techniques.
   3) Educate about disease process and prognosis.
   4) Offer spiritual support.
   5) Identify support groups.
   6) Offer counseling.
   7) Encourage lifestyle changes (SIGN, 2002):
      a) Returning to work
         (1) The decision to return to work should be made with the cardiologist.
         (2) Returning to work depends on the patient's stamina, postoperative complications, and job demands.
      b) Resuming sexual activity (AHA, 2007l)
         (1) Be well rested.
         (2) Wait until at least 30 minutes after a meal.
         (3) Stay relaxed.
         (4) Avoid straining the upper arms and sternum; try new positions.
         (5) Avoid sexual activity in hot, humid, or very cold conditions.
         (6) Cease activity if angina occurs and call cardiologist.

Figure 12-4. Physical Activity Teaching Guide

General Guidelines

Check with physician before beginning an exercise program.

Follow appropriate physical guidelines, which vary according to the type and extent of heart disease.

Gradually increase exercise.

Do warmup exercises.

Pace exercise efforts so as to not tire too quickly; build to target heart rate gradually.

Schedule rest breaks into program.

Follow guidelines for heart rhythm and rate, blood pressure, and body signals.

Drink water before, during, and after unless fluids are limited by type of heart disease.

Choose activities that improve flexibility, build muscle strength and endurance, and involve large muscles of the legs and arms (e.g., brisk walking, hiking, stair climbing, swimming, rowing, bicycling, cross-country skiing, dancing, jogging).

Target Heart Rate

If unable to count heart rate:
Conversation pace is the pace at which one can walk and talk at the same time, indicating adequate pace.

Becoming short of breath quickly indicates working too hard.

If able to count heart rate:
(For the deconditioned patient, a target heart rate may be set by the physical therapist or physician.)

Measure pulse periodically while exercising and staying within 50%–85% of maximum recommended heart rate or target heart rate.

Maximum heart rate is about 220 minus your age.

Gradually build up from 50% in first few weeks of program to 85% after 6 months.

Examples of target and maximum heart rates:
20 years: Target heart rate (50%–85%) = 100–170 beats per minute (bpm), maximum heart rate (100%) = 200 bmp.

50 years: Target heart rate = 85–145 bpm, maximum heart rate = 170 bpm.

70 years: Target heart rate = 75–128 bpm, maximum heart rate = 150 bpm.

Body signals for rest:
Shortness of breath, diaphoresis, fatigue, nausea, dizziness, chest pain.

Sources consulted

American Heart Association (AHA). (2007o). *Top 10 tips for starting a physical activity program.* Retrieved July 17, 2007 from http://www.american-heart.org/print_presenter.jhtml?identifier=528

American Heart Association (AHA). (2007n). *Target heart rates.* Retrieved July 17, 2007 from http://www.americanheart.org/print_presenter.jhtml?identifier=4736

American Heart Association (AHA). (2007j). *Physical activity.* Retrieved July 17, 2007 from http://www.americanheart.org/print_presenter.jhtml?identifier=4563

8) Teach cardiopulmonary resuscitation (CPR).
g. Control weight.
2. Invasive interventions
a. Percutaneous transluminal coronary angioplasty (PTCA) (AHA, 2007m; WebMD, 2006c)
1) PTCA is an invasive nonsurgical therapeutic procedure performed via a catheter introduced into the coronary artery.
2) Patency is restored to the coronary artery by inflating and deflating a balloon at the distal end of the catheter to compress plaques in the arteries.
a) Atherectomy: A rotary device slices or pulverizes plaques in the arterial lumen.
b) Stent placement: After angioplasty, a small metal stent is inserted to maintain patency of the arterial lumen (Saint Joseph's Regional Medical Center, 1996).
3) Laser angioplasty is similar to PTCA except that a laser is used to open the artery.
b. Surgical procedures
1) Open heart:
a) Coronary artery bypass graft (CABG): New passages for blood are created from other vessels of the body attached from the heart vessels to the aorta. CABGs were performed in 1995 at a cost of $44,820 per procedure (AHA, 1996) (see Figure 12-5).
b) Valve replacement
c) Minimally invasive heart surgery, alternative to "open" surgery, to restore circulation to the heart
2) Heart transplantation
3) Pacemaker or automatic implantable cardioverter–defibrillator placement
4) Ablation: laser procedure that focuses on an area of the heart, causing a dysrhythmia;

the area is lysed to stop the cycle.
5) Correction of congenital defects
3. Medications, which can be used alone or in combination (depending on the CVD and the severity of symptoms) (AHA, 2007b; WebMD, 2005)
a. Vasodilators
b. Beta-adrenergic blocking agents
c. Angiotensin-converting enzyme inhibitors
d. Anticoagulation and antiplatelet medications
e. Antiarrhythmics
f. Calcium antagonists
g. Antihyperlipidemic agents
h. Stool softeners
i. Cardiac glycosides
j. Diuretics
k. Nitrates
l. Oxygen
G. Nursing Process
1. Assessment
a. Subjective elements
1) Palpitations, dizziness, lightheadedness, syncope, shortness of breath, fatigue, poor appetite, insomnia, restlessness, anxiety and fear, denial, nausea, jaw pain, indigestion (especially in older adults)
2) Chest discomfort: quality, location, precipitating factors, duration, alleviating factors

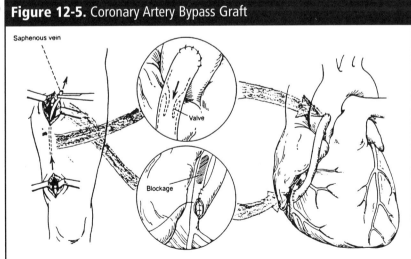

Figure 12-5. Coronary Artery Bypass Graft

Reprinted with permission of Mosby from Huang, S., Kessler, C., McCulloch, C., & Dasher, L. (1989). Cardiac rehabilitation of the myocardial patient. In *Coronary care nursing* (2nd ed., p. 408). Philadephia: W.B. Saunders.

b. Objective elements
   1) Skin: pallor, diaphoresis
   2) Cardiac output: tachycardia, bradycardia, irregular heart rhythm, heart murmur, hypotension, hypertension, confusion, decreased urine output, peripheral edema, sacral or genital edema, weight gain, abdominal distention, electrocardiogram changes, elevated cardiac serum enzymes (creatine kinase myocardial band) and muscle proteins (T[cTNT] and 1[cTN1])
   3) Pulmonary status: crackles; wheezes; dyspnea; labored breathing; frothy, blood-tinged sputum; cyanosis
   4) Nutritional: anorexia, decreased skin turgor and integrity
c. History
   1) Health habits
   2) Medical
   3) Social support
   4) Previous independence level
   5) Medications

2. Diagnoses (North American Nursing Diagnosis Association [NANDA], 1999)
   a. Activity intolerance
   b. Pain
   c. Impaired home maintenance management
   d. Altered nutrition (less than body needs)
   e. Altered thought processes
   f. Altered tissue perfusion (cardiopulmonary)
   g. Anxiety
   h. Fluid volume excess
   i. Knowledge deficit: disease process, medications, self-care, compliance
   j. Impaired gas exchange
   k. Impaired skin integrity
   l. Ineffective individual coping
   m. Ineffective family coping (compromised)
   n. Self-care deficits (e.g., feeding, bathing, grooming, dressing, toileting)
   o. Noncompliance with therapeutic regimen

3. Plan: goals for patient and family
   a. Demonstrate understanding of exercise plan and verbalize understanding of activity intolerance by modifying activity and rest to prevent fatigue, palpitations, shortness of breath, and diaphoresis.
   b. Verbalize pain relief after measures are taken and reduced symptoms of angina, dyspnea, and fatigue.

c. Demonstrate understanding of and participation in self-care management, including activities of daily living (ADLs), exercise programs, dietary management, and lifestyle changes.
d. Maintain adequate nutritional status to lower risks of further cardiac events and promote healing.
e. Maintain adequate urine output, mentation, heart rate, and rhythm.
f. Demonstrate decreased anxiety and verbalize understanding of disease, procedures, and expected outcomes.
g. Identify stressors and develop strategies to decrease stress.
h. Verbalize an understanding of the importance of taking medications as prescribed, actions of medications, how to administer medications, and potential side effects.
i. Maintain skin integrity without breakdown.
j. Verbalize and demonstrate an understanding of the importance of following therapeutic and medical treatment recommendations.
k. Verbalize improved health-related quality of life.
l. Reduce hospitalizations and use of medical resources (AACVPR, 2005).

4. Implementation
   a. Activity intolerance
      1) Monitor activities that aggravate condition: type of activity, intensity, and frequency of symptoms.
      2) Monitor blood pressure, heart rate, and respiratory rate before, during, and after exercise, staying within target heart rate parameters.
      3) Incorporate rest periods into program.
      4) Increase activities gradually.
   b. Cardiac pain management
      1) Administer vasodilators for chest pain as ordered.
      2) Administer oxygen therapy as ordered to increase oxygen to myocardium.
      3) Monitor vital signs.
      4) Assess effectiveness of analgesia.
   c. Nutrition
      1) Consult with dietitian for special dietary instructions and meal planning.
      2) Weigh daily.

3) Offer caloric supplements.
4) Offer measures to improve appetite (e.g., appropriate environment, good oral care, small, frequent meals).
5) Administer antiemetics before meals.
6) Administer medications so they do not interfere with meals.

d. Tissue perfusion
1) Monitor level of consciousness, signs and symptoms of hypoxemia.
2) Monitor laboratory values of blood urea nitrogen, creatinine, electrolytes.
3) Monitor vital signs for changes.
4) Have baseline electrocardiogram available.
5) Document changes in the patient's condition.

e. Anxiety
1) Explain procedures, disease process, and expected outcomes.
2) Allow patient to express feelings.
3) Involve family, significant other, and spiritual counselor.
4) Encourage participation in decision-making process and lifestyle changes.
5) Offer information about support groups, social services, and vocational counseling.

f. Fluid volume excess
1) Administer diuretics as ordered and monitor their effectiveness (e.g., increased urine output, decreased edema, clear lung sounds).
2) Monitor weight daily and report weight gain of 2 lb in 24 hours.
3) Restrict sodium and fluid intake.

g. Knowledge deficit
1) Instruct about disease process and expected outcomes.
2) Instruct about medications: purpose, dosage, how to administer, potential side effects, take only as prescribed (do not use previous medications unless approved by physician), and the importance of follow-up with physician.
3) Practice energy conservation techniques, teaching signs and symptoms of overexertion.
4) Instruct on dietary restrictions and infection prevention.
5) Offer counseling for school, sports, employment, genetics, marriage, childbearing, contraceptive use, resuming sexual relations, and learning CPR.

6) Instruct about oxygen safety.
7) Instruct about proper protection of sternum and grafts if the patient has had open-heart surgery (see Figure 12-6).
8) Instruct on modification of risk factors.
9) Include significant other and family members in all instructions.

h. Gas exchange
1) Monitor chest X-ray.
2) Elevate head of the bed.
3) Monitor breath sounds and respiratory function.
4) Encourage coughing and deep breathing.

i. Self-care
1) Perform ADLs in seated position to conserve energy.
2) Teach proper incisional care for surgical patients.

j. Compliance
1) Assess patient's and family members' readiness to learn and follow therapeutic regimen.
2) Stress importance of administering medications as prescribed, reporting untoward reactions or responses to medications and difficulties in obtaining recommended medications (e.g., expenses, accessibility).
3) Assess understanding and willingness to comply.

5. Evaluation
a. Patient and family should achieve goals set with the nurse.
b. If goals are not met as originally designed, then reassessment should be done and revisions to the plan of care developed.

II. Pulmonary Disease

A. Types
1. Obstructive pulmonary diseases (ALA, 2006a)
a. COPD: persistent airway obstruction that decreases the lung's capacity to take in and excrete oxygen
1) Chronic bronchitis: excessive secretion of bronchial mucus, obstructing air flow and causing chronic coughing and scarring of the bronchial tissue.
2) Emphysema: abnormal alterations of the air spaces distal to the terminal bronchiole; damaged alveoli are less

Figure 12-6. Instructions for Open-Heart Surgical Patients

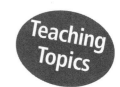

Incision Care

Wash the incisions every day with warm water and antibacterial soap.

Wash hands first and use separate clean washcloths for each incision to prevent cross infections.

Do not use lotions, creams, or oils on the incisions (they can cause infection).

Watch the incisions daily and report any signs of infection (e.g., change in amount or color of drainage, bright red color, increased swelling or tenderness, or edges that pull apart) to the surgeon.

Bathing

Take a shower at home if it has been approved by the occupational therapist.

Have the water stream on the back, not directly on the incisions.

Wait to take tub baths for at least 3 weeks after the operation and then only if the therapist thinks it is safe.

Leg Elevation

Wear antiembolism hose until the follow-up visit with the surgeon.

Put hose on in the morning, take them off at night, and clean them on a daily basis.

Have someone help put them on.

Put legs up on a stool when resting if the ankles and feet begin to swell and at frequent intervals throughout the day.

Incentive Spirometer

Use the incentive spirometer every 2 hours while awake (this helps to prevent pneumonia or other breathing problems).

Check with the surgeon at follow-up visits about continuing use.

Diet

If using a specific diet before surgery, continue it at home; however, adhere to any modifications made by the dietitian or speech therapist.

Be aware that loss of appetite is normal after surgery and that it will gradually return.

Bowel Activity

Prevent constipation by eating fresh fruits, vegetables, and whole-grain foods.

Exercise.

Avoid straining.

Drink adequate amounts of water.

Add prune juice to breakfast.

Call the family physician if no bowel movement for 3 days.

Activity

Follow the home exercise program described by the physical and occupational therapists.

Walk as an excellent form of exercise.

Alternate periods of activity with rest.

Stop and rest if experiencing extreme fatigue, excessive sweating, shortness of breath, light-headedness, nausea, or a pounding heart.

Do not lift more than 10 lb to protect the breastbone and the grafts on the heart while they heal.

Smoking

Please quit smoking: Smoking decreases the oxygen in the blood, damages the arteries and the new bypass grafts, and increases the risk for needing another bypass operation.

Driving

Do not drive until the physiatrist or surgeon recommends it: Conditions requiring patients to come to the rehabilitation unit may put them at risk for injury.

Remember that it is okay to be a passenger.

Continue to use seatbelts; pad the shoulder strap if necessary.

Warning Signs

Call the surgeon if any of the following occur: a temperature of 101° or higher, chills, shortness of breath, abnormal pain, changes in pulse rate, palpitations, a weight gain of 2 lb or more in 1 day, signs of infection at the incision sites, diarrhea for more than 24 hours.

Emotions

Realize that being emotional or having difficulty concentrating or remembering is common after surgery: This should improve each day and disappear as strength is regained (within about 4–6 weeks).

Source consulted

Carbone, L. (1999). An interdisciplinary approach to the rehabilitation of open-heart surgical patients. *Rehabilitation Nursing, 24*(2), 55–61.

able to transfer oxygen to the blood, causing shortness of breath; lung tissue loses flexibility, making it difficult to exhale (ALA, 2006a).

  b. Asthma: inflammation of the trachea and bronchi lining in response to various stimuli, causing narrowing of the airway passages, tightening of the muscles, and increased mucus secretions in the airways (ALA, 2004)

  c. Cystic fibrosis (CF): genetic disorder of the exocrine glands, causing secretion of abnormally thick mucus that obstructs glands and ducts of various organs, most commonly the respiratory, pancreatic, and sweat glands, causing respiratory infections and malabsorption (ALA, 2006b)

  d. Alpha1-antitrypsin (a1AT) deficiency

  e. Bronchiectasis

  f. Bronchiolitis obliterans

2. Restrictive pulmonary diseases (ALA, 2007)

  a. Interstitial lung disease (ILD)

    1) Description: Damaged lung tissue causes the walls of the air sacs to become inflamed. The inflammation leads to scarring or fibrosis (pulmonary fibrosis) of the interstitium, causing the lung to become stiff.

    2) Examples: interstitial pulmonary fibrosis, occupational lung disease, sarcoidosis.

  b. Neuromuscular and neurologic conditions: Parkinson's disease, postpolio syndrome, amyotrophic lateral sclerosis (ALS), multiple sclerosis (MS), Guillain–Barré syndrome, myasthenia gravis, Duchenne's muscular dystrophy, spinal cord injury, diaphragm dysfunction

  c. Chest wall diseases: kyphoscoliosis, spondylitis

3. Other conditions

  a. Lung cancer

  b. Lung transplantation

  c. Morbid obesity

  d. Primary pulmonary hypertension

  e. Thoracic surgery

  f. Sleep apnea

  g. Ventilator dependency

  h. Volume reduction surgery

B. Epidemiology

1. Obstructive pulmonary diseases

  a. COPD (includes chronic bronchitis and emphysema) (ALA, 2006a)

    1) Fourth leading cause of death in the United States

    2) 122,283 deaths in 2003, with women surpassing men in the United States.

    3) 24 million Americans live with impaired lung function.

    4) In 2004, $37.2 billion in total healthcare costs, with $20.9 billion in direct costs, $7.4 billion in indirect morbidity, and $8.9 billion indirect mortality costs.

    5) 80%–90% of deaths from COPD are caused by smoking.

  b. Asthma (ALA, 2004)

    1) In 2004, 20.5 million Americans had asthma.

    2) After a steady increase in deaths related to asthma, deaths have plateaued or declined.

    3) As of 2004, asthma costs $11.5 billion annually in direct care and $4.6 billion in indirect care, with another $5 billion in prescription drugs (Connors & Hilling, 1998).

    4) 14.5 million lost work days for adults in 2004

  c. CF (ALA, 2006b)

    1) Second most common life-threatening inherited pulmonary disease of children

    2) Incidence is higher in white children than in other races.

    3) More than 10 million Americans are symptomless carriers of the CF gene.

    4) More than 80% are diagnosed by the age of 3.

    5) In 2004, 41% of CF patients were adults.

    6) Although survival rates have improved, the leading cause of death is respiratory failure.

    7) Seen in one of every 2,000 live births.

2. Lung cancer (ALA, 2006c)

  a. Lung cancer is the most common cause of cancer death in men and women.

  b. Incidence is decreasing in men and increasing in women.

  c. Lung cancer is a more common cause of cancer death in some European countries whose legal smoking age is younger than that of the United States.

C. Causes
1. Obstructive pulmonary diseases (ALA, 2006a)
   a. Chronic bronchitis
      1) Smoking
      2) Recurrent infections
      3) Environmental irritants: coal mines, industrial pollutants, grain handlers, metal molders, dust
   b. Emphysema
      1) Smoking
      2) Recurrent infections
      3) Environmental irritants
      4) a1AT is an inherited form of emphysema.
   c. Asthma (ALA, 2004)
      1) Exercise-induced: occurs during exercise and may be related to heat or water loss from bronchioles
      2) Occupational: triggered by agents found in the workplace and occurs within a few weeks to many years after exposure to the irritant
      3) Cardiac: bronchospasm associated with CHF
      4) Medication-induced: may be caused by medications (e.g., beta-blocking agents, aspirin, nonsteroidal anti-inflammatory drugs, histamine, methacholine, acetylcysteine, nebulized medications)
      5) Environmental irritants: cigarette smoke, air pollution, sudden change in temperature, animal dander
      6) Genetic: CF (ALA, 2006b)
2. Restrictive pulmonary diseases (ALA, 2007)
   a. ILD: inflammation
      1) Occupational and environmental irritants
      2) Sarcoidosis
      3) Drugs
      4) Radiation
      5) Connective tissue or collagen diseases
         a) Rheumatoid arthritis
         b) Systemic sclerosis
      6) Genetics
   b. Neuromuscular and neurologic disease: amyotrophic lateral sclerosis, diaphragm dysfunction, multiple sclerosis, Parkinson's disease, postpolio syndrome
3. Other conditions
   a. Lung cancer (ALA, 2006c)
      1) Smoking and second-hand smoke
      2) Exposure to radon

3) Exposure to occupational carcinogens such as asbestos, uranium, arsenic, and some petroleum products
   b. Lung transplantation related to ILD, emphysema, a1AT, CF

D. Pathophysiology
1. Obstructive pulmonary diseases
   a. COPD
      1) Chronic bronchitis
         a) Hypertrophy and hypersecretion of goblet and mucous gland cells in bronchioles extending into terminal bronchioles.
         b) Increased secretions cause bronchial congestion and narrowing of the bronchioles and small bronchi.
         c) Lower respiratory tract becomes colonized by bacteria and stimulates secretions by leukocytes.
         d) Leukocytes cause swelling and tissue destruction of the bronchial walls so that they become granulated and fibrotic, leading to stenosis and obstruction that impair the exchange of oxygen to and from the lungs.
            (1) Acute: not associated with fever
            (2) Chronic: mucus-producing cough most days of the month for 3 months out of a year for 2 successive years without underlying disease
            (3) May precede or accompany emphysema (ALA, 2006a)
      2) Emphysema (ALA, 2006a)
         a) Recurrent infections, history of smoking, and exposure to environmental irritants cause deficiency in the protease inhibitor a1AT.
         b) Elastase, a neutral protease, which is produced by leukocytes and alveolar macrophages, proliferates and destroys lung elastin as it becomes uninhibited because of the deficiency of a1AT.
         c) Alveoli are destroyed, creating permanent holes in the lower lung tissues.
         d) Oxygen–carbon dioxide transfer in the blood is inhibited.

e) Lungs lose their elasticity and bronchial tubes collapse, trapping air in the lungs.

   3) Asthma (WebMD, 2006a)

     a) Irritants stimulate bronchoconstriction of the smooth muscles that line the bronchial tubes, causing fluid to leak from blood vessels and stimulating inflammation.

     b) The inflammation narrows the airways and mucus becomes so thick that the cilia are unable to remove it from the airways effectively.

     c) This impairs oxygen delivery to the blood and lungs, trapping carbon monoxide.

  b. CF (ALA, 2004)

    1) Genetic disorder of the exocrine glands

    2) Dysfunctional exocrine gland production of abnormal secretions of mucus

    3) Involves thick mucoproteins that coagulate in glands and ducts, causing obstruction in multiple organs, especially the lungs and digestive tract

2. Restrictive pulmonary disease: ILD (ALA, 2007)

  a. There are a variety of chronic lung disorders—some with known causes and some with unknown causes (idiopathic)—whose progress and symptoms vary from one person to another.

  b. All ILDs begin with inflammation. Areas of inflammation heal and may lead to permanent scarring of the lung tissue, causing pulmonary fibrosis. The fibrosis causes permanent loss of the tissue's ability to transport oxygen.

    1) Bronchiolitis: inflammation of the bronchioles

    2) Alveolitis: inflammation of the alveoli

    3) Vasculitis: inflammation of the capillaries of the lungs

3. Lung cancer ((ALA, 2006c; National Cancer Institute [NCI], 2002a)

  a. Develops when the genes responsible for sequential cell division, proto-oncogenes, change to oncogenes

    1) This causes cells to divide indiscriminately.

    2) Division and proliferation occur

without regard to the needs of the body.

    3) These undifferentiated cells do not function normally and impede the functions of healthy cells.

  b. Types of lung cancer (NCI, 1998; Wilson & Thompson, 1990)

    1) Non–small cell

     a) Adenocarcinoma

      (1) Occurs in 40% of cases

      (2) Begins along periphery of lungs and under the lining of bronchi

      (3) Affects peripheral lung tissue or areas scarred by pulmonary infarct, infection, or fibrosis

      (4) Affects more women and nonsmokers

     b) Squamous cell carcinoma

      (1) Occurs 30% of cases

      (2) Begins in bronchi

      (3) Occludes airways and causes lungs to collapse

      (4) Spreads to intrathoracic sites

     c) Large cell carcinoma

    2) Small cell or oat cell carcinoma

     a) Occurs in 20% of cases

     b) Spreads quickly to nodes, intrathoracic structures, and other organs

E. Residual Effects

1. Obstructive pulmonary diseases

  a. COPD: chronic bronchitis and emphysema (ALA, 2006a)

    1) Factors that worsen the condition

     a) Acute bronchitis

     b) Pneumonia

     c) Pulmonary embolus

     d) Left ventricular failure

     e) Smoking

    2) Common complications

     a) Pulmonary hypertension

     b) Cor pulmonale

     c) Chronic respiratory failure

    3) Symptoms

     a) Shortness of breath

     b) Cough

     c) Sputum production

     d) Weight loss (with emphysema)

     e) Obesity (with chronic bronchitis) (Tierney et al., 1994)

    4) Decreased quality of life

    5) Shortness of breath necessitating supplemental oxygen

    6) Limited ability to work, participate

in social and family activities, sleep restfully

b. Asthma (WebMD, 2006a)
   1) Wheezing
   2) Bronchitis
   3) Coughing
   4) Chest tightness
   5) Respiratory failure
   6) Shortness of breath
   7) Trouble sleeping
   8) Pneumonia
   9) Respiratory infections

c. CF
   1) Systemic effects
      a) Reproductive tract: causes sterility by obstructing the vas deferens in men and producing thick cervical secretions in women, blocking sperm from entering the uterus
      b) Pancreatic duct obstruction: inability of pancreatic enzymes to be released, causing malabsorption, nutritional deficiencies, diabetes mellitus
      c) Bile duct obstruction: causes portal hypertension and liver failure
      d) Blocked sweat glands: decrease absorption of sodium and chloride, leading to dehydration, salty-tasting skin (ALA, 2006c)
      e) Bronchial obstruction: causes infections, respiratory disease, cor pulmonale, coughing, wheezing, and shortness of breath
   2) Intestinal obstruction and gastrointestinal malabsorption (excessive appetite with poor weight gain and greasy, bulky stools)
   3) Esophageal varices
   4) Pulmonary hypertension
   5) Cor pulmonale
   6) Lung abscess
   7) Pulmonary insufficiency
   8) Atelectasis
   9) Pneumonia

2. Restrictive pulmonary disease: ILD, respiratory distress

3. Lung cancer (ALA, 2006c)
   a. Chronic cough
   b. Hemoptysis
   c. Wheezing
   d. Chest pain

e. Hoarseness
f. Weight loss and loss of appetite
g. Fever of unknown cause
h. Shortness of breath
i. Repeated bronchitis or pneumonia
j. Residual effects of treatments (NCI, 2002b)
   1) Surgical treatment: weakened arm and chest muscles; fluid may build up in space left after resection.
   2) Radiation therapy: loss of appetite related to nausea, vomiting, loss of taste, oral and throat sores affecting swallow, weight loss, pulmonary fibrosis, and dry, itching, tender skin.
   3) Chemotherapy: immunosuppression, decreased clotting time, fatigue, alopecia, nausea, vomiting, and oral sores affecting appetite.

F. Management Measures
   1. For all respiratory diseases
      a. Maximize breathing.
      b. Maintain or improve functional status.
      c. Enhance coping skills, identify stressors, and modify behavior.
      d. Maintain or improve nutritional status.
      e. Educate about disease process and prognosis.
      f. Use mechanical ventilation as needed.
      g. Identify irritants.
   2. For specific diseases
      a. Obstructive pulmonary disease
         1) COPD (ALA, 2006a)
            a) Goal: to stop the progression of the disease; maximize breathing; reduce airway secretions, inflammation, and bronchospasm; and prevent complications.
            b) Identify and manage precipitating factors.
            c) Encourage smoking cessation.
            d) Encourage prevention and early treatment of airway infections and vaccinations against influenza and pneumococcal disease (Tierney et al., 1994).
            e) Encourage use of chest physiotherapy techniques (see Figure 12-7).
            f) Provide medications:
               (1) Bronchodilators
               (2) Antibiotics
               (3) Systemic glucocorticosteroids

g) Use supplemental oxygen.

h) Pulmonary rehabilitation for stable patients

i) Lung transplantation

j) Lung volume reduction for some with emphysema

2) Asthma (ALA, 2004; WebMD, 2006a)

a) Include interventions as above, except chest physiotherapy

b) Control environmental and emotional triggers

c) Medications

(1) Bronchodilators

(2) Anticholinergics

(3) Theophylline

(4) Corticosteroids

(5) Antimediators: cromolyn sodium

(6) Use of peak flow meter

(a) Inexpensive handheld device that measures air flow from the lungs

(b) Benefits: asthma management, medication adjustment, indication of worsening or improvement of symptoms, reassurance

3) CF (ALA, 2006b)

a) Goal: Early diagnosis and comprehensive interdisciplinary therapy are important in lengthening survival time and alleviating symptoms.

b) Psychological, genetic, and occupational counseling

c) Chest physiotherapy

d) Medications:

(1) Treat infections based on results of culture and sensitivity testing.

(2) Expectorants

(3) Bronchodilators

(4) Anti-inflammatories

(5) Agents that help digest carbohydrates, fats, and proteins (e.g., pancreatin with meals or snacks, pancrelipase before or with meals or snacks)

(6) Immunizations against influenza and pneumonia.

e) Oxygen therapy

f) Surgical procedures:

(1) Pulmonary lavage or bronchial washing

(2) Resection of blebs and pleural scars

(3) Lung transplantation

b. Restrictive pulmonary disease (ALA, 2007)

1) Goal: prevent inflammation and relieve symptoms

2) Medications

a) Corticosteroids or combination therapy of drugs with corticosteroids

b) Immunizations against influenza and pneumonia

3) Oxygen therapy

c. Lung cancer (ALA, 2006c)

1) Surgery: lobectomy, pneumonectomy, segmental resection

2) Radiation therapy

3) Chemotherapy

4) Strengthening program

5) Weight loss management

6) Infection prevention

G. Nursing Process (AARC, 2002)

Figure 12-7. Patient Teaching for Home Management of Chest Physiotherapy

General Information

Chest physiotherapy (e.g., postural drainage, chest percussion, coughing) may be recommended by the physician for patients with chronic bronchitis, emphysema, or cystic fibrosis to help loosen and remove mucus from the lungs.

Techniques may be done in the morning, before bedtime, or when secretions are more than usual, as recommended by the physician. Oral fluids will help to thin the mucus.

Postural Drainage

Lie on bed with chest over side, resting head on a pillow on the floor.

For 10–20 minutes each, lie on stomach, left side, then right side.

Chest Percussion (requires a second person)

While the patient is in the postural drainage position, the second person cups his or her hands and rhythmically pats the patient's back, alternating hands for 3–4 minutes.

Cough

While in the postural drainage position, take slow deep breath through the nose

Open the mouth and, while breathing out, cough three times to help bring up the mucus.

Repeat several times.

Cough mucus out of the mouth because swallowing may cause nausea.

Contraindications

Cyanosis or dyspnea caused by technique, increased pain or discomfort, prolonged bleeding or clotting times, extreme obesity, predisposition to pathological fractures.

Sources consulted

Loeb, S. (Ed.). (1992). *Teaching patients with chronic conditions*. Bethlehem Pike, PA: Springhouse Corp.

Wilson, S.F., & Thompson, J.M. (1990). *Respiratory disorders*. St. Louis: Mosby.

Teaching Topics

---

1. Assessment
   a. Medical and family history
      1) Use of supplemental oxygen, medical devices, and knowledge of appropriate usage
      2) Medications: allergies and drug intolerance
      3) Triggers in work and home environments
      4) Lifestyle
         a) Smoking history
         b) Work and home activities
      5) Recent illnesses: complete blood cell count to monitor white blood cells for signs of infection and hematocrit to follow anemia, bleeding, cirrhosis, and dehydration
      6) Self-care skills
      7) Knowledge and use of medications
      8) Test results: pulmonary function, blood tests, electrocardiogram, chest radiography
   b. Physical (AARC, 2002)
      1) Exercise
         a) Physical limitations (e.g., strength, functional ability, orthopedic limitations)
         b) Exercise tolerance, need for supplemental oxygen, cardiac function
      2) Neurological: cognition changes, lethargy, restlessness
      3) Pulmonary: dyspnea, tachypnea, wheezes, crackles, rhonchi, decreased breath sounds, cough, hoarseness, clubbed fingers, chest retractions, barrel chest, decreased chest wall movement, productive thick sputum that may be odorous, hemoptysis, postnasal drainage
      4) Cardiovascular: tachycardia, dysrhythmia, fatigue, chest pain, edema
      5) Gastrointestinal
         a) General: weight loss or gain, appetite, oral sores, constipation, dehydration, reflux
         b) Special gastrointestinal considerations for CF patients: bulky, foul-smelling, pale, or watery stool; intestinal obstruction, fecal impaction, and tarry stools if bleeding; jaundice; ascites; abnormal liver function; laboratory results
      6) Skin: decreased skin turgor with dehydration, diaphoresis
   c. Nutritional: weight loss, lack of appetite, loss of taste, swallowing difficulties, constipation, hydration, serum albumin
   d. Psychosocial
      1) Support systems
      2) Individual and family coping
      3) Psychosocial: fear of suffocation, sleep disturbance, depression, anxiety
      4) Willingness to participate in program, health-changing behavior
      5) Symptoms of depression
   e. Knowledge of disease process, description and interpretation of medical tests
2. Diagnoses (NANDA, 1999)
   a. Ineffective breathing pattern
   b. Ineffective airway clearance
   c. Impaired gas exchange
   d. Activity intolerance
   e. Altered nutrition (less than body needs)
   f. Risk for constipation
   g. Risk for infection
   h. Sleep pattern disturbance
   i. Risk for spiritual distress
   j. Ineffective individual coping
   k. Ineffective family coping (compromised)
   l. Anxiety
   m. Sexual dysfunction
   n. Self-care deficits (e.g., feeding, bathing, grooming, dressing, toileting)
   o. Impaired home maintenance management
   p. Knowledge deficit
   q. Ineffective management of therapeutic regimen (individual or family)
3. Plan (AARC, 2002; Bernier & Leonard, 2001)
   a. Goals for the patient
      1) Demonstrate effective breathing patterns without fatigue and energy conservation measures.
      2) Demonstrate improved airway clearance through use of postural drainage when appropriate, coughing, deep breathing, and taking medications as directed.
      3) Demonstrate resolution of cognitive changes if they have not become permanent; resolve cyanosis.
      4) Demonstrate ability to do ADLs using compensation measures when necessary to prevent dyspnea or fatigue; for children, demonstrate

ability to participate in normal activities using preactivity medications.

5) Demonstrate stable weight for age and size, take adequate caloric intake daily, and have a normal albumin level.

6) Have regular bowel movements without constipation or dehydration and take in adequate amounts of fluid daily.

7) Remain free of infection and prevent influenza and pneumonia.

8) Demonstrate adequate sleep patterns for rest and rejuvenation.

9) Verbalize decreased spiritual distress, increasing sense of integrity while living with chronic disease.

10) Demonstrate and verbalize reduction of disability and use of medical resources (Bernier & Leonard, 2001).

b. Goals for the family

1) Demonstrate support for the person with the disability and verbalize resources available for family support.

2) Acknowledge fear and anxiety and demonstrate ways to decrease anxiety (e.g., hobbies, social activities, relaxation techniques).

3) Verbalize understanding of compensation measures while engaging in sexual activity.

4) Verbalize knowledge of disease process, precipitating factors of respiratory difficulties and how to avoid or minimize effects, how to administer medication and oxygen therapy properly, and when to call the physician.

5) Verbalize and demonstrate understanding of the therapeutic regimen and the importance of self-monitoring and compliance with therapeutic recommendations.

4. Interventions (AARC, 2002)

a. Observe respiration depth and rate, dyspnea, nasal flaring.

b. Inspect thorax or symmetry of respiratory movement, chest muscle retractions, changes in skin color and capillary refill, changes in mentation or behavior.

c. Auscultate lungs for adventitious sounds.

d. Administer oxygen, bronchodilators,

Figure 12-8. Breathing Tips and Exercises

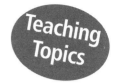
Teaching Topics

Things to Avoid to Help Make Breathing Easier

Heavy traffic and smog.

Aerosol spray.

Products that produce fumes.

Cold weather.

Very dry air.

Exercise.

Pursed-Lip Breathing

Can be done anywhere.

Helps get rid of air trapped in the lungs.

Slows breathing to make it more efficient.

Must be practiced so that when an episode of shortness of breath occurs, the exercise is familiar.

Technique

Breathe in slowly through the nose, holding for 3 seconds.

Purse the lips as if whistling.

Breathe out slowly through the pursed lips for 6 seconds.

Abdominal Breathing

Must be done lying down.

Slows breathing to become more efficient.

Helps relax the body.

Technique

Lie on back in a comfortable position with a pillow under the head.

Place one hand on abdomen below the ribs and the other on the chest.

Slowly breathe in and out through the nose, using abdominal muscles.

Watch the hand on the abdomen, which should rise and fall with breathing, and the hand on the chest, which should remain still.

Sources consulted

Connors, G., & Hilling, L. (Eds.). (1998). *Guidelines for pulmonary rehabilitation programs: American Association of Cardiovascular and Pulmonary Rehabilitation—Promoting health and preventing disease* (2nd ed.). Champaign, IL: Human Kinetics.

Wilson, S.F., & Thompson, J.M. (1990). *Respiratory disorders*. St. Louis: Mosby.

antibiotics, corticosteroids, and other medications as directed.

e. Teach breathing techniques and exercises to conserve energy (see Figure 12-8).

f. Identify ways to conserve energy in daily activities.

g. Adapt ways to increase endurance and conserve energy.

h. Slowly increase activity as tolerance allows, promoting as much independence as possible.

i. Encourage adherence to a regular exercise program with planned rest periods between activities. Teach patients receiving intermittent, continuous, or nocturnal ventilator support to do the following:

1) Strengthen skeletal muscles that have atrophied from critical illness, suboptimal nutritional support, or corticosteroid use.

2) Strengthen skeletal muscles by beginning exercises during periods while the patient is receiving ventilator support, adjusting ventilator settings as needed, and including strengthening techniques (e.g., free weights, gravity, manual resistance, elastic bands).

3) Improve nutritional support through supplements, considering the possibility of using a feeding tube to increase muscle strength and endurance. Patients with a tracheotomy have limited speech and are at risk of aspiration.

   a) Assist with speech through the use of cuffless or fenestrated tracheotomy tubes or Passy–Muir valves.

   b) Prevent aspiration by teaching compensatory swallowing techniques.

j. Provide uninterrupted periods of rest.

k. Identify sources of irritants (ALA, 2002):

   1) Triggers

      a) Air particles (indoor and outdoor)

      b) Cold air or sudden temperature change

      c) Tobacco or smoke from burning wood or leaves

      d) Perfume, paint, hairspray

      e) Strong odors or fumes

      f) Allergens (e.g., dust mites, pollen, pollution, animal dander)

      g) Common cold, flu, or respiratory illness

      h) Vigorous exercise

      i) Stress or excitement

      j) Certain foods

   2) Control measures (ALA, 2002)

      a) Do a skin test to identify allergens.

      b) Keep an asthma diary to list triggers.

      c) Use pillow and mattress covers.

      d) Remove carpets.

      e) Use air-filtering devices or air conditioning.

      f) Wash pets (especially dogs) weekly.

      g) Ensure early detection of respiratory infections.

      h) Manage nasal disorders.

      i) Stop smoking.

l. Monitor pollution index and adjust outdoor activities accordingly.

m. Avoid exposure to colds and flu and encourage vaccinations against influenza and pneumonia.

n. Promote caloric intake to support adequate growth.

o. Provide frequent small meals to lessen fatigue.

p. Provide appropriate food consistency to enhance energy conservation during meals.

q. Offer antiemetics before meals to reduce nausea.

r. Maintain good oral care.

s. Monitor for swallowing difficulties and risk for aspiration.

t. Monitor for nutritional risk:

   1) Weight loss (weigh daily), dehydration (keep records of intake and output and skin turgor)

   2) Appetite (count calories)

   3) Loss of taste, oral sores, nausea, or vomiting

   4) Monitor albumin levels and offer protein supplements as needed for healing and weight maintenance.

   5) Administer vitamins and pancreatic enzymes for patients with CF as ordered.

u. Monitor stools:

   1) Be alert for constipation:

      a) Encourage fluids, fiber, stool softeners, or laxatives.

      b) Encourage ambulation.

   2) Note color, amount, consistency, consistency, frequency, and presence of blood.

v. Teach about medications:

   1) Explain usage and symptoms of effectiveness, ineffectiveness, and toxicity.

   2) Monitor theophylline levels.

   3) Maintain inhalation equipment.

   4) Teach about safe oxygen use in the home (ALA, 2005).

      a) Explain that oxygen is very combustible.

         (1) Keep away from open flames and heat.

         (2) Stay away from smokers.

         (3) Stay out of rooms with a running gas stove or gas or kerosene space heater.

      b) Prevent leakage:

(1) Keep tank upright.

(2) Turn off system when not in use.

(3) Do not place anything over the tubing.

(4) Keep an all-purpose fire extinguisher available.

(5) In case of fire, turn off the oxygen and leave the home.

(6) Notify the fire department that there is oxygen in the home. Many fire departments offer free safety inspections.

c) Watch for symptoms of not enough or too much oxygen:

(1) Difficult, irregular, or slow breathing

(2) Restlessness or anxiousness

(3) Tiredness or drowsiness

(4) Difficulty waking up

(5) Persistent headache

(6) Confusion, difficulty concentrating, or slurred speech

(7) Cyanotic fingertips or lips

d) Teach the patient to notify the physician if any of these symptoms occur. Never change the flow rate without guidance from the physician.

w. Teach about diagnostic tests, disease process, prognosis, and therapies.

x. Assist the patient and family with coping and stress reduction:

1) Develop trust with patient and family, encourage family members to express feelings, assist in problem solving, identify support systems, offer support network as needed.

2) Promote normal growth and development.

3) Discuss financial concerns and make appropriate referrals.

4) Encourage personal control.

5) Maintain privacy.

6) Teach relaxation and stress reduction techniques.

y. Consult with chaplain or the patient's spiritual guide to offer spiritual support.

z. Offer education on sexual and other physical activity (ALA, 1999; Tierney et al., 1994):

1) Determine knowledge of effects of illness and treatment on sexual functioning.

2) Provide an atmosphere to discuss sexual concerns.

3) Perform airway clearance therapies 1 hour before sexual activity.

4) Help the patient plan sexual activity at optimal times.

5) Avoid sexual activity after meals.

6) Encourage alternative positions that are less stressful.

7) Encourage frequent rest during sexual activity to minimize pulmonary compromise while increasing partner satisfaction by prolonged stimulation.

aa. Stress the importance of adhering to the medical and therapeutic regimen. Ensure that the patient and family understand and follow through with the treatment plan.

5. Evaluation

a. Remember that patient follow-up is very important.

b. Evaluate the patient's understanding of instructions and how the interventions are affecting them, positively or negatively.

c. Revise goals and interventions with the patient and the physician as needed.

References

Adams, J., Nuss, T., Banks, C., Hartman, J., Segrest, W., Spears, J., et al. (2007). Risk factor outcome comparison between exercise-based cardiac rehabilitation, traditional care, and an educational workshop. *Journal of Continuing Education in Nursing, 28*(2), 83–88.

Ades, P.A. (2001). Cardiac rehabilitation and secondary prevention of coronary heart disease. *New England Journal of Medicine, 354*(12), 892–902.

Aldana, S., Whitmer, W., Freenlaw, R., Avins, A., Salberg, A., Barnjurst, M., et al. (2003, November–December). Cardiovascular risk reductions associated with aggressive lifestyle modification and cardiac rehabilitation. *Heart and Lung*, pp. 374–382.

American Association of Cardiovascular and Pulmonary Rehabilitation (AACVPR). (2005). *Fast facts: Referral/ resource pages.* Retrieved May 25, 2007 from http://www.aacvpr.org/dmtf/cardiacspecific.cfm.

American Association for Respiratory Care (AARC). (2002). AARC clinical practice guideline: Pulmonary rehabilitation. *Respiratory Care, 47*(5), 617–625.

American Heart Association (AHA). (1996). *Coronary artery calcification: Pathophysiology and epidemiology.* Retrieved May 25, 2007 from http://www.americanheart.org/presenter.jhtml?identifier=1684.

American Heart Association (AHA). (2007a). *Adults with congenital heart disease.* Retrieved May 25, 2007 from http://www.americanheart.org/presenter.jhtml?identifier=11062.

American Heart Association (AHA). (2007b). *Cardiac medications at a glance.* Retrieved May 25, 2007 from http://www.americanheart.org/presenter.jhtml?identifier=3038846

American Heart Association (AHA). (2007c). *Cardiomyopathy.* Retrieved May 25, 2007 from http://www.americanheart.org/presenter.jhtml?identifier=4468

American Heart Association (AHA). (2007d). *Causes of heart failure.* Retrieved May 25, 2007 from http://americanheart. org/presenter.jhtml?identifier=324.

American Heart Association (AHA). (2007e). *Congenital heart defects in children.* Retrieved May 25, 2007 from http://www. americanheart.org/presenter.jhtml?identifier=12012.

American Heart Association (AHA). (2007f). *Heart attack.* Retrieved May 25, 2007 from http://americanheart.org/ presenter.jhtml?identifier=120000.

American Heart Association (AHA). (2007g). *Heart disease and stroke statistics: 2007 update.* Retrieved May 25, 2007 from http://circ.ahajournals.org/cgi/content/full/CIRCULATIONAH A.106.179918#SEC13.

American Heart Association (AHA). (2007h). *Heart failure.* Retrieved May 25, 2007 from http://americanheart.org/ presenter.jhtml?identifier=1486.

American Heart Association (AHA). (2007i). *Lifestyle and exercise.* Retrieved May 25, 2007 from http://americanheart. org/presenter.jhtml?identifier=1543.

American Heart Association (AHA). (2007j). *Physical activity.* Retrieved May 25, 2007 from http://www.americanheart.org/ print_presenter.jhtml?identifier=4563.

American Heart Association (AHA). (2007k). *Physical activity and a healthy heart.* Retrieved May 25, 2007 from http:// americanheart.org/presenter.jhtml?identifier=1518.

American Heart Association (AHA). (2007l). *Sex and heart failure.* Retrieved May 25, 2007 from http://americanheart. org/presenter.jhtml?identifier=359.

American Heart Association (AHA). (2007m). *Surgery and other treatments.* Retrieved May 25, 2007 from http://www. americanheart.org/presenter.jhtml?identifier=501#cardiac_ procedures.

American Heart Association (AHA). (2007n). *Target heart rates.* Retrieved May 25, 2007 from http://www.americanheart.org/ print_presenter.jhtml?identifier=4736.

American Heart Association (AHA). (2007o). *Top 10 tips for starting a physical activity program.* Retrieved May 25, 2007 from http://www.americanheart.org/print_presenter. jhtml?identifier=528.

American Heart Association (AHA). (2007p). *What your cholesterol levels mean.* Retrieved June 23, 2007 from http:// www.americanheart.org/presenter.jhtml?identifier=183.

American Lung Association. (ALA). (1999). *Exercise and keep active.* Retrieved June 23, 2007 from http://www.lungusa.org/ site/apps/s/content.asp?c=dvLUK9O0E&b=34706&ct=67330.

American Lung Association. (ALA). (2002). *Home control of asthma & allergies.* Retrieved June 23, 2007 from http://www. lungusa.org/site/pp.asp?c=dvLUK9O0E&b=22591.

American Lung Association. (ALA). (2004). *Asthma in adults fact sheet.* Retrieved June 23, 2007 from http://www. lungusa.org/site/apps/nl/content3.asp?c=dvLUK9O0E& b=2058817&content_id={39966A20-AE3C-4F85-B285- 68E23EDC6CA8}&notoc=1.

American Lung Association. (ALA). (2005). *Tips on oxygen use.* Retrieved June 23, 2007 from http://www.lungusa.org/site/ apps/s/content.asp?c=dvLUK9O0E&b=34706&ct=1471537.

American Lung Association. (ALA). (2006a). *Chronic obstructive pulmonary disease (COPD) fact sheet.* Retrieved June 23, 2007 from http://www.lungusa.org/site/apps/nl/content3. asp?c=dvLUK9O0E&b=2058819&content_id={EE451F66- 996B-4C23-874D-BF66586196FF}&notoc=1.

American Lung Association. (ALA). (2006b). *Cystic fibrosis (CF) fact sheet.* Retrieved June 23, 2007 from http://www. lungusa.org/site/apps/nl/content3.asp?c=dvLUK9O0E&b =2058829&content_id={2C5B0EF6-D044-4306-AF93- 416DE1C89DE8}&notoc=1.

American Lung Association. (ALA). (2006c). *Facts about lung cancer.* Retrieved June 23, 2007 from http://www. lungusa.org/site/apps/nl/content3.asp?c=dvLUK9O0E&b =2058829&content_id={62C3D98B-887D-4C19-B7AA- C558C240D450}&notoc=1.

American Lung Association. (ALA). (2007). *Interstitial lung disease and pulmonary fibrosis.* Retrieved June 23, 2007 from http://www.lungusa.org/site/apps/nl/content3.asp?c=dvLU K9O0E&b=2060321&content_id={4350F20F-98E4-403B- A33B-68B20A3C2FBA}&notoc=1.

Bernier, M.J., & Leonard, B. (2001). Pulmonary rehabilitation after acute COPD exacerbation. *Critical Care Nursing Clinics of North America, 13*(3), 375–387.

Carbone, L. (1999). An interdisciplinary approach to the rehabilitation of open-heart surgical patients. *Rehabilitation Nursing, 24*(2), 55–61.

Centers for Disease Control (CDC). (2007). *Metabolic equivalent (MET) level.* Retrieved June 23, 2007 from http://www.cdc. gov/nccdphp/dnpa/physical/measuring/met.htm.

Connors, G., & Hilling, L. (Eds.). (1998). *Guidelines for pulmonary rehabilitation programs: American Association of Cardiovascular and Pulmonary Rehabilitation—Promoting health and preventing disease* (2nd ed.). Champaign, IL: Human Kinetics.

Huang, S., Kessler, C., McCulloch, C., & Dasher, L. (1989). Cardiac rehabilitation of the myocardial patient. In *Coronary care nursing* (2nd ed.).Philadelphia: W.B. Saunders.

Krau, S., Ward, K., & Parsons, L. (2001). Living the healthy heart path: Rehabilitation after a cardiac event. *Critical Care Nursing Clinics of North America, 13*(3), 389–397.

Loeb, S. (Ed.). (1992). *Teaching patients with chronic conditions.* Bethlehem Pike, PA: Springhouse Corp.

National Cancer Institute (NCI). (1998). *General information about lung cancer.* Retrieved June 23, 2007 from http://www. healthtouch.com/level1/leaflets/nci/nci062.htm.

National Cancer Institute. (2002a). *Understanding lung cancer.* Retrieved June 23, 2007 from http://www.cancer.gov/ cancertopics/wyntk/lung/page4.

National Cancer Institute. (2002b). *Side effects.* Retrieved from http://www.cancer.gov/cancertopics/wyntk/lung/page12.

Ninot, G., Fortes, M., Poulain, M., Brun, A., Desplan, J., Prefaut, C., et al. (2006). Gender difference in coping strategies among patients enrolled in an inpatient rehabilitation program. *Heart and Lung, 35*(2), 130–136.

North American Nursing Diagnosis Association (NANDA). (1999). *Nursing diagnoses: Definitions and classification 1999–2000.* Philadelphia: Author.

Saint Joseph's Regional Medical Center. (1996). *The beat goes on: Educational materials for the cardiac patient and family.* South Bend, IN: Author.

Scottish Intercollegiate Guidelines Network (SIGN). (2002). *Cardiac rehabilitation: A national clinical guideline.* Edinburgh, Scotland: SIGN Executive.

Tierney, L.M., McPhee, S.J., & Papadakis, M.A. (Eds.). (1994). *Current medical diagnosis and treatment* (33rd ed.). Norwalk, CT: Appleton & Lange.

WebMD. (2004a). *Dilated cardiomyopathy: Topic overview.* Retrieved June 23, 2007 from http://www.webmd.com/heart-disease/tc/Dilated-Cardiomyopathy-Topic-Overview.

WebMD. (2004b). *Restrictive cardiomyopathy: Topic overview.* Retrieved June 23, 2007 from http://www.webmd.com/heart-disease/Heart-Failure/tc/Restrictive-Cardiomyopathy-Topic-Overview.

WebMD. (2005). *Medications.* Retrieved June 23, 2007 from http://www.webmd.com/heart-disease/Heart-Failure/tc/Heart-Failure-Medications.

WebMD. (2006a). *Asthma in children: Overview.* Retrieved June 23, 2007 from http://www.webmd.com/asthma/tc/Asthma-in-Children-Overview.

WebMD. (2006b). *Coronary artery disease: Overview.* Retrieved June 23, 2007 from http://www.webmd.com/heart-disease/tc/Coronary-Artery-Disease-Overview.

WebMD. (2006c). *Heart disease: Procedures and surgeries.* Retrieved June 23, 2007 from http://www.webmd.com/heart-disease/guide/heart-disease-procedures-surgeries.

WebMD. (2007). *Heart failure: The basics.* Retrieved June 23, 2007 from http://www.webmd.com/heart-disease/Heart-Failure/heart-failure-basics.

Wilson, S.F., & Thompson, J.M. (1990). *Respiratory disorders.* St. Louis: Mosby.

Suggested Resources

Brennan, P.F., Moore, S.M., Bjornsdottir, G., Jones, J., Visovsky, C., & Rogers, M. (2001). Heartcare: An Internet-based information and support system for patient home recovery after coronary artery bypass graft (CABG) surgery. *Journal of Advanced Nursing, 35*(5), 699–708.

Clark, A.M., Whelan, H.K., Barbour, R., & MacIntyre, P.D. (2005). A realist study of the mechanisms of cardiac rehabilitation. *Journal of Advanced Nursing, 52*(4), 362–371.

Covey, M.K., & Larson, J.L. (2004). Exercise and COPD: Aerobic and strengthening exercises are crucial in patients with chronic obstructive pulmonary disease. *American Journal of Nursing, 104*(5), 40–43.

Ford, C.M., Pruitt, R., Parker, V., & Reimels, E. (2004). CHF: Effects of cardiac rehabilitation and brain natriuretic peptide. *The Nurse Practitioner, 29*(3), 36–39.

Franklin, B.A., Swain, D.P., & Shephard, R.J. (2003). New insights in the prescription of exercise for coronary patients. *Journal of Cardiovascular Nursing, 18*(2), 116–123.

Gassner, L., Dunn, S., & Pillar, N. (2003). Aerobic exercise and the post myocardial infarction patient: A review of the literature. *Heart and Lung, 32*(4), 258–264.

MacMillan, J., Davis, L., Durham, C., & Matteson, E. (2006). Exercise and heart rate recovery. *Heart and Lung, 35*(6), 383–390.

Pederson, A., Early, M.B., Fenner, D., Postlewaite, C., & Scott, A. (2001). How to build a cardiac surgery program. *Nursing Management, 32*(10), 46–48, 50.

Phillips, L., Harrison, T., & Houck, P. (2005). Return to work and the person with heart failure. *Heart and Lung, 34*(2), 79–88.

Chapter 13

Understanding Acute and Chronic Pain

Dalice Hertzberg, MSN RN ARNP BC

Pain is a symptom of tissue damage or illness that signals the organism to institute protective steps. When pain occurs, the homeostasis of the body is disrupted, producing stress. In response, the body initiates a complex sequence of events that involves neural, hormonal, and behavioral systems in an attempt to restore homeostasis. The presence and degree of pain are subjective and are not necessarily equal to the amount of tissue damage or physiological dysfunction. The sensation of pain is entwined with emotional and psychological factors and the person's past experience of pain. Although current imaging techniques can indicate brain activity in response to pain, the person's self-report of pain presence, nature, and intensity remains the most reliable method of assessing pain (Bushnell & Apkarian, 2006; Flor & Turk, 2006; Janig & Levine, 2006; Melzack, 1999; U.S. Department of Health and Human Services, 2005).

"The goal of the pain management rehabilitation nurse is to improve the level of functioning and the quality of life for those affected by pain" (Association of Rehabilitation Nurses [ARN], 1994). Effective pain management continues to be a challenge for nurses and healthcare providers in all settings. Rehabilitation nurses must evaluate the patient's pain in its entirety, including the effects on the patient's personal, family, and community roles. By considering the global picture, nurses can achieve the pain management outcomes anticipated by the patient.

I. Overview

A. Definitions

1. Pain is "an unpleasant, sensory and emotional experience associated with actual or potential tissue damage" (The Taxonomy Committee of the International Association for the Study of Pain, 1979, as cited in Bond, 2006, p. 259).

2. Acute pain is the expected response to a noxious stimulus from surgery, injury, or illness. It is characterized as a rapid response to the insult, with a short duration, lasting from less than 1 month to as much as 6 months (Carr & Goudas, 1999).

3. Chronic pain has a number of characteristics that distinguish it from acute pain:
   a. It persists past the healing period.
   b. The underlying disorder is insufficient in proportion to the symptoms.
   c. It no longer protects from harm.
   d. It diminishes health, causes disability, and reduces quality of life (American Pain Society [APS], 2006).

B. Epidemiology

1. Pain management is becoming a higher priority in the United States, as evidenced by health policy makers, health professionals, regulators, and the public becoming more knowledgeable about pain management (American Academy of Pain Medicine [AAPM] & American Pain Society [APS], 1997).

2. One quarter of all adult Americans (about 76.5 million) experience some type of pain lasting at least 24 hours (National Center for Health Statistics, 2006).

3. "Sixty-five million Americans suffer from painful disabilities each year" (Menard, 1999, p. 1).

4. Children are more likely to experience undertreatment of pain than adults, particularly very young children (Alexander & Manno, 2003).

C. Effects of Pain on Family and Society

1. Effects on the family
   a. Chronic pain results in significant role changes within the family.
   b. Rehabilitation nurses involve the family in care (with the patient's permission) whenever possible.
   c. The family's support can reinforce positive outcomes the patient has established (Lubkin & Jeffrey, 1998).

2. Effects on society
   a. Almost half of the U.S. population experiences chronic or recurrent pain at some time (ABC News Health, 2005).
   b. Lost work productivity due to pain complaints has been estimated at more than $61 billion (Stewart, Ricci, Chee,

Morganstein, & Lipton, 2003).

   c. The most common cause of long-term disability is chronic pain (APS, 2006).

D. Cultural Considerations

   1. Increasing immigration, heterogeneity of immigrants coming from the same geographic area, differences in language and dialect, long stays in refugee camps, and the experience of war and genocide combine to increase the cultural differences between patients and caregivers (Lasch, 2000).

   2. Health disparities experienced by members of minority groups extend to pain management, especially in the undertreatment of cancer pain (Bernabeia et al., 1998; Intercultural Cancer Council, 2003).

   3. Culture influences health beliefs, including those about the nature and meaning of pain, expression of pain, and treatment of pain (Lasch, 2000).

   4. An understanding of the impact of culture on the patient's pain experience is crucial. Rehabilitation nurses review research, learn through personal and professional experience, and ask patients and their families about their cultural beliefs about pain.

   5. Rehabilitation nurses use culturally sensitive care principles in evaluating the patient's pain and designing a collaborative care plan.

E. Gender

   1. Physiological, psychosocial, and cultural differences exist in pain and pain management.

   2. Women experience a disproportionate amount of pain and painful syndromes, such as headache and migraine, carpal tunnel syndrome, irritable bowel syndrome, and fibromyalgia (Holdcroft & Berkley, 2006).

   3. Men are less likely to complain about pain or to seek health care to remediate it (Holdcroft & Berkley, 2006).

   4. Gender differences exist in the efficacy of many medications used to treat pain, such as nonsteroidal anti-inflammatory drugs, opioids, anticonvulsants, and antidepressants (Holdcroft & Berkley, 2006).

F. Etiology

   1. Acute pain is the result of trauma or injury (e.g., accidents, falls, burns), disease processes, or surgical interventions, which "diminishes with healing, and disappears when healing is complete" (U.S. Department of Health and Human Services, 2005, p. 2).

   2. Chronic (neuropathic) pain may occur as a result of the aforementioned processes or unknown processes and does not have a protective function (U.S. Department of Health and Human Services, 2005).

G. Pathophysiology

   1. Categories of pain

     a. Nociceptive pain is detected by the peripheral nervous system and transmitted to the brain via the spinal cord. Examples include surgical pain, trauma, cancer pain, and pain from inflammation, such as arthritis (U.S. Department of Health and Human Services, 2005).

       1) Somatic pain is "well localized, constant, and described as sharp, aching, throbbing, or gnawing" (U.S. Department of Health and Human Services, 2005, p. 2).

       2) Visceral pain may be described as "cramping or squeezing in nature" (U.S. Department of Health and Human Services, 2005, p. 2).

     b. Neuropathic pain is chronic, results from long-term changes in the nervous system, and lacks a recognized physiological function (U.S. Department of Health and Human Services, 2005). Neuropathic pain may be central or peripheral.

       1) Peripheral neuropathic pain is the most common and results from damage to the peripheral nerves, such as diabetic neuropathy (Huether & DeFriez, 2006).

       2) Central neuropathic pain is less common, as occurs with multiple sclerosis (Herret al., 2006).

   2. Origin of the stimulus

     a. Nociceptors are specialized nerve endings found at the ends of small unmyelinated and myelinated afferent neurons that respond to a stimulus, such as heat, pressure, or other tissue damage (Barber, 1997; Meyer, Ringkamp, Campbell, & Raja, 2006).

     b. Nociceptors may be polymodal, responding to many different types of stimulus such as heat, chemical, or mechanical, or they may be more specialized and may share both afferent and efferent functions (Meyer et al., 2006).

   3. Stimulus transmission

     a. Two types of fibers transmit pain impulses. Myelinated A-delta fibers transmit rapidly and are responsible for the initial pain response, and unmyelinated C-fibers produce a slower response and are felt after an injury (e.g., if you touch a hot stove, A-delta fibers cause you to withdraw your hand before C-fibers transmit the burning pain sensation) (Barber, 1997).

1) The primary afferent nerves connect with the laminae, or layers of the gray matter of the dorsal horn.

2) The majority of the nociceptive afferents connect with spinal lamina II, or the substantia gelatinosa.

3) In the dorsal horn, second-order neurons transmit to the brain, other neurons, or motor cells or to impulse-moderating inhibitory interneurons.

4) The synapses between the primary afferents and the neurons in the substantia gelatinosa and other laminae of the dorsal horn compose the gate described by the gate control theory of pain and modulate the message of pain being sent to the brain (Huether & DeFriez, 2006).

5) The modulation of nociceptive input involves descending pathways and ascending pathways (APS, 2006).

b. The transmission of impulses in primary afferent nerves is facilitated by neurotransmitters, particularly glutamate.

1) Other neurotransmitters include aspartate, neuropeptides such as substance P, and calcitonin gene-related peptide (Julius & McKleskey, 2006).

2) The initial stimulus causes a release of inflammatory mediators (e.g., bradykinin, serotonin, histamine, arachidonic acids, and cytokines), resulting in a flare response that sensitizes surrounding nociceptors to further stimuli (Meyer et al., 2006).

3) The inflammatory mediators affect pain processing in the central nervous system and in the damaged tissue itself (McMahon, Bennett, & Bevan, 2006).

c. Ascending pain impulses are then transmitted contralaterally to pathways in the dorsal horn of the spinal cord (Bradley & McKendree-Smith, 2002).

d. Most afferent impulses ascend via the lateral spinothalamic tract and spinoreticular tract (Bradley & McKendree-Smith, 2002).

e. The impulses then ascend to the thalamus and reticular formation in the brain and on to the cortex (Bradley & McKendree-Smith, 2002).

4. Perception and response to pain

a. The limbic system (the thalamus and reticular formation) activates protective responses to the pain, releasing stress hormones and causing the fight-or-flight reaction (Huether & DeFriez, 2006, p. 450).

b. In response to the impulses, the perception of pain is formed in the primary and secondary somatosensory cortex, the insular cortex, and other parts of the limbic forebrain (Bradley & McKendree-Smith, 2002).

c. The somatosensory cortex formulates the "affective expression of pain (how . . . pain looks to an observer)" (Huether & DeFriez, 2006, p. 450).

5. Psychosocial influences on pain

a. The threat presented by acute and especially chronic pain is based in part on the effect on daily activities, ability to cope with the pain, and potential long-term consequences of the pain or its cause (Bond, 2006).

b. Personality, environmental factors (e.g., presence or absence of social support), and affective disorders (e.g., depression or anxiety) or other psychiatric conditions also affect the person's expression of pain and behaviors surrounding the pain experience (Bond, 2006).

II. Pain Theories

A. Gate Control Theory

1. The most widely accepted theory of pain

2. Postulates a gating mechanism in the spinal cord (The Gate Control Model, 1998)

a. Nociceptor impulses are transmitted from specific skin sites via large A-delta and small C-fibers to the spinal cord, terminating in the substantia gelatinosa.

b. The cells of the substantia gelatinosa function as the gate. The large, fast-conducting fibers close the gate, and the small, slower cells open the gate.

1) The closed gate results in a decrease in the stimulation of trigger cells, a decrease in pain impulses, and a decrease in pain perception. If persistent stimulation of the large fibers occurs, it results in adaptation.

2) The opposite occurs with an open gate. Stimulation of trigger fibers, transmission of impulses, and pain perception increase when the substantia gelatinosa opens the gate.

c. In addition to the substantia gelatinosa control of the gate, the central nervous system may open, close, or partially close the gate (The Gate Control Model, 1998) (see Figure 13-1).

B. The Neuromatrix Theory. The neuromatrix theory, developed by Melzack and Wall, proposes an explanation for pain that does not correlate with actual injury or with a specific cause.

1. Consistent with the gate control theory, developed by Melzack (1999), this theory suggests that the central nervous system contains a built-in body–self neuromatrix, which is capable of generating nerve impulses that represent the multidimensional somatosensory experience (Huether & DeFriez, 2006).

2. These nerve impulses, called the neurosignature patterns, may be activated by peripheral sensory stimulation or by brain processes to produce persistent pain.

a. Phantom limb pain is an example of this activation; there is no real body part to feel pain, yet the brain perceives that the limb is both present and painful (Huether & DeFriez, 2006; Melzack, 1999).

b. The neuromatrix provides an explanation for chronic pain, which may exist with no discernible cause or stimulus (Huether & DeFriez, 2006; Melzack, 1999).

III. Clinical Manifestations of Pain

A. Acute Pain

1. Somatic pain

a. Refers to the skin or surface area of the body

b. Presents symptoms such as sharp and well-localized pain or dull, aching, poorly localized pain (Huether & DeFriez, 2006)

2. Visceral pain

a. Originates in cutaneous tissues, deep somatic tissue, or organs (viscera)

b. May be categorized as "(1) acute somatic, (2) acute visceral, and (3) referred" (Huether & DeFriez, 2006, p. 456)

c. May be accompanied by "nausea and vomiting, hypotension, restlessness, and, in some cases, shock." The pain may radiate or be referred to another site (Huether & DeFriez, 2006, p. 457).

1) Referred pain is perceived in a part of the body distant from the original stimulus.

2) Pain is said to radiate when the sensation "spreads away from the actual site of the pain" (Huether & DeFriez, 2006, p. 457).

3. Manifestations

a. Physiological responses (in response to a warning of or actual tissue damage)

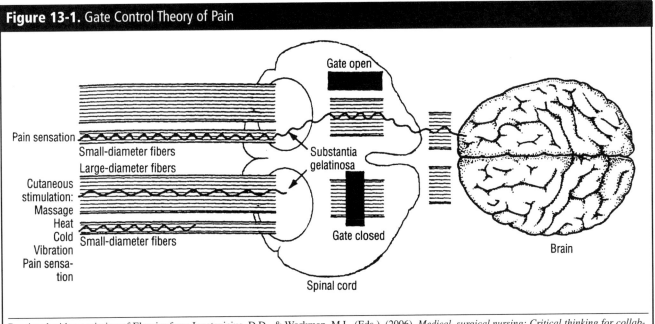

Figure 13-1. Gate Control Theory of Pain

Reprinted with permission of Elsevier from Ignatavicius, D.D., & Workman, M.L. (Eds.). (2006). *Medical–surgical nursing: Critical thinking for collaborative care* (5th ed., p. 66). St. Louis: Elsevier Saunders.

1) Increased heart rate, respiratory rate, blood pressure, and blood sugar level
2) Decreased gastric acid secretion and motility and blood flow to the viscera and skin
3) Pallor and flushing, dilated pupils, and diaphoresis

b. Psychological responses: fear, anxiety, and uneasiness while the person waits for information about the cause, treatment options, and prognosis of acute pain

c. Behavioral responses: vocalizations (moaning, crying), motor responses (touching or rubbing the affected area), attention-seeking behavior in order to relieve the pain (Huether & DeFriez, 2006)

B. Chronic Pain

1. Defined as extended duration of pain past the healing period of 3 months or longer (Huether & DeFriez, 2006).

2. Suspected nervous system alterations may cause "misinterpretation of nociceptive input" (Huether & DeFriez, 2006, p. 458). Physiological factors that may contribute to chronic pain include the following:

   a. A decreased level of endorphins
   b. Alterations in the neuronal sensitivity
   c. Spontaneous impulses arising from regenerating peripheral nerves
   d. Changes in dorsal root ganglia
   e. Reduced pain inhibition in the spinal cord (Huether & DeFriez, 2006).

3. Manifestations.

   a. Physiological
      1) Intermittent pain imitates acute pain.
      2) Persistent pain allows physiological adaptation, resulting in lack of the typical pain symptoms without pain relief (Huether & DeFriez, 2006).

   b. Psychological
      1) Depression
      2) Disturbances in sleep, such as insomnia
      3) Changes in appetite and food intake
      4) Potential for the person to become focused on the pain (Huether & DeFriez, 2006)

   c. Behavioral
      1) The person may be overwhelmed by the pain, to the exclusion of other life experiences.
      2) The person may deny the pain's effects, trying to prevent the pain from taking over (e.g., the person

may refuse to discuss the pain or may participate in activities that place him or her at risk for harm) (Huether & DeFriez, 2006).

IV. **Variations in Pain Across the Lifespan**

A. Role of the Rehabilitation Nurse

1. Systematically assess the various dimensions of pain and their impact on the person's functional capacity and quality of life.

2. Acknowledge that pain is a multidimensional problem that affects the person's functioning level, psychological well-being, social interactions, and family and friends.

3. Give high priority to the patient's self-report, the family's report, observed behaviors (e.g., verbal, vocal, and body language), and physiological measures (McCaffery, 1997) (see Table 13-1).

4. Consider that children generally lack an understanding of magnitude and serial order, which is necessary to use most pain scales, and that observation of behavior and caregiver report must be relied on instead of self-report (Voepal-Lewis, Malviya, & Tait, 2005).

5. Remember that the perception of pain crosses all age ranges, and special attention must be focused on young people and older adults.

B. Infants

1. Infants experience pain but can't express where they hurt or how they feel (Assessment of Pain in Children, 1999).

2. It is essential to perform a thorough assessment to assess pain in infants and children.

   a. Identify possible sources of pain (e.g., disease, injury, infection, procedures).

   b. Pain is generally indicated by a disturbance in infant behavior, such as a change in vocal or facial expression or body movement (Herr et al., 2006).
      1) A cry that is not relieved by feeding, changing, or comforting
      2) A change in facial expression: lowered and drawn-together eyebrows, a vertical bulge between the brows in the forehead, tightly closed eyes, an open mouth, or chin quivers
      3) Harsh, high-pitched cries
      4) Behaviors indicative of chronic pain in infants include posturing,

Table 13-1. Pain Assessment Tool

Physiological	Pain History	Observed Behaviors	Family Involvement	Role Changes
Complete physical	Causal factor	Nonverbal behavior	Is there family support?	Home
Diagnostics	Onset	Facial expressions	Does the family reinforce pain behaviors?	School
Psychosocial history	Location	Body language	Is the family supportive of the patient's recovery?	Work
Past history	Intensity		What are the family's financial concerns?	Church
Family history	Variation over 24 hours			Community
Review of records	What aggravates it			
Collaboration with colleagues	What eliminates it			
	Current treatments			
	Medication regime			
	Adjunct therapies			
	Sleep patterns			
	Appetite changes			
	Coping patterns			
	Mood			
	Substance use			
	Activities and exercise			
	Family functioning			
	Cultural influences			
	Education of diagnosis			

Sources consulted

McCaffery, M. (1979). *Nursing management of the patient with pain* (2nd ed.). Philadelphia: Lippincott. Swartz, M.H. (1998). Caring for patients in a culturally diverse society. In M.H. Swartz (Ed.), *Textbook of physical diagnosis: History and examination* (3rd ed., pp. 43-69). Philadelphia: W.B. Saunders. U.S. Department of Health and Human Services, The Office on Women's Health. (2005). Breakthroughs and challenges in the pharmacologic management of common chronic pain conditions. *Clinician, 23*(3), retrieved from https://www.aapainmanage.org/education/EducationLit/PainCLINICIANmonograph11.29.05.pdf

unwillingness to be moved, and withdrawal (Herr et al., 2006).

3. Consider using a behavioral pain assessment tool (see Table 13-1).

4. Parents are the advocates when an infant, child, or adolescent with physical or cognitive impairments cannot communicate. Parents may benefit from explanations of behavior scales for pain to assist them in quantifying their child's response (Herr et al., 2006).

C. Toddlers

1. Toddlers may express pain through crying, facial expressions (as in infants), agitation, aggression, rocking, and rubbing or guarding a body part with their hands.

2. Typically developing 2-year-olds may be able to indicate pain; typically developing 3-year-olds may be able to use simple pain scales (Herr et al., 2006).

3. Delays in healing and changes in the child's sleep, appetite, or play schedule may develop if pain is left untreated (O'Connor-Von, 1999).

D. Preschoolers

1. May be able to indicate the presence of pain but not identify its location

2. May use descriptors such as "hurt," "owie," or "boo-boo" to refer to pain (Hockenberry, Wilson, Winkelstein, & Kline, 2003). Rehabilitation nurses collaborate with parents to determine the language used at home to identify pain.

3. Can express the amount of pain they are experiencing by using their hands: Putting the hands together (as if praying) indicates little or no pain, whereas holding the hands far apart indicates the most pain (O'Connor-Von, 1999)

4. Can begin to use formal instruments to indicate where they have pain (see Figures 13-2 and 13-3)

   a. Faces scale: A series of faces from happy (*no pain*) to very upset (*the worst pain possible*) are shown to the child, who is asked to point to the face that most resembles how he or she feels.

   b. Number scales: The child is asked to rate the pain, with 0 representing *no pain* and higher numbers representing *the worst pain*. Scales of 0–5 or 0–10 are used.

c. Poker chip tool: Can be instrumental at this age because it is well validated and concrete.
   1) Four poker chips are placed in front of the child. The chips are described as pieces of hurt.
   2) The first chip is described as "just a little hurt," the second is "a little more hurt," the third chip is "more hurt," and the fourth chip is "the most hurt you could have."
   3) The child is asked, "How many pieces of hurt do you have?"
d. Body outlines: The child colors in the area on the picture to show where the pain is (Hockenberry et al., 2003).
e. The FLACC (face, legs, activity, cry, consolability) scale is a tool for assessing

---

Figure 13-2. Pain Diagram

Pain Diagram

Mark the areas on this body where you feel the described sensations.
Use the appropriate symbols.
Mark areas of radiation.
Include all affected areas.

Numbness	Pins & Needles	Burning	Aching	Stabbing
- - - - -	00000	xxxxx	*****	/ / / / /
- - - - -	00000	xxxxx	*****	/ / / / /
- - - - -	00000	xxxxx	*****	/ / / / /

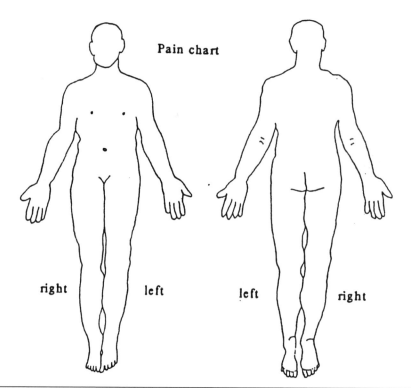

Pain chart

right   left   left   right

Reprinted with permission of Aspen from Skogsbergh, D.R., & Chapman, S.A. (1994). Dealing with the chronic patient. *Topics in Clinical Chiropractic,* *1*(4).

postoperative pain in young children with cognitive impairment, which is scored by the nurse based on body position and behavior (Voepal-Lewis, Merkel, Tait, Trzcinka, & Malviya, 2002).

E. School-Aged Children

   1. Can use some descriptors (e.g., *shooting, stabbing, burning*)

   2. Can use the faces and number scales

F. Adolescents and Adults

   1. Can provide a self-report of their pain using various instruments such as word descriptors and numerical scales

   2. Are able to participate in a full assessment

   3. The American Chronic Pain Association (2003) Quality of Life Scale is a useful tool to evaluate the effect of a person's pain on his or her life.

G. People with Intellectual Disability or Cognitive Impairment

   1. Includes people with mental retardation, traumatic brain injury, severe mental illness, and dementia.

   2. Cognitive impairment affects behavior related to pain and the ability to communicate pain.

      a. Depending on the level of cognitive impairment, different tools may be necessary to determine pain level.

      b. One study found that in people with cognitive impairment, using facial expression or a tool based solely on facial expression (the Modified Facial Action Coding System) was less reliable in accurately detecting pain behaviors than a tool using facial expression, vocalization, body movements, and physiological measurements (the Non-Communicating Children's Pain Checklist–Revised). This study suggests that using a variety of evaluation measures is most successful in evaluating the level of pain in people with cognitive impairment (Defrin, Lotan, & Pick, 2006).

H. Older Adults

   1. Older adults are at high risk for pain and face a number of obstacles to adequate treatment.

   2. Although pain sensitivity may differ, an assumption that less pain is experienced is incorrect.

   3. Several factors may inhibit appropriate pain management in older adults.

      a. Fear of addiction to or side effects of pain medications

      b. A belief that pain is the inevitable consequence of aging or that reporting pain may indicate that something more serious is wrong (e.g., if the healthcare provider does not ask about the pain, the older patient may perceive that it should not exist)

      c. A belief that if they admit to pain, family or providers will label them as "bad patients" (Hanks-Bell, Halvey, & Paice, 2004)

   4. Healthcare providers may not manage an older adult's pain properly because of the inaccurate perception that older adults experience less pain.

      a. Healthcare providers may believe that if the patient does not report pain, he or she is not experiencing it.

      b. Older adults' sensitivity to the side effects of pain medications, especially narcotics, may indicate that these medications should be avoided. Older adults experience diminishing renal and liver function, which affects metabolism of medications commonly used for pain and its sequelae, such as opiates, benzodiazepines, and anticholinergics.

      c. Nurses may lack the ability to evaluate pain in people with cognitive impairment (Hanks-Bell et al., 2004).

      d. Pain that is undertreated may result in significant medical problems, such as pneumonia or deep vein thrombosis, and diminish quality of life (APS, 2006).

   5. As in other populations, self-reports of pain are the most reliable.

   6. It is important for rehabilitation nurses to do the following when assessing an older adult's pain:

      a. Provide a quiet milieu.

      b. Proceed at a slow pace.

      c. Allow sufficient time for the person to respond.

      d. Use direct and focused questioning.

      e. Exchange information at a volume the person can hear.

      f. Use enlarged written information.

      g. Ask the family or caregiver to fill in details of the person's condition, especially if the person is fatigued or has cognitive deficits (e.g., deficits in memory, attention span, language [aphasia], visuospatial skills, or fatigue) (Todd, 1997).

h. Use age-appropriate questions.
   1) Where do you hurt?
   2) Does the pain stay there or move around?
   3) Is the pain always there?
   4) Does the pain interrupt your sleep or prevent you from falling asleep?
   5) What are you unable to do because of the pain (e.g., activities of daily living, shopping, housekeeping, visiting with friends, going to church)?
   6) What has worked in relieving your pain in the past?
   7) What has not worked in the past (Kruse, 1999)?
i. Use assessment tools, including word scales with descriptors (e.g., *mild, moderate,* or *severe*), the 0–10 number scale, the pain thermometer (picture of a thermometer with degrees of pain), and the faces pain scale (see Figure 13-3). The faces scale may be most appropriate for people with dementia or aphasia (Hanks-Bell et al., 2004; Todd, 1997).

V. Pain Assessment and Management

A. Process: Pain assessment and management is a complex biological, psychological, social, spiritual, and cultural process.

B. Assessment of Pain
   1. Pain behaviors vary from individual to individual.
      a. Verbal indicators (i.e., what the patient reports) are considered the most useful.
      b. Nonverbal indicators (i.e., observable behaviors) often complement verbal ones and inform an individualized treatment plan, particularly in children or nonverbal patients.
   2. Simon and McTier (1996) outlined a scale with 10 indicators that was developed and is used at the University of Alabama at Birmingham in which the healthcare professional observes the patient's pain.
      a. Verbal vocal complaints
      b. Nonverbal vocal complaints
      c. Down time (i.e., time spent lying down each day between 8 am and 8 pm because of pain)
      d. Facial grimaces
      e. Standing posture (e.g., stooped, favoring one side of the body)
      f. Mobility (e.g., limping, slow pace)

g. Body language (e.g., clutching or rubbing site of pain)
h. Use of visible supportive equipment (e.g., braces, crutches, cane)
i. Stationary movement (e.g., squirming, restlessness)
j. Use of medication

   3. Frequent use of the healthcare system (e.g., scheduled office appointments, emergency room visits, doctor shopping) is another indicator to consider (Simon & McTier, 1996).
   4. Rehabilitation nurses work with the patient and family to teach about the diagnosis and available treatment options (see Table 13-2) and to help the patient establish realistic goals (ARN, 1994).
   5. Because most chronic pain is not curable, the goal is to help the patient improve his or her quality of life and return to enjoyable activities.

C. Using an Outcome Approach to Pain Management.
   1. Description: Patients, healthcare professionals, and the insurance industry continue to note inconsistent and ineffective pain management (Barnason, Merboth, Pozehl, & Tietjen, 1998).
   2. Roles of the rehabilitation nurse: The determination of the patient's pain status and the extent of its communication through nursing interventions are necessary steps toward improving patient outcomes (Malek & Olivieri, 1996).
      a. Assess the patient.
      b. Observe all cues (verbal, nonverbal, family report).
      c. Diagnose the patient's pain.
      d. Coordinate and facilitate appropriate interventions for better pain management.
      e. Establish rapport with the patient.
      f. Educate the patient on the various resources available and advocate for their implementation.
      g. Help the patient and other healthcare providers address the myths that may compromise pain management (see Figures 13-4 and 13-5).

D. Applying the Nursing Process to Pain Management.
   1. Assess the patient: Interview the patient, communicate, observe, and collect, verify, and organize the data.

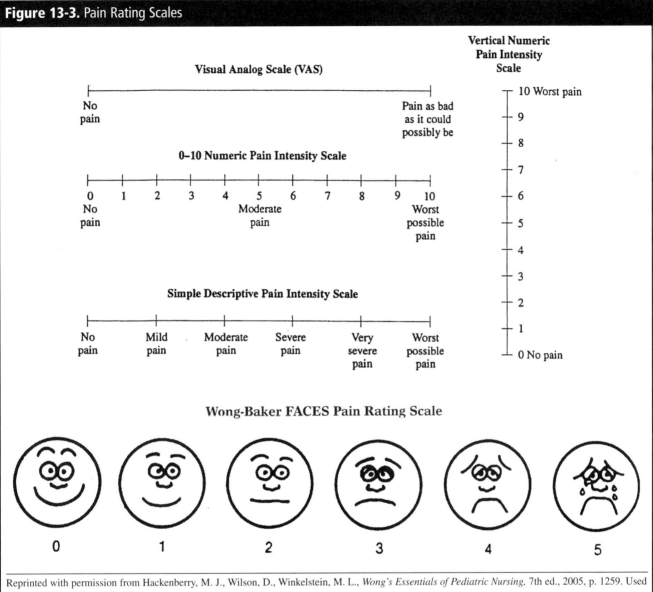

Figure 13-3. Pain Rating Scales

Visual Analog Scale (VAS)

No pain — Pain as bad as it could possibly be

0–10 Numeric Pain Intensity Scale

0 No pain | 1 | 2 | 3 | 4 | 5 Moderate pain | 6 | 7 | 8 | 9 | 10 Worst possible pain

Simple Descriptive Pain Intensity Scale

No pain — Mild pain — Moderate pain — Severe pain — Very severe pain — Worst possible pain

Vertical Numeric Pain Intensity Scale

10 Worst pain
9
8
7
6
5
4
3
2
1
0 No pain

Wong-Baker FACES Pain Rating Scale

0   1   2   3   4   5

Reprinted with permission from Hackenberry, M. J., Wilson, D., Winkelstein, M. L., *Wong's Essentials of Pediatric Nursing,* 7th ed., 2005, p. 1259. Used with permission. Copyright Mosby.

2. Diagnose: State the actual or potential healthcare problems.

3. Plan: Set healthcare priorities based on the patient's input and develop goals for nursing interventions.

4. Implement the plan: Collect data on an ongoing basis and revise the plan as needed to help the patient reach the highest level of wellness.

5. Evaluate the outcomes: Determine whether goals are achieved.

6. Manage care: Build rapport with the patient and family, advocate for appropriate services, collaborate with colleagues, and contain costs through early intervention.

E. Methods of Pain Management.

1. Pharmacological pain management

a. Includes nonprescription and prescription medications (see Table 13-2).

b. Local anesthetics, including lidocaine patches and epidural or intrathecal administration of anesthesia.

c. Joint injections of substances such as corticosteroids and hyaluronic acid may be helpful in managing pain from osteoarthritis.

d. Interventional techniques such as chemical or surgical rhizotomy (Hanks-Bell et al., 2004).

2. Nonpharmacological pain management

a. Used more often by older adults who fear medication side effects

Table 13-2. Pharmacological and Nonpharmacological Pain Management

Medication Class	Examples	Indicators	Action	Major Adverse Effects*
Nonopioid analgesics	Acetaminophen	Mild to moderate pain	Blocks pain impulses by inhibiting prostaglandin synthesis, possibly by inhibition of cyclooxygenase-3	Liver dysfunction, renal damage
Nonopioid analgesics: nonsteroidal anti-inflammatory drugs Oral	Aspirin, diclofenac NA (Voltaren), ibuprofen (Motrin), ketoprofen, naproxen NA (Naprosyn, Aleve)	Inflammatory pain, bone and joint pain, and menstrual pain	Inhibits prostaglandin synthesis; antipyretic	Bleeding, gastrointestinal ulceration, renal dysfunction, hypertension
Nonopioid analgesics: cyclooxygenase-2 inhibitors Oral	Celecoxib (Celebrex)	Inflammatory pain, bone pain, postsurgical pain	Selectively blocks cyclooxygenase-2 to inhibit prostaglandin	Gastrointestinal upset, cardiovascular problems
Co-analgesics: antidepressants Oral	Tricyclics: amitriptyline, nortriptyline	Neuropathic pain, fibromyalgia	Inhibits serotonin uptake	Anticholinergic side effects, cardiovascular effects
	Selective serotonin reuptake inhibitors: fluoxetine HCl, sertraline HCl	Neuropathic pain, less effective than tricyclics	Inhibits serotonin uptake	Gastrointestinal upset, suicidal ideation, serotonin syndrome
	Bupropion	Back pain, neuropathic pain	Blocks norepinephrine and dopamine	Seizures, suicidal ideation
	Duloxetine (Cymbalta)	Neuropathic pain, fibromyalgia	Blocks norepinephrine and serotonin	Gastrointestinal upset, suicidal ideation, serotonin syndrome
Co-analgesics: anticonvulsants Oral	Phenytoin NA, gabapentin, divalproex NA, carbamazepine	Neuropathic pain, trigeminal and postherpetic neuralgia	Decreases abnormal impulses in the nervous system	Sedation, nausea, liver damage, thrombocytopenia, hyponatremia, drug toxicity
Muscle relaxants Oral and intrathecal	Baclofen (Lioresal)	Skeletal muscle pain and spasticity	Decreases impulse transmission from spinal cord to skeletal muscle	Sedation; avoid abrupt discontinuation
Opioids: mixed opioid Oral	Tramadol HCl (Ultram)	Moderate to severe pain	Binds opioid receptors, inhibits uptake of serotonin and norepinephrine	Lower seizure threshold, sedation, respiratory depression; habit forming
Opioids Oral and topical (fentanyl)	Codeine, meperidine, hydrocodone, fentanyl, oxycodone (Percocet; OxyContin [long acting]), morphine sulfate (MS-Contin [oral, long acting])	Moderate to severe pain, cancer pain	Binds with opiate receptors in the central nervous system, altering the perception and emotional response to pain	Sedation, confusion, respiratory depression, habit forming
Anesthetic agents Topical	Lidocaine patch	Postherpetic pain, neuropathic pain	Block sodium and calcium channel transmissions	Skin irritation, few adverse effects

*This is a partial list of adverse effects; please consult a reliable drug reference source for complete information.

Sources consulted

American Chronic Pain Association (ACPA). (2005). ACPA medications and chronic pain: Supplement 2005. Available: http://www.theacpa.org
American Pain Society (APS). (2006). *Pain: Current understanding of assessment, management, and treatments.* Available: http://www.ampainsoc.org/ce/enduring.htm

Hanks-Bell, M., Halvey, K., & Paice, J.A. (2004). Pain assessment and management in aging. *Online Journal of Issues in Nursing, 9*(3). Available: www.nursingworld.org/ojin/topic21/tpc21_6.htm

Harris, J.A. (2000). Understanding acute and chronic pain. In P.A. Edwards (Ed.), *The specialty practice of rehabilitation nursing: A core curriculum* (4th ed., pp. 263–278). Glenview, IL: Association of Rehabilitation Nurses.

b. Includes cognitive–behavioral methods (e.g., guided imagery, education, and prayer)

c. Physical methods, including physical therapy and the application of heat, cold, and bracing and physical movement such as tai chi (Hanks-Bell et al., 2004)

d. Complementary and alternative medicine such as chiropractic, massage, acupuncture, and herbal treatments (Wirth, Hudgins, & Paice, 2005)

F. North American Nursing Diagnosis Association Diagnoses for Pain.

1. Exchanging: risk for injury

2. Relating: social isolation

3. Valuing: spiritual distress

4. Choosing: ineffective individual coping, ineffective coping in the community, ineffective or compromised family coping, and ineffective management of therapeutic regimen

5. Moving: activity intolerance, impaired home maintenance management, and impaired physical mobility

6. Perceiving: hopelessness and powerlessness

7. Knowing: knowledge deficit

8. Feeling: anxiety and fear (Carpenito-Moyet, 2005)

VI. Rehabilitation Nursing Roles in the Management of Acute and Chronic Pain

A. Professional Rehabilitation Nurse

1. Uses evidence-based guidelines and standards

2. Applies knowledge of clinical nursing care

3. Uses understanding of physiology, pathophysiology, psychosocial factors, and pharmacologic and nonpharmacologic methods in order to

a. Implement the nursing process to prevent, identify, and alleviate pain

b. Work collaboratively with the rehabilitation team, the patient, and the family

c. Facilitate the restoration of function for the patient

4. Advocates for the patient and coordinates the plan of care with the patient, family, and rehabilitation team

a. Provides patient and family education

b. Promotes patient comfort, well-being, and safety (American Society for Pain Management Nursing, 2005; ARN, 1994).

5. Functions in the acute care setting, in the freestanding rehabilitation center, and in the community to provide direct patient care

B. Advanced Practice Rehabilitation Nurse: uses advanced assessment and diagnostic skills, prescriptive authority, and an expanded scope of practice

1. Clinician

a. Identifying pain management issues and strategizing solutions

b. Providing primary care and preventive services to rehabilitation patients

c. Providing health-promoting activities that reduce or alleviate pain

d. Prescribing pharmacological and nonpharmacological methods of pain relief and providing long-term patient management

e. Functioning independently (per state practice acts) and collaboratively

2. Educator

a. Providing staff and rehabilitation team with education on pain

b. Providing nursing education in the university setting

c. Providing comprehensive patient and family about regarding health promotion and disease states to enable the patient to improve functional capacity and minimize the effect of pain on his or her life

3. Rehabilitation nursing leader

a. In state and national professional and interdisciplinary organizations, such as the Association of Rehabilitation Nurses and the American Pain Society

b. As a change agent affecting systems of care on behalf of rehabilitation patients and those experiencing pain

c. Providing leadership in clinical care of the rehabilitation patient experiencing pain

4. Consultant

a. Acting as a resource for nurses, patients, and other healthcare professionals

b. Providing specialty consultation on pain in rehabilitation patients

c. Functioning independently and as a member of the rehabilitation or pain management team

5. Researcher

a. Identifying critical questions in assessment and management of pain in rehabilitation patients

Figure 13-4. Myths About Pain

Healthcare providers are the authority on the existence and extent of the patient's pain.

The patient is not in pain if he or she does not report it.

Pain is an unavoidable process of aging.

As a person ages, his or her perception of pain decreases.

For pain to be real, it must have an associated physical cause.

Everything that can be done for the pain is always done.

Addiction is perceived when a person repeatedly requests something else for pain.

When pain is reported, it automatically implies a progression of the disease or some other problem.

By requesting additional medication or assistance, the person in pain is making a nuisance of himself or herself.

The pain a person is experiencing is not worthy of being reported.

Sources consulted
Barnason, S., Merboth, M., Pozehl, B., & Tietjen, M.J. (1998). Utilizing an outcomes approach to improve pain management by nurses: A pilot study. *Clinical Nurse Specialist, 12*(1), 28–36.
Malek, C.J., & Olivieri, R.J. (1996). Pain management: Documenting the decision making process. *Nursing Case Management, 1*(2), 64–73.

Figure 13-5. Nursing Interventions for Pain

Establish a rapport with the patient so he or she can understand the nurse's role in pain management.

Teach the patient that he or she is the most accurate reporter of the pain experience.

Instruct the patient that all people experience pain and that pain is individualized.

Educate the patient about pharmacological and adjunct interventions in pain management and determine the patient's preferences.

Evaluate the patient's response to pharmacological interventions, determine whether an adjunct intervention or additional medication is indicated, and facilitate the intervention.

Collaborate with other healthcare professionals to advocate for the interventions necessary to help the patient manage his or her pain.

Educate the patient on lifelong interventions and facilitate appropriate referrals in managing cost-effective and timely outcomes.

b. Validating assessment tools and methods

c. Contributing to the evidence base in nursing science (American Society for Pain Management Nursing, 2005; ARN, 1994).

C. Evidence-Based Practice

1. Evidence-based practice regarding pain assessment in the cognitively impaired adult

   a. Rehabilitation nurses often are required to assess acute or chronic pain in people with cognitive impairment.

   b. Literature suggests that a multidimensional assessment, evaluating more than one aspect of pain response, such as physiological and behavioral, is more representative of the actual pain experience of the cognitively impaired patient (McLennon, 2005).

2. Clinical question: What is the most effective method of assessing pain in the cognitively impaired adult?

3. Appraisal of evidence

   a. In the guideline *Persistent Pain Management,* McLennon (2005) reported that no Level I evidence exists that cognitively impaired older adults experience less pain than people who are not impaired but that the cognitive impairment may influence the patient's ability to "interpret and report" pain (McLennon, 2005, p. 5).

   b. McLennon further reported that three

main methods of assessing pain are represented in the literature: proxy reports (by nurse or caregiver), observational methods (by nurse or other caregiver), and analgesia trials (although little evidence exists on this method).

   c. The Verbal Descriptor Scale was recommended by Chibnall and Tait (2001) and Taylor, Harris, Epps, and Herr (2005) for assessment of pain in older adults with mild to moderate cognitive impairment (Level IV evidence).

   d. African American and Hispanic older adults with cognitive impairment preferred the Faces Pain Scale–Revised (Ware, Epps, Herr, & Packard, 2006) (Level VI evidence).

   e. For people with severe cognitive impairment, the Pain Assessment Checklist for Seniors with Limited Ability to Communicate, an observational tool, can indicate the presence of pain (Fuchs-Lacelle & Hadjistavropoulos, 2004) (Level IV evidence).

   f. Herr et al. (2006) recommended using a variety of strategies for assessing the presence and intensity of pain in cognitively impaired adults (Level I evidence).

4. Recommendation for best rehabilitation nursing practice

   a. Evidence suggests that nurses should use a variety of strategies to assess pain in adults with cognitive impairment.

   b. Because no specific tool has been found to be superior to another, tool selection should take into account individual levels of cognitive impairment and the patient's medical conditions, cultural background, and rehabilitation setting.

c. Whichever assessment strategy the nurse chooses for the individual patient, that tool should be used consistently for the same patient (Herr et al., 2006; McLennon, 2005).

References

ABC News Health. (2005, May 9). Poll: *Americans searching for pain relief.* Retrieved March 19, 2007, from http://abcnews.go.com/Health/PainManagement/story?id=732395

Alexander, J., & Manno, M.(2003). Underuse of analgesia in very young pediatric patients with isolated painful injuries. *Annals of Emergency Medicine, 41*(5).

American Academy of Pain Medicine (AAPM) & American Pain Society (APS). (1997). The use of opioids for the treatment of chronic pain: A consensus statement. *The Clinical Journal of Pain, 13*(1), 6–8.

American Chronic Pain Association (ACPA). (2003). *The ACPA quality of life scale: A measure of function for people with pain.* Retrieved March 19, 2007, from http://www.theacpa.org/managingyourrisk/Quality_of_Life_Scale.pdf

American Chronic Pain Association (ACPA). (2005). *ACPA medications and chronic pain: Supplement 2005.* Available: http://www.theacpa.org

American Pain Society (APS). (2006). *Pain: Current understanding of assessment, management, and treatments.* Available: http://www.ampainsoc.org/ce/enduring.htm

American Society for Pain Management Nursing. (2005). *Pain management nursing: Scope and standards of practice.* Lenexa, KS: American Society for Pain Management Nursing and American Nurses Association.

Assessment of pain in children: Pediatric. (1999, March). Available: http://pedspain.nursing.uiowa.edu/Assess/Assessme.htm

Association of Rehabilitation Nurses (ARN). (1994). *The pain management rehabilitation nurse: Role description* [Brochure]. Skokie, IL: Author.

Barber, D. (1997). The physiology and pharmacology of pain: A review of opioids. *Journal of PeriAnesthesia Nursing, 12*(2), 95–99.

Barnason, S., Merboth, M., Pozehl, B., & Tietjen, M.J. (1998). Utilizing an outcomes approach to improve pain management by nurses: A pilot study. *Clinical Nurse Specialist, 12*(1), 28–36.

Bernabeia, R., Gambassi, G., Lapane, K., Landi, F., Gatsonis, C., Dunlop, R., et al. (1998). Management of pain in elderly patients with cancer. *Journal of the American Medical Association, 279,* 1877–1882.

Bond, M.R. (2006). Psychiatric disorders and pain. In A.B. McMahon & M. Koltzenburg (Eds.), *Wall and Melzack's textbook of pain* (5th ed., pp. 259–266). Philadelphia: Elsevier.

Bradley, L.A., & McKendree-Smith, N. (2002). Central nervous system mechanisms of pain in fibromyalgia and other musculoskeletal disorders: Behavioral and psychologic treatment approaches. *Current Opinion in Rheumatology, 14*(1), 45–51.

Bushnell, M.C., & Apkarian, A.V. (2006). Representation of pain in the brain. In A.B. McMahon & M. Koltzenburg (Eds.), *Wall and Melzack's textbook of pain* (5th ed., pp. 107–124). Philadelphia: Elsevier.

Carpenito-Moyet, L.J. (2005). *Nursing diagnosis in the nursing process.* Philadelphia: Lippincott Williams & Wilkins.

Carr, D.B., & Goudas L.C. (1999). Acute pain. *Lancet, 353*(9169), 2055–2058.

Chibnall, J.T., & Tait, R.C. (2001). Pain assessment in the cognitively impaired and unimpaired older adult. A comparison of four scales. *Pain, 92*(1–2), 173–186.

Defrin, R., Lotan, M., & Pick, C.G. (2006). The evaluation of acute pain in individuals with cognitive impairment: A differential effect of the level of impairment. *Pain, 124*(3), 112–120.

DiLima, S.N., & Niemyer, S. (Eds.). (1995). *Pain management: Patient education manual.* Gaithersburg, MD: Aspen.

Flor, H., & Turk, D.C. (2006). Cognitive and learning aspects. In A.B. McMahon & M. Koltzenburg (Eds.), *Wall and Melzack's textbook of pain* (5th ed., pp. 241–258). Philadelphia: Elsevier.

Fuchs-Lacelle, S., & Hadjistavropoulos, T. (2004). Development and preliminary validation of the Pain Assessment Checklist for Seniors with Limited Ability to Communicate (PACSLAC). *Pain Management Nursing, 5*(1), 37–49.

The gate control model opens a new era in pain research. (1998). Available: http://www.library.ucla.edu/libraries/biomed/his/PainExhibit.

Hanks-Bell, M., Halvey, K., & Paice, J.A. (2004). Pain assessment and management in aging. *Online Journal of Issues in Nursing, 9*(3). Available: www.nursingworld.org/ojin/topic21/tpc21_6.htm

Harris, J. (1998). Protocols for an interdisciplinary rehabilitation approach to pain management. *Inside Case Management, 5*(2), 8–10.

Harris, J.A. (2000). Understanding acute and chronic pain. In P.A. Edwards (Ed.), *The specialty practice of rehabilitation nursing: A core curriculum* (4th ed., pp. 263–278). Glenview, IL: ARN.

Herr, K., Coyne, P.J., Key, T., Manworren, R., McCaffery, M., Merkel, S., et al. (2006, Junc). Pain assessment in the nonverbal patient: Position statement with clinical practice recommendations. *Pain Management Nursing, 7*(2), 44–52.

Hockenberry, M.J., Wilson, D., Winkelstein, M.L., & Kline, N.E. (2003). *Wong's nursing care of infants and children* (7th ed.). St. Louis: Mosby.

Holdcroft, A., & Berkley, K.J. (2006). Sex and gender differences in pain and its relief. In A.B. McMahon & M. Koltzenburg (Eds.), *Wall and Melzack's textbook of pain* (5th ed., pp. 1181–1194). Philadelphia: Elsevier.

Huether, S.E., & DeFriez, C.B. (2006). Pain, temperature regulation, sleep, and sensory function. In K.L. McCance & S.E. Huether (Eds.), *Pathophysiology: The biologic basis for disease in adults and children* (5th ed., pp. 447–490). Philadelphia: Elsevier Mosby.

Ignatavicius, D.D., & Workman, M.L. (Eds.). (2006). *Medical–surgical nursing: Critical thinking for collaborative care* (5th ed., p. 66). St. Louis: Elsevier Saunders.

Intercultural Cancer Council. (2003, November). *Fact sheet: Pain and cancer.* Retrieved April 5, 2007, from http://iccnetwork.org/cancerfacts/cfs7.htm

Janig, W., & Levine, J.D. (2006). Autonomic–endocrine–immune interactions in acute and chronic pain. In A.B. McMahon & M. Koltzenburg (Eds.), *Wall and Melzack's textbook of pain* (5th ed., pp. 205–218). Philadelphia: Elsevier.

Julius, D., & McKleskey, E.W. (2006). Cellular and molecular properties of primary afferent neurons. In A.B. McMahon & M. Koltzenburg (Eds.), *Wall and Melzack's textbook of pain* (5th ed., pp. 35–48). Philadelphia: Elsevier.

Kruse, L. (1999, May). *Gerontology assessment: Healthcare professional version.* Available: http://www.nursing.uiowa.edu/sites/Adultpain/GenePain/Geraas.

Lasch, K.E. (2000). Culture, pain and culturally sensitive pain care. *Pain Management Nursing, 1*(3, Suppl. 1), 16–22.

Lubkin, I.M., & Jeffrey, J. (1998). Chronic pain In L.B. Ames (Ed.), *Chronic illness: Impact and interventions* (pp. 149–180). Toronto: Jones and Bartlett.

Malek, C.J., & Olivieri, R.J. (1996). Pain management: Documenting the decision making process. *Nursing Case Management, 1*(2), 64–73.

McCaffery, M. (1979). *Nursing management of the patient with pain* (2nd ed.). Philadelphia: Lippincott.

McCaffery, M. (1997). Pain management handbook. *Nursing 97, 27*(4), 42–45.

McLennon, S.M. (2005). *Persistent pain management.* Iowa City: University of Iowa Gerontological Nursing Interventions Research Center, Research Translation and Dissemination Core.

McMahon, S.B., Bennett, D.L., & Bevan, S. (2006). Inflammatory mediators and modulators of pain. In A.B. McMahon & M. Koltzenburg (Eds.), *Wall and Melzack's textbook of pain* (5th ed., pp. 49–72). Philadelphia: Elsevier.

Melzack, R. (1999). From the gate to the neuromatrix. *Pain* (Suppl. 6), S121–S126.

Menard, R.G. (1999). *A patient's guide to pain management* [Brochure]. Glenview, IL: American Academy of Pain Medicine.

Meyer, R.A., Ringkamp, M., Campbell, J.N., & Raja, S.N. (2006). Peripheral mechanisms of cutaneous nociception. In A.B. McMahon & M. Koltzenburg (Eds.), *Wall and Melzack's textbook of pain* (5th ed., pp. 3–34). Philadelphia: Elsevier.

National Center for Health Statistics. (2006). Health, United States. In *Chartbook on trends in the health of Americans* (pp. 68–71). Hyattsville, MD: Author.

O'Connor-Von, S. (1999, March). *Pain assessment in children: Parent and family version.* Available: http://pedspain.nursing.uiowa.edu/Assess/Chiasst.htm

Pasero, C.L., & McCaffery, M. (1996). Managing postoperative pain in the elderly. *American Journal of Nursing, 96*(10), 39–45.

Potter, P.A., & Perry, A.G. (1989). *Fundamentals of nursing: Concepts, process, and practice.* St. Louis: Mosby.

Simon, J.M., & McTier, C.L. (1996). Development of a chronic pain assessment tool. *Rehabilitation Nursing, 21*(1), 13–19.

Skogsbergh, D.R., & Chapman, S.A. (1994). Dealing with the chronic patient. *Topics in Clinical Chiropractic, 1*(4).

Stewart, W.F., Ricci, J.A., Chee, E., Morganstein, D., & Lipton, R. (2000). Lost productive time and cost due to common pain conditions in the US workforce. *JAMA, 290*(18), 2443–2454.

Swartz, M.H. (1998). Caring for patients in a culturally diverse society. In M.H. Swartz (Ed.), *Textbook of physical diagnosis: History and examination* (3rd ed., pp. 43–46). Philadelphia: W.B. Saunders.

Taylor, L.J., Harris, J., Epps, C.D., & Herr, K. (2005). Psychometric evaluation of selected pain intensity scales for use with cognitively impaired and cognitively intact older adults. *Rehabilitation Nursing, 30*(2), 55–61.

Todd, C. (1997). *Pain in the elderly, Part 1: Assessing a complex population.* Available: http://www.nurse.ceu.com/geri.htm.

U.S. Department of Health and Human Services, the Office on Women's Health. (2005). Breakthroughs and challenges in the pharmacologic management of common chronic pain conditions. *Clinician, 23*(3). Retrieved February 17, 2007 from https://www.aapainmanage.org/education/EducationLit/PainCLINICIANmonograph11.29.05.pdf

Voepal-Lewis, T., Malviya, S., & Tait, A.R. (2005, December). Pain in children with cognitive impairment. *Pain Management Nursing, 6*(4), 168–174.

Voepal-Lewis, T., Merkel, S., Tait, A.R., Trzcinka, A., & Malviya, S. (2002). The reliability and validity of the face, legs, activity, cry, consolability observational tool as a measure of pain in children with cognitive impairment. *Anesthesia and Analgesia, 95*(5), 1224–1229.

Ware, L.J., Epps, C.D., Herr, K., & Packard, A. (2006). Evaluation of the Revised Faces Pain Scale, Verbal Descriptor Scale, Numerical Rating Scale, and Iowa Pain Thermometer in older minority adults. *Pain Management Nursing, 7*(3), 117–125.

Wirth, J.H., Hudgins, J.C., & Paice, J.A. (2005). Use of herbal therapies to relieve pain: A review of efficacy and adverse effects. *Pain Management Nursing, 6*(4), 145–167.

Chapter 14

Specific Disease Processes Requiring Rehabilitation Interventions

Karen (Cervizzi) Manning, MSN RN CRRN CNA • Patricia A. Haldi, MN RN CRRN CDE

Life with a chronic illness is still life.

Rehabilitation nurses play an important role in caring for people with a wide variety of chronic illnesses and disabilities. This chapter covers the following specific disease processes that warrant rehabilitation interventions:

- Diabetes mellitus
- Multiple sclerosis
- Parkinson's disease
- HIV and AIDS
- Burns
- Cancer
- Alzheimer's disease

Coping with a chronic condition is very stressful, and rehabilitation nurses are the ideal practitioners to provide and coordinate patient and family education and interventions to help the patient integrate the illness into daily life and become as independent as possible. It is important for rehabilitation nurses to have current knowledge and the requisite skills to prevent complications and modify the effects of chronic conditions regardless of the practice setting.

I. Diabetes Mellitus (DM)

A. Overview

1. A group of diseases marked by high fasting, preprandial, or postprandial blood glucose levels resulting from defects in insulin production, insulin action, or both. Requires a partnership between the client and health professional for medical care and self-management. Diabetes care is complex and entails addressing many issues beyond glycemic control. A large body of evidence supports a range of interventions to control the disease and lower the risk of complications.

2. The treatment and management of diabetes have made great progress in the past 30 years, and even as this is being written many new options for treatment are being researched and marketed. New products and new medications are becoming available. Examples include real-time continuous glucose monitoring systems, noninvasive blood glucose testing devices, artificial pancreases, new and safer oral medications, new and safer insulin and administration systems, and the search for the cure for Type 1 diabetes.

3. Involves an increasing number of people who need rehabilitation nursing care:

   a. DM is a comorbid condition commonly treated in rehabilitation (along with stroke, heart disease, amputation, renal failure) and is a major management issue.

   b. Optimal recovery from any of these conditions relies primarily on the control of acute and chronic hyperglycemia.

4. Rehabilitation nurses can make a difference in patient outcomes by using current standards of care in diabetes management and effective patient teaching to empower behavior changes (e.g., lifestyle changes in diet, exercise, stress management, and medication administration).

B. Types (Centers for Disease Control and Prevention [CDC], 2005)

1. Type 1

   a. Previously known as insulin-dependent diabetes mellitus or juvenile-onset diabetes

   b. Affects 5%–10% of the total number of people with diabetes

2. Type 2

   a. Previously known as non–insulin-dependent diabetes mellitus, or adult-onset diabetes

   b. Affects 90%–95% of the total number of people with diabetes

3. Gestational diabetes (National Institutes of Health, 2006b)

   a. Hyperglycemia that first appears in pregnancy and usually resolves at birth.

b. An estimated 200,000 American women, approximately 5% of total pregnancies, are diagnosed with gestational diabetes annually (one out of every 100 pregnancies).

4. Other types
    a. Result from specific genetic conditions (e.g., maturity-onset diabetes of youth), surgery, drugs, malnutrition, infections, and other illnesses
    b. Accounts for 1%–5% of all diagnosed cases (CDC, 2005)

5. Prediabetes
    a. Affects 41 million adults in the United States and raises the risk of developing Type 2 diabetes, heart disease, and stroke.
    b. People with prediabetes have blood glucose levels higher than normal but not high enough to be classified as diabetes.

C. Epidemiology and Incidence (CDC, 2005)
1. Diabetes is a global epidemic and burden, with more than 230 million people worldwide having diabetes, and this number is estimated to increase to 350 million by 2050.
2. In the United States a total of 20.8 million people (7.0% of the population) have diabetes: 14.6 million with diagnosed diabetes and 6.2 million with undiagnosed diabetes.
3. CDC predicts the prevalence of diabetes in the United States will double by 2050 and affect more than 48 million people (or 12% of the population).
4. Ethnic minorities and older adults are expected to be disproportionately affected by the increase, with the number of Hispanics with diabetes predicted to rise almost 6-fold.
5. People aged 65 years or older account for almost 40% of the population with diabetes.
6. Diabetes is the sixth most common cause of death in the United States and is the leading cause of adult blindness, chronic renal failure, and nontraumatic lower extremity amputations.
7. People with diabetes have 2 to 4 times the risk of atherosclerosis and are 3 times more likely to have a heart attack or stroke than those who do not have diabetes.
8. The direct and indirect costs of diabetes are staggering, totaling more than $132 billion a year; however, the full burden of diabetes is hard to measure because death records often fail to reflect the role of diabetes, and the costs related to undiagnosed diabetes are unknown.

9. Diabetes is the fourth most common comorbid condition in hospital discharges.
10. Martz et al. (2006) reported a 31% prevalence of known diabetes in hospitalized stroke patients and an additional 16% of patients with unrecognized diabetes and hospital-related hyperglycemia.

D. Etiology (American Diabetes Association [ADA], 2006a)
1. Type 1 diabetes is an autoimmune disorder involving B-cell destruction by islet cell antibodies leading to absolute insulin deficiency.
2. Type 2 is caused primarily by any one or a combination of the following: islet cell malfunction; diminished insulin release pre– and post–insulin receptor; cellular resistance to insulin in fat, liver, and muscle; loss of first-place insulin release (i.e., insulin released within 10 minutes of eating).
3. Gestational diabetes is a form of glucose intolerance diagnosed during pregnancy that uncontrolled puts both mother and baby at risk for complications during the pregnancy and for the mother to have a 20%–50% chance of developing diabetes in the next 5–10 years.
4. Other types of diabetes result from specific genetic conditions (e.g., maturity-onset diabetes of youth, surgery, drugs, malnutrition, infections, and other illnesses) and may account for 1%–5% of all diagnosed cases of diabetes.
5. Prediabetes (ADA, 2006b):
    a. Prediabetes is an elevated risk of developing diabetes as indicated by an impaired fasting glucose (IFG) or impaired glucose tolerance (IGT).
    b. IFG is a condition in which the fasting blood sugar level is elevated (100–125 mg/dl) after an overnight fast but is not high enough to be classified as diabetes.
    c. IGT is a condition in which the blood sugar level is elevated (140–199 mg/dl) after a 2-hour oral glucose tolerance test but is not high enough to be classified as diabetes.
    d. Progression to diabetes among those with prediabetes is not inevitable because weight loss and increased physical activity may prevent or delay diabetes and may return blood glucose levels to normal.

e. People with prediabetes are already at increased risk for other adverse health outcomes such as heart disease and stroke.

E. Risk Factors for Diabetes

   1. Type 1

      a. Family history of diabetes

      b. Age: usually associated with children and young adults, although disease onset can occur at any age

      c. Environmental factors

   2. Type 2

      a. Obesity: body fat of more than 25% for men and more than 30% for women.

      b. Physical inactivity

      c. Environmental factors

      d. Family history of diabetes

      e. Race or ethnicity: African Americans, Hispanic and Latino Americans, American Indians, and some Asian Americans and Native Hawaiians or other Pacific Islanders are at particularly high risk for Type 2 diabetes and its complications.

      f. Age: usually associated with older adults, but type 2 diabetes in children and adolescents is being diagnosed more frequently, particularly in the nonwhite populations listed above.

F. Pathophysiology

   1. Impaired release of insulin from the pancreas

      a. Normal

         1) Phase 1: Stored insulin from beta cells is released within the first 5 minutes after glucose ingestion.

         2) Phase 2: More insulin is released and newly synthesized by beta cells.

      b. In diabetes

         1) Type 1: Endogenous insulin release is deficient.

         2) Type 2: Endogenous insulin release may be normal, inefficient, or deficient.

   2. Insulin resistance

      a. The condition in which normal amounts of insulin are inadequate to produce a normal insulin response from fat, muscle, and liver cells.

      b. Insulin resistance in fat cells results in hydrolysis of stored triglycerides, which elevates free fatty acids in the blood plasma.

      c. Insulin resistance in muscle reduces glucose uptake, whereas insulin resistance in liver reduces glucose storage, with both effects elevating blood glucose.

      d. High plasma levels of insulin and glucose caused by insulin resistance often lead to the metabolic syndrome and Type 2 diabetes.

      e. Leads to insulin deficiency as the pancreas works harder to meet the increasing need to overcome the resistance

   3. Insulin deficiency

      a. Primary problem in Type 1 diabetes

      b. Common in thin people with Type 2 diabetes

      c. Increases in Type 2 diabetes with longevity of the disease

   4. Clinical manifestations (see Table 14-1)

G. Diagnostic Criteria: Results are confirmed 2 different days (ADA, 2006b). For Type 1 or Type 2, any one of the following tests, plus symptoms of diabetes (e.g., polyuria, polydipsia, polyphagia, unexplained weight loss, blurry vision, slow healing, weight loss, numbness or tingling in the hands and feet)

   1. Casual nonfasting plasma glucose (any time of day without consideration of last meal) greater than 200 mg/dl

   2. Fasting plasma glucose (no food for at least 8 hours) greater than 126 mg/dl (preferred method)

   3. 2-hour oral glucose tolerance test, 75-g glucose load test greater than 200 mg/dl (not routinely used because of inconvenience and cost)

H. HbA1c (glycosylated hemoglobin test, also called the A1c test)

   1. Measurement of average glycemic levels in a time scale of 6–9 weeks, which reflects the lifespan of red blood cells (Leahy, Clark, & Cefalu, 2000)

   2. Use of point-of-care testing for HbA1c (A1c) allows timely therapy decisions.

   3. The A1c goal for patients in general is less than 7% (ADA, 2006c).

   4. The A1c goal for the individual patient is an A1c as close to normal (less than 6%) as possible without significant hypoglycemia (ADA, 2006c).

   5. Two studies, the Diabetes Control and Complications Trial and the United Kingdom Prospective Diabetes Study, found that lowering HbA1c levels dramatically reduces

Table 14-1. Symptomatic Manifestations of Diabetes Mellitus

Primary Symptoms	Secondary Symptoms	Tertiary Symptoms
Poor wound healing	Infection, chronic ulceration, limb amputation	Dysfunctional denial
Skin and feet	Dryness and cracking, callus formation, ulceration, deformities (e.g., Charcot's foot)	Dysfunctional grief
		Body image crisis
		Social isolation
Peripheral neuropathy (e.g., numbness, tingling, pain, decreased sensation in extremities)	Cold intolerance, rest and sleep disturbance, inadequate hand and finger movement (e.g., carpal tunnel syndrome)	Ineffective coping with anxiety, reactive depression, anger
Gastroparesis (e.g., bowel, bladder, sexual dysfunction)	Constipation, urinary retention, urinary tract infections, gastroparesis, vaginal dryness, decreased libido and orgasmic ability	Marital conflict or divorce
		Loss of job, financial stability, self–esteem, and self–worth
		Loss of ability to provide adequate self–care, causing loss of independence and control over life, living situation, location (i.e., often needing nursing home placement if unable to do self–insulin management)
Blurred vision, cataracts, blindness, retinopathy	Errors with insulin drawing and mixing, declining ability to visually inspect skin and feet	Falls, accidents
Hypoglycemia	Mild symptoms (sweating, trembling, impaired concentration, dizziness), severe symptoms (mental confusion, lethargy, unconsciousness)	End-stage renal disease
		Microvascular disease
		Macrovascular disease
Hyperglycemia	Specific symptoms (polyuria, polydipsia, blurred vision, polyphagia, weight loss), nonspecific symptoms (weakness, malaise, lethargy, headaches), gastrointestinal symptoms (nausea, vomiting, abdominal pain), respiratory symptoms (Kussmaul's, ketonuria, metabolic acidosis, hyperventilation, coma)	
Weight changes (i.e., more or less than ideal body weight)	Obesity (body fat more than 25% in men and 30% in women) central adipose tissue accumulation, inadequate nutrition	
Chronic systemic dysfunction	Orthostatic hypertension, cardiac denervation, hypoglycemia unaware, proteinuria	

the risks of complications in patients with Type 1 and 2 diabetes (Genuth, 2006).

I. Management Options

1. Medical nutritional therapy (ADA, 2006c)

   a. Eliminate the sugar-restricted diet and the idea that only "diabetic" food can be consumed; focus on serving size and total carbohydrates.

   b. Eliminate predetermined nutrition prescriptions based on ADA caloric formulas and shift to individualized meal plans based on the patient's needs and preferences.

   c. Have a registered dietitian individualize meal plans with specific amounts of carbohydrates, fats, and protein according to height, weight, eating habits, food preferences, lipid profile, blood protein, and other medical conditions (e.g., end-stage renal disease).

   d. Emphasize that both the amount (grams) of carbohydrate and the type of carbohydrate in a food influence blood glucose level.

   e. Monitoring total grams of carbohydrate, whether by use of exchanges or carbohydrate counting, remains a key strategy in achieving glycemic control.

   f. The use of the glycemic index or glycemic load may provide an additional benefit over that observed when total carbohydrate is considered alone.

   g. Low-carbohydrate diets (restricting total carbohydrate to less than 130 g/day) are not generally recommended in the management of diabetes.

   h. To reduce the risk of neuropathy, protein intake should be limited to the recommended dietary allowance (0.8 g/kg) in those with any degree of chronic kidney disease.

   i. Saturated fat intake should be less than 7% of total calories.

   j. Intake of trans fat should be minimized.

k. Weight loss is recommended for all overweight (body mass index 25.0–29.9 kg/m2) or obese (body mass index greater than 30.0 kg/m2) adults who have or are at risk for developing Type 2 diabetes.

l. The primary approach for achieving weight loss is therapeutic lifestyle change: reduction in energy intake and increase in physical activity plus a moderate decrease in caloric balance, supplying at least 1,000 kcal/day for women and 1,200 kcal/day for men, resulting in slow but progressive weight loss (1–2 lb/week).

m. Nonnutritive sweeteners are safe when consumed within the acceptable daily intake levels established by the U.S. Food and Drug Administration (FDA).

n. Alcohol use should be limited to a moderate amount (1 drink per day or less for adult women and 2 drinks per day or less for adult men); 1 drink is defined as 12 oz beer, 5 oz wine, or 1.5 oz distilled spirits.

o. Routine supplementation with antioxidants, such as vitamins E and C and beta-carotene, is not advised because of lack of evidence of efficacy and concern over long-term safety.

p. Benefit of chromium supplementation in people with diabetes or obesity has not been conclusively demonstrated.

2. Exercise therapy

a. Initial physical activity recommendations should be modest and based on the patient's willingness and ability, gradually increasing the duration and frequency to 30–45 minutes of moderate aerobic activity 3–5 days per week (goal at least 150 min/week).

b. Greater activity levels of at least 1 hour a day of moderate (e.g., walking) or 30 minutes a day of vigorous (e.g., jogging) activity may be needed to achieve successful long-term weight loss.

c. Exercise options and strategies for self-directed exercise can be identified by a physical therapist.

d. Benefits, effects, risks, and precautions vary depending on:
   1) Age and type of diabetes
   2) Physical conditioning and presence of other chronic diseases
   3) Presence of ketonuria

3. Medication therapy (Chitre & Burke, 2006)

a. Oral agents:
   1) Classifications of oral antidiabetic agents include first- and second-generation sulfonylureas (tolazamide, glyburide, glipizide, glimepiride), biguanides (metformin), meglitinides or nonsulfonylurea secretagogues (repaglinide, nateglinide), alpha-glucosidase inhibitors (acarbose, miglitol), thiazolidinediones (pioglitazone, rosiglitazone), and the newest class, dipeptidyl-peptidase 4 inhibitors (sitagliptin).
   2) Each class of drugs differs in its modes and sites of action, advantages, and disadvantages, and the choice of agent for each person should be made in consideration of the person's overall health status.
   3) Oral antidiabetic agents may act by stimulating pancreatic insulin production and secretion; decreasing hepatic glucose production; decreasing intestinal glucose absorption; increasing insulin sensitivity; inhibiting glucagon release; reducing rate of gastric emptying; or mediating satiety centrally, resulting in reduced food intake (e.g., biguanide works in the liver, small intestine, and peripheral tissues to decrease hepatic glucose production and intestinal glucose absorption and improves insulin sensitivity; sitagliptin slows the inactivation of incretin hormones and improves pancreatic beta cell insulin synthesis and release, lowers pancreatic alpha cell glucagon secretion, and reduces hepatic glucose production [Merck & Co., 2006]).
   4) Medication regimens can be simple or complex, with options for monotherapy or polytherapy with dual agents or triple agents.
   5) Complexity of regimen is increased by addition of insulin therapy to oral therapy (e.g., bedtime insulin and daytime orals) when oral therapy alone is no longer effective.
   6) Evidence supports combination of biguanides with insulin to improve weight management and glycemic control and reduce congestive heart disease risk.

b. Injectable agents other than insulin (Odegard, Setter, & Iltz, 2006):

1) Exenatide (Byetta, 2007), an incretin mimetic for the treatment of Type 2 DM in patients experiencing inadequate glycemic control with oral DM medications, is not approved to be used with insulin. It reduces fasting and postprandial glucose concentrations though glucose-dependent insulin secretion, restores first-phase insulin response, regulates glucagon secretion, delays gastric emptying, reduces appetite, and helps to lower weight (McKennon & Campbell, 2007; Odegard et al., 2006).
2) Pramlintide, synthetic analog of the hormone amylin found to be deficient in Type 1 DM, used as an adjunct therapy with mealtime insulin, slows gastric emptying, curbs appetite, suppresses postprandial plasma glucagon and hepatic glucose output, and helps mediate satiety centrally, resulting in decreased caloric intake and promoting weight loss; approved for people with Type 1 DM and Type 2 DM taking insulin (Odegard et al., 2006).

c. Insulin types usually address basal insulin (e.g., fasting) and bolus (e.g., preprandial glucose level and postprandial excursion) (LaSalle, 2006):
1) Traditional basal insulin (e.g., neutral protein Hagedorn [NPH] insulin), onset 2–4 hours, peak 4–10 hours, duration 10–16 hours)
2) Traditional bolus insulin (Novolin R, Humulin R), onset 30–60 minutes, peak 2.5–5 hours, duration 6–8 hours
3) Analog basal insulin (e.g., glargine [Lantus], detemir [Levemir]), onset 1 hour, duration 21–24 hours, no peak, mimics continuous insulin infusion
4) Analog bolus insulin (preferred because of improvements over traditional insulins: more rapid onset and more consistent in absorption rate, increases flexibility in meal and activity timing (e.g., glulisine [Apidra], lispro [Humalog], aspart [NovoLog]), average onset 10–15 minutes, peak 30–45 minutes, duration, 2–4 hours

d. Insulin regimens are numerous, ranging from simple to complex, and will challenge the rehabilitation nurse; the following is limited to the basic regimens because the ideal is a individualized program suited to the person's needs, lifestyle, and resources (Diabetes Health, 2006).

e. Combination regimens:
1) Daily routine doses of long-lasting insulin (basal) (e.g., NPH, glargine, or detemir) may be combined with a secretagogue with or without additional oral sensitizer.
2) Premixtures (e.g., NPH 50/regular 50, NPH 70/regular 30, Humulin R 70/70 or Novolin R 70/30, NPH 75/lispro 25, Humalog mix 75/25, NPH 70/aspart 30, Novolog mix 70/30) twice daily with or without oral sensitizers normally used for convenience and to improve compliance.

f. Intensive conventional therapy (LaSalle, 2006):
1) Multiple daily injections 0.2–0.6 initial units per kilogram with or without oral sensitizers, 50% bolus (rapid-acting insulin) at meals, and 50% basal insulin (i.e., NPH, glargine, or detemir) once or twice a day
2) Daily routine doses of basal insulin (i.e., NPH, glargine, or detemir) once or twice daily with fast-acting insulin boluses using carbohydrate/insulin ratios calculated according to future carbohydrate consumption
3) Provides flexibility (e.g., a meal can be delayed and less consumed because the bolus amount is determined by the amount of food eaten compared to having to take the right amount of food at the right time to match the action of the traditional insulin, such as NPH)

g. Correction dose (previously called sliding scale): bolus dose of rapid- or fast-acting insulin calculated on actual blood glucose level

h. Injection therapy (LaSalle, 2006):
1) Absorption rates differ between sites and types of insulins: The abdomen is the fastest, followed by the arms, thighs, and buttocks, less absorption variability with the analog insulin.
2) Lipohypertrophy usually slows absorption, less of a problem with the analog insulins.
3) Exercise increases the rate of

absorption by providing increased blood flow to the injection site, less of a problem with the analog insulin.

i. Inhaled insulin therapy (LifeMed Media, 2006):

1) Inhaled powder form of recombinant human insulin (rDNA) that is administered into the mouth through an inhaler device

2) Rapid-acting insulin only, causing the continued need for injections of a basal (long-acting) insulin

3) Peak insulin levels can be achieved at 49 minutes (range 30–90 minutes) with inhaled insulin, compared with 105 minutes (range 60–240 minutes) with regular insulin

4) In Type 1 diabetes, inhaled insulin may be added to longer-acting insulin as a replacement for short-acting bolus injections taken with meals.

5) In Type 2 diabetes, inhaled insulin may be used alone, with oral medications that control blood sugar, or with longer-acting insulin.

6) Inhaled insulin is not recommended for smokers, people who recently stopped smoking (within the last 6 months), or people with asthma, bronchitis, or emphysema.

7) Baseline tests for lung function are recommended after the first 6 months of treatment and every year thereafter.

j. Insulin pump therapy (Scheiner, 2006; Unger & Marcus, 2004):

1) Insulin pumps are devices used for administering insulin, consisting of controls, processing module, batteries, insulin reservoir, and a catheter to carry the insulin into the subcutaneous tissue.

2) Insulin pumps make it possible to deliver continuous small amounts of fast-acting (basal) and a mealtime bolus dose, providing tighter control over blood sugar and reducing the chance of long-term complications (i.e., blindness, amputation, renal disease).

3) Costs can run into the thousands of dollars for initial setup and continued maintenance including the costs of insulin, batteries, and infusion catheter sets.

4) Insurance and Medicare may pay up to 80% of the costs of pump therapy.

5) Numbers of insulin pump users continue to rise, and pump features continue to advance.

6) Patients using their pumps often rebel against forced removal.

7) Rehabilitation nurses must be prepared to deal with the patient who continues to use the pump during an inpatient stay.

8) Pump use may be helpful in achieving glycemic control by its ability to match the typical insulin pattern of a person without diabetes.

9) Transitioning on and off a pump can entail a complex series of insulin management plans and orders from the physician and coordination of pharmacy and nursing staff.

10) A comprehensive plan should be in place for the safe use of an insulin pump using the Joint Commission standards regarding a facility's responsibility for the cleanliness and maintenance of any home medical equipment and the competency of staff responsible for overseeing the equipment.

J. Hospital Inpatient Diabetes and Glycemic Control (ADA, 2006a)

1. Poorly controlled blood glucose levels are associated with increased morbidity and mortality and with higher healthcare costs caused by increased length of stay, complications, and readmissions.

2. Both undertreatment and overtreatment of hyperglycemia are safety issues in the hospitalized patient and considered errors of omission because hyperglycemia creates an unsafe setting for the treatment of illness and diabetes.

3. Use of intensive insulin therapy to achieve glucose levels of 80–110 mg/dl reduced mortality by 34%, sepsis by 46%, renal failure by 41%, and need for blood transfusion by 50% (Bloomgarden & Mechanick, 2007; Van den Berghe et al., 2001).

4. New glucose guidelines for hospitalized patients established by the American Association of Clinical Endocrinologists and the ADA: 80–110 mg/dl for intensive care units and 110–180 mg/dl other units with or without a diagnosis of diabetes; modify for unstable cardiac disease, hypoglycemia unawareness, or recurrent hypoglycemia (Bloomgarden & Mechanick, 2007).

5. ADA targets for most adults with diabetes: premeal 90–130 mg/dl and postmeal (1–2 hours after eating) less than 180 mg/dl.

6. Lower or higher targets may be recommended for certain people who are at lower or higher risk for hypoglycemia, especially patients going to physical therapy as part of their rehabilitation program.

7. Protocols or algorithms and order sets guide the management of hyperglycemia and hypoglycemia (i.e., Portland insulin drip protocol, Providence Health System, 2004).

K. Acute Problems Associated with Diabetes

1. Hypoglycemia

   a. Not eating, too much insulin or oral diabetes medication, extra exercise, alcohol, certain cancers, critical illnesses such as kidney, liver, or heart failure, hormonal deficiencies

   b. Symptoms
      1) Mild: sweating, trembling, difficulty concentrating, lightheadedness, blurred vision
      2) Specific: inability to self-treat, mental confusion, lethargy, unconsciousness
      3) Hypoglycemia unawareness may be present due to autonomic neuropathy, with loss of warning neuroglycopenic symptoms resulting from deficient sympathetic neuronal (norepinephrine) and adrenomedullary (epinephrine) responses to falling glucose levels.
      4) Some medications may mask symptoms (e.g., beta blockers).

   c. Treatment options
      1) Begin with administration of 10–15 g (5–10 g for children) fast-acting carbohydrate (e.g., three glucose tablets or 1 small tube of glucose gel, two tablespoons raisins, 8 oz lowfat milk, half a can of regular soda).
      2) Retest blood glucose level after 15 minutes.
      3) Give an additional 15 g carbohydrate if blood glucose is still less than 70 mg/dl.
      4) Consider preference, allergies, and food intolerance when making treatment choices (e.g., glucose gel for patients with dysphagia).
      5) Patients taking glucosidase inhibitors (acarbose or nateglinide) must use glucose (dextrose) tablets or, if

unavailable, milk or honey (Prandase, 2001).
      6) Be careful not to overtreat and cause rebound hyperglycemia.
      7) Using a food with added fat (e.g., chocolate bar) is not recommended because fat may slow down the body's absorption of the carbohydrate.
      8) The use of protein to keep blood glucose up after a low is not necessary and may add calories and promote weight gain.
      9) Follow the treatment with a snack or scheduled meal if 2 hours before the next meal.
      10) Severe hypoglycemia may be treated with glucagon injection or intravenous glucose.
      11) Prevention of low blood glucose is the best treatment (e.g., not skipping meals, eating 6 small meals a day instead of 3 large ones, taking the fast-acting bolus insulin after a meal instead of before, reducing amount of insulin or oral diabetes medications before exercise, frequent monitoring of blood glucose before and after exercise, and taking a snack if indicated before exercising) (Feigenbaum, 2006).

2. Hyperglycemia

   a. Causes: eating too much food; not enough insulin or oral diabetes medication; physical stress such as a cold, infection, or the flu; emotional stress such as family conflict; problems with the insulin; or medications (e.g., corticosteroids, phenytoin)

   b. Symptoms
      1) Specific: polyuria, polydipsia, blurred vision, dysphagia, weight loss
      2) Nonspecific: weakness, malaise, lethargy, headache
      3) Gastrointestinal: nausea, vomiting, abdominal pain
      4) Respiratory: Kussmaul's breathing, metabolic acidosis, hyperventilation

   c. Treatment: insulin and fluids

   d. Prevention of hyperglycemia: eating correct number and portion sizes of carbohydrates established per individual needs, taking medications on time, limiting snacking, treating infections and illness, controlling stress, increasing exercise, limiting fats

3. Other complications associated with diabetes

   a. Cardiovascular disease is the major cause of mortality for people with diabetes (ADA, 2006c).

   b. Diabetes is an independent risk factor for macrovascular disease and its common coexisting conditions (e.g., hypertension and dyslipidemia).

   c. Other complications (e.g., Charcot's foot, amputations, neuropathy, gastroparesis, depression, retinopathy, nephropathy, and autonomic nerve disease, which affects nerves that control heartbeat, digestion, and other automatic functions).

4. Self–blood glucose testing and diabetes medication administration

   a. The rehabilitation nurse often is responsible for initiating self-monitoring of blood glucose and self-medication administration (e.g., self-administering of insulin) for newly diagnosed patients and ensuring that those with previous skills are competent, knowledgeable, and safe.

   b. Facilities that follow Joint Commission standards and allow patients to use their own glucose monitors and provide new monitors for education purposes should review the home medical equipment standards from the Joint Commission.

   c. The rehabilitation nurse may find it helpful to refer the patient learning diabetes self-management skills to a certified diabetes educator on staff or in the community (American Association of Diabetes Educators, 2006).

   d. Adding the specialty practice of diabetes education is a possibility for every rehabilitation nurse; information about this additional specialty can be obtained from the American Association of Diabetes Educators (http://www.aadenet.org).

   e. Facilities need written policies, procedures, and medical staff approval to ensure the safety and legality of the self-monitoring and self-medication administration programs.

L. Nursing Process

   1. Assessment

      a. Gather objective data: Determine type of diabetes and classification. Patients with hyperglycemia can be classified into one of three categories: previously diagnosed DM, unrecognized DM, or hyperglycemia related to hospitalization (ADA, 2003, 2006b).

      b. Gather subjective data: Determine the patient's self-perceived compliance with medical and nutritional prescriptions for medication administration, blood glucose monitoring, meal planning, exercise, foot and skin care, sick day management, and treatment and preventive methods for high and low glucose levels.

      c. Determine the patient's acceptance of the disease, the effect on his or her lifestyle, and perceived social and economic barriers to compliance.

      d. Observe the patient's functional ability and physical and psychological barriers (e.g., verbal and nonverbal communication, mobility, vision, cognition).

      e. Observe the patient's ability in self–glucose testing, self–insulin drawing and administration, and foot and skin care.

   2. Plan of care

      a. Nursing diagnoses

         1) Ineffective individual coping related to denial and depression

         2) Knowledge deficit related to disease cause, progression, and treatments

         3) Self-care deficits related to the following:

            a) Physical, social, economic, and psychological barriers and limitations (e.g., medication administration, self–glucose testing)

            b) Neuropathy, limited mobility, and poor vision (e.g., foot and skin care)

            c) Lack of knowledge of target blood glucose levels

            d) Lack of financial and social support systems

            e) Lack of knowledge of follow-up needs and prevention of further complications related to the disease process

         4) Altered nutritional intake (more or less than body needs) related to lack of awareness about serving sizes, limited self-discipline, and noncompliance with dietary guidelines

         5) Sensory–perceptual alterations related to neuropathy

         6) Sexual dysfunction related to

microvascular and macrovascular impairment

b. Goals
1) State barriers to and develop methods of effective coping with diabetes.
2) Increase level of independent self-administration of medication and glucose testing.
3) Perform or direct daily foot checks and skin care.
4) Identify adequate nutritional intake according to ADA guidelines.
5) Practice selecting proper serving sizes of favorite foods.
6) Identify ways to compensate for altered sensory–perceptual sensations.
7) Identify individual concerns with and compensate for sexual dysfunction.
8) Learn normal and target blood glucose levels.
9) Identify variances of blood glucose levels, corrective actions, and when to call for help.
10) State sick day care.
11) Identify and obtain needed adaptive equipment (e.g., talking meters, insulin bottle holders, dose-dialing insulin syringes, premixed syringes, magnifying guides).
12) Identify and obtain insurance and Medicare, Medicaid benefits for diabetes education and equipment (e.g., meters, strips, lancets, therapeutic shoes).

3. Interventions
a. Teach coping strategies (e.g., stress management, humor, breathing exercises).
b. Provide opportunities for assisted practice with self-medication program (e.g., drawing, mixing, and injecting insulin).
c. Direct daily self–foot checks and skin care (e.g., using skin cream).
d. Promote identification and selection of proper number and size of carbohydrate servings for individualized meal programs (e.g., 4 carbohydrate servings would total 60 g carbohydrate, 15 g carbohydrate times 4 food choices).
e. Suggest ways to compensate for altered sensory–perceptual sensations (e.g., wear diabetic socks at night to increase warmth, circulation, and comfort).
f. Teach compensation for sexual dysfunction (e.g., cream for vaginal dryness, enhancer medications and pumps for men).
g. Teach problem-solving skills to treat and prevent blood glucose variances and to know when and how to get help.
h. Teach use of adaptive equipment (e.g., talking meters, insulin bottle holders).
i. Teach survival skills and suggest follow-up education and self-management support as needed after dismissal from the hospital.
j. Discuss insurance and Medicare, Medicaid benefits for education, equipment, and continued assistance (e.g., nursing home or assisted living placement, support groups).
k. Discuss follow-up care (e.g., annual eye exam, HbA1c test, kidney function test).
l. Teach sick day management (e.g., increase frequency of blood glucose testing, when to call the doctor).

II. Multiple Sclerosis (MS)

A. Overview
1. A chronic neuroimmunologic condition that affects the white matter of the central nervous system (CNS).
2. Affects primarily adults in the prime years of life
3. Characterized by numerous etiologic possibilities, an uncertain prognosis, and a course that consists of episodes of remission and relapse
4. An unpredictable disease that can result in diverse neurologic impairments and necessitates a collaborative approach to care
5. A degenerative progressive disease characterized by inflammation, demyelination (loss of the myelin sheath that surrounds the nerve fiber tracts), and scarring of the myelin sheath in the CNS
6. Involves partial or complete destruction of the myelin sheath followed by sclerotic plaques or scar tissue formation
7. Is associated with various signs and symptoms caused by the loss of myelin sheath integrity that interferes with the efficiency of nerve impulse conduction in the CNS
8. The name *multiple sclerosis* signifies that myelin is lost in multiple areas, leaving scar tissue.

B. Epidemiology
1. Incidence

a. Currently there are approximately 350,000–500,000 people affected with MS in the United States and 2.5 million people worldwide (Multiple Sclerosis Foundation, 2006; National Multiple Sclerosis Society, 2005).

b. Approximately 200 people are diagnosed every week (National Multiple Sclerosis Society, 2005).

c. A major cause of disability and economic hardship in young adults between the ages of 20 and 40.

d. Occurs more often in women than men, in people who live in colder northern latitudes, in Caucasians, and in people who have first-degree relatives with MS (Monahan, Sands, Neighbors, Marek, & Green, 2007).

e. The number of children with MS is climbing, and statistics suggest there may be 20,000 undiagnosed children in the United States with MS because healthcare providers do not typically associate MS with children (Steefel, 2006).

2. Disease patterns

a. Relapsing–remitting MS: the most typical pattern of the disease
   1) Defined by episodes with clear relapses (also known as exacerbations or acute attacks) followed by either complete or partial recovery periods (remission) free of disease progression
   2) Involves no disease progression between relapses

b. Secondary progressive MS
   1) Can begin as a relapsing–remitting course followed by progression that is unpredictable
   2) Involves acute attacks that can result in a progressive worsening level of disability

c. Primary progressive MS: identified by a slow but continuous worsening of the patient's disability but with no actual relapses or remissions

d. Progressive relapsing MS
   1) Marked by disease progression from the onset with definite acute relapses
   2) Involves disease progression that continues to escalate between relapses

C. Etiology

1. The specific cause remains unknown.

2. Factors that may be involved in causing MS are viral, immunologic, and genetic susceptibility.

a. A latent viral infection may either cause inflammation of white matter or trigger an autoimmune reaction that precipitates demyelination.

b. Although there is no specific genetic pattern of transmission for MS, researchers support a multigenic predisposition that makes certain people susceptible to the disease (Lewis, Heitkemper, & Dirksen, 2004; National Multiple Sclerosis Society, 2006).

c. Various stressors such as emotional stress, fatigue, pregnancy, viral infection, extreme physical exertion, trauma, and secondary illness have been suggested as triggers for MS.

D. Pathophysiology

1. Overview

a. Normally, an intact blood–brain barrier protects the brain from immune cell activity. In MS, the protective barrier is breached as activated T cells migrate into the CNS, triggering antibody–antigen reaction, resulting in inflammation, leading to loss of myelin, disappearance of oligodendrocytes, and proliferation of astrocytes or scavenger cells that remove the damaged myelin, forming scar tissue over the affected area (Lewis et al., 2004; Monahan et al., 2007).

b. Inflammation and oligodendrocyte loss are found in MS, but which comes first has been a focus of some recent research (Lewis et al., 2004).

c. Demyelination appears as diffuse and discrete lesions (plaques) throughout the brain and spinal cord.
   1) Although natural healing (remyelination) by oligodendrocytes may restore some myelin function, the characteristic plaque formation or sclerosis interferes with normal nerve conduction.
   2) Nerve impulses slow down initially; eventually, with permanently damaged nerve fibers the impulses are completely blocked.
   3) Sites of demyelination can occur anywhere in the CNS, producing a wide range of signs and symptoms; however, progressive scarring leads to progressive deterioration in

neurological function (Lewis et al., 2004; White & Duncan, 2002).

2. Clinical manifestations (see Table 14-2)

   a. Primary symptoms

      1) Occur as the result of the nerve conduction deficits caused by demyelination and plaque formation

      2) Reflect a specific area of dysfunction in the CNS

      3) Symptoms may range from mild to severe; symptoms are unpredictable and vary from person to person and from time to time in the same person.

   b. Secondary symptoms

      1) Occur as a consequence of primary symptoms

      2) Include problematic complications resulting from decreased neurologic function

   c. Tertiary symptoms

      1) Evolve as the cumulative and detrimental effects of the disease affect all aspects of the person's life

      2) Include psychosocial, vocational, financial, and emotional problems

3. Diagnosis

   a. There is no specific laboratory or radiologic test to definitively diagnose MS.

   b. Because MS can mimic other diseases and the initial symptomatic presentation varies and fluctuates so greatly in severity, the diagnosis of MS is a challenge and a process of eliminating all other possibilities.

   c. A diagnosis of MS is based on a history of episodic neurologic disability and actual signs of neurologic dysfunction on physical examination. Basic rule for diagnosis: Two attacks (relapses or exacerbations) occur at least 1 month apart, and the location of the lesions must be in at least 2 distinct sites in the CNS (Barker, 2002; Lewis et al., 2004).

   d. Diagnostic tests that can support a suspected MS diagnosis include the following:

      1) Magnetic resonance imaging (MRI)

         a) Extremely sensitive to white matter lesions and useful in identifying demyelinated plaque in the CNS

         b) Is used to distinguish between old and new lesions and to monitor disease progression

      2) Cerebrospinal fluid analysis: reveals elevated immunoglobulin G and the presence of oligoclonal (immunoglobulin G) bands and increased protein (Barker, 2002; Lazoff, 2005)

      3) Evoked potential studies (somatosensory, auditory, visual): demonstrate a slow, absent, or abnormal response in electrical impulse conduction

E. Management Options

   1. Goal: to decrease the number and frequency of relapses, enhance recovery from exacerbations, alleviate symptoms, maintain independence, and ensure the highest quality of life (Lewis et al., 2004; Monahan et al., 2007)

   2. Pharmacotherapy (see Figure 14-1)

      a. Involves the potential use of drugs from different classes, such as anti-inflammatory agents, immunomodulators, immunosuppressants, and others for symptom management

Table 14-2. Symptomatic Manifestations of Multiple Sclerosis

Primary Symptoms	Secondary Symptoms	Tertiary Symptoms
Muscle weakness, paralysis, spasticity, and hyperreflexia	Falls, fractures, skin breakdown, contractures, and other injuries	Loss of job
Mild to disabling fatigue	Marked reduction in carrying out all aspects of self-care	Complete change in roles
Visual impairments (e.g., diplopia, scotoma, decreased acuity)	Decreased safety caused by decreased visual input	Social isolation
	Interruption in rest and disrupted sleep	Divorce
Numbness, tingling, pain, and tremors	Urinary tract infections, bowel and bladder incontinence or retention, and marked decline in libido and orgasmic ability	Ineffective coping with anxiety, denial, anger, reactive depression, and suicide
Bowel, bladder, and sexual dysfunction		
Ataxia, nystagmus, dysarthria (scanning speech), and dysphagia	Problems affecting a safe gait pattern, communication ability, and swallowing function	Loss of financial stability, self-esteem, and self-worth
Cognitive changes (e.g., memory loss, impaired judgment), emotional lability, and depression	Marked decline in healthy and effective coping strategies	

The Specialty Practice of Rehabilitation Nursing: A Core Curriculum, 5th Ed.

b.	Is most often used to treat spasticity and tremor, urinary retention or frequency, chronic pain, fatigue, and depression

3.	Alternative approaches (e.g., bee venom therapy, massage, herbal treatment, dietary modifications)

4.	Use of a collaborative team of professionals, including physicians, physical and occupational therapists, spiritual advisers, social workers, psychologists, vocational rehabilitation specialists, legal advisers, and nurses

5.	Exercise

a.	Aquatic or water therapy gives buoyancy to the body, allowing performance of activities that otherwise would not be possible.

b.	Yoga and tai chi can be beneficial.

c.	Avoid exercises that are fatiguing.

6.	Nutritional therapy

a.	A high-protein, low-fat, and low-cholesterol diet with supplemental vitamins is recommended (Lewis et al., 2004; Multiple Sclerosis Foundation, 2006).

b.	Natural fiber is encouraged to promote bowel regularity.

F.	Nursing Process

1.	Assessment

a.	Obtain a complete health history and information about current symptoms, time of onset, and past history of relapses, including recent or past viral infections or vaccinations, physical or emotional stress, pregnancy, or exposure to extremes of heat and cold.

b.	Pay particular attention to mental state and overt coping abilities.

c.	Determine how the disease has affected the patient's lifestyle and family.

d.	Observe the patient's overall appearance.

e.	Investigate physical mobility, urinary elimination, self-care activities, and safety concerns.

f.	Assess for spasticity, weakness, incontinence, and visual impairments.

g.	Investigate use of and compliance in taking prescription medications and alternative approaches.

2.	Plan of care

a.	Nursing diagnoses

1)	Impaired physical mobility related to neuromuscular impairment (weakness, spasticity, and tremor)

Figure 14-1. Pharmacotherapeutic Agents Used to Treat MS

Treatment of Acute Relapses
Short course of anti-inflammatory corticosteroids
• Methylprednisolone (Solu-Medrol)
• Adrenocorticotropic hormone
• Prednisone

Treatment to Reduce the Frequency of Relapses
Parenteral injections of immunomodulators (effective for only one or two MS disease patterns)
• Interferon beta-1b (Betaseron)
• Interferon beta-1a (Avonex, Rebif)
• Glatiramer acetate (Copaxone)

Treatment of Disease Progression
Immunosuppressants that halt disease progression
• Azathioprine (Imuran)
• Methotrexate (Rheumatrex)

Treatment of Spasticity and Tremor
• Baclofen (Lioresal)
• Dantrolene (Dantrium)
• Tizanidine (Zanaflex)
• Diazepam (Valium)
• Clonazepam (Klonopin)
• Botulinum toxin (Botox)

Treatment of Urinary Retention
• Bethanechol chloride (Urecholine)

Treatment of Urinary Frequency and Urgency
• Propantheline (Pro-Banthine)
• Oxybutynin (Ditropan)

Treatment of Chronic Pain, Fatigue, and Depression
• Carbamazepine (Tegretol)
• Pemoline (Cylert)
• Amitriptyline (Elavil)
• Imipramine (Tofranil)
• Fluoxetine (Prozac)

---

2)	Fatigue related to the MS disease process

3)	Self-care deficits (e.g., bathing, dressing, feeding, toileting) related to weakness, spasticity, and tremor

4)	Altered urinary elimination (e.g., retention, frequency, urgency) related to spinal cord involvement and decreased functional ability

5)	Knowledge deficit related to the variable nature of symptoms and multifaceted treatment options

6)	Ineffective individual coping related to the variability of the disease course, cognitive impairments, decreased independence, and changes in family and vocational roles

7)	Sensory perception alterations: visual, related to optic nerve involvement (diplopia, nystagmus, blurred vision)

8) Chronic pain related to neuropathy
b. Goals
   1) Maintain maximal level of mobility.
   2) Demonstrate safety in mobility and recognize the need for appropriate assistive devices.
   3) Conserve energy and verbalize understanding of ways to integrate energy conservation principles into daily activities.
   4) Attain maximal level of function in activities of daily living (ADLs).
   5) Maintain continence and identify symptoms of urinary tract infection.
   6) Verbalize understanding of the disease process, significant implications, and prescribed regimens.
   7) Verbalize appropriate plans for coping with stress.
   8) Attain maximal visual functioning and demonstrate satisfactory use of compensatory measures when needed.
   9) Verbalize satisfactory pain relief.

3. Nursing interventions
   a. Improve mobility and neuromuscular function.
      1) Encourage progressive, resistive exercises according to the prescribed physical therapy program to maintain function of the uninvolved nerves.
      2) Gradually build up tolerance through a daily exercise program.
      3) Use assistive devices (e.g., walker, cane, wheelchair, motorized scooter).
      4) Avoid physical and emotional stressors.
      5) Avoid exposure to extreme heat and schedule activities to occur in the cooler part of the day; ensure that air conditioning is available in warm weather.
   b. Conserve energy.
      1) Avoid vigorous exercise.
      2) Ensure that the patient gets adequate sleep and rests frequently.
      3) Space out activities and allow rest periods.
   c. Maintain independence in ADLs.
      1) Encourage a balance between assisted and independent activities.
      2) Encourage the use of assistive devices to promote patient's independence.
      3) Avoid extremes in body temperature and use air conditioning when needed.
   d. Improve bladder function and prevent complications.
      1) Avoid giving the patient caffeinated beverages and encourage high daily fluid intake (approximately 3,000 ml per day).
      2) Administer medications to improve muscle tone of bladder and facilitate emptying and instruct patient on effective use of medication.
      3) Teach intermittent self-catheterization or external catheter procedures.
      4) Use Crede's maneuver or manual reflex stimulation for emptying reflexic bladder (unless contraindicated by complications such as detrusor sphincter dyssynergia).
      5) Instruct the patient to identify and prevent urinary tract infections.
   e. Improve knowledge.
      1) Provide information to help manage the disease on a continuous basis.
      2) Encourage the patient to ask questions.
      3) Review educational information with the patient and family.
   f. Develop effective coping strategies to adjust to the illness.
      1) Encourage the patient and family to verbalize feelings and concerns.
      2) Refer the patient and family to support groups (e.g., Multiple Sclerosis Association of America, National Multiple Sclerosis Society).
      3) Make referrals for psychological counseling as necessary.
   g. Maintain visual functioning.
      1) Administer treatment as needed (eye patch or occluder, medications).
      2) Instruct the patient to rest eyes when fatigue is noticed.
      3) Advise patient of availability of large-type material and talking books.
   h. Promote comfort.
      1) Provide medication as ordered for pain control and instruct patient on effective use of medications and precautions.
      2) Encourage use of alternative pain relief measures (distraction, relaxation, imagery, music, massage).

3) Assess effectiveness of pain relief measures.

III. Parkinson's Disease (PD)

A. Overview

1. PD is a slowly progressive neurodegenerative disease of the brain.

2. PD involves manifestations that occur when there is significant damage to or destruction of dopamine-producing neurons in the substantia nigra within the basal ganglia of the brain.

3. PD begins insidiously and is characterized by a prolonged course of illness.

4. Loss of dopamine causes neurons to fire out of control, leading to marked disability with the initiation and execution of smooth coordinated voluntary movements and balance.

5. There is no known way to stop or cure the disease.

6. PD is one of the more common chronic diseases of the nervous system.

B. Types

1. Primary PD

a. A chronic debilitating disease caused by an idiopathic dopamine deficiency in the basal ganglia of the brain

b. Characterized by tremor, rigidity, bradykinesia, and postural instability

2. Secondary parkinsonism or parkinsonism syndrome: a group of symptoms (e.g., tremors, stiffness, slow movements) where there is a known cause of injury to the dopamine-producing cells

C. Epidemiology and Incidence

1. 1.5 million Americans have PD. The disease shows no socioeconomic or cultural preferences (Parkinson's Disease Foundation, 2005).

2. Approximately 40,000–50,000 new cases are diagnosed annually in the United States (Monahan et al., 2007; Springhouse, 2002).

3. PD occurs in men slightly more often than women.

4. PD most commonly occurs after age 50. With an aging population, the prevalence of PD is likely to increase.

5. Approximately 10% of people with PD are younger than age 40, however the incidence in younger persons has been growing (Monahan et al., 2007).

D. Etiology

1. Primary PD is idiopathic.

2. A number of theories of causation for PD are being tested, including viral, vascular, metabolic, environmental, event, and genetic, although PD is currently believed to be associated with a combination of genetic and environmental factors (e.g., viruses, toxins, free radical exposure) (Monahan et al., 2007).

3. Secondary parkinsonism may be linked to a variety of causes: response to antipsychotic, antihypertensive, or neuroleptic agents or illicit drug use; response to brain trauma, tumors, ischemia, encephalitis infections, and arteriosclerosis; response to neurotoxins such as cyanide, manganese, carbon monoxide, and pesticides (Monahan et al., 2007).

E. Pathophysiology

1. Overview

a. Degenerative changes in several areas in the basal ganglia deplete the inhibitory neurotransmitter dopamine, normally provided to the basal ganglia by the neurons in the substantia nigra.

1) Dopamine is a neurotransmitter essential for the functioning of the extrapyramidal system, which includes control of upright posture, support, and voluntary motion.

2) Normally, there is a balance between the neurotransmitters dopamine and acetylcholine (ACh), which are responsible for controlling and refining motor movements and have opposing effects.

b. An increase in the excitatory effects of ACh caused by depletion of dopamine causes the manifestations of PD and prevents affected brain cells from performing their normal inhibitory function in the CNS.

c. A shift in the balance of neurotransmitter activity is responsible for the patient's difficulty in controlling and initiating voluntary movements (Lewis et al., 2004).

d. As the disease progresses, dopamine receptors in the basal ganglia are reduced.

2. Clinical features: classic manifestations (Barker, 2002; Monahan et al., 2007)

a. Tremor:

1) Occurs in the tongue, lips, jaw, chin, head, and limbs

2) May involve a pill-rolling movement of the thumb and finger
3) Is present at rest and diminishes with active movement

b. Rigidity or cogwheeling: resistance to movement caused by constant contraction of opposing muscle groups due to abnormal muscle stiffness and jerky movements with passive motion

c. Bradykinesia or akinesia: inability to initiate movement or change movement, which results in abnormal slowness

d. Postural instability, which causes a stooped-over, flexed posture, no arm swing with a shuffling propulsive gait. Diminished postural reflexes lead to frequent falls that are associated with balance and coordination problems.

e. Other symptoms: masklike facial appearance; difficulty with chewing, swallowing, and voice changes; autonomic disturbances (e.g., orthostatic hypotension, constipation, excessive perspiration, oily skin); and numerous cognitive losses (e.g., memory, problem solving, depression)

3. Diagnosis (Monahan et al., 2007)

a. Diagnosis is made clinically from the patient's history and presenting symptoms.

b. No specific laboratory or radiologic studies are available to support a positive diagnosis.

c. Positron emission tomography scan may detect low levels of dopamine (not typically done because of high cost and unavailability).

d. Definitive diagnosis may be confirmed after assessment of the patient's response to antiparkinson medications.

F. Management Options

1. General notes

a. Currently, there is no known treatment that halts or reverses neuronal degeneration.

b. Current options provide symptom relief and improve the quality of life.

2. Types of treatment

a. Pharmacotherapy involves the use of drugs from various classes (e.g., monoamine oxidase B inhibitor, levodopa, dopamine agonist, antiviral, anticholinergic, and catechol-O-methyltransferase inhibitor) (Barker, 2002; Monahan et al., 2007) (see Table 14-3).

b. Surgical interventions offer selected patients relief from some symptoms; however, they cannot improve the disease course or guarantee long-lasting disease improvement (Barker, 2002; Monahan et al., 2007):

1) Pallidotomy and thalamotomy destroys groups of brain cells of the thalamus or basal ganglia to prevent involuntary movement, some of the most distressing symptoms.

2) Thalamic or deep brain stimulators have been approved by the FDA to treat tremor.

a) Electrodes are surgically implanted into the thalamus, globus pallidus, or subthalamic nuclei and connected to a neurostimulator (pulse generator) implanted under the skin of the chest (like a pacemaker).

b) Once the system is in place, the device is programmed to deliver electrical stimulation sent from the neurostimulator up along the

Table 14-3. Drugs Prescribed for Symptomatic Control of Parkinson's Disease

Drug Category and Name	Action
Monoamine oxidase B inhibitor: selegiline (Eldepryl)	Used in the early stages of PD to delay the breakdown of naturally occurring dopamine
Carbidopa–levodopa (Sinemet)	Is the first-line, gold-standard therapy that restores deficient dopamine to the brain without causing extreme, uncomfortable peripheral side effects
Dopamine agonists: bromocriptine (Parlodel), pergolide (Permax), pramipexole (Mirapex), ropinirole (ReQuip)	Directly stimulates the dopamine receptors in the brain to produce more dopamine
Antiviral: amantadine (Symmetrel)	Acts by releasing dopamine from neuronal storage sites
Anticholinergic: benztropine (Cogentin), trihexyphenidyl (Artane)	Counteracts the action of acetylcholine in the central nervous system
Catechol-O-methyltransferase inhibitor: tolcapone (Tasmar)	Used in combination with Sinemet to block the enzyme that metabolizes levodopa, thus allowing more levodopa to be available for conversion to dopamine

extension wire and the lead and into the brain to targeted areas that control movement, blocking the abnormal nerve signals that cause tremor and PD symptoms.

    c) The patient can self-activate the device.

    d) Currently, the procedure is used only for patients whose symptoms cannot be adequately controlled with medications.

    e) Many patients experience reduction of their PD symptoms after undergoing deep brain stimulation and are able to greatly reduce their medications.

c. Transplantation: Still in experimental stages, transplantation of fetal neural tissue into the brain is designed to provide dopamine-producing cells in the brain, allowing these cells to grow and process dopamine with a goal of either halting or reversing disease process (Barker, 2002; Lewis et al., 2004).

d. Nutritional intervention:

    1) Diet should contain adequate roughage and fruit to prevent constipation.

    2) Low-protein diet with less fat and more carbohydrates; foods high in protein can decrease absorption of levodopa (Lewis et al., 2004).

    3) Food should be cut into bite-size pieces and ample time should be planned for eating.

G. Nursing Process

  1. Assessment

    a. Obtain a complete health history and information about current symptoms, time of onset, and progression, including CNS trauma, exposure to metals, carbon dioxide, encephalitis, and use of tranquilizers or antipsychotic medications.

    b. Pay particular attention to mental status, ability to answer questions, and overt coping abilities.

    c. Determine how the disease has affected the patient and family and ask about what aspects of the disease are most troublesome.

    d. Observe overall appearance, posture, and gait pattern.

    e. Determine level of extremity stiffness, tremors, and ability to move.

    f. Investigate safe mobility, self-care

activities, nutritional intake, and verbal communication.

  2. Plan of care

    a. Nursing diagnoses (Monahan et al., 2007)

      1) Ineffective individual coping related to depression and increasingly severe physical limitations

      2) Knowledge deficit related to disease progression, treatment, ongoing adaptations, and availability of support systems

      3) Impaired physical mobility related to tremor, rigidity, bradykinesia, and postural instability

      4) Self-care deficits (e.g., bathing, dressing, feeding, toileting) related to tremor, rigidity, bradykinesia, and postural inability

      5) Inadequate nutrition related to difficulty with chewing, swallowing, and drooling

      6) Impaired verbal communication related to low voice, slow speech, and difficulty moving facial muscles

      7) Risk of injury (falling) related to tremors, bradykinesia, and altered gait

    b. Goals

      1) Verbalize appropriate plans for coping with stress.

      2) Verbalize understanding of the disease process, significant implications, and prescribed regimen.

      3) Maintain maximal level of mobility.

      4) Attain maximal level of function in ADLs.

      5) Verbalize understanding of diet management and achieve adequate hydration and nutritional balance.

      6) Communicate effectively.

      7) Demonstrate safety in mobility and recognize the need for appropriate assistive devices.

  3. Interventions

    a. Develop positive coping mechanisms:

      1) Allow the patient to freely verbalize feelings and concerns.

      2) Encourage participation in support groups (e.g., Parkinson's Disease Foundation, Parkinson's Support Groups of America, National Parkinson Foundation).

      3) Encourage the patient to establish realistic, attainable goals.

      4) Support the use of prescribed psychotherapy and medication to combat depression.

b. Develop a sound knowledge base about the disease and treatments:
   1) Teach the patient about the common signs, symptoms, and progression of PD.
   2) Discuss aspects of the disease that are unique to PD and the use of antiparkinson drugs (e.g., "on–off," "wearing off," and "freezing" phenomena).
   3) Educate the patient and family about the desired effects and side effects of prescribed medications and surgical treatments.
   4) Offer suggestions to make living with PD easier.
   5) Inform the patient and family of local and national support groups for assistance and education.
c. Improve mobility and maximize neuromuscular function:
   1) Encourage active and passive range of motion (ROM) exercises according to the prescribed physical therapy program.
   2) Allow time for rest after activity and avoid rushing.
   3) Administer medications as prescribed to avoid exacerbation of symptoms.
   4) Use warm baths and massage to help relax muscles.
   5) Teach the patient to concentrate on walking erect by consciously using a wide-based gait and deliberately swinging the arms; teach the patient to pretend to cross over an imaginary line or rock side to side to initiate leg movement to help deal with "freezing" while walking.
   6) Provide muscle stretching and massage to reduce rigidity.
d. Maintain independence in ADLs:
   1) Encourage the use of devices to make self-care easier (e.g., raised toilet seats, trapeze bar, grab bars, long-handled shoehorns, elastic shoelaces).
   2) Allow adequate time to accomplish self-care.
   3) Make environmental modifications to enhance safety and independence.
e. Achieve satisfactory hydration and nutritional status:
   1) Encourage the patient to sit upright for all meals.
   2) Offer semisolid foods and thickened liquids if choking occurs.

   3) Use stabilized plates, plate guards, nonspill cups, and large-handled utensils.
   4) Augment caloric intake with supplementary feedings.
   5) Monitor weight weekly.
f. Improve verbal communication:
   1) Reinforce exercises prescribed by the speech and language therapist.
   2) Inform family and friends to wait for the patient to answer questions.
   3) Encourage the patient to engage in conversation and read aloud.
g. Maintain safety:
   1) Modify the environment to remove hazards and improve lighting.
   2) Install devices for safety (e.g., grab bars, raised toilet seat).
   3) Change position slowly with orthostatic hypotension.

IV. Human Immunodeficiency Virus (HIV) and Acquired Immunodeficiency Syndrome (AIDS)

A. Overview
   1. AIDS was first recognized in 1981 as a serious life-threatening illness and has since become a worldwide epidemic.
   2. In 1985 the causative agent HIV was identified, and AIDS was determined to be the end stage of the HIV infection.
   3. Although significant breakthroughs in prevention, treatment, and diagnosis have increased survival times, the long-term prognosis for people with HIV and AIDS remains poor.
   4. Drug therapy to treat the infection became available in 1987 and has since expanded, but despite research and new developments, no cure or vaccine is available, and the HIV epidemic is far from over (Lewis et al., 2004).
   5. An estimated 1 million people in the United States were living with HIV or AIDS at the end of 2003, with about one-fourth of those with HIV undiagnosed and unaware of their infection (Centers for Disease Control and Prevention [CDC], 2006d).
   6. It is estimated that 25 million people worldwide have died of AIDS since the start of the epidemic, including 500,000 Americans (CDC, 2006f).
   7. Avoiding behaviors that put a person at risk of infection is the only way to prevent the infection.

8. Nurses play a vital role in caring for people with HIV and AIDS and are challenged to stay up to date on the most current research because information in this area is constantly developing.

B. Types

1. AIDS: The most advanced stage of a progressive immune function disorder caused by the retrovirus HIV

2. HIV

    a. Attacks the immune system and leaves the body defenseless to numerous infections and health problems

    b. Involves two strains that cause AIDS but have differing geographic distributions

        1) HIV-1: Accounts for the majority of infections worldwide

        2) HIV-2: Appears to be prevalent in Western African countries but has only limited distribution in other areas

C. Epidemiology

1. Globally, between 34.6 and 42.3 million people are living with HIV or AIDS and 5 million are newly diagnosed (Monahan et al., 2007; Ohio State University Medical Center, 2006).

2. An estimated 5 million new HIV infections occurred worldwide in 2003, or about 14,000 new infections each day (Ohio State University Medical Center, 2006).

3. AIDS is a leading killer of African American men ages 25–44, and an increasing number of African-American women and children are being affected by HIV and AIDS (National Institute of Allergy and Infectious Diseases [NIAID], 2005).

4. Although advances in treatment slowed the progression of HIV infection to AIDS, leading to dramatic decreases in AIDS deaths, the number of AIDS diagnoses increased between 2000 and 2004 (CDC, 2006d).

D. Etiology

1. The origin of HIV is unknown.

2. The causative agent of HIV infection is HIV, a retrovirus.

3. A person with HIV may be asymptomatic for many years and not even know that he or she is infected; however, as the immune system weakens, the person will become ill more often.

4. HIV is one continuous disease process that ranges from asymptomatic to AIDS, which is characterized by potentially life-threatening opportunistic infections (OIs) (CDC, 2006d; Monahan et al., 2007).

    a. Primary infection or early chronic infection: period from infection with HIV to the development of HIV-specific antibodies, which results in viremia (large amounts of virus in the blood)

        1) Onset is 0–12 weeks from initial infection.

        2) Virus infects white blood cells called CD4+ T-lymphocytes (T-helper cells), which are the master coordinators of the immune system.

        3) Immune system clears virus to lymphatic organs.

        4) The CD4+ T-cell count declines and is greater than or equal to 500 cells/mm3.

        5) Physical characteristics are similar to those of flu or mononucleosis (e.g., fever, fatigue, headache, arthralgia, myalgia, generalized lymphadenopathy, pharyngitis, anorexia, weight loss, and night sweats). Symptoms usually disappear after a week to a month.

    b. Chronic asymptomatic infection

        1) Onset is 12 weeks–12 years or more from initial infection.

        2) Anti-HIV antibodies have been produced around 12 weeks and can be detected by antibody screening.

        3) The virus is present primarily in lymphatic tissue and slowly spreads throughout the body.

        4) Clinical symptoms usually are absent or mild. Vague symptoms include fatigue, headache, lymphadenopathy, and night sweats.

        5) As the viral load increases, the CD4+ T-cell count gradually declines (200–499 cells/mm3).

    c. AIDS

        1) As the immune system fails, symptoms increase, and the illnesses that occur become more severe.

        2) Signs and symptoms progress from mild to moderate (e.g., chills, frequent fever, night sweats, dry productive cough, dyspnea, lethargy, confusion, stiff neck, seizures, headaches, malaise, oral lesions, generalized lymphadenopathy, skin rashes, abdominal discomfort, chronic diarrhea, weight loss, fatigue,

short-term memory loss, tuberculosis, oral hairy leukoplakia, shingles, thrombocytopenia, pelvic inflammatory disease in women that does not respond to treatment, developmental delays and failure to thrive in children) to life-threatening OIs.

3) CD4+ T-cell counts continue to decline to less than 200 cells/mm3.

4) One or more OIs or diseases (AIDS indicator conditions) develop (Figure 14-2). Children may get the same OI or disease as do adults, but they also have severe forms of the typically common childhood bacterial infections, such as conjunctivitis, ear infections, and tonsillitis (NIAID, 2005).

5) Clinical manifestations involve the loss of lean body mass and wasting syndrome.

6) Without treatment, death occurs in 3–5 years and usually results from infection, cancer, or wasting syndrome.

E. Pathophysiology

1. Overview (Lewis et al., 2004; Monahan et al., 2007)

a. HIV is a retrovirus that consists of RNA virus that contains a special viral enzyme called reverse transcriptase, which allows the virus to replicate backward, going from RNA to DNA, and then integrate and take over a cell's own genetic material.

b. HIV cannot replicate unless it is inside a living cell.

c. HIV interacts with human cells that have CD4 receptors on their surface membrane, which include lymphocytes, monocytes, macrophages, astrocytes, and oligodendrocytes (white blood cells that fight infections); once attached, HIV virus enters the cell.

d. Once the virus enters the cell, viral RNA is transcribed into DNA with the assistance of the enzyme reverse transcriptase, becoming a permanent part of the cell's genetic structure and replicated during normal cell processes.

e. It uses the cell to make copies of itself and produces new HIV retroviruses and kills primarily CD4+ T-lymphocytes because they have more CD4+ receptor–bearing cells.

f. Viral load increases (number of circulating HIV retroviruses in the person's serum).

g. Antibodies are produced and detectable between 6 weeks and 6 months after infection; however, these antibodies are not able to fight the infection.

h. Millions of CD4+ T-cells are destroyed every day, but the bone marrow and thymus are able to produce enough CD4+ T-cells to replace the destroyed cells for many years.

i. Once the ability of HIV to destroy CD4+ T-cells exceeds the body's ability to make them, they will not be able to regulate immune responses, resulting in the most serious stage of HIV infection, AIDS, with OIs.

j. Immune problems start to occur when the CD4+ T-cell count drops to 200–499 cells/mm3; severe problems develop with fewer than 200 CD4+ T-cells/mm3.

2. Transmission

a. HIV is transmitted from human to human through exposure of infected body fluid (e.g., blood, semen, vaginal secretions, breast milk).

b. No evidence has been found that HIV is transmitted through tears, sweat, saliva, vomit, urine, or feces.

c. Common modes of transmission:

1) Sexual contact (e.g., oral, vaginal, anal)

2) Sharing a needle or syringe (e.g., intravenous drug use, tattooing, body piercing)

3) Blood transfusion (risk extremely small because of blood screening and heat treatment)

4) Tissue or organ donation

5) Prenatal contact from mother to

Figure 14-2. Opportunistic Infections (OIs) Associated with AIDS

Viral: Cytomegalovirus disease, herpes simplex, pneumonitis or esophagitis

Bacterial: *Mycobacterium* tuberculosis, recurrent pneumonia, recurrent *Salmonella* septicemia

Protozoal: *Pneumocystis carinii* pneumonia (PCP), toxoplasmosis of the brain

Fungal: Candidiasis of bronchi, trachea, lungs, or esophagus

Neurological: Dementia, headaches

Neoplastic processes: Lymphoma, Kaposi's sarcoma (KS), cervical carcinoma

Wasting syndrome: Chronic diarrhea, weakness, weight loss, constant or intermittent fever for at least 30 days

infant before or during birth or during breastfeeding
6) Occupational exposure (e.g., needle stick)

d. HIV is not spread through casual contact (e.g., touching, hugging, shaking hands, sharing eating utensils, eating food prepared by a person with HIV, coughing, sneezing, using restrooms, touching animals or insects, working or attending school with an HIV-infected person).

3. Clinical manifestations
   a. Common signs and symptoms of HIV infection include chills, fever, fatigue, weight loss, dry productive cough, sore throat, rash, night sweats, shortness of breath, stiff neck, headache, yeast infection, lymphadenopathy, gastrointestinal distress, diarrhea, pain, and dementia (Monahan et al., 2007).
   b. People with AIDS are susceptible to OIs, which are life-threatening illnesses caused by organisms that are normally fought off by a healthy immune system (CDC, 2006d).
      1) OIs can affect every organ and body system.
      2) Diagnosis and treatment of OIs are essential to increase longevity.
      3) Children are susceptible to OIs, conjunctivitis, ear infections, and tonsillitis.

4. Diagnosis
   a. Early testing and routine voluntary testing for HIV will alert the HIV-infected person to avoid high-risk behavior, reducing HIV transmission, and enable appropriate treatment, resulting in improved health, extended life, and prevention of OIs (CDC, 2006a).
   b. Recommendations for HIV testing (CDC, 2006a):
      1) Routine HIV screening for patients 13–64 years of age in all healthcare settings after the patient is notified that the testing will be performed unless patient declines (opt-out screening)
      2) HIV testing at least once per year for people at high risk unless the patient declines (opt-out screening)
      3) HIV screening included in panel of prenatal screening tests for all pregnant women and repeat screening in the third trimester in certain areas with elevated HIV

infection rates unless patient declines (opt-out screening)
   c. Written consent is not recommended, and HIV screening should be incorporated into the general consent for medical care (CDC, 2006a).
   d. Prevention and pretest counseling is encouraged but not required for diagnostic testing as part of routine screening programs in healthcare settings (CDC, 2006a).
      1) Pretest counseling
         a) Review test procedures.
         b) Explain the meaning of positive and negative test results.
         c) Provide information on HIV and AIDS.
         d) Set a plan for risk reduction.
         e) Describe the importance of follow-up care.
         f) Prepare the patient for potential psychological and emotional reactions to a positive test result.
      2) Posttest counseling
         a) If the test is negative, provide advice on retesting (if the person engages in high-risk behavior) and preventing the spread of HIV.
         b) If the test is positive, evaluate the person's potential for suicide; provide crisis intervention if needed and information on symptoms of HIV and AIDS; teach health maintenance; refer for medical follow-up and tuberculosis screening, support groups, clinical trials, or experimental protocols; and discuss potential discrimination.
   e. Confidentiality with HIV testing is very important because disclosure may result in discrimination.
   f. Diagnostic tests available (CDC, 2006a; Monahan et al., 2007)
      1) Antibody testing (rapid test [20 minutes], enzyme-linked immunosorbent assay, Western blot)
         a) Detects the presence of antibodies to HIV.
         b) Involves a delay (window period) of 3 weeks to 6 months before a detectable antibody is produced.
         c) A positive test should be repeated and then confirmed by alternative method, usually Western blot.
      2) Antigen testing

a) Detects the virus (HIV RNA) in the blood

b) Is detectable 1 week earlier than antibody testing but is labor intensive and costly

c) May be performed if an antibody test is negative and the person is highly likely to be positive

3) Viral load: measures plasma HIV RNA levels in a sample of blood, indicating the amount of virus in the person's serum, how well the immune system is controlling the virus, or whether the medication regimen is working

a) No antiretroviral medication: viral load every 3–4 months

b) With antiretroviral medication: viral load 2–8 weeks after initiation of treatment and then every 3–4 months to make sure drug is still working

4) CD4 cell count: used to measure the extent of immune damage that has occurred, to stage HIV infection and prognosis, and to determine whether medication regimen is working

5) Drug resistance testing: determines whether a person's HIV strain is resistant to any anti-HIV medication

F. Management Options

1. Early intervention allows the person to survive longer. Research has focused on antiretroviral agents to inhibit disease progression, prophylactic therapy to prevent OIs, therapy to restore the damaged immune system, and vaccine development (Monahan et al., 2007).

2. Goal: to halt the spread of infection, decrease HIV RNA level, maintain or increase CD4+ T-cell count to more than 200 cell/mm3, and delay the development of HIV related symptoms.

3. The U.S. FDA has approved a number of drugs for treating HIV infection (Monahan et al., 2007; U.S. Department of Health and Human Services [USDHHS], 2006a, 2006b):

a. Nucleoside analog reverse transcriptase inhibitors:

1) Interrupt the early stage of the virus making copies of itself by competitively binding with reverse transcriptase and block the elongation of the DNA chain, resulting in a slowing of the spread of HIV and delaying the start of OIs

2) Include azidothymidine (AZT), zalcitabine (ddC), didanosine (ddI), stavudine (d4T), lamivudine (3TC), abacavir (Ziagen), tenofovir (Viread), and emtricitabine (Emtriva)

b. Nonnucleoside reverse transcriptase inhibitors:

1) Prevent viral replication through competitive binding of reverse transcriptase but do not terminate DNA chain

2) Include delavirdine (Rescriptor), nevirapine (Viramune), and efavirenz (Sustiva)

c. Nucleotide reverse transcriptase inhibitors:

1) Competitively bind to reverse transcriptase and block the elongation of DNA

2) Include tenofovir disoproxil fumarate and emtricitabine (Emtriva)

d. Protease inhibitors:

1) Prevent the virus from making long protein molecules necessary to create a new virus, thus halting replication

2) Include ritonavir (Norvir), saquinavir (Invirase), indinavir (Crixivan), nelfinavir (Viracept), lopinavir (Kaletra), atazanavir (Reyataz), and fosamprenavir (Lexiva)

e. Fusion inhibitors

1) Interfere with HIV-1's ability to enter cells by blocking the merging of the virus with the cell membrane

2) Include enfuvirtide or T-20 (Fuzeon)

4. The most effective treatment strategy is combination drug therapy, which can attack viral replication in several different ways, attack different stages of the HIV life cycle, produce a more sustained antiviral effect in a person with HIV, and decrease the likelihood of drug resistance.

a. Factors in deciding when to start treatment include symptoms of advanced HIV disease, CD4+ T-cell count below 200 cells/mm3, and viral load of 100,000 copies/ml or more (USDHHS, 2006b).

b. USDHHS recommends a combination of 3 or more medications in a regimen called highly active antiretroviral therapy (HAART):

1) Researchers have credited HAART as a major factor in reducing the number of deaths from AIDS in this country (NIAID, 2005).

2) HAART is not a cure but reduces the

amount of virus circulating in the bloodstream.

    3) Access, response, and adherence to antiretroviral drug therapy affects whether or when HIV progresses to AIDS (NIAID, 2005).

5. A number of treatments are available for some opportunistic diseases [e.g., radiation and chemotherapy for Kaposi's sarcoma and other forms of cancer, foscarnet and ganciclovir to treat cytomegalovirus eye infections, fluconazole to treat yeast and other fungal infections, pentamidine or trimethoprim/sulfamethoxazole to treat *Pneumocystis carinii pneumonia* (PCP)].

    a. Adults with HIV whose CD4+ T-cell counts drop below 200 cells/mm3 are given prophylactic treatment to prevent PCP if they exhibit unexplained fever for 2 weeks or longer and have a history of oropharyngeal candidiasis. Those who have survived an episode of PCP are given medications to prevent recurrence (Monahan et al., 2007).

    b. Cannabinoid drugs (marijuana) or megestrol may offer relief from wasting syndrome and help stimulate the appetite.

6. Influenza vaccine is recommended; people with advanced HIV disease may have a poor response to immunization and should be given antiviral medications if they are likely to be exposed to other people with influenza.

7. Alternative and complementary therapies include therapeutic touch, massage therapy, meditation, imagery, tai chi, and herbal medicine.

8. Health promotion and disease prevention can be effective in preventing the spread of infection.

    a. Promote a lifestyle that prevents or decreases the risk of HIV infection:

        1) Abstain from sexual activity or use a condom for all insertive sexual practices with a partner who has or may have HIV.

        2) Stop using intravenous drugs, stop sharing needles and equipment, use a clean needle and syringe or disinfect them after each use, decrease the number of injections, and avoid engaging in risky sexual activity.

        3) Early testing and routine screening for all patients 13–64 years of age.

        4) Screen all potential blood donors for high-risk behaviors and signs

and symptoms of AIDS and test all human tissue for transplantation for HIV antibodies.

        5) Adhere to safety guidelines to prevent occupational exposure.

    b. Promote a healthy lifestyle in people who are already infected:

        1) Decrease high-risk behavior.

        2) Attend regular medical and psychiatric evaluations and follow-ups.

        3) Maintain proper nutrition and diet (high calorie, high protein to prevent weight loss), which improve immune function.

        4) Maintain food safety by keeping food at the proper temperature, cooking food thoroughly, avoiding foods that may be contaminated or harbor bacteria, and washing fruits and vegetables before eating (because people with HIV infection are vulnerable to foodborne illness).

        5) Remove fresh flowers and plants from room.

        6) Avoid cleaning the litter box.

        7) Ask visitors to wear a mask if they have a cold.

        8) Maintain proper handwashing.

        9) Reduce and control stress.

        10) Avoid or limit cigarettes, alcohol, and drugs.

        11) Exercise regularly.

G. Nursing Process

    1. Assessment

        a. Obtain a complete history of current high-risk behaviors that could put other people at risk and signs and symptoms that may indicate the progression of HIV and the presence of OIs.

        b. Perform neurological evaluation.

        c. Perform psychosocial evaluation (e.g., support systems, financial state, coping strategies).

        d. Observe the patient's overall health and appearance and conduct a complete physical and functional assessment because any body system can be affected.

        e. Investigate nutritional status, energy level, preventive strategies to protect others and self from further infectious insult.

        f. Assess for weight loss, fever, skin lesions, short-term memory loss, and cold symptoms.

        g. Assess compliance with treatment,

effectiveness of treatment regimen, and side effects.

2. Plan of care
   a. Nursing diagnoses
      1) Hopelessness related to terminal disease process
      2) Fear related to possible death
      3) Anticipatory grieving related to terminal diagnosis
      4) Ineffective individual coping or compromised family coping related to diagnosis
      5) Inadequate nutrition related to the disease process, wasting syndrome, and side effects of treatment regimen
      6) Pain related to disease process
      7) Fatigue related to poor nutrition, disease process, and muscle weakness
      8) Activity intolerance related to weakness, poor nutrition
      9) Risk for infection related to deficient immune system
      10) Knowledge deficit related to diagnosis, prognosis, and long-term care
   b. Goals (Lewis et al., 2004)
      1) For asymptomatic stage
         a) Demonstrate healthy lifestyle.
         b) Verbalize understanding of measures to prevent further HIV transmission.
         c) Identify and use effective strategies for coping with stressful situations and adjustment to illness.
         d) Verbalize understanding of the disease process, significant implications, and treatment options.
      2) For symptomatic stage
         a) Verbalize understanding of the prevention and treatment of OIs.
         b) Verbalize understanding of and appropriately manage problems caused by HIV infection.
         c) Maintain maximal level of function.
         d) Verbalize understanding of and adhere to drug regimen to keep the viral load as low as possible for as long as possible.
      3) For terminal stage
         a) Maintain a desired level of comfort.
         b) Verbalize wishes and declare

preferences regarding treatment options.
         c) Experience a dignified and comfortable death.

3. Interventions
   a. Asymptomatic stage
      1) Provide education about the diagnosis of HIV, prevention of the spread of HIV, disease progression, and treatment options.
      2) Use strategies to prevent infection.
      3) Provide education for HIV-negative people who are at risk for contracting HIV and prevent the HIV-infected person from transmitting the virus to others.
      4) Empower patient to take control over preventive measures.
      5) Encourage patient to maintain social and community activities.
      6) Monitor for signs and symptoms of infection, which may indicate disease progression.
      7) Provide emotional support, include significant others in plan of care, and help identify additional sources of financial and emotional support.
      8) Assess psychological response to situations.
   b. Symptomatic stage
      1) Provide education about medications and adverse effects.
      2) Assess effectiveness of treatment regimen (viral load, CD4+ T-cell count), adverse reactions, and compliance with medication regimens.
      3) Educate about changing treatment options and encourage continued adherence.
      4) Monitor weight and provide high-calorie, high-protein diet and nutritional supplements as necessary.
      5) Manage and treat HIV-related symptoms with antibiotics, antifungal or antiviral medication for infection, antiemetics for nausea, analgesics for pain, antidiarrheal medication for diarrhea.
      6) Balance energy with rest to maintain normal or nearly normal activity level and use assistive devices (wheelchair, cane) to conserve energy.
      7) Encourage verbalization of fears and concerns.

The Specialty Practice of Rehabilitation Nursing: A Core Curriculum, 5th Ed.

c. Terminal stage
1) Assist with end-of-life, comfort measures in a suitable care setting and appropriate services (e.g., hospice).
2) Administer pain medication to relieve pain and discomfort.
3) Administer anti-anxiety medication for anxiety and restlessness.
4) Promote calm environment.
5) Provide emotional and spiritual support to patient and significant others.
6) Maintain patient's dignity and wishes throughout the dying process.
7) Instruct significant others on dying process.
8) Provide bereavement counseling for significant others.
4. Evaluation: Modify care according to the stage of HIV and the patient's response to nursing interventions.

V. Burns

A. Overview
1. Burns
   a. A burn is tissue damage resulting from exposure to flames or hot liquids, contact with an electrical current, or exposure to radiation, strong acids, or alkali chemicals.
   b. On average in the United States in 2005, someone died in a fire every 2 hours, and someone was injured every 29 minutes (Karter, 2006).
   c. Death rates from serious burns have declined because of advances in fluid resuscitation, nutritional support, skin replacement, topical antimicrobials to prevent infection, early surgical interventions, and improvement in the management of inhalation injury and hypermetabolism (National Institutes of Health, 2006a).
   d. Rehabilitation of the patient with burns requires interdisciplinary teamwork to achieve restoration of function and reintegration into the community.
   e. Rehabilitation nurses must be knowledgeable in wound management and healing and in the pathophysiology and psychological components associated with burn injuries.
2. Skin
   a. The skin is the largest organ of the body.
   b. The skin's major functions are to protect internal organs from infection and trauma, prevent the fluid loss, and regulate body temperature.
   c. Exposure to heat above 120° F will damage the skin, interfere with its primary functions, and cause burn injuries.

B. Epidemiology
1. More than 1.1 million burn injuries warrant medical assistance in the United States each year, and approximately 45,000 of these warrant hospitalization. The exact number of burn injuries is unknown because not all states are required to report burn injuries (CDC, 2006a, 2006b; Karter, 2006; Office of Statistics and Programming, 2006).
2. As many as 75% of burn injuries may be preventable (Monahan et al., 2007).
3. Approximately 4,500 people die of burn injuries each year in the United States; fires and burns are the fifth most common cause of unintentional injury death in the United States (CDC, 2006b, 2006c).
4. Children, older adults, and disabled are the high-risk groups for burn injuries (CDC, 2006c).
5. Most common burn injuries are caused by scalds, building fires, and flammable liquids and gases (National Institute of General Medical Sciences, 2006).

C. Etiology
1. Thermal:
   a. Flame (e.g., house fire, burning leaves)
   b. Scald (stream or hot liquid, e.g., boiling water)
   c. Flash (e.g., flame burn associated with explosion)
   d. Contact (e.g., hot metal or hot tar)
2. Chemical: Strong acids or alkalis compounds (e.g., common household cleaning agents) that are ingested or inhaled or come in contact with skin or mucous membranes. The amount of damage depends on the concentration and quantity of the agent, duration of skin contact, and degree of penetration into the tissue (Lewis et al., 2004).
3. Electrical: Exposure to electrical current. The amount of damage depends on the type of circuit, voltage and amperage, the pathway of the current through the body, and the duration of contact.
   a. Exposed or faulty wiring

b. High-voltage power lines

c. Strikes of lightning

4. Radiation:

a. Sunburn

b. Therapeutic radiation for cancer treatment

c. Nuclear radiation accidents

5. Smoke and inhalation: Directly inhaled smoke, hot air, or flames damage the tissues of the respiratory tract and can also contain chemicals that poison the body's cells, such as carbon monoxide.

D. Pathophysiology

1. Severity of burn injury

a. Degree of burn (see Figure 14-3).

b. Extent of burn:

1) Total body surface area: Percentage of the burn injury compared with healthy tissue.

2) Rule of 9: a formula that divides the body into anatomical sections, each representing 9% or a multiple of 9% (hands and neck = 9%, arms = 9% each, anterior trunk = 18%, posterior trunk = 18%, legs = 18% each, and the perineum = 1%). Calculations are modified for infants and children younger than 10 years because of their larger head and smaller body size.

c. Level of skin damage (Hettiaratchy & Dziewulski, 2004; Lewis et al., 2004):

1) Minor burns

a) Can be managed on an outpatient basis

b) Less than 15% partial-thickness (second-degree) burn; less than 2% full-thickness (third-degree) burn

2) Moderate (uncomplicated) burns: 15%–25% partial-thickness (second-degree) burn; less than 10% full-thickness (third-degree) burn

3) Major burns

a) More than 25% partial-thickness (second-degree) burn; more than 10% full-thickness (third-degree) burn; all fourth-degree burns.

b) Electrical burns: Despite minimal skin damage, interior damage can be extensive and damage the heart.

c) Inhalation injury.

d) Includes all burns of the eyes, face, ears, feet, hands, and perineum (regardless of the

---

Figure 14-3. Levels of Burn Severity

First Degree (partial thickness)
Does not extend below the epidermis

Is dry and very painful

Heals in a matter of days

Second Degree
Involves the epidermis and part of the dermis

May be superficial (moist, painful, blisters) or deep thickness (less painful); may have a white or red base

Superficial burns heal in 1–2 weeks; deep thickness burns heal in 3 weeks or more

Third Degree (full thickness)
Extends into dermis

Is dry and involves no pain, because sensory nerves are damaged; can be any color (e.g., white, black, yellow, brown)

Autograft is the usual form of treatment

Fourth Degree
Extends beyond fat and into the muscle and bone

Involves no pain and has variable color

Amputation of extremity is often necessary; autografting is the primary method for healing

---

estimated percentage).

e) Complicated burn injury such as circumferential burn around extremity or neck or other injuries sustained at time of burn.

d. Age: Burn victims younger than 2 years of age and older than 60 years have a higher mortality rate than other age groups with similar burn injuries. In both groups, the skin is thin and more prone to infection.

e. Preexisting conditions: Cardiovascular, respiratory, or renal disease, DM, peripheral vascular disease, sickle cell anemia, or hepatic disease (Lewis et al., 2004).

2. Clinical manifestations

a. Local: Capillaries of the injured tissue become leaky; plasma is lost, drawing water with it, resulting in edema of the involved tissue and pain.

b. Systemic responses: A major burn can affect all body systems and can cause serious complications through excessive fluid loss and tissue damage (see Figure 14-4).

c. Complications from burn surface:

1) Pain related to exposed nerve endings in partial-thickness burns and donor sites.

2) Scars:

a) Hypertrophic scars are red, thick,

and raised above the level of normal skin but are within the boundaries of the burn wound and result from an imbalance between collagen synthesis and collagen lysis.

b) Keloid scars are thick, nodular, and ridged scar tissue that grows beyond the site of injury; can become binding and limit mobility if the keloids are extensive (Burn Survivor Resource Center, 2002b).

c) Scar tissue affects thermal regulation. Shivering is not possible with full-thickness scar with extensive grating. A cool environment is preferred.

3) Contractures: tightening and shortening of the tendons and muscles, resulting in immobility and decreased ROM. Prevention is the most effective treatment (e.g., splinting, exercising, positioning, using pressure garments). Surgery may be needed, depending on the severity and location of contractures.

4) Heterotopic ossification: abnormal deposit of new bone in soft tissue surrounding a joint that does not normally ossify.

5) Surgical interventions may be needed if mobility is limited.

6) Altered sensation: diminished or absent response to sharp–dull, hot–cold; caution is needed to avoid further injury.

7) Pruritus or itching as the wound heals.

E. Management Options

1. Prevention (Herndon, 2002)

a. House fires:

1) Use a smoke detector on each floor, replace batteries at least once a year, and test them monthly.

2) Have a fire extinguisher in the kitchen.

3) Use a cooking timer with a loud alarm.

4) Install a sprinkler system.

5) Place firefighting decals on the window of children's bedrooms.

6) Make sure address is clearly visible on the outside of the house.

7) Keep matches and lighters out of reach of children.

Figure 14-4. Systemic Responses to Burn Injury

Vascular Alterations

Vasoconstriction results from exposure to heat and from stress response, resulting in decreased blood flow.

Dilation of adjacent vessels and capillaries and increased capillary permeability occur after the initial vasoconstriction.

Sodium pump is disturbed.

Fluid shifts from the vascular space into the extracellular space, resulting in edema. (If edema is not corrected, ischemia in the underlying tissues can occur.)

Cardiac output is decreased as a result of hypovolemia.

Fluid resuscitation must be initiated to prevent cell shock and to maintain cardiac output and renal and tissue perfusion. (Adults with burns of a total body surface area greater than 15% need fluid resuscitation.)

Pulmonary Alterations

Obstruction can occur when damage around the neck area becomes tight or when superheated air, steam, gases, flames, or smoke is inhaled.

Depending on the severity, treatment can range from humidified air to mechanical ventilation.

Hematologic Alterations

Destruction of red blood cells in the burned area results in anemia.

Hematocrit level increase blood flow decreases as the fluid shifts to the extravascular space, resulting in possible ischemia of underlying tissue and thrombosis.

Immune Response

Immune responses decrease because of damage of the protective skin layer, stress, protein and caloric malnutrition, and side effects of immunosuppressant medication and steroids.

The individual is highly susceptible to infection.

Gastrointestinal Alterations

Ileus is due to vasoconstriction.

Parenteral route is used if an ileus is present.

Nutritional Alterations

Metabolic rate increases, resulting in increased caloric need of about two times normal (Wilson, 1996).

The metabolic rate will slowly return to normal when the wound is healed (Wilson, 1996).

Blood glucose rises.

Nutritional support may include oral supplements, tube feeding, intravenous supplements, or total parenteral nutrition.

---

8) Have a fire escape plan, know two ways out of every room, and practice fire drills and meeting at a designated space (a safe distance outside away from the house).

b. Hotels and workplace:

1) Become familiar with exits and posted evacuation plan.

2) Learn location of building exits.

3) Respond to every alarm as if it were a real fire.

c. Hot water:

1) Do not exceed a maximum temperature of 120° F.

---

2) Turn handles of pots and pans inward while cooking.

3) Place cold water in bathtub first then add hot water to appropriate temperature.

d. Chemical: Lock all flammable and caustic substances out of reach of children.

e. Electrical:
1) Cover outlets with plastic protectors.
2) Do not use appliances with frayed or worn cords.

f. Ultraviolet rays of sun:
1) Avoid long exposure to sun.
2) Wear hats and sunscreen with a minimum sun protector factor (SPF) of 15.

g. Static electricity:
1) Leave cell phone inside vehicle or turn it off during refueling.
2) Do not reenter vehicle during refueling.
3) If you need to reenter vehicle during refueling, close door after getting out, and make contact with metal before pulling out nozzle to discharge static from body.

h. Disabled:
1) Keep wheelchair or assistive device close to bed.
2) Keep whistle to alert rescuers of location.
3) Place sticker on bedroom window.
4) Do not smoke if using oxygen.

2. Acute phase: airway management, fluid resuscitation, wound care, pain management, nutritional therapy, and psychosocial care

3. Management of burn surface

a. Burn location and severity determine treatment: Wound care should focus on cleaning the wound and removing debris until healthy tissue is present.

b. Wound management includes moist dressing, infection control, debridement of necrotic tissue (i.e., removal of dead tissue), or surgical care.
1) Nonsurgical care
a) Apply a topical antimicrobial agent (e.g., Silvadene cream, mafenide acetate cream, silver nitrate 5% solution) and leave the wound open to air or apply a sterile occlusive or semiocclusive dressing to cover the wound.
b) For facial wound or people allergic to sulfa drugs, use bacitracin or another antibiotic.
c) Expose the area to light and maintain a cool environment.
d) Use daily hydrotherapy, which promotes cleansing and removes bacteria.
e) Debride the wound (manually or enzymatically) to remove contaminated tissue and eschar.

2) Surgical care (Burn Survivor Resource Center, 2006)
a) Surgical excision of damaged tissue
b) Escharotomy: cutting through the burnt tissue until healthy tissue is reached to relieve pressure from circumferential wounds that go around the whole chest, leg, arm, or digits
c) Dermabrasion: to smooth scar tissue by shaving or scraping off the top layers of the skin to improve or minimize the appearance of scars, restore function, and correct disfigurement resulting from an injury
d) Grafting: to close deep partial-thickness or full-thickness wounds and protect the skin as it heals on its own
(1) Autograft: use of the patient's own skin from another site.
(a) The donor site is the harvested area of the patient's own skin.
(b) Partial-thickness wounds require an absorbent dressing because of excessive drainage.
(c) Cultured epithelium: Take small piece of unburned skin from patient and grow skin under special tissue culture conditions until it forms confluent sheets that can be used as skin graft.
(2) Cadaver skin: obtained through a graft bank.
(a) Allograft: from another living or dead person
(b) Xenograft: usually pigs because their skin is

most similar to human skin

(3) Artificial skin: synthetic product used to replace burned skin but only as a temporary fix; the use of artificial skins means a thinner skin graft, which allows the donor site and the patient to heal faster with fewer surgeries.

4. Management of complications

a. Begin positioning and splinting immediately on admission to maintain the functional position of joints and prevent contractures. After the graft is stable, the splint should be worn continuously for at least 3 months.

b. Use pressure garments against the skin to reduce scar formation and deformities for 23 hours per day for 1–2 years until the scar is fully mature, removing for bathing and cleaning of garment only.

c. Use topical scar treatment gel and massage therapy to limit scar tissue formation.

d. Manage pain by administering over-the-counter analgesics, nonsteroidal anti-inflammatory drugs (NSAIDs), and narcotics and using diversional activities (e.g., music, imagery, relaxation techniques) during dressing changes.

e. Infection control: Apply topical antimicrobial cream.

f. Nutritional therapy: Increase protein and increase calories, with vitamin supplements.

F. Nursing Process

1. Assessment:

a. Begin with a history:
1) Cause of burn and any contributing factors
2) Pain (e.g., location, quality, duration, intensity)
3) Dietary evaluation
4) Psychosocial evaluation (e.g., support systems, coping strategies)

b. Perform a complete physical and functional assessment, including the amount of burn area involved and the depth, severity, and any complications from the injury.

c. Use a body diagram to document the location and appearance of burns, grafted areas, and donor sites.

2. Plan of care:

a. Nursing diagnoses
1) Alteration in comfort related to pain and itching
2) Self-care deficit related to burn, contracture, wound care, splitting, or pressure garment
3) Impaired skin integrity related to burn injury
4) Impaired physical mobility related to burn injury, contracture, wound care, splitting, or pressure garment
5) Risk of infection related to loss of skin integrity
6) Inadequate nutrition related to diuresis, metabolic response to burn injury, inactivity, and self-care deficit (inability to self-feed)
7) Anxiety related to treatment regimen
8) Body image disturbance related to burn injuries, contractures, and scarring
9) Ineffective coping related to burn injury, pain, prognosis, and long-term outcome
10) Knowledge deficit related to burn process, treatment regimen, and signs and symptoms of complication

b. Goals
1) Report pain relief as a result of pain management interventions.
2) Maintain independence or demonstrate progression toward independence in performing ADLs.
3) Show signs of wound healing.
4) Maintain full ROM.
5) Remain free of complications caused by burn injuries such as extensive scarring or contracture.
6) Remain free of signs and symptoms of infection.
7) Maintain present weight and maintain fluid hydration.
8) Verbalize feelings about change in appearance and develop a realistic body image.
9) Develop effective coping strategies to adjust to burn injury.
10) Verbalize understanding about the healing process, treatment options, and signs and symptoms of complications.

3. Interventions:

a. Provide pain relief with prescribed analgesics, especially before wound care, elevate legs, and use nonpharmacological methods of pain control (imagery, distraction, relaxation, music).

b. Use therapeutic positioning, splints, and ROM exercises to maintain proper position and prevent contractures.

c. Provide assistive devices for use in performing ADLs.

d. Provide care for the wound and the development of healing tissue.

e. Use pressure garment to prevent or minimize scarring.

f. Prevent infection by applying topical antimicrobial cream, adhering to strict handwashing protocols, maintaining aseptic technique, and monitoring for signs and symptoms of infection.

g. Ensure adequate hydration and nutrition (high protein, high calories, with vitamin supplements for wound healing).

h. Provide psychological support and health education regarding health status, treatments, nutritional needs, prevention of infections, and support groups.

i. Provide education on healing process, treatment options, pain relief measures, and complications.

4. Evaluation: Modify care according to the patient's response to nursing interventions.

VI. Cancer

A. Overview

1. Cancer encompasses a group of diseases characterized by the growth and spread of abnormal cells that result in death if not controlled.

2. Cancer is the second most common cause of death in the United States, and smoking alone causes one-third of all cancer deaths (American Cancer Society [ACS], 2006c).

3. Prostate, breast, lung, and colorectal cancers are the most common cancers in the United States (Springhouse, 2002).

4. Remarkable progress against cancer has been made, and the death rates are leveling off or decreasing except for an increasing rate of death from lung cancer in women (Lewis et al., 2004).

5. Major types of cancer:

a. Carcinoma: malignancy of internal and external linings of the body (e.g. skin, lungs, breast, pancreas, and other organs and glands)

b. Sarcoma: malignancy of connective tissue

origin (e.g., bone, skeletal muscle, fibrous tissue, or cartilage)

c. Myeloma: malignancy of plasma cells of bone marrow

d. Lymphoma: cancer of cells in the glands or nodes of the lymphatic system

e. Leukemia: malignancy that affects the blood-forming elements of the bone marrow

f. Mixed type: cancer composed of a mixture of different tissue types

6. Early detection and treatment improve chances of the cancer being cured.

B. Epidemiology and Incidence

1. More than 1 million people each year are diagnosed with cancer (ACS, 2006i).

2. One out of every 2 American men and one out of every 3 American women will develop cancer during their lifetime (ACS, 2006i).

3. 77% of all cancers are diagnosed in people 55 years and older (ACE, 2006h).

4. Cancer is the second leading cause of death in the United States; 1 of every 4 deaths is caused by cancer.

5. More than 500,000 Americans die each year from cancer, and this number is expected to increase with the aging population (Monahan et al., 2007).

C. Etiology and Risk Factors

1. The exact cause of cancer remains a mystery.

2. Development of cancer is a multistep process that is influenced by many independent variables causing damage to DNA, resulting in mutation within the genes of cells.

3. These mutations can be caused by chemicals or physical agents called carcinogens or occur spontaneously and may be passed down from one generation to the next.

4. Risk factors:

a. Age: The risk of nearly all cancers increases with age.

b. Genetic factors: Some cancers are inherited and create a significant predisposition to cancer.

c. Hormonal factor: Evidence suggests that hormones may be connected with the development of certain cancers.

d. Exposure to environmental factors:
   1) Tobacco smoke is the most lethal known carcinogen.
   2) Radiation: Ionizing and ultraviolet radiation (sunlight) can cause cancer.

3) Nutrition, obesity, and inactivity: Research shows that approximately one-third of all cancer deaths are related to unhealthy diet and lack of physical activity in adulthood (ACS, 2006g).
   a) Grilled meats on the barbecue may be more risky than those prepared by baking or broiling (Aetna InteliHealth, 2006).
   b) People who have diets high in saturated fats have a higher cancer risk than those with lower-fat diets.
   c) Inactivity has been linked to a higher risk of colon cancer.
4) Certain viruses: A number of cancers have been linked to viruses (sexually transmitted disease organisms) that suppress the immune system.
5) Occupational exposure: Exposure to carcinogens (e.g., drugs, chemicals, radiation) increases the risk of cancer.
6) Alcohol: Drinking alcohol has been linked with an increased risk of cancer of the esophagus, oral cavity, pharynx, and larynx (ACS, 2006c).

   e. Precancerous lesions: Benign lesions and tumors (polyps of colon and rectum, certain pigmented moles) exhibit a tendency toward progression to cancer.

   f. Psychosocial factors: Extreme stress activates the body's endocrine (hormone) system, which in turn can cause changes in the immune system.

D. Pathophysiology
1. Overview: Cancer develops when a number of mechanisms, either alone or in combination, cause abnormalities in cell growth and multiplication.
2. Cancer cells:
   a. Characteristics
      1) Variable size and shape
      2) Loss of capacity for specialized function
      3) Continued growth after division
         a) Normal cells usually die after 50–60 divisions; however, cancer cells continue in an uncontrolled growth pattern.
         b) Cancer cells continue to grow despite a diminished concentration of growth hormones.
   b. Tumor growth

1) Cancer cells accumulate and form a mass of abnormal cells (or tumors) that may compress, invade, and destroy normal tissues.
2) Most cancers form tumors, but not all tumors are cancerous.
   a) Benign: noncancerous tumors that stop growing and do not spread to other parts of the body
   b) Malignant: cancerous tumors

   c. Carcinogenesis
      1) The process through which cancer develops and abnormal cells grow and proliferate out of control.
      2) Change or mutation in the nucleus of a cell: Millions of cells in the human body die and are replaced every second. The body's immune system typically recognizes mutant cells and destroys them before they multiply, but some mutant cells survive and cause cancer (Corner & Bailey, 2001).
      3) May occur after exposure to carcinogens, which are substances that start or promote the process (e.g., various chemicals, gases, and other substances found in the air, water, foods, pesticides, and industrial settings; tobacco smoke; cleaning products; paints; certain viruses [HIV, hepatitis B, Epstein–Barr]).

   d. Metastasis
      1) Abnormal cells that multiply out of control.
      2) The spread of a tumor from the original site to another site via the lymphatic system or blood vessels.
      3) This uncontrolled growth and spread of cancer cells can eventually interfere with vital organs or functions, resulting in a variety of other tissue changes in the body such as pain, cachexia, lowered immunity, anemia, leukopenia, and thrombocytopenia, and if not controlled can result in death.
      4) The primary sites of cancer metastasis are the bone, the lymph nodes, the liver, the lungs, and the brain.
      5) Note: Cancer is classified by the body part where it started.

3. Symptoms that may signal the presence of cancer (ACS, 2006b):
   a. A change in the size, color, shape, or thickness of a wart, mole, or mouth sore

b. A sore that resists healing

c. Persistent cough, hoarseness, or sore throat

d. Thickening or lumps in the breasts, testicles, or elsewhere

e. A change in bowel or bladder habits

f. Any unusual bleeding or discharge

g. Chronic indigestion or difficulty swallowing

h. Persistent headaches

i. Unexplained loss of weight or appetite

j. Persistent fatigue, nausea, or vomiting

k. Persistent low-grade fever, either constant or intermittent

l. Repeated instances of infection

4. Diagnosis:

a. Noninvasive: radiological studies, computed tomography (CT), MRI, ultrasonography, nuclear medicine studies, laboratory studies, and tumor markers (i.e., substances measurable in the blood that are not produced or are produced in a lesser amount in healthy people).

b. Invasive procedures: biopsy (ranges from needle biopsy to surgical procedure), endoscopy.

c. Staging:

1) The process used to describe the extent of the disease or the spread of cancer from the original site.

2) The tumor–node–metastasis (TNM) staging system is a uniform system used worldwide that assesses tumors in three ways to determine a "stage" (i.e., I, II, III, IV) (Monahan et al., 2007).

a) T: extent of the primary tumor. The numbers T1–T4 describe the size or level of invasion into nearby structures (the higher the T number, the larger the tumor).

b) N: absence or presence of regional lymph node involvement. The numbers N1–N3 describe the size, location, or number of lymph nodes involved. The higher the N number, the more involved the lymph nodes are.

c) M: absence or presence of metastases. M0 means there are no known distant metastases, and M1 means that distant metastases are present.

d. Pap smear: Cells found in body secretions are spread, stained, and examined for tissue classification.

e. Tumor marker blood test: measures for the presence of tumor markers or proteins associated with specific cancers (e.g., CA-125 for ovarian cancer, prostate-specific antigen for prostate cancer).

f. Screening examinations by healthcare professionals can help detect cancer of the breast, colon, rectum, cervix, prostate, testis, oral cavity, and skin.

g. Self-examination for breast and skin cancer may result in early detection of tumors.

E. Management Options

1. Prevention measures:

a. Do not smoke or chew tobacco. Tobacco is believed to play a role in approximately 30% of all cancer deaths in the United States and 85% of all lung cancer deaths (Aetna InteliHealth, 2006; Monahan et al., 2007).

b. Limit alcohol intake. According to the ACS (2006g), alcohol increases the risk of cancers of the mouth, pharynx, larynx, esophagus, liver, and breast and probably of the colon and rectum.

c. Eat a well-balanced diet:

1) Studies suggest that people who eat more fruits and vegetables, which are rich sources of antioxidants, may have a lower risk for some types of cancer (ACS, 2006g).

2) Reduce the intake of fat.

3) Avoid processed, smoked, cured, fried, or barbecued foods.

4) Balance caloric intake with physical activity.

5) Maintain a healthy weight and avoid excessive weight gain throughout life.

d. Protect skin from the sun's rays:

1) Stay out of the sun between 10:00 am and 3:00 pm.

2) Use sunscreen with an SPF of 15 or higher outdoors or wear a hat and shirt when in the sun.

3) Wear ultraviolet light–filtering sunglasses.

4) Do not use tanning booths.

e. Exercise regularly. Exercise reduces the risk of several types of cancer (e.g., breast, colon, endometrium, prostate) and reduces the risk of other health problems (e.g., heart disease, high blood pressure, diabetes, osteoporosis).

    f. Follow occupational hazard guidelines if exposed to carcinogens:
       1) Limit exposure to carcinogens at home.
       2) Avoid using aerosol cleaning products.
       3) Wear gloves when using carcinogenic chemicals.
       4) Follow safety warnings when using paint, solvents, pesticides, household cleaners, and other carcinogenic chemicals.

    g. Remove precancerous adenomatous polyps to prevent colon cancer.

2. Cancer treatment modalities are used to cure, control, or provide palliation; options depend on the stage of the tumor and the level of metastasis.

    a. Surgery: the oldest form of treatment; offers the greatest chance for cure for many types of cancer.
       1) Biopsy: Obtain specimens of suspected tissue.
       2) Curative resection: Resect lesions.
       3) Palliation: Relieve symptoms to improve quality of life.

    b. Radiation: A stream of high-energy particles or waves is used to destroy or damage cancer cells in a specific area.
       1) Used before surgery to shrink a tumor so it can be removed more easily
       2) Used after surgery to stop the growth of cancer cells that remain
       3) Side effects: irritation to the overlying skin, nausea, vomiting, anorexia, bone marrow depression, anemia, thrombocytopenia, leukopenia

    c. Chemotherapy is the use of drugs to treat cancer by interfering with the stages of the dividing cell cycle, used to treat cancer cells that have metastasized.
       1) Anticancer drugs are more powerful when used in combination. More than 50 anticancer drugs are currently in use.
         a) Drugs of different actions can work together to kill more cancer cells.
         b) Use of multiple drugs can reduce the chance of developing a resistance to one particular drug.
       2) Side effects: nausea, vomiting, fatigue, temporary hair loss, mouth sores or dryness, difficulty swallowing, diarrhea, increased vulnerability to infection.

    d. Bone marrow transplantation (BMT):
       1) Autologous BMT: Patient's own bone marrow is used.
       2) Allogenic BMT: Patient receives a donor's bone marrow.
         a) Syngenic: Donor is an identical twin.
         b) Related: Donor is a relative.
         c) Unrelated: Donor is not a relative.

    e. Hormone therapy consists of drug treatment that interferes with hormone production or action to kill or slow the growth of cancer cells.

    f. Biologic therapies (immunotherapy or biologic response modifier therapy) manipulate the immune system through the use of naturally occurring biologic substances or genetically engineered agents that promote or support the immune system's response to cancer.

    g. Gene therapy manipulates genetic material inside cancerous cells to make them easier to destroy or prevent their growth and in some approaches targets healthy cells to increase their ability to fight cancer (National Cancer Institute, 2006b).

    h. Alternative and complementary therapy are unconventional therapies that have not been scientifically tested but may complement conventional care, may help relieve certain symptoms and side effects, and may include vitamins, herbs, dietary supplements, or procedures such as acupuncture.
       1) Body work promotes relaxation and reduces cancer-related fatigue (e.g., massage, reflexology).
       2) Exercise controls fatigue, muscle tension, and anxiety.
       3) Mind–body medicine improves quality of life through behavior modification (e.g., guided imagery, hypnotherapy, biofeedback, art or music therapy).
       4) Acupuncture has been found to be effective in the management of chemotherapy-associated nausea and vomiting and in controlling pain associated with surgery (National Cancer Institute, 2006a).

i. Nutrition and diet can play a role in cancer prevention, but no diet can cure cancer. A proper diet with vitamins, minerals, and other nutrients may inhibit the development of cancer by neutralizing carcinogens, ensuring proper immune function, and preventing tissue and cell damage.

3. Treatment of side effects:

a. Pain: The goal of pain management is to relieve suffering and control pain.
   1) Medication
      a) For mild to moderate pain: nonopioids, including aspirin, acetaminophen, and NSAIDs such as ibuprofen
      b) For moderate to severe pain:
         (1) Opioids, including morphine, hydromorphone, oxycodone, hydrocodone, codeine, fentanyl, and methadone. A prescription is needed for these medicines. Nonopioids may also be used along with opioids for moderate to severe pain.
         (2) Adjunct medications.
      c) For tingling and burning pain: antidepressants, including amitriptyline, imipramine, doxepin, and trazodone; antiepileptics, including gabapentin.
      d) For pain caused by swelling: steroids, including prednisone and dexamethasone
   2) Other methods: relaxation techniques, imagery, distraction, music, humor, biofeedback, hypnosis
   3) Invasive techniques: surgery, nerve block, acupuncture

b. Nausea: Eat light snacks throughout the day rather than heavy meals.
   1) Avoid gas-forming foods.
   2) Eat small, frequent meals to keep the stomach from feeling too full.
   3) Ginger candy, tea, or capsules.
   4) Bland foods such as rice, applesauce, crackers, toast.
   5) Cold or room-temperature foods.
   6) Relaxation, imagery, and distraction techniques.
   7) Antiemetics: dronabinol (Marinol), ondansetron (Zofran).
   8) Antiulcer medications: ranitidine (Zantac), sucralfate (Carafate), metoclopramide (Reglan).
   9) Lorazepam (Ativan) may produce adjunct antiemetic therapy.

c. Increased risk for infection:
   1) Arises from underlying disease, side effects of treatment (e.g., neutropenia, immune suppression), disruption of mucous membranes or skin, presence of long-term venous access device, impaired nutrition, and prolonged hospitalization
   2) Can be managed via prevention; prompt recognition of suspected infection; treatment of skin complications; administration of antibiotics, antifungals, or antiviral agents; fever management; or platelet or blood transfusion for bleeding

d. Fatigue:
   1) Minimize symptoms that interfere with sleep.
   2) Avoid stimulants.
   3) Pace activities to save energy.
   4) Exercise.

e. Weight loss:
   1) Can be caused by treatment side effects that impair nutritional status, uncontrolled pain that impairs appetite, or fatigue that affects the ability to obtain and eat food
   2) Can be treated according to the cause of the weight loss and the overall goals
   3) Can be treated with oral or parenteral nutritional supplementation

f. Pruritus:
   1) Systemic histamine
   2) Topical corticosteroids cream may reduce localized urticaria; antifungal cream can be used for fungal infections.
   3) Tepid bath with aloe vera or oatmeal
   4) Creams containing aloe vera or lanolin for radiation dermatitis
   5) Stop medications suspected of causing pruritus.

g. Arm care precautions for women after breast or axillary surgery:
   1) Perform ROM exercises:
      a) Ensures full use and flexibility of the arm to help alleviate damage to the nerves and muscles that accompanies breast cancer surgery
      b) Reduces the risk and severity of lymphedema (i.e., the

accumulation of lymph fluid in the tissues of the upper extremity after breast cancer surgery), which occurs most commonly in women with breast cancer who had axillary node dissection followed by radiation

2) Avoid sunburn and burns while cooking, baking, or smoking.

3) Wear protective gloves while gardening.

4) Wear loose-fitting watches, jewelry, and clothing.

5) Treat cuts immediately and monitor for signs of infection.

6) Use the unaffected arm for intravenous access, blood draws, and blood pressure; avoid getting chemotherapy in the affected arm.

7) Avoid carrying heavy objects with the affected arm.

h. Monitor for oncologic emergencies: hypercalcemia, disseminated intravascular coagulation, alterations in blood-clotting mechanisms, septic shock, pleural effusion, spinal cord compression, neoplastic cardiac tamponade, superior vena cava syndrome, elevated intracranial pressure, airway obstruction, urinary obstruction., massive hemoptysis (Monahan et al., 2007).

F. Clinical Management of Cancers Necessitating Rehabilitation

1. Brain tumors

a. Brain cancer is the second leading cause of cancer death in people less than 20 years old and accounts for 2% of all malignancies and 2.5% of all cancer deaths (Vogel, Wilson, & Melvin, 2004).

b. Metastasis to the brain is more common, with an incidence 10 times that of primary brain cancer (Vogel et al., 2004).

c. Exposure to chemicals, such as pesticides, herbicides, fertilizers, petrochemicals, and viruses; bioelectromagnetic fields and cellular telephones have been studied as potential contributors to brain cancer (Muscat et al., 2000; Vogel et al., 2004).

d. Glioma is the most common CNS tumor and represents two-thirds of CNS tumors (Vogel et al., 2004).

e. Brain tumors have better outcomes in children than in adults.

f. Clinical manifestations vary according to the location and size of the tumor but

may include headache, seizure activity, nausea and vomiting, memory deficit, and changes in speech, motor skills, and vision.

g. Diagnosis: neurologic assessment, CT, MRI, biopsy.

h. Treatment:

1) Types: surgery, radiation therapy, chemotherapy

2) Complications of CNS surgery: intracranial bleeding, cerebral edema, infection, neuromotor deficits, thrombosis, and hydrocephalus

2. Spinal cord tumors

a. Most tumors that affect the vertebrae have spread to the spine from another site in the body.

b. Cancerous tumors that originate in the bones of the spine are far less common and include osteosarcomas (osteogenic sarcomas), the most common type of bone cancer in children, and Ewing's sarcoma, a particularly aggressive tumor that affects young adults.

c. Many cases of spinal cord tumors run in families.

d. Intradural–extramedullary tumors develop in the spinal cord's arachnoid membrane (meningiomas), in the nerve roots that extend out from the spinal cord (schwannomas and neurofibromas), or at the spinal cord base (filum terminale ependymomas (Mayo Clinic, 2006).

e. Intramedullary tumors begin in the supporting cells within the spinal cord. Most are either astrocytomas, which affect mainly children and adolescents, or ependymomas, the most common type of spinal cord tumor in adults (Mayo Clinic, 2006).

f. Clinical manifestations are related to the site and size of tumor and may include pain, weakness, sensory loss (numbness, decrease skin sensitivity to temperature), muscle spasms, and loss of bowel and bladder control. If left untreated, symptoms may progress to include muscle wasting and paralysis.

g. Diagnosis: neurologic assessment, CT, MRI, biopsy

h. Treatment: surgery, radiation therapy, chemotherapy

3. Bone cancer

a. Cancer that originates in the bone (primary bone cancer) is rare; however, cancer that spreads to the bones (metastatic cancer) from other parts of the body is more common.

1) Primary bone cancer generally attacks young people and is more likely to occur in bones that have been fractured or infected in the past.
2) The likelihood of a cure for primary bone cancer depends on how early it is detected and how rapidly it spreads.
3) Primary bone cancers make up a small percentage of all cancer.
4) In 2006 there were an estimated 2,760 new cases of cancer of the bones and joints in the United States (ACS, 2006f).

b. Symptoms: a hard lump felt on the surface of the bone, pain (especially at night), swelling in bones and joint, spontaneous bone fracture, fever, weight loss, fatigue, and impaired mobility (Monahan et al., 2007).

c. Diagnosis: X-rays, other imaging tests, biopsy.

d. Treatment:
1) Surgical removal when possible. If the cancer is in the arm or leg, amputation usually is avoided and the bone is reconstructed with a metal prosthesis.
2) Radiation and chemotherapy:
   a) May be given before surgery to reduce the size of the tumor
   b) May be used after surgery to kill remaining cells
   c) Used to treat inoperable bone cancer
3) Therapy should begin as soon as possible to avoid stiffness and improve mobility and, if amputation was unavoidable, to help the patient learn how to use the prosthesis.

e. Common types (ACS, 2006a):
1) Osteosarcoma
   a) Tends to affect people between 10 and 30 years of age
   b) Makes up approximately 35% of all primary bone cancers
   c) Has an incidence rate that is twice as high in men as in women
   d) Starts most often in bones of the arms, legs, or pelvis
2) Chondrosarcoma
   a) Tends to attack middle-aged adults; not often found in people younger than 20
   b) Originates in the cartilage cells
   c) Most common sites: pelvic bone, long bones, scapula
3) Ewing's family of tumors
   a) Tend to occur in children and teenagers; not common in adults after 30 years of age.
   b) Occur most often in the Caucasian population and are extremely rare in African American and Asian populations (ACS, 2006d).
   c) About 60% of Ewing tumors start in bone, but others are found outside the bone in soft tissue (ACS, 2006e).
   d) Most common place is the pelvis.
4) Fibrosarcoma
   a) Originates in soft tissue around the bones (ligaments, tendons, fat, and muscle)
   b) Tends to occur in older and middle-aged adults
   c) Originates most often in legs, arms, or jaw

G. Nursing Process
1. Assessment:
   a. History
   1) Signs and symptoms of underlying disease and side effects of treatment
   2) Pain: quality, location, duration, intensity, relieving factors
   3) Dietary evaluation with food preferences
   4) Use of complementary therapies
   5) Psychosocial evaluation (e.g., support systems, coping strategies)
   b. Complete physical and functional assessment to determine the degree of loss of function
2. Plan of care:
   a. Nursing diagnoses
   1) Risk of impaired skin integrity related to skin irritation during radiotherapy
   2) Pain related to tumor causing pressure on nerves, metastases, and reaction from cancer therapy
   3) Fatigue related to poor nutrition, disease progression, and reaction to cancer treatment
   4) Risk of inadequate nutrition related to side effects of cancer therapy
   5) Risk of infection related to effects of

therapy on bone marrow production of white blood cells and platelets

    6) Anxiety related to diagnosis, prognosis, treatment, and pain

    7) Ineffective individual coping related to diagnosis, fear, treatment, and pain

    8) Ineffective family coping related to diagnosis, treatment, and fear

    9) Fear related to prognosis and possible death

    10) Anticipatory grieving related to cancer diagnosis and prognosis

    11) Spiritual distress related to cancer diagnosis and prognosis

  b. Goals, according to phase of illness

    1) Acute phase

      a) Demonstrate healthy lifestyle and remain free of signs and symptoms of infection.

      b) Identify and use effective strategies for coping with stressful situations and adjustment to illness.

      c) Verbalize understanding of the disease process and significant implications.

      d) Verbalizes understanding of treatment regimen and side effects.

      e) Verbalize discomfort.

    2) Intermittent or chronic phase

      a) Verbalize understanding of the prevention and management of side effects of treatment regimen.

      b) Maintain maximal level of function.

      c) Demonstrate safety in mobility and use assistive devices as needed.

      d) Verbalize understanding of diet management, maintain present weight, and maintain fluid hydration.

      e) Verbalize relief from discomfort.

    3) Palliative phase

      a) Maintain a desired level of comfort.

      b) Verbalize wishes and declare preferences regarding treatment options.

      c) Experience a dignified and comfortable death.

3. Interventions:

  a. Acute phase: to attain remission and prevent and control side effects of treatment

    1) Educate the patient and family about the diagnosis, prognosis, treatment, side effects and symptoms, nutritional needs, risk of injury caused by immunosuppression medication, prevention of infections, and support groups.

    2) Provide emotional support by helping the patient and family express grief.

    3) Minimize infection and use strategies to prevent infection.

    4) Provide education on pain relief measures and complications.

    5) Maximize comfort and provide pain relief with prescribed analgesics, accepting the patient's report of pain, using a consistent method or scale to evaluate pain, and providing nonpharmacological methods of pain control (imagery, distraction, relaxation, music).

    6) Assess psychological response to situations and provide emotional support by helping the patient and family express grief.

    7) Ensure adequate hydration and nutrition with vitamin supplements.

  b. Intermittent or chronic stage: to address side effects of treatment and complications

    1) Provide assistive devices for use in performing ADLs.

    2) Balance rest with activities to conserve energy.

    3) Prevent infection, adhering to strict handwashing protocols, maintaining aseptic technique, and monitoring for signs and symptoms of infection, administering antimicrobial therapy as needed.

    4) Assess response to pain management and maintain comfort.

  c. Palliative and end-of-life care: to provide comfort, emotional support, and symptom management and promote peaceful death

    1) Neither hasten nor postpone death.

    2) Assist with end-of-life, comfort measures in a suitable care setting and appropriate services (e.g., hospice).

    3) Help patient achieve as full a life as possible with relief from pain and other symptoms; administer pain medication to relieve pain and discomfort, antianxiety medication for anxiety and restlessness, antiemetic for nausea and vomiting.

---

4) Offers support systems to help patient live as actively as possible until death.
5) Promote calm environment.
6) Provide emotional and spiritual support to patient and significant others.
7) Maintain patient's dignity and spiritual beliefs and wishes throughout the dying process.
8) Educate patient and significant others about dying process.
9) Provide bereavement counseling for significant others.

4. Evaluation: Modify care according to the patient's response to nursing interventions, focusing on quality of life and comfort.

VII. Alzheimer's Disease (AD)

A. Overview

1. A chronic degenerative disease of the brain that destroys brain cells and advances at widely different rates

2. Most common form of dementia (a group of conditions that gradually destroy brain cells and lead to progressive decline in mental function), accounting for more than half of all dementias (Springhouse, 2002)

3. AD is not a normal part of aging.

4. The duration of the illness varies from 3 to 20 years, and eventually the person with AD will need complete care.

5. AD is a devastating disorder of the brain with a subtle progression that impairs memory, thinking, and behavior and leads to death (Alzheimer's Association, 2006c).

6. Currently there is no cure for AD, but research has also shown that effective care and support can improve quality of life for patients and their caregivers over the course of the disease from diagnosis to the end of life (Alzheimer's Association, 2006c).

7. AD significantly affects patients, families, and the U.S. healthcare system medically, socially, and economically.

B. Epidemiology and Incidence

1. Approximately 4–5 million Americans have AD, and that number is estimated to rise to 11–16 million by 2050 unless a cure or method of prevention is found (Alzheimer's Association, 2006b; Hebert, Scherr, Bienias, Bennett, & Evans, 2003).

2. The number of people with AD has more than doubled since 1980 (Hebert et al., 2003).

3. Women are more likely than men to develop AD because they live longer.

4. Annual costs of caring for people with AD are at least $100 billion (Alzheimer's Association, 2006b).

5. Approximately half of all nursing home residents have AD (Alzheimer's Association, 2006b).

6. Approximately 100,000 people die each year from AD (Monahan et al., 2007).

C. Etiology

1. Progressive brain cell death and tissue loss occur; the cause of cell failure remains unknown, but plaques and tangles throughout the brain are found.

2. Abnormal beta-amyloid protein theory (amyloid precursor protein is not broken down but accumulates in large concentrations in the brain,), genetic predisposition, slow-virus theory, aluminum toxicity theory (based on the findings of aluminum deposits in the brain), inflammatory processes, and neurotransmitter deficiency have been implicated.

3. Familial AD is inherited and caused by deterministic genes, and many family members in multiple generations are affected.

D. Risk Factors (Alzheimer's Association, 2006b)

1. Increasing age is the greatest risk factor; the likelihood of developing AD doubles every 5 years after the age of 65 years.

2. Family history: The likelihood of developing AD increases if a parent, sibling, or child had AD. The risk increases more if more than one family member had AD.

3. Genetics: There is a clear pattern of family history, and two categories of genes can play a role in determining whether a person develops AD.
    a. Apolipoprotein E-e4 (APOE-e4):
        1) Those who inherit one copy of the gene APOE-e4 have a higher risk of developing AD.
        2) Inheriting two copies of the gene APOE-e4 raises the risk of developing AD further.
    b. Deterministic genes: Scientists have found rare genes that directly cause AD (guaranteeing that anyone who inherits them will develop the disorder) in less than 5% of cases (familial AD).

4. Head injury: There is a strong link between

serious head injury and future risk of AD.

5. Heart–head connection: There is strong evidence linking brain health to heart health, and the risk of developing AD appears to be increased by many conditions that damage the heart or blood vessels.

6. Down's syndrome: The amyloid precursor protein gene is located on chromosome 21, of which there is an extra copy in Down's syndrome.

E. Pathophysiology

1. Overview (Barker, 2002; Monahan et al., 2007)

   a. Senile plaques form when protein pieces called beta-amyloid (chemically "sticky" minute areas of tissue degeneration) clump together and build up between nerve cells.

   b. Protein called tau (helps the tracks of the vital cell transport system stay straight) collapses into twisted strands called tangles (neurofibrillary tangles) so that nutrients and other essential supplies can no longer move through the cells, which eventually fall apart and disintegrate.

   c. Plaques, neurodegeneration with a loss of the ACh neurotransmitter from synapses, and tangles within neurons spread through the cortex in a predictable pattern as AD progresses. Within the plaques between neurons are dying nerve terminals, aluminum deposits, and abnormal protein fragments.

   d. The immune system cells are activated, triggering inflammation and devouring disabled cells.

   e. In the earliest stages, cell-to-cell signaling is blocked at synapses, resulting in a decrease in functioning neurons, which accounts for a decline in cognition, memory, and thought.

   f. In mild to moderate stages, there is increased nerve cell death and tissue loss, and the brain shrinks dramatically, affecting memory, thinking, and planning in ways serious enough to interfere with work or social life.

   g. In advanced AD, most of the cortex is seriously damaged and shrivels, affecting areas involved in thinking, planning, and remembering, resulting in the loss of ability to care for self, communicate, and recognize family members and loved ones.

   h. Hippocampus shrinks, damaging area that plays a key role in formation of new memories.

   i. As the brain shrinks, the ventricles enlarge.

   j. Usually death results from infection.

2. Warning signs

   a. Progressive memory loss: forgets recently learned information

   b. Difficulty performing familiar tasks

   c. Problems with language: forgets simple words or substitutes unusual words, making speech and language harder to understand

   d. Disorientation to time and place: forgets where he or she is and how he or she got there and does not know how to get home

   e. Poor or decreased judgment: may dress inappropriately for the weather or give large sums of money away to telemarketers

   f. Problems with abstract thinking: difficulty performing complex mental tasks

   g. Misplacing things: may put things in unusual places (e.g., keys in the refrigerator)

   h. Changes in mood or behavior: rapid mood swings, from calm to tears to anger

   i. Changes in personality: can change drastically to confused, suspicious, or fearful

   j. Loss of initiative: may become very passive, not wanting to do usual activities

   k. Inability to concentrate

   l. Loss of eye contact

3. Staging (Alzheimer's Association, 2006a)

   a. Stage 1: no impairment (normal function). No memory problems are evident to a healthcare professional during a medical interview.

   b. Stage 2: very mild cognitive decline. Patient forgets familiar words or names or location of keys, eyeglasses, or other everyday objects.

   c. Stage 3: mild cognitive decline. Friends, family, and coworkers begin to notice deficiencies, and medical intervention may detect some problems with memory or concentration.

      1) Word finding problem

      2) Losing or misplacing valuable objects

      3) Decline in ability to plan or organize

4) Word finding problems noticeable to family or close associates
5) Performance problems in social or work settings noticeable to family, friends, or coworkers

d. Stage 4: moderate decline (mild or early stage). Friends, family, and healthcare providers detect clear-cut deficiencies.
   1) Decreased knowledge of recent occasion or event
   2) Impaired ability to perform challenging mental arithmetic
   3) Decreased capacity to perform complex tasks such as paying bills
   4) May withdraw from social or mentally stimulating situations

e. Stage 5: moderately severe decline (moderate or mid-stage). Major gaps in memory and deficits in cognitive function emerge, and assistance with day-to-day activities becomes essential.
   1) Unable to recall current address, telephone number, or the name of former school
   2) Confused about current location and the date, day of the week, or season
   3) Trouble with simple mental arithmetic (e.g., counting backward from 20 by 2s)
   4) Needs help choosing proper clothing for weather
   5) Independent with eating and toileting
   6) Remembers name and family members

f. Stage 6: severe decline (moderately severe or mid-stage). Memory problem worsens, significant personality changes may emerge, and patient needs extensive help with ADLs.
   1) At times forgets the name of spouse or primary caregiver but generally can distinguish familiar from unfamiliar faces
   2) Need assistance with ADLs, getting dressed properly and toileting (increased episodes of urinary or fecal incontinence)
   3) Loses awareness of most recent experiences and events and of surroundings; wanders and becomes lost
   4) Disrupted sleep–wake cycle
   5) Personality changes and behavioral symptoms, including suspiciousness and delusions, hallucinations, or compulsive, repetitive behaviors such as hand-wringing or paper shredding

g. Stage 7: severe decline (severe or late stage). Loses ability to respond to the environment, ability to speak, and ability to control movement.
   1) Loses capacity for recognizable speech, although words or phrases may occasionally be understood
   2) Dependent with all ADLs
   3) Loses the ability to walk without assistance, then the ability to sit without support, the ability to make facial expression, and the ability to hold head up
   4) Abnormal reflexes and stiff, rigid muscles
   5) Impaired swallowing, with increased risk of aspiration

4. Diagnosis
   a. No single test can diagnose AD.
   b. Accurate history from a reliable family member
   c. Complete physical and neurological examination evaluating overall health and identifying any conditions that could affect how the mind works, including nutrition, alcohol, and medication
   d. Mental status evaluation:
      1) Mini–Mental State Exam is commonly used to assess mental functioning by asking a series of questions designed to test a range of everyday mental skills.
      2) Mini-cog: involves 2 tasks:
         a) Remembering and a few minutes later repeating names of 3 common objects
         b) Drawing a face of a clock showing all 12 numbers in the right places and a specified time given by examiner
   e. Brain imaging studies (X-ray, CT scan, MRI, positron emission tomography scan) rule out other causes, show brain atrophy and enlarged vesicles in advanced stage.
   f. Lab tests: Blood tests rule out infections, blood disorders, chemical abnormalities, metabolic disorders, and hormonal disorders that could cause cognitive impairment.
   g. Spinal tap: Analysis of cerebrospinal fluid rules out certain other brain conditions that can cause dementia.
   h. A definitive diagnosis of AD is confirmed by the presence of neurofibrillary tangles and plaques at autopsy.

F. Management Options

1. Goal: Support remaining abilities and compensate for those that are lost while enhancing safety and security and planning for the future.

2. Treatment could delay onset by 5 years and could reduce the number of people with Alzheimer's disease by nearly 50% after 50 years of age (Alzheimer's Association, 2006b).

3. Pharmacological:

   a. Medication to slow progression of AD or control symptoms (Monahan et al., 2007):

      1) Cholinesterase inhibitors aim to preserve and enhance the physiological effects of ACh by increasing its synaptic levels to close to nondiseased concentrations, thereby slowing the progression of AD. Include tacrine (Cognex), donepezil (Aricept), rivastigmine (Exelon), and galantamine (Reminyl).

      2) N-methyl-D-aspartate (NMDA) receptor antagonists protect brain's nerve cells against excessive glutamate (chemical in the brain that acts on NMDA receptors), which is released by damaged cells in AD. Include memantine (Namenda).

      3) NSAIDs are hypothesized to improve cognition in AD because inflammation is associated with plaques and tangles and is thought to play a part in their formation.

   b. Antipsychotics or neuroleptics control behavior such as agitation, uncooperativeness, anger, hallucinations and delusions, and insomnia caused by AD. Include risperidone (Risperdal), olanzapine (Zyprexa), and haloperidol (Haldol).

   c. Antidepressants and anxiolytics treat depression, anxiety, restlessness, and resistance in patients with AD.

   d. Anticonvulsants used as mood stabilizers can help decrease behavioral problems in AD. Include carbamazepine (Tegretol), gabapentin (Neurontin), levetiracetam (Keppra), topiramate (Topamax), and oxcarbazepine (Trileptal).

   e. Sedatives: used for insomnia.

4. Complementary and alternative therapy:

   a. Vitamin E is a natural antioxidant found in oils from soybeans, sunflower seeds, corn, cottonseed, whole-grain foods, fish liver oils, and nuts, which can slow the progression of AD from moderate to late stage by protecting the nerve cells from the effects of beta-amyloid.

   b. Ginkgo biloba is a naturally occurring substance extracted from the maidenhair tree, used to enhance memory. It is useful mainly in combination with other treatments.

   c. Huperzine A is a moss extract used in traditional Chinese medicine for centuries and promoted as a treatment of AD.

   d. Ubiquinone (coenzyme Q) is produced by the human body and is necessary for the basic functioning of cells. It has been found to decrease with age and to be low in patients with some chronic diseases such as AD. Coenzyme Q supplementation slows the progression of AD.

   e. Music therapy improves memory recall and mood, decreases agitation and anxiety, and improves pain management in people with AD.

5. Nonpharmacologic measures:

   a. Simplify the environment.

   b. Simplify tasks and routines.

   c. Allow adequate rest periods.

   d. Use labels as cues and reminders.

   e. Make sure the person stops driving when he or she forgets how to locate familiar places, fails to observe traffic signals, makes slow or poor decisions, drives at an inappropriate speed, or becomes angry and confused while driving.

   f. Ensure that the home has adequate lighting and handrails on stairways and in bathroom and remove scattered rugs.

   g. Equip doors and gates with safety locks or alarms.

   h. Remove guns.

   i. Remove poisonous plants from the home.

   j. Keep furniture in the same place and remove excessive clutter.

   k. Use appliances that have an automatic shut-off function.

6. Health promotion and disease prevention:

   a. There is no known way to prevent AD, but being alert for warning signs may allow earlier diagnosis and treatment.

   b. Postmenopausal women who take estrogen have a lower incidence of AD. It is believed that estrogen increases ACh production, prevents plaque formation, and plays a role in the functioning of the hippocampus (Monahan et al., 2007).

c. Some experts think that intellectual challenge may have a protective effect against the disease. People with low levels of education and mental activity are said to be at a higher risk for dementia or AD.

d. Protect head from head injury by buckling seatbelt, wearing a proper helmet for sports, and fall-proofing homes.

e. The risk of developing AD or vascular dementia appears to be increased by conditions that damage the heart or blood vessels (heart–head connection).

   1) Preventing and controlling high blood pressure, heart disease, stroke, diabetes, and high cholesterol may decrease risk.

   2) A recent study reported that atorvastatin (Lipitor) slows the progression of AD (Alzheimer disease, 2004).

f. Collaborate with doctor to monitor heart health and treat any problems that arise.

g. Overall healthy aging may help keep the brain healthy and may even offer some protection against developing AD; strategies include keeping weight within recommended guidelines, avoiding tobacco and excess alcohol, staying socially connected, and exercising both body and mind.

G. Nursing Process

1. Assessment

   a. Obtain a complete health history and information about current symptoms, time of onset, and past history of head trauma, stroke, exposure to metals, previous CNS infection, and family history of dementia or AD.

   b. Pay particular attention to memory difficulties, impaired judgment, communication difficulties, personality changes, sleep disturbances, anxiety, wandering, lack of energy, and inability to perform ADLs.

   c. Determine how the disease has affected the patient's lifestyle and family's coping abilities.

   d. Observe the patient's overall appearance.

   e. Investigate physical mobility, urinary elimination, self-care activities, and safety concerns.

   f. Assess for signs of infection, signs of malnutrition, ability to swallow, neurological deficits such as strength, gait, and flexibility and other warning signs of AD.

   g. Investigate use of and compliance in taking prescription medications and use of complementary and alternative therapy.

2. Plan of care

   a. Nursing diagnoses

      1) Risk of injury related to memory loss, impaired judgment, disorientation, and tendency for wandering

      2) Risk of caregiver role strain related to challenges and demands of caring for a person with AD

      3) Impaired physical mobility related to progressive cognitive decline and loss of initiative

      4) Self-care deficits (e.g., bathing, dressing, feeding, toileting) related to inability to perform familiar tasks, loss of initiative, and progressive cognitive decline

      5) Urinary and bowel incontinence related to disturbed thought processes

      6) Knowledge deficit related to the diagnosis, treatment options, safety, prevention, and prognosis

      7) Impaired verbal communication related to memory loss, cognitive decline, and personality changes

      8) Inadequate nutrition related to impaired ability to swallow

   b. Goals: patient and family

      1) Demonstrate safety and recognize the need for structured environment, supervision, and assistive devices.

      2) Verbalize understanding of disease progress, significant implications, complications, and treatment regimen.

      3) Verbalize appropriate plans for coping with stressful situations and progression of illness.

      4) Attain maximal level of function in mobility for as long as possible.

      5) Attain maximal level of function in ADLs for as long as possible.

      6) Verbalize understanding of diet management and prevention of complications (choking, aspiration pneumonia, dehydration).

      7) Maintain continence and follow a bathroom schedule to maintain

bladder and bowel function and prevent complications.

8) Achieve a desired level of comfort.

9) Verbalize wishes and declare preferences regarding treatment options.

10) Verbalize available options to prevent mental and physical exhaustion of caregiver.

11) Experience a dignified and comfortable death.

3. Nursing interventions

   a. Mild stage

     1) Provide education about safety, disease progression, and treatment options to slow progression of AD and to control symptoms.

     2) Encourage activities such as visiting family and friends, listening to music, and participating in hobbies.

     3) Encourage exercise and participation in ADLs to help maintain independence and mobility.

     4) Advise the family to establish durable power of attorney and advanced directives.

     5) Provide clues for home, establish a routine, determine specific locations where essential items are kept, and label drawers, cabinets, and faucets (hot and cold) for safety.

     6) Register with Safe Return, a program established by the Alzheimer's Association to locate people who wander from their homes.

     7) Advise the family to make plans for future care options, finances, and personal preferences for care.

     8) Refer patient and family to social service and community resources for legal and financial support and for support groups (e.g., Alzheimer's Foundation of America, Alzheimer's Association).

   b. Moderate stage

     1) Install door locks for patient safety.

     2) Provide a regular schedule for toileting to reduce incontinence.

     3) Develop strategies such as distraction and diversion to cope with behavioral problems.

     4) Identify and reduce potential behavioral problem triggers (e.g., reduce stress, extreme noise, extreme heat).

     5) Provide medication for behavioral symptoms.

     6) Provide memory triggers such as pictures of family and friends.

     7) Help family develop effective coping strategies to adjust to the illness, encourage them to verbalize feelings and concerns, and help them focus on their loved one's remaining strengths.

     8) Educate the family about avoiding caregiver burnout by scheduling time for self, support groups, and personal interests such as exercise, massage, yoga, hobbies, journaling, and art.

     9) Involve patient in decision making, if still capable of providing input regarding wishes related to future care and end-of-life issues.

   c. Late stage

     1) Provide protective wear for urinary and fecal incontinence.

     2) Provide care to meet total care needs, including oral care and skin care.

     3) Monitor weight, diet, and fluid intake to ensure their adequacy.

     4) Monitor for swallowing difficulties and signs and symptoms of aspiration.

     5) Provide education to the family regarding dysphagia and alternative nutritional and hydration therapy options.

     6) Continue communication through talking and touching.

     7) Provide education regarding care options including respite and long-term facilities when total care becomes too difficult.

     8) Assist with decisions about end-of-life care in a suitable care setting (home, assistive living, long-term care) with access to palliative care with appropriate services (e.g., hospice).

     9) Provide music interventions to promote wellness, manage stress, decrease agitation, alleviate pain, enhance memory, improve communication, and provide opportunities for interaction.

     10) Help patient achieve as full a life as possible with relief from pain and other symptoms; administer pain medication to relieve pain and discomfort, antianxiety medication for anxiety, antipsychotic medication for agitation, and sedatives for insomnia.

     11) Maintain patient's dignity and spiritual beliefs and wishes

throughout the advanced stage of AD and the dying process.

12) Respect patient's and family's rights to refuse treatment.

13) Educate patient and family on dying process.

VIII. Advanced Practice for Specific Disease Processes That Warrant Rehabilitation Interventions

A. Clinician

1. Goal of treatment is to prevent onset of disease process or injury through education about healthy living, reduction of risk factors, support and treatment of symptoms, and prevention of further complications.

2. Assess history, clinical presentation, and current treatment.

3. Complete a physical examination.

4. Assess effectiveness of treatment and medications.

5. Assess psychosocial and economic factors that may influence the management of disorder or injury.

6. Assess coping mechanisms and available support systems.

7. Follow up with the patient as needed according to the progression of the disease, complications, and effects of current treatment.

B. Educator

1. Educate the patient, family, and significant others regarding the disease process, course, signs and symptoms, and treatment options.

2. Provide education about prescribed medications and adverse effects.

3. Discuss prevention strategies, emphasizing the need to reduce risk factors that can be changed.

4. Educate and encourage participation in local and national support groups.

5. Teach the patient, family, and significant others to assist with active and passive exercises to prevent further complications and maintain independence in mobility and ADLs.

6. Teach the importance of eating a nutritious diet according to disorder and injury.

7. Encourage regular rest periods and daily activity and teach the patient to balance rest with activity to prevent fatigue.

C. Leader

1. Provide in-service education to interdisciplinary staff in acute care about specific disease processes, clinical manifestations, interventions, and treatment options.

2. Provide community education about disease prevention, healthy living, specific disease processes, treatment options, and prevention of further complications.

3. Update protocols and procedures and implement changes in practice reflecting evidence-based practice.

4. Participate in research and translate research into practice.

5. Actively participate in specialty nursing organization focusing on policy and practice.

D. Consultant

1. Refer to or consult with specialist (neurologist, urologist, oncologist, burn specialist, HIV and AIDS specialist, endocrinologist) for evaluation and complete workup.

2. Refer to national organization or chapters for education and support:

a. American Diabetes Association: http://www.diabetes.org/home.jsp

b. American Association of Diabetes Educators: http://aadenet.org/

c. National Diabetes Education Program: http://www.ndep.nih.gov/

d. CDC National Diabetes Fact Sheets: http://www.cdc.gov/diabetes/pubs/factsheet.htm

e. National Multiple Sclerosis Society: http://www.nationalmssociety.org/

f. Multiple Sclerosis Foundation: http://www.msfocus.org/

g. National Parkinson Foundation: http://www.parkinson.org/

h. American Parkinson Disease Association: http://www.apdaparkinson.org/

i. National Association of People with AIDS: http://www.napwa.org/

j. CDC HIV/AIDS: http://www.cdc.gov/hiv/

k. American Burn Association: http://www.ameriburn.org/

l. Burn Survivor Resource Center: http://www.burnsurvivor.com/

m. American Cancer Society: http://www.cancer.org/

n. American Association for Cancer Research: http://www.aacr.org/

o. National Cancer Institute: http://www.cancer.gov/

p. Alzheimer's Association: http://www.alz.org/

q. Alzheimer's Foundation of America: http://www.alzfdn.org/

3. Refer to and collaborate with the rehabilitation team for therapy.

4. Refer patient and family for psychological counseling to help them cope with the diagnosis and prognosis.

E. Researcher

1. Evidence-based practice related to music as a treatment modality:

   a. Studies demonstrate that music is being used to reduce agitation in confused patients, increase focus and concentration, improve mood, facilitate communication, reduce pain reduction in cancer and postsurgical patients, decrease dyspnea and anxiety in chronic obstructive pulmonary disease patients, decrease anxiety for patients undergoing invasive procedures, and reduce nonadaptive behaviors in patients with AD.

   b. Current trends suggest that many facilities are using music for therapeutic purposes.

   c. More music therapists are being used in rehabilitation, long-term care, and home care with the goal of assisting in the physical recovery and health maintenance of patients.

2. Clinical question: Can music therapy improve patient outcomes in AD?

3. Appraisal of evidence:

   a. Three level I articles with good evidence (Goodall & Etters, 2005; Sherratt, Thornton, & Hatton, 2004; Sung & Chang, 2005)

   b. Two level III articles with good evidence (Gerdner, 2005; Wilkins & Moore, 2004)

   c. Two level VI articles with good evidence (Hicks-Moore, 2005; Kydd, 2001)

   d. One level VII article with good evidence (Tow, 2007)

4. Recommendation for best rehabilitation nursing practice:

   a. The evidence supports the use of music and music therapy to increase or maintain physical, mental, and social and emotional functioning.

   b. Like other therapies, music therapy typically is preapproved for coverage or reimbursement and is found to be reimbursable when deemed medically necessary to reach the treatment goals of the individual patient.

   c. Integrate music as part of patient's daily experience and use music to calm patients with AD as an alternative to chemical or physical restraints.

   d. Introduce soothing music at mealtime in the long-term care facility as part of the patients' daily experience to decrease eating and weight loss problems.

   e. Music based on the patient's individual preference has an especially calming effect on agitation.

References

Aetna InteliHealth. (2006). *Causes of cancer.* Retrieved December 1, 2006, from http://www.intelihealth.com/IH/ihtIH/WSIHW000/8096/24516/294899.html?d=dmtContent

Alzheimer disease: New study results show benefit for AD patients taking Lipitor. (2004, May 21). *Drug Week,* p. 26. Retrieved December 2, 2006, from LexisNexis Academic database.

Alzheimer's Association. (2006a). Stages of Alzheimer's disease. Retrieved December 1, 2006, from http://www.alz.org/AboutAD/stages.asp

Alzheimer's Association. (2006b). *Statistics about Alzheimer's disease.* Retrieved December 1, 2006, from http://www.alz.org/AboutAD/Statistics.asp

Alzheimer's Association. (2006c). *What is Alzheimer's?* Retrieved December 1, 2006, from http://www.alz.org/AboutAD/WhatIsAD.asp

American Association of Diabetes Educators. (2006). *Who we are.* Retrieved December 2, 2006, from http://aadenet.org/

American Cancer Society. (2006a). Detailed guide: *Bone cancer—What is bone cancer?* Retrieved December 2, 2006, from http://www.cancer.org/docroot/CRI/content/CRI_2_4_1X_What_Is_bone_cancer_2.asp?sitearea=CRI

American Cancer Society. (2006b). *Detailed guide: Cancer (general information)—Signs and symptoms of cancer.* Retrieved December 2, 2006, from http://www.cancer.org/docroot/CRI/content/CRI_2_4_3X_What_are_the_signs_and_symptoms_of_cancer.asp?sitearea=

American Cancer Society. (2006c). *Detailed guide: Cancer (general information): What are the risk factors for cancer?* Retrieved December 2, 2006, from http://www.cancer.org/docroot/CRI/content/CRI_2_4_2x_What_are_the_risk_factors_for_cancer_72.asp?sitearea=

American Cancer Society. (2006d). *Detailed guide: Ewing's family of tumors—What are the key statistics about the Ewing family of tumors?* Retrieved December 2, 2006, from http://www.cancer.org/docroot/CRI/content/CRI_2_4_1X_What_are_the_key_statistics_for_Ewings_Family_of_tumors_48.asp?sitearea=

American Cancer Society. (2006e). *Detailed guide: Ewing's family of tumors: What is the Ewing family of tumors?* Retrieved December 2, 2006, from http://www.cancer.org/docroot/CRI/content/CRI_2_4_1X_What_is_Ewings_Family_of_tumors_48.asp?sitearea=

American Cancer Society. (2006f). *Overview: Bone cancer—How is bone cancer treated?* Retrieved December 2, 2006, from http://www.cancer.org/docroot/CRI/content/CRI_2_2_4x_How_Is_Bone_Cancer_Treated.asp?sitearea=

American Cancer Society. (2006g). *Prevention and early detection: Common questions about diet and cancer.* Retrieved December 2, 2006, from http://www.cancer.org/docroot/PED/content/PED_3_2X_Common_Questions_About_Diet_and_Cancer.asp

American Cancer Society. (2006h). *Statistics detailed guide: Cancer (general information)—Who gets cancer?* Retrieved December 1, 2006, from http://www.cancer.org/docroot/CRI/content/CRI_2_4_1x_Who_gets_cancer.asp?sitearea=STT

American Cancer Society. (2006i). *Statistics for 2005.* Retrieved December 2, 2006, from http://www.cancer.org/docroot/STT/stt_0_2005.asp?sitearea=STT&level=1

American Diabetes Association. (2003). Follow-up report on the diagnosis of diabetes mellitus. *Diabetes Care, 26,* 3160–3167. Retrieved September 13, 2006, from http://care.diabetesjournals.org/cgi/content/full/26/11/3160

American Diabetes Association. (2006a). American College of Endocrinology and American Diabetes Association consensus statement on inpatient diabetes and glycemic control: A call to action. *Diabetes Care, 29,* 1955–1962. Retrieved February 18, 2007, from http://care.diabetesjournals.org/cgi/content/full/29/8/1955

American Diabetes Association. (2006b). Standards of medical care in diabetes: 2006. *Diabetes Care, 29,* S4–S42. Retrieved February 16, 2007, from http://care.diabetesjournals.org/cgi/content/full/29/suppl_1/s4

American Diabetes Association. (2006c). Summary of revisions for the 2006 clinical practice recommendations. *Diabetes Care, 29,* S3. Retrieved February 18, 2007, from http://care.diabetesjournals.org/cgi/content/extract/29/suppl_1/s3?maxtoshow=&amp

Barker, E. (2002). *Neuroscience nursing: A spectrum of care* (2nd ed.). St. Louis, MO: Mosby.

Bloomgarden, Z., & Mechanick, J.I. (2007). Acute glycemic control in hospitalized patient: Evidence published since the American College of Endocrinology position statement. *Insulin: A Clinical Journal for Health Care Professionals, 2*(1), 12–21.

Burn Survivor Resource Center. (2002). *Medical care guide: Types of scars.* Retrieved December 2, 2006, from http://www.burnsurvivor.com/scar_types.html

Burn Survivor Resource Center. (2006) Surgical procedures. Retrieved July 18, 2007 from http://www.burnsurvivor.com/surgicalprocedure.html

Byetta (exenatide injection) [package insert]. (2007). San Diego, CA: Amylin Pharmaceuticals, Inc. Retrieved February 18, 2007, from http://pi.lilly.com/us/byetta-pi.pdf

Centers for Disease Control and Prevention. (2005). *National diabetes fact sheet: General information and national estimates on diabetes in the United States, 2005.* Retrieved December 2, 2006, from http://www.cdc.gov/diabetes/pubs/factsheet05.htm

Centers for Disease Control and Prevention. (2006a). *CDC HIV/AIDS science facts: CDC releases revised HIV testing recommendations in healthcare settings.* Retrieved December 2, 2006, from http://www.cdc.gov/hiv/topics/testing/resources/factsheets/healthcare.htm

Centers for Disease Control and Prevention. (2006b). *Emergency preparedness & response mass casualty: Burns.* Retrieved December 2, 2006, from http://www.bt.cdc.gov/masscasualties/burns.asp

Centers for Disease Control and Prevention. (2006c). *Fire deaths and injuries: Fact sheet overview.* Retrieved December 2, 2006, from http://www.cdc.gov/ncipc/factsheets/fire.htm

Centers for Disease Control and Prevention. (2006d). *Overview.* Retrieved December 2, 2006, from http://www.cdc.gov/hiv/topics/testing/index.htm

Centers for Disease Control and Prevention. (2006e, June 23). Rapid HIV test distribution: United States 2003–2005. *Morbidity and Mortality Weekly Report, 55,* 673–676. Retrieved December 2, 2006, from http://www.cdc.gov/mmwr/preview/mmwrhtml/mm5524a2.htm?s_cid=mm5524a2_e

Centers for Disease Control and Prevention. (2006f). *Spotlight: Commemorating 25 years of HIV/AIDS.* Retrieved December 2, 2006, from http://www.cdc.gov/hiv/spotlight.htm

Chitre, M.M., & Burke, S. (2006). Treatment algorithms and the pharmacological management of Type 2 diabetes. *Diabetes Spectrum, 19,* 249–255. Retrieved February 18, 2006, from http://spectrum.diabetesjournals.org/cgi/content/abstract/19/4/249

Corner, J., & Bailey, C. (2001). *Cancer nursing: Care in context.* London: Blackwell Science.

Diabetes Health. (2006, June). Your complete insulin reference guide from *Diabetes Health. Diabetes Health,* pp. 38–41.

Edlich, R.F., Drake, D.B., & Long, W.B., III. (2006). *Burns, thermal*. Retrieved December 2, 2006, from http://www.emedicine.com/plastic/topic518.htm

Feigenbaum, K. (2006). Treating gastroparesis. *Diabetes Self-Management, 23*(5), 24–32.

Genuth, S. (2006, January–February). Insights from the Diabetes Control and Complications Trial/Epidemiology of Diabetes Interventions and Complications study on the use of intensive glycemic treatment to reduce the risk of complications of Type 1 diabetes. *Endocrine Practice, 12*(Suppl. 1), 34–41. Retrieved February 17, 2006, from http://www.ncbi.nlm.nih.gov/entrez/query.fcgi?db=pubmed&cmd=Retrieve&dopt=AbstractPlus&list_uids=16627378&query_hl=6&itool=pubmed_docsum

Gerdner, L.A. (2005). Use of individualized music by trained staff and family: Translating research into practice. *Journal of Gerontological Nursing, 31*(6), 22–30.

Goodall, D., & Etters, L. (2005). The therapeutic use of music on agitated behavior in those with dementia. *Holistic Nursing Practice, 19*(6), 258–262.

Hebert, L.E., Scherr, P.A., Bienias, J.L., Bennett, D.A., & Evans, D.A. (2003). Alzheimer disease in the U.S. population: Prevalence estimates using the 2000 census. *Archives of Neurology, 60*, 1119–1122.

Herndon, D. (2002). *Total burn care* (2nd ed.). London: W.B. Saunders.

Hettiaratchy, S., & Dziewulski, P. (2004). ABC of burns: Pathophysiology and types of burns. *British Medical Journal, 328*, 1427–1429. Retrieved December 2, 2006, from http://www.bmj.com/cgi/content/full/328/7453/1427

Hicks-Moore, S.L. (2005). Relaxing music at mealtimes in nursing homes: Effects on agitated patients with dementia. *Journal of Gerontological Nursing, 31*(12), 26–32.

Karter, M.J., Jr. (2006). U.S. fire loss for 2005. Residential fires accounted for 77.5 percent of all structure fires in 2005 [Electronic version]. *National Fire Prevention Association Journal*. Retrieved December 2, 2006, from http://www.nfpa.org/publicJournalDetail.asp?categoryID=1302&itemID=30183&src=NFP

Kydd, P. (2001). Using music therapy to help a client with Alzheimer's disease adapt to long-term care. *American Journal of Alzheimer's Disease and Other Dementias, 16*, 103–108.

LaSalle, J. (2006). New insulin analogs insulin detemir and insulin glulisine. *Practical Diabetology, 25*(3), 34–44.

Lazoff, M. (2005). Multiple sclerosis. Retrieved December 2, 2006, from http://www.emedicine.com/emerg/topic321.htm

Leahy, J.L., Clark, N.G., & Cefalu, W.T. (Eds.). (2000). *Medical management of diabetes mellitus*. Burlington: University of Vermont College of Medicine.

Lewis, S.M., Heitkemper, M.M., & Dirksen, S.R. (2004). Medical–surgical nursing. In *Assessment and management of clinical problems* (6th ed.). St. Louis: Mosby.

LifeMed Media, Inc. (2006). Ask an expert: About inhaled insulin. Retrieved December 2, 2006, from http://www.dlife.com/dLife/do/ShowContent/inspiration_expert_advice/expert_columns/campbell_qa.html

Martz, K., Keresztes, K., Tatschl, C., Nowotny, M., Dachenhausen, A., Brainin, M., et al. (2006). Disorders of glucose metabolism in acute stroke patients: An underrecognized problem. *Diabetes Care, 29*, 792–797. Retrieved February 18, 2007, from http://care.diabetesjournals.org/cgi/content/abstract/29/4/792

Mayo Clinic. (2006). *Nervous system: Spinal tumor*. Retrieved December 2, 2006, from http://www.mayoclinic.com/health/spinal-tumor/DS00594/DSECTION=3

McKennon, S.A., & Campbell, R.K. (2007). The physiology of incretin hormones and the basis for DPP-4 inhibitors. *The Diabetes Educator, 33*(1), 55–46.

Merck & Co. (2006). FDA-approved patient labeling package insert (p. 5). Whitehouse Station, NJ: Merck & Co.

Monahan, F.D., Sands, J.K., Neighbors, M., Marek, J.F., & Green, C.J. (2007). *Phipps' medical–surgical nursing: Health and illness perspectives* (8th ed.). St. Louis: Mosby Elsevier.

Multiple Sclerosis Foundation. (2006). FAQs: *What is multiple sclerosis?* Retrieved December 2, 2006, from http://www.msfacts.org/info_faq.php

Muscat, J.E., Malkin, M.G., Thompson, S., Shore, R.E., Stellman, S.D., McRee, D., et al. (2000). Handheld cellular telephone use and the risk of brain cancer. *Journal of the American Medical Association, 284*, 3001–3007.

National Cancer Institute. (2006a). *Complementary and alternative medicine in cancer treatment: Questions and answers*. Retrieved December 2, 2006, from http://www.cancer.gov/cancertopics/factsheet/therapy/CAM

National Cancer Institute. (2006b). *Gene therapy for cancer: Questions and answers*. Retrieved December 2, 2006, from http://www.cancer.gov/cancertopics/factsheet/Therapy/gene

National Institute of Allergy and Infectious Diseases. (2005, March). *HIV infection and AIDS: Overview*. Retrieved December 2, 2006, from http://www.niaid.nih.gov/factsheets/hivinf.htm

National Institute of General Medical Sciences. (2006). *Fact sheet: Trauma, shock, burn, and injury—Facts and figures*. Retrieved December 2, 2006, from http://publications.nigms.nih.gov/factsheets/trauma_burn_facts.html

National Institutes of Health. (2006a, September). *Fact sheet: Burns and traumatic injury*. Retrieved December 2, 2006, from http://www.nih.gov/about/researchresultsforthepublic/BurnsandTraumaticInjury.pdf

National Institutes of Health. (2006b, April). *What I need to know about gestational diabetes*. No. 06-5129. Retrieved February 18, 2007, from http://www.nichd.nih.gov/health/topics/Diabetes_During_Pregnancy.cfm

National Multiple Sclerosis Society. (2005). *About MS: Who gets MS?* Retrieved December 2, 2006, from http://www.nationalmssociety.org/Who%20gets%20MS.asp

National Multiple Sclerosis Society. (2006). *Library and literature: Genetics*. Retrieved December 2, 2006, http://www.nationalmssociety.org/Sourcebook-Genetics.asp

Odegard, P.S.D., Setter, S.M., & Iltz, J.L. (2006). Update in the pharmacologic treatment of diabetes mellitus focus on pramlintide and exenatide. *The Diabetes Educator, 32*, 693–712.

Office of Statistics and Programming, National Center for Injury Prevention and Control. (2006). *Overall fire/burn nonfatal injuries and rates per 100,000 2005, United States, all races, both sexes, all ages disposition: All cases*. Retrieved December 2, 2006, from http://webappa.cdc.gov/sasweb/ncipc/nfirates2001.html

Ohio State University Medical Center. (2006). *What is AIDS?* Retrieved December 2, 2006, from http://medicalcenter.osu.edu/patientcare/healthinformation/diseasesandconditions/infectious/aids/

Parkinson's Disease Foundation. (2005). *Ten frequently asked questions about Parkinson's disease*. Retrieved December 2, 2006, from http://www.pdf.org/Publications/factsheets/PDF_Fact_Sheet_1.0_Final.pdf

Prandase (acarbose) [product monograph]. (2001). Toronto, ON: Bayer. Retrieved February 16, 2007, from http://meriter.staywellsolutionsonline.com/RelatedItems/26,2

Providence Health System. (2004). *Portland protocol: Floors and ICU*. Retrieved October 20, 2006, from http://www.providence.org/resources/oregon/PDFs/Protocol80120.pdf#search='portland%20protocol,%20insulin%20drip'

Scheiner, G. (2006, November–December). *Diabetes Self-Management*, pp. 12–13.

Sherratt, K., Thornton, A., & Hatton, C. (2004). Music interventions for people with dementia: A review of the literature. *Aging & Mental Health, 8*(1), 3–12.

Springhouse. (2002). *Disease management for nurse practitioners.* Philadelphia: Author.

Steefel, L. (2006, May 22). Not just for grown-ups: The number of children with multiple sclerosis is climbing at an alarming rate. *Nursing Spectrum,* 16–17.

Sung, H., & Chang, A.M. (2005). Use of preferred music to decrease agitated behaviors in older people with dementia: A review of the literature. *Journal of Clinical Nursing, 14*(9), 1133–1140.

Tow, D. (2007). Music is a magic for residents with Alzheimer's. *Nursing Home: Long-Term Care Management, 55*(11), 40–41.

Unger, J., & Marcus, A.O. (2004). Glucose control in the hospitalized patient. *Emergency Medicine, 36*(9), 12–18. Retrieved November 1, 2006, from http://www.emedmag.com/html/pre/fea/features/091504.asp

U.S. Department of Health and Human Services. (2006a). *HIV and its treatment: What you should know—Health information for patients.* Retrieved December 2, 2006, from http://www.aidsinfo.nih.gov/ContentFiles/HIVandItsTreatment_cbrochure_en.pdf

U.S. Department of Health and Human Services. (2006b). *Recommended HIV treatment regimens.* Retrieved December 2, 2006, from http://www.aidsinfo.nih.gov/ContentFiles/RecommendedHIVTreatmentRegimens_FS_en.pdf

Van den Berghe, G., Wouters, P., Weekers, F., Verwaest, C., Bruyninckx, F., Schetz, M., et al. (2001). Intensive insulin therapy in the critically ill patients. *New England Journal of Medicine, 345,* 1359–1367.

Vogel, W.H., Wilson, M.A., & Melvin, M.S. (2004). *Advanced practice oncology and palliative care guidelines.* Philadelphia: Lippincott Williams & Wilkins.

White, L., & Duncan, G. (2002). *Medical–surgical nursing: An integrated approach* (2nd ed.). Albany, NY: Delmar Thompson Learning.

Wilkins, M.K. & Moore, M.L. (2004). Music intervention in the intensive care unit: A complementary therapy to improve patient outcomes. *Evidence-Based Nursing, 7*(4), 103–104.

Wilson, R.E. (1996). Care of the burn patient. *Ostomy/Wound Management, 42*(8), 16–34.

Suggested Reading

American Diabetes Association. (2004). Hospital admission guidelines for diabetes (position statement). *Diabetes Care, 27*(Suppl. 1), S103.

American Diabetes Association. (2006b). Frequently asked questions about pre-diabetes. Retrieved August 13, 2006, from http://www.diabetes.org/utils/printthispage.jsp?PageID=ALLABOUTDIABETES_233172

Burn Survivor Resource Center. (2002a). *Medical care guide: Surgical procedures.* Retrieved December 2, 2006, from http://www.burnsurvivor.com/surgical_procedure.html

Ewend, M.G., Carey, L.A., Morris, D.E., Harvey, R.D., & Hensing, T.A. (2001). Brain metastases. *Current Treatment Options in Oncology, 2,* 537–547.

Hieronymus, L., & Hood, G. (2006). Navigating your way to optimal health. *Diabetes Self-Management, 23*(5), 76–78, 80–84.

Jancin, B. (2006). Cystic fibrosis-related diabetes on the increase. *Clinical Endocrinology News, 1,* 10.

Section IV

Rehabilitation Nursing
Across the Life Continuum

· ·

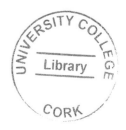

Chapter 15

Developmental Theories and Tasks Across the Lifespan: Individuals and Families

Linda L. Pierce, PhD RN CNS CRRN FAHA

Developmental theories provide the backdrop for understanding the process of human development. Each theory provides a framework for relating life history and past circumstances to the client's or family's tasks of functioning, engaging in healthy relationships, and developing ways to understand the world. Developmental theories propose that people grow and change and master the tasks of living across the lifespan through increasing levels of separation, mastery, and independence.

This chapter reviews two types of developmental theories:
- Individual human development from intrapsychic, interpersonal, social learning, cognitive, behavioral, and interactionist perspectives
- Family development and functioning

I. Individual Human Development Theories

A. Overview

1. Complex factors and forces foster the development of human beings.

2. Human traits are built and exist as enduring behavioral patterns.

3. Unique individual personal dispositions and preferences are demonstrated through behavioral patterns.

4. Behavior patterns lead to successful or unsuccessful management of life and its circumstances.

5. Nursing assessment, diagnosis, intervention, and resultant evaluation depend on a firm understanding of human developmental theories (Whiting, 1997).

B. Theories (see Table 15-1)

1. Intrapsychic theory: Freud (1959) the early and long-dominant theorist in the field of personality development, is responsible for intrapsychic theory (Thornton, 2006).

a. Individuals experience conflict between their natural instincts and society's restrictions on them.

b. Conflict experienced in childhood influences one's adult personality.

c. Libidinal or instinctual drives influence behavior and are related to the individual's attempt to gain pleasure

through the mouth, anus, or genitalia (Glod, 1998; Jarvis, 1996; Whiting, 1997).

1) Oral phase

a) Occurs in the first year of life.

b) Involves exploring the world through the mouth. Mouth, lips, and tongue are the center of existence for the infant.

c) Begins development of the infant's personality, which depends on the mother's (or mothering person's or caretaker's) sense of personal security in self and satisfaction in the mother role.

d) Involves maternal experiences, which are taken on by the infant. The infant experiences whatever the mothering person feels.

e) Leads to the infant being vulnerable (e.g., if mother's anxiety is pervasive and infant begins life with a deficit in adaptive abilities).

2) Anal phase

a) Occurs from about 18 months to 3 years of age

b) Centers on buildup and release of tension in the orifices; involves experiencing pleasure in expelling urine and feces

The Specialty Practice of Rehabilitation Nursing: A Core Curriculum, 5th Ed.

c) Is challenging for parents' coping ability in allowing child to move away, to seek freedom or a greater sense of self

d) Brings psychological problems to the forefront during toilet training and other experiences related to rules of culture and custom

e) Involves ambivalence

    (1) Complying through proper elimination on the part of the infant and interjecting the values of the parents

    (2) Complying through retention or inappropriate discharge of feces or urine by the infant, which brings retribution and further anxiety

    (3) Holding on and letting go responses by the infant lead to various behaviors known as anal characteristics

f) Involves approaching the issue of toilet training by the parents and the infant's corresponding response, which can govern adult personality

3) Phallic phase

  a) Occurs from about 3 to 6 years of age

  b) Draws on the foundation that has been established in the previous 2 stages

  c) Involves becoming aware of individuals' separateness; learning gender or how males and females differ; sex-typing

    (1) Having a romantic attraction to the parent of the opposite sex (Oedipus complex)

    (2) Having a rivalry with the same-sex parent

    (3) Producing guilt and fear from attraction and rivalry

    (4) Resolving guilt and fear by identifying with the same-sex parent

    (5) Repressing sexual urges and imitating the sex-related behaviors, attitudes, and beliefs of the parent of the same sex

    (6) Sex-typing, which has a broader scope than just learning appropriate sex roles in that children learn,

assimilate, and internalize their parents' ideals and values

d) Familiarizes the child with the standards of society (by the parents' words and deeds) and leads to the development of the conscience

4) Latent and genital phase

  a) Occurs from 6 to 12 years (latent) and from puberty (genital)

  b) Involves hiding sexuality, which happens in 6- to 12-year-olds as they engage in the larger world and are absorbed by its challenges; the libidinal drive seems to be less important and receives less attention

  c) Involves reawakened oedipal strivings during adolescence

  d) Rechannels energy toward peers of the opposite sex in an effort to rework the libidinal drive

  e) Involves individuals' responses during the preceding stages, which may cause serious adjustment problems if brought into adulthood

  f) Can involve feelings of constant jeopardy, in which the person is unable to turn energy away from the self to a more productive activity and may produce sexual problems

  g) Results in self-absorption and defensiveness to protect the self or ego

  h) Brings out defensive measures used in earlier phases of development (e.g., repression, introjection, projection, denial, isolation, ambivalence, regression, sublimation) (Freud, 1959; Glod, 1998; Jarvis, 1996; Whiting, 1997)

2. Interpersonal theory: Sullivan (1956, 1971), one of psychiatry's most influential thinkers, developed interpersonal theory.

a. Sullivan's theory departed from Freudian concepts.

b. The term *integrating tendencies* describes behavior by which one person moves toward another person.

c. Healthy development is based on repeated experiences between parents or caretakers and children that lead to the development

Table 15-1. Summary of Individual Development and Function Theories

Theory and Theorist	Description	Infancy (0–12 months)	(Birth–2 years old)	Toddler (12–36 months)	(2–7 years old)
Intrapsychic (Freud, 1959)	Conflict between individuals' natural instincts and society's restrictions on them experienced in childhood influence individuals' adult personality; children are thought to progress through four stages of psychosexual development (Glod, 1998; Whiting, 1997).	Oral	N/A	Anal	N/A
Interpersonal (Sullivan, 1956, 1971)	Repeated experiences between parents or caretakers and children lead to development of a good self and a bad self, which is the basis for healthy development; six stages represent processes by which an individual's identity develops in the context of relationships (Glod, 1998; Whiting, 1997).	Infancy	N/A	Childhood	N/A
Social Learning (Erikson, 1963)	Interaction between parents or caretakers and child is essential to healthy psychological growth; each phase of normal development requires the individual to accomplish age-appropriate developmental tasks through eight phases of development from infancy to older adulthood (Glod, 1998).	Trust vs. mistrust	N/A	Autonomy vs. shame and doubt	N/A
Behavioral (Pavlov, 1927; Skinner, 1953)	Individuals' development is influenced by stimulus–response interaction; individuals' behavior is shaped through the consistency of responding; two attributes of the human brain—flexibility and plasticity—allow for a developmentally significant variety of adaptive sequences (Glod, 1998).	N/A	N/A	N/A	N/A
Interactional (Schaie, 1981)	Development of individuals in a progressive direction occurs when goodness of fit (consonance) exists; poorness of fit (dissonance) involves discrepancies between individuals and their environment, which results in distorted development and maladaptive functioning; starting with dependency in infancy, interference with development of independence in adolescence is likely to inhibit the establishment of interdependence in adulthood (Schaie, 1981; Whiting, 1997).	Dependency	N/A	N/A	N/A
Cognitive (Piaget, 1952)	Motor activity involving concrete objects results in the development of mental functioning; children move through four general periods of cognitive development in the same sequence although not according to the same timetable (Glod, 1998).	N/A	Sensorimotor	N/A	Preoperational

Major Points

- Human development is a complex, interactive, and multifaceted process that involves a variety of forces.

- Some older theories of development (Freud, 1959; Piaget, 1952) emphasize completion of development early in childhood.

- Other theories (Pavlov, 1927; Skinner, 1953) are not age-specific but allow for a developmentally significant diversity of adaptive sequences.

*Many theories (Erikson, 1963; Schaie, 1981; Sullivan, 1956, 1971) view individual development as a continuous process that unfolds throughout the lifespan rather

of a good self and a bad self (Glod, 1998; Whiting, 1997).

d. Seven stages of development represent processes by which the person's identity develops in the context of relationships.
   1) Infancy
      a) Developing both good and bad self-representations
      b) Beginning to realize a sense of sequential time in which things are causally related
   2) Childhood: beginning to develop interpersonal relationships with

peers, language skills, and gender identity
   3) Juvenile: expanding interactions to social, group, and societal relationships
   4) Preadolescence
      a) Forming peer relationships with people of the same sex
      b) Developing the ability to form a meaningful nondependent relationship
   5) Early adolescence: developing sexuality and gender identity
   6) Late adolescence: beginning to

Preschooler (3–5 years old)	School age (5–12 years old)	(7–11 years old)	(11–15 years old)	Childhood (1–12 years old)	Adolescence (12–18 years old)	Early adulthood (18–25 years old)	Adulthood (26–65 years old)	Older adulthood (older than 65 years old)
Phallic, oedipal	Latent and genital	N/A	N/A	N/A	N/A	N/A	N/A	N/A
Childhood, juvenile	Juvenile, preadolescence	N/A	N/A	N/A	Early to late adolescence	Adulthood	Adulthood (continues)	Adulthood (continues)
Initiative vs. guilt	Industry vs. inferiority	N/A	N/A	N/A	Identity vs. role confusion	Intimacy vs. isolation	Generativity vs. stagnation	Integrity vs. despair
N/A	N/A	N/A	N/A	N/A	N/A	N/A	N/A	N/A
N/A	N/A	N/A	N/A	Decreasing dependency	Dependency to independence	Interdependency (adulthood)	Interdependency (adulthood) (continues)	Interdependency (adulthood) (continues)
N/A	N/A	Concrete operational	Formal operational	N/A	N/A	N/A	N/A	N/A

ess that is limited to a few early years in relationships with limited numbers of people (Glod, 1998; Whiting, 1997).

assume responsibility

7) Adulthood: containing these interpersonal themes that continue to emerge in new relationships

e. Personality is shaped by previous relationships.

f. Difficulties in development are viewed as manifestations of disordered interpersonal relationships (Glod, 1998; Sullivan, 1956, 1971; Whiting, 1997).

3. Social learning theory: Erikson (1963) was one of the first developmental theorists to suggest that the interaction between parent or caretaker and child is essential to healthy psychological growth (i.e., parents raise the child, and the child influences the parents).

a. Through satisfactory completion of the developmental task of each psychosocial stage, individuals become ready to move through the stages of development from infancy to adulthood (Glod, 1998; Luggen, 1998; Whiting, 1997).

b. There are 8 sequential psychosocial stages:

1) Trust versus mistrust (infancy)

a) Viewing the universe as reliable

b) Seeing relationships as stable and available
2) Autonomy versus shame and doubt (toddlerhood)
   a) Understanding control over one's body and thinking
   b) Understanding disappointment in self and others
3) Initiative versus guilt (preschool years): dealing with predominantly genital issues
4) Industry versus inferiority (school age): dealing with latency, school, and relationships outside the family
5) Identity versus role confusion (adolescence)
   a) Clarifying personal identity
   b) Depersonifying internal representations
6) Intimacy versus isolation (young adulthood)
   a) Rediscovering attachment
   b) Developing mature bonding
7) Generativity versus stagnation (middle adulthood)
   a) Being creative and productive
   b) Carrying out parental responsibilities (Erikson, 1963; Glod, 1998; Whiting, 1997)
8) Integrity versus despair (older adulthood): feeling a sense of completeness, based on an integrated philosophy of one's unique life (Erikson, 1963; Glod, 1998; Luggen, 1998; Whiting, 1997)

4. Behavioral theories: Pavlov (1927) and Skinner (1953) studied how behavior is affected by its consequences.
   a. Overview
      1) Behavior is developed through the stimulus–response interaction.
      2) Behavior is shaped through consistency of responding.
      3) Two attributes of the human brain—flexibility and plasticity—allow a developmentally significant variety of adaptive sequences (Glod, 1998).
      4) Human behavior is derived from behavioral principles and aversive childhood experiences (Glod, 1998; Whiting, 1997).
   b. Classical conditioning theory (Pavlov, 1927)
      1) Conditioning occurs when a once-neutral stimulus becomes analogous with a response, after they have been associated with each other (Glod, 1998; Pavlov, 1927).
      2) Derived in part from Pavlov's work with dogs, behavioral theory suggests that internal responses can be changed by modifying behavior.
   c. Environmental consequences of behavior theory (Skinner, 1953)
      1) Skinner's theory extends Pavlovian theory to human beings.
      2) Learning is influenced by the effect of individuals' behaviors.
      3) During development, actions are weakened or strengthened.
      4) Shaping behavior occurs with positive and negative reinforcers, which are events that increase or decrease the likelihood that a given action will result; these action responses also reflect learning (Glod, 1998; Skinner, 1953).

5. Interactional model: Schaie (1981) was concerned with how people develop and change from young adulthood to old age.
   a. Development focuses on the concept of goodness of fit and the related ideas of consonance and dissonance.
   b. Many outcomes may be influenced by the development that occurs during childhood and adolescence (Whiting, 1997).
      1) Development occurs when consonance (or goodness of fit) exists.
         a) Involves having environmental demands and expectations in accord with one's capacity to respond
         b) Results in a sense of comfort or consonance, which makes progressive, optimal development possible
            (1) The progression from dependence to interdependence occurs through each developmental stage.
            (2) Adaptation results in and corresponds with the demands of the child's chronological age and particular interests.
               (a) Developing dependency in infancy (0–1 year of age)
               (b) Developing decreasing dependency in

childhood (1–12 years of age)

      (c) Experiencing conflict in dependency in early adolescence, struggling toward independence in middle adolescence, and attaining independence in late adolescence (older than 13 years of age)

      (d) Achieving interdependency in adulthood (older than 21 years of age)

  2) Development of dissonance (or poorness of fit) involves discrepancies between the individual and the environment.

    a) Results in distorted development from the discrepancies

    b) Results in maladaptive functioning from the discrepancies (Schaie, 1981; Whiting, 1997)

6. Cognitive theory: Piaget (1952) studied the development of children's understanding.

  a. The major focus of this theory is to understand how children evolve ways of knowing and how they develop right and wrong answers (Glod, 1998).

  b. Every child passes through stages of cognitive development in the same sequence, although not according to a given timetable.

  c. Every child develops strategies for interacting with the environment and knowing the environment's properties.

  d. A gradual progression takes place from one period of cognitive development to another; acquisition of each new operation builds on existing ones.

  e. Differentiation and complexity occur and are matched by increasing integration and coordination of schemata in this process of development (Drucker, 1979; Ricci-Balich & Behm, 1996).

  f. Infants possess both fixed and flexible reflexes that enable them to develop abstract, intelligent behavior (Glod, 1998).

  g. Children move through 4 general periods of cognitive development:

    1) Sensorimotor

      a) Occurs from 0 to 2 years of age

      b) Development proceeds from reflex activity to representation and sensorimotor learning.

        (1) Feelings and actions are inseparable.

        (2) Sucking and touching actions by infants are innate at first.

        (3) Individuals begin to understand how personal behavior affects the world and become involved in trial-and-error actions.

    2) Preoperational

      a) Occurs from 2 to 7 years of age

      b) Development proceeds from sensorimotor representation to prelogical thought.

        (1) By maintaining stable and consistent images, children are able to create a representational world.

        (2) Children begin to fantasize and use symbols to represent objects and feelings.

    3) Concrete operational

      a) Occurs from 7 to 11 years of age

      b) Development proceeds from prelogical thought to logical, concrete thought.

        (1) Rules are devised to govern behavior.

        (2) Trial-and-error is replaced by the ability to problem solve.

    4) Formal operational

      a) Occurs from 11 to 15 years of age

      b) Development proceeds from logical, concrete thought to logical solutions to all kinds or categories of problems.

        (1) Reasoning and abstract conceptualizations are used to help guide future actions.

        (2) The ability to "walk in another's shoes" is gained.

        (3) Deductive logic is used (Glod, 1998; Piaget, 1952; Whiting, 1997).

7. Moral theories: Kohlberg's (1963, 1976) and Gilligan's (1982) theories of moral development are outgrowths of Piaget's (1952). A comparison of Kohlberg's and Gilligan's theories is presented in Table 15-2.

  a. Overview

    1) Focus on adolescents' moral development

    2) Can be applied to ethical situations

Table 15-2. A Comparison of Kohlberg's (1963, 1976) and Gilligan's (1982) Theories of Moral Development

	Kohlberg's Theory	Gilligan's Theory
Development of the self	Autonomy, individuality, independence.	Connections with others, interdependence.
Others	Objective concern for others; treats others fairly in terms of equality.	Concern for others; helping, caring.
Relationships	Reciprocity between separate individuals with a focus on fulfilling duties and obligations.	Responsiveness to others in the context of their situation and on their own terms.
Morality	Use of a "justice" approach: Moral problems are resolved by the use of impartial, abstract rules, principles, and standards of society, especially fairness.	Use of a "care" approach: Moral problems are resolved by reflecting or responding to the problem in the context of the individual; use of relativism and situational ethics; concern for maintaining relationships and interdependence.

Gilligan, C. (1982). *In a different voice: Psychological theory and women's development.* Cambridge, MA: Harvard University Press.

Kohlberg, L. (1963). Moral development and identification. In H. Stevenson (Ed.), *Child psychology.* Chicago: University of Chicago Press.

Kohlberg, L. (1976). Moral stages and moralization: The cognitive-developmental approach. In T. Lickona (Ed), *Moral development and behavior: Theory, research and social issues.* New York: Holt, Rinehart & Winston.

b. Kohlberg's (1963, 1976) theory of moral development
  1) Background
    a) Extends the work of Piaget, who developed a conceptual framework on moral development from childhood through adulthood
    b) Has a theoretical model based on responses to hypothetical moral dilemmas
    c) Did not include women in the study sample
  2) Stages of moral development
    a) Stage 1: A punishment and obedience orientation in children aged 5–6, in which decisions are based on avoidance of punishment by an authority figure
    b) Stage 2: Instrumental–relativist orientation in children age 7–10, in which decisions are based on perceived benefits to the self in return for agreeing to a rule. The focus is on reciprocity (i.e., the right action consists of satisfying one's own needs by seeking out rewards for good behavior).
    c) Stage 3: Good boy–nice girl orientation in early adolescence, in which decisions are based on seeking approval and on helping and pleasing others
    d) Stage 4: Law-and-order orientation in adolescents to young adulthood, in which decisions are based on adhering to rules for the sake of maintaining social order

    e) Stage 5: Social contract, legalistic orientation in adults, in which decisions are based on justice and fairness to others. The emphasis is on the possibility of changing laws in order to maintain social utility.
    f) Stage 6: A universal ethical principle orientation in adults, in which decisions are based on a person's self-chosen ethical principles such as the universal principles of justice, equality of human rights, and respect for the individuality of human beings as people

c. Gilligan's (1982) moral development theory
  1) Background
    a) Based on a study of female adolescents, which differs from Kohlberg's work, based on findings from an all-male sample
    b) Consists of broad developmental patterns of orientation to care
    c) Does not have a stage hierarchy
  2) Basic elements of moral judgment
    a) A definition and development of the self: Individuals define themselves in terms of their ability to form meaningful relationships or connections with others and their ability to care for others.
    b) A description of others in relation to the self: This concept focuses on the self's interdependence with others.
    c) Relationships with others: The

focus is on the helping and caring relationship with others.

d) Moral decision making: This is based on the context of the situation, but exceptions to rules are allowed. The focus is on responsibility and on caring for others and maintaining relationships with others.

C. Critique

1. Older theories of development emphasize completion of development early in childhood; some were based only on study findings from males.

2. Today, theories assert that individual human development is complex and cannot be classified and categorized.

3. Two attributes of the human brain—flexibility and plasticity—allow a developmentally significant variety of adaptive sequences.

4. Although early life experiences and influences are significant, they are not the only producers of healthy or negative outcomes (Whiting, 1997).

II. Family Development and Function Theories (see Table 15-3)

A. Overview

1. The family is a group of people in varying stages of development.

2. There is a family group stage of development.

3. Family life stages of development can be useful to rehabilitation nurses who are assessing and intervening with families across the lifespan.

4. The needs of the family can be anticipated, depending on the family's developmental stage (Hogarth & Weeks, 1997).

B. Theories

1. Family life cycle: Duvall (1977) was among the first to apply developmental theories to the study of families.

a. Basic tasks of families

1) Keeping the family together: physical maintenance

2) Allocating resources: meeting the family's needs and allocating goods, facilities, space, and authority

3) Dividing the work within the family: division of labor

4) Teaching family members active participation in society: socialization of family members

5) Providing for reproduction: recruitment and release of family members

6) Maintaining order: keeping structure and organization within the family

7) Placing family members into society

8) Maintaining motivation and morale: giving encouragement and affection, meeting personal and family crises, refining a philosophy of life and a sense of family loyalty through use of rituals (Hogarth & Weeks, 1997; Youngblood, 1999)

b. Stages of family development

1) Marriage and the joining of families

a) Establishing an identity as a couple

b) Establishing relationships with extended families

c) Making decisions about parenthood

2) Families with infants

a) Maintaining the couple's relationship while bonding with and integrating the infant into the family

b) Maintaining the couple's relationship while assuming the parenting role

3) Families with preschool children

a) Teaching socialization to children

b) Learning to adjust to the children being with babysitters or other adults

4) Families with school children

a) Helping the children develop peer relationships

b) Adjusting to longer periods of separation by both parents and children

5) Families with teenagers

a) Adjusting to increased autonomy, which the children are developing

b) Focusing on midlife issues

6) Families as launching centers

a) Adjusting to the children leaving home and becoming independent adults

b) Adjusting the couple's relationship as they need to do less parenting

7) Families of middle years (empty nesters)

Table 15-3. Summary of Family Development and Function Theories

Theory	Description	Stage 1	1–10 years	Stage 2
Duvall's (1977) Family Life Cycle	Family development is an 8-stage division that allows differentiation of the family's changes over time and an analysis of the relationship between the family and the individual's developmental tasks. These cycles begin with the establishment of the marital relationship and are based primarily on the age or school placement of the eldest child. Successful accomplishment of the tasks in each stage promotes growth and provides a basis for success in the next developmental stage. On the other hand, failure to successfully complete each stage's developmental tasks may result in unhappiness, societal disapproval, and difficulties in accomplishing the tasks in the next stage (Hogarth & Weeks, 1997; Youngblood, 1999).	Marriage and the joining of families	N/A	Families with infants
Stevenson's (1977) Family Life Cycle	Four stages of family development are identified that are based on the couple's relationship over time. Success or failure of the family depends on the developmental tasks accomplished in each stage beginning in the first year of the relationship. The last stage ends with the death of one partner and the remaining partner grieving and continuing to grow (Hogarth & Weeks, 1997; Stevenson, 1977).	N/A	The emerging family	N/A

Major Points

- Family life cycle is defined as the existence of a nuclear family unit (i.e., mother, father, child) from its inception to its dissolution.
- Family life cycle stages are viewed as the amount of time needed to complete each stage of family development.
- The family is a task-performance group that also has specific stage-related behaviors.
- A family evolves over time. The life history of a family is divided into expected stages of development.
- Each stage of development is characterized by relevant tasks and predictable crises associated with the achievement or nonachievement of specific developmental
- The life cycles defined by Duvall (1977) and Stevenson (1977) are based on a traditional nuclear family form. Neither theory reflects today's lifestyle changes and va
- Duvall's theory assumes that an intact family (i.e., marriage and children) has universal tasks as well as specific developmental tasks that must be accomplished by
- Stevenson's four stages of family development are based on the length of the couple's relationship and specific developmental task completion throughout the

a) Adjusting to living alone again as a couple as the last child leaves home
b) Beginning to prepare for retirement
c) Developing new relationships with adult children and grandchildren

8) Families in retirement (retirement to death)
 a) Beginning to prepare for death of spouse
 b) Adjusting to loss of family members and friends (Duvall, 1977; Hogarth & Weeks, 1997)

2. Family life cycle: Stevenson (1977) based the stages of family development on the length of the couple's relationship.
 a. The emerging family (years 1–10 of the relationship)
  1) Initiating work and career paths by the couple
  2) Deciding to have and having children
 b. The crystallizing family (years 11–25 of the relationship)
  1) Dealing with adolescent children, a

2-way relationship between parents and children
  2) Launching children into independent status
  3) Continuing to grow as a couple
  4) Beginning participation in community life by the couple
 c. The integrating family (years 26–40 of the relationship)
  1) Renewing and enhancing the couple's relationship
  2) Continuing work roles by the couple
  3) Developing leisure activities by the couple
  4) Making adjustments on the part of the children to aging parents
 d. The actualizing family (more than 40 years of living together)
  1) Continuing development by the couple
  2) Dealing with aging, chronic illness and disease, dying spouse or parents, and death
  3) Grieving and continuing to grow if one partner dies (Hogarth & Weeks, 1997; Stevenson, 1977)

Stage 3	Stage 4	Stage 5	Stage 6	11–25 years	Stage 7	26–40 years	Stage 8	More than 40 years
Families with preschool children	Families with school children	Families with teenagers	Families as launching centers	N/A	Families of middle years (empty nesters)	N/A	Families in retirement (retirement to death)	N/A
N/A	N/A	N/A	N/A	The crystallizing family	N/A	The integrating family	N/A	The actualizing family

types of families (e.g., divorce, alternative marriage, single parenting).

family at eight different stages.

relationship (Carter & McGoldrick, 1989; Youngblood, 1999).

C. Critique

1. Theories such as Duvall's (1977) and Stevenson's (1977) that describe family life stages can be useful for those who study families and for practicing rehabilitation nurses because the needs of the family can be anticipated depending on the stage of the family.

2. Because the life cycles defined by both Duvall and Stevenson are based on the traditional nuclear family form, caution is needed when rehabilitation nurses assess nontraditional families.

3. Duvall's and Stevenson's work cannot be used to describe many of the families in today's society that reflect varying lifestyles and forms (e.g., divorce, alternative marriage, single parenting) (Carter & McGoldrick, 1989; Youngblood, 1999).

III. Advanced Practice

A. Clinician:

1. Developmental theories link the determinants of health and illness across the lifespan.

a. Providing a construct for interpreting how individuals' and families' experiences in their early years influence their later health and functioning

b. Aiding in understanding individuals' and families' health and well-being for nurses providing direct care

2. Developmental theories and tasks across the lifespan provide paradigms for clinical issues.

a. Assessing and diagnosing healthcare needs

b. Planning, implementing, and evaluating proactive health and illness interventions when working with individuals and families in various settings

B. Educator:

1. Developmental theories and tasks of individuals and families must be taken into account in teaching clients:

a. Assessing, such as determining the most appropriate teaching strategy based on the developmental stage or life point of the client and family

b. Planning and implementing the

educational intervention, such as choosing the best presentation method or teaching material to fit the needs of the client and family

    c. Evaluating informal and formal educational programs related to developmental needs of the client and family

  2. Developmental theories and tasks of individuals and families must be taken into account in teaching professional and nonprofessional staff members:

    a. Assessing individuals' and group's readiness for learning

    b. Planning and implementing educational content, such as in-service offerings

    c. Evaluating informal and formal educational offerings

C. Leader and Consultant: Developmental theories and frameworks serve as a foundation for integrating child and adult health policies by emphasizing the potential for social and biologic processes early in life to find clinical expression in adult-onset disease. Applying this knowledge to reduce the heavy human and economic costs precipitated by health inequities can involve the following:

  1. Setting policy at the federal, state, and local government levels

  2. Setting policy at the organizational, nursing administration, and interdisciplinary team levels

D. Researcher:

  1. In general, theoretical frameworks depict or explain relationships between concepts of interest in a study.

  2. Developmental theories may form a base for research studies that advanced practice nurses design or participate in or for programs of research that nurse scientists develop and direct. Examples:

    a. Asking the burning clinical question and collecting the most relevant and best evidence so that it can be applied to practice: the National Children's Study (2006):

      1) Improving the health and well-being of children is the purpose of this study.

      2) Examining the effects of environmental influences (defined as natural and human-made environment factors, biological and chemical factors, physical surroundings, social factors, behavioral influences and outcomes, genetics, cultural and family influences and differences, and geographic locations) on the health and development of more than 100,000 children across the United States, following them from before birth until age 21.

  b. Critically appraising and synthesizing the evidence:

    1) Analyzing how these elements interact with each other and what helpful or harmful effects they might have (in this case, on children's health).

    2) By studying children through their different phases of growth and development, researchers will be better able to understand the role of these factors on health and disease and inform best practices.

References

Carter, B., & McGoldrick, M. (1989). *The changing family life cycle: A framework for family therapy.* Needham Heights, MA: Allyn & Bacon.

Drucker, J. (1979). Development from one to two years: Ego development. In J. Noshpitz (Ed.), *Basic handbook of child psychiatry* (Vol. 1, pp. 157–165). New York: Basic Books.

Duvall, E. (1977). *Marriage and family development* (5th ed.). Philadelphia: Lippincott.

Erikson, E. (1963). *Childhood and society* (2nd ed.). New York: Norton.

Freud, S. (1959). Inhibitions, symptoms, and anxiety. In J. Strachey (Ed.), *The standard edition of the complete psychological works of Sigmund Freud* (Vol. 18, pp. 1–64). London: Hogarth.

Gilligan, C. (1982). *In a different voice: Psychological theory and women's development.* Cambridge, MA: Harvard University Press.

Glod, C. (1998). Developmental and psychological theories of mental illness. In C. Glod (Ed.), *Contemporary psychiatric–mental health nursing* (pp. 64–72). Philadelphia: F.A. Davis.

Hogarth, C., & Weeks, S. (1997). Families and family therapy. In B. Johnson (Ed.), *Psychiatric–mental health nursing: Adaptation and growth* (4th ed., pp. 277–298). Philadelphia: Lippincott.

Jarvis, C. (1996). Assessment of the whole person. In C. Jarvis (Ed.), *Physical examination and health assessment* (pp. 1–46). Philadelphia: W.B. Saunders.

Kohlberg, L. (1963). Moral development and identification. In H. Stevenson (Ed.), *Child psychology.* Chicago: University of Chicago Press.

Kohlberg, L. (1976). Moral stages and moralization: The cognitive-developmental approach. In T. Lickona (Ed.), *Moral development and behavior: Theory, research and social issues.* New York: Holt, Rinehart & Winston.

Luggen, A. (1998). Developmental theories. In A. Luggen, S. Travis, & S. Meiner (Eds.), *NGNA core curriculum for gerontological advanced practice nurses* (pp. 7–9). Thousand Oaks, CA: Sage.

The National Children's Study. Retrieved September 5, 2006, from http://www.nationalchildrensstudy.gov/

Pavlov, I. (1927). *Conditioned reflexes: An investigation of the physiological activity of the cerebral cortex.* New York: Oxford University Press.

Piaget, J. (1952). *Origins of intelligence in children.* New York: International Universities Press.

Ricci-Balich, J., & Behm, J. (1996). Pediatric rehabilitation. In S. Hoeman (Ed.), *Rehabilitation nursing: Process and application* (2nd ed., pp. 660–682). St. Louis: Mosby.

Schaie, K. (1981). Psychological changes from midlife to early old age: Implications for the maintenance of mental health. *American Journal of Orthopsychiatry, 51*(4), 199–218.

Skinner, B.F. (1953). *Science and human behavior.* New York: Macmillan.

Stevenson, J. (1977). *Issues and crises during middlescence.* New York: Appleton-Century-Crofts.

Sullivan, H. (1956). *Clinical studies in psychiatry.* New York: Norton.

Sullivan, H. (1971). *The fusion of psychiatry and social science.* New York: Norton.

Thornton, S. (2006). *The Internet encyclopedia of philosophy.* Retrieved September 1, 2006, from http://www.iep.utm.edu/f/freud.htm

Whiting, S. (1997). Development of the person. In B. Johnson (Ed.), *Psychiatric–mental health nursing: Adaptation and growth* (4th ed., pp. 357–373). Philadelphia: Lippincott.

Youngblood, N. (1999). Family-centered care. In P. Edwards, D. Hertzberg, S. Hays, & N. Youngblood (Eds.), *Pediatric rehabilitation* (pp. 129–143). Philadelphia: W.B. Saunders.

Suggested Resources

Armour, M. (1995). Family life cycle stages: A context for individual life stages. *Journal of Family Social Work, 1*(2), 27–42.

Atherton, J. (2005). *Piaget.* Retrieved September 1, 2006, from http://www.learningandteaching.info/learning/piaget.htm

Cronau, H., & Brown, R. (1998). Growth and development: Physical, mental, and social aspects. Primary Care: *Clinics in Office Practice, 25*(1), 23–47.

Davis, D., & Clifton, A. (2006). *Psychosocial theory: Erikson.* Retrieved September 1, 2006, from http://www.haverford.edu/psych/ddavis/p109g/erikson.stages.html

Developmental psychology: Lifespan theories. (2006). Retrieved September 1, 2006, from http://www.geocities.com/psychtheory/lifespan.html#synopsis

Grant, G., Nolan, M., & Keady, J. (2003). Supporting families over the life course: Mapping temporality. *Journal of Intellectual Disability Research, 47*(4–5), 342–351.

Harrison, T. (2003). Women aging with childhood onset disability: A holistic approach using the life course paradigm. *Journal of Holistic Nursing, 21*(3), 242–259.

Quinn, A. (1993). Commentary on Erik Erikson: Ages, stages, and stories [Original article by S. Weiland]. AWHONN's *Women's Health Nursing Scan, 7*(6), 4.

Schroots, J.J.F., van Dijkum, C., & Assink, M.H.J. (2004). Autobiographical memory from a life span perspective. *International Journal of Aging & Human Development, 58*(1), 69–85.

Weiland, S. (1993). Erik Erikson: Ages, stages, and stories. *Generations, 17*(2), 17–23.

Westermeyer, J.F. (2004). Predictors and characteristics of Erikson's life cycle model among men: A 32-year longitudinal study. *International Journal of Aging & Human Development, 58*(1), 29–48.

Wise, P.H. (2003). Framework as metaphor: The promise and peril of MCH life-course perspectives. *Maternal & Child Health Journal, 7*(3), 151–156.

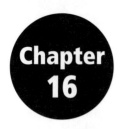

Chapter 16

Pediatric Rehabilitation Nursing

Patricia A. Edwards, EdD RN CNAA • Dalice Hertzberg, MSN RN ARNP BC • Lyn Sapp, BSN RN CRRN

This chapter brings together a unique body of knowledge specific to the care of children and adolescents with disabilities and chronic conditions and their families. It provides a reference for nurses in a variety of settings across the continuum of care, from hospital to home and community. The emphasis is on the roles of the pediatric rehabilitation nurse in relation to care coordination and provision, health teaching and promotion, leadership, collaboration, advocacy, and professional practice.

Family-centered care and developmental assessment and intervention are addressed in this chapter in an interdisciplinary approach. Specific diagnoses are outlined, including accidents and trauma, congenital diseases and birth defects, and chronic conditions. Long-term planning, including community services, home health care, school, and early intervention programs and transition to adulthood are presented.

I. Overview

A. Definitions

1. Pediatric rehabilitation nursing: "Pediatric rehabilitation nursing is the specialty practice committed to improving the quality of life for children and adolescents with disabilities and their families. The mission is to provide, in collaboration with the interdisciplinary team, a continuum of nursing care from onset of injury or illness to productive adulthood. The goal of the rehabilitation process is for children, regardless of their disability or chronic illness, to function at their maximum potential and become contributing members of both their families and society" (Association of Rehabilitation Nurses [ARN], 2007, pp. 1–2).

2. Habilitation: needing new skills and abilities to meet maximum potential (i.e., children usually have not learned some skills as they continue to progress through the developmental levels).

3. Rehabilitation: relearning skills and abilities or adjusting existing function to meet age-related developmental expectations.

B. Roles of the Pediatric Rehabilitation Nurse

1. Advocacy
2. Coordination of care
3. Leadership and consulting
4. Care provision
5. Health teaching and promotion
6. Team participation
7. Research

8. Professional practice, education, and evaluation (ARN, 2007, pp. 1–2)

C. Practice Settings

1. Pediatric rehabilitation hospitals (inpatient and outpatient)
2. Pediatric rehabilitation units in rehabilitation hospitals
3. Subacute and postacute rehabilitation units
4. Day treatment programs
5. Medical homes
6. Freestanding pediatric outpatient therapy centers
7. Health department outpatient services
8. State children's rehabilitation services
9. School or day care centers
10. Home health agencies
11. Family homes

D. General Principles

1. Family-centered care: a philosophy of care that recognizes the role of the family in the lives of children.
   a. All children are part of a family even if the family is not considered traditional in American culture.
   b. Including the family in care ensures that family members and the child receive support in coping with the child's disability or chronic illness.
2. Community-based delivery systems: services that are delivered in the child's environment (e.g., early intervention center, medical home, school, day care, pediatric outpatient therapy center, home).

3. Medical home: "A medical home is not a building, house, or hospital, but rather an approach to providing health care services in a high-quality and cost-effective manner" (American Academy of Pediatrics, 2007). Pediatric healthcare professionals and parents act as partners in a medical home to identify and access all the medical and nonmedical services needed to help children and their families achieve the maximum potential for the child. A medical home for a child usually is part of a pediatrician's office but may be part of a comprehensive outpatient program.

4. Human development:
   a. Pediatric rehabilitation nurses must have in-depth knowledge of developmental theories, normal development, and related assessment skills and knowledge of interventions that promote developmental milestones. [Refer to Chapter 15 for more information about developmental theories.]
   b. Understanding family life stages of development can be useful in assessing and intervening with children and families.

5. Developmental levels: The child's developmental level should be considered in determining the rehabilitation plan and interventions.
   a. Infant and toddler (1–3 years old)
   b. Preschooler (3–5 years old)
   c. School-age child (6–12 years old)
   d. Adolescent (12–21 years old)

6. Assessment: Each child should be assessed for the following items, regardless of his or her disability or illness.
   a. Current developmental level
   b. Delays related to developmental level for child's age
   c. The impact of the child's disability on his or her developmental level
   d. Plans for transition into adult services

7. Interventions: Physical, emotional, social, cultural, educational, developmental, and spiritual dimensions are all considered in a holistic approach to care.
   a. Focus on helping the child meet his or her developmental milestones as much as possible.
   b. Investigate alternative ways to achieve tasks if developmental milestones cannot be met through therapy or assistive devices.
   c. Attempt to map the future by being proactive rather than reactive.
   d. Facilitate adaptation to the disability and treatment.
   e. Promote community integration.
   f. Provide resources and referrals to meet transitional needs when the child is no longer eligible for pediatric services.
   g. Incorporate appropriate recreational activities, toys, and fun as well as therapeutic interventions. Play, the means by which children learn about the world, is an integral part of the rehabilitation plan.

8. Interdisciplinary team approach (nursing, medicine, physical and occupational therapy, speech, nutrition, psychology, education, social work, orthotics, and support services, e.g., vision and dental):
   a. Recognize the child's intellectual and physical abilities.
   b. Coordinate the plan of care to maximize potential.
   c. The family plays a vital role in advocating for the child and is a core part of the rehabilitation team.
   d. Provide parent education and training.
   e. Develop appropriate experiences to enrich quality of life.

II. Specific Pediatric Diagnoses

A. Accidents and Trauma

1. Traumatic brain injury (TBI)
   a. Definition: an insult to the brain from noncongenital trauma, associated with an altered state of consciousness, causing permanent neurologic impairment (Dawodu, 2007).
      1) Children may experience deficits in physical, psychosocial, and cognitive functioning.
      2) Children differ from adults with TBI. Physiologic differences in children lead to differences in acute care management:
         a) Response to injury, such as more diffuse cerebral edema after injury, makes acute management of increased intercranial pressure paramount.
         b) Maintenance of adequate cerebral perfusion is critical to a more positive outcome in children (Hackbarth et al., 2002).
         c) Characteristics of injury, such as delays in treatment, particularly

in young children, can lead to increased ischemic injury.

d) Causes of injury differ (e.g. in young children falls or child abuse are likely causes, whereas in older children motor vehicle accidents are common causes, and in adolescents and young adults sports-related head injuries are more prevalent).

e) Outcomes of injury are affected in part by age at the time of injury; infants are more likely to have worse outcomes (Giza, Mink, & Madikians, 2007; Dawodu, 2007).

3) Differences between children and adults lead to differences in rehabilitation management and outcome:

a) Children are more likely to survive TBI than adults.

b) Predictors of outcome in children and adolescents include Glasgow Coma Scale rating, intracranial pressure, length of time in coma, and severity of injury (Chung et al., 2006; Giza et al., 2007).

c) Children continue to grow and develop after TBI; this puts them at an additional disadvantage with regard to future learning.

d) There is even more impact on the family because caregiving often is extended beyond childhood.

e) The cost to family and society is greater because the child with TBI generally has more years to live.

f) The school system and special education are critical pieces in the rehabilitation of children with TBI, yet programs often lack expertise with these children (Agency for Health Care Policy and Research, 1999).

b. Epidemiology:

1) TBI in children from birth to 14 years of age results in 2,685 deaths, 37,000 hospitalizations, and 435,000 emergency department visits (National Center for Injury Prevention and Control [NCIPC], 2006).

2) Of children with head injury, about 30,000 experience long-term disability (NCIPC, 2006; National Dissemination Center for Children

with Disabilities, 2006).

3) Adolescents, young adults, and very young children are at highest risk for TBI.

4) As with adults, males are more likely to experience TBI than females.

c. Outcomes of TBI in children may include the following:

1) Speech and language disorders

2) Motor deficits

3) Dysphagia and feeding problems; some children need gastrostomy feedings temporarily or in the long term (Morgan, Ward, Murdoch, Kennedy, & Murison, 2003).

4) Behavioral problems: impulsivity, secondary attention deficit disorder, aggression, and personality changes

5) Cognitive deficits (executive function disorders, processing disorders, memory deficits) leading to need for special education and school services

6) Social problems, caused in part by cognitive deficits and behavioral disorders

7) Seizure disorder

8) Vision and hearing deficits (Agency for Health Care Policy and Research, 1999)

d. Assessment:

1) Physical assessment for common postinjury problems

a) Neurologic deficit: level of consciousness, intercranial pressure, Glasgow Coma Scale (Chung et al., 2006), Rancho Los Amigos Scale

b) Respiratory deficit: adequate oxygenation, some children need tracheostomy or ventilation initially, and those with more severe injury may be discharged on mechanical ventilation.

c) Cardiovascular: hemodynamic instability

d) Endocrine deficit (e.g. syndrome of inappropriate antidiuretic hormone, diabetes insipidus, hyperglycemia)

e) Gastrointestinal and nutritional assessment: nasogastric tube, gastrostomy tube, oral stimulation, oral feedings, choking risk (Blissit, 2006)

2) Developmental assessment: cognitive abilities, premorbid functioning

3) Functional assessment: WeeFIM™

instrument [Refer to Chapter 19.] (Rice et al., 2005)

4) Communication and language
5) Family assessment: coping, guilt, ability to care for child, financial concerns, siblings (Swift et al., 2003; Wade et al., 2004)

e. Rehabilitation issues
1) Independence level appropriate for developmental level
2) Cognitive rehabilitation
3) Speech and language therapy
4) Prevention of further injury and complications
5) Family involvement
6) Behavioral problems, personality changes, need for increased supervision
7) Special education, integration into school, planning with school staff
8) Discharge planning: daily care of child at home, therapy and medical appointments, equipment and planning for an emergency, respite care, community resources (Agency for Health Care Policy and Research, 1999; Tomlin, Clarke, Robinson, & Roach, 2002)
9) Community integration

f. Family and child education topics
1) Methods of promoting development and independence; "normalization"
2) Use and care of equipment and assistive devices
3) Prevention of further injury and use of protective equipment
4) Behavior modification strategies
5) Service coordination and advocacy
6) Teaching strategies that may include play therapy

2. Spinal cord injury (SCI) [Refer to Chapter 10 for in-depth discussion of SCI.]

a. Before puberty, children have unique physical and developmental characteristics that distinguish them from adults. These characteristics predispose them to SCI from lap-belt injuries, injuries related to birth and child abuse, SCI without radiologic abnormalities (more common in children <8 years old), delayed onset of neurologic deficits, high cervical injuries, and potential for additional common associated brain, chest, and limb injuries (Launay, Leet, & Sponseller, 2005; Martin, Dykes, & Lecky, 2004; Vogel, Hickey, Klaas, &

Anderson, 2004). Injuries occur at all ages, including in utero, during delivery, and throughout childhood (Brand, 2006; Massagli, 2000; Vogel et al., 2004).

b. Assessment components:
1) Health history
2) Functional and cognitive levels.
3) Spinal stability
4) Developmental levels: Rehabilitation goals are dynamic, to be adjusted with growth and development of the child
5) Skin integrity
6) Bladder and bowel function
7) Psychosocial issues
8) Family history
9) Respiratory status (especially in tetraplegia and upper level thoracic injury)
10) Home environment accessibility

c. Rehabilitation issues:
1) Neurogenic bladder and bowel management
2) Skin care: Adolescents may be at risk for pressure ulcers, related to body image and peer embarrassment, challenge of taking time to check skin, and distraction by teen activities (Vogel et al., 2004).
3) Mobility: Immobilization and spine stabilization with bracing, functional dependent to independent mobility activities (power mobility for children as young as 3 years of age)
4) Pulmonary function, mechanical ventilation (if injury is at C3 and above): Infants and younger children with tetraplegia are at risk of incipient respiratory failure. Sleep studies are recommended for history of excessive daytime sleepiness or prominent snoring (Vogel et al., 2004).
5) Risk for heterotopic ossification
6) Risk for autonomic dysreflexia (injuries at level T6 and above): 20–40 mmHg above baseline in adults, 15–20 mmHg above baseline in adolescents, 15 mmHg above baseline in children (Vogel et al., 2004). Recommendation: Child should wear medical alert bracelet and have autonomic dysreflexia information card and care supplies in his or her school backpack.
7) Risk for spasticity and contractures: range of motion and splinting for pediatrics.

8) Risk for sexual dysfunction
9) Risk for osteopenia
10) Risk for deep vein thrombosis: prophylactic treatment follows adult practice.
11) Prevention of further injury
12) Plans for return to home, school, and community
13) Orthopedic complications: scoliosis and hip instability
14) Hypercalcemia
15) Latex sensitivity, related to longevity of exposure. It is best to be in a latex-free environment to prevent development of latex sensitivity and allergy (Vogel et al., 2004).

d. Patient education topics: Dramatic developmental changes occur as children grow. Developmentally appropriate educational methods and family-centered care are essential because of dependency on caregivers. An individualized educational SCI program is essential, incorporating parental and child education adjustment from dependence to independence as the child grows into adulthood (Vogel et al., 2004).
1) Bladder and bowel program: considerations of learning self–clean intermittent catheterization (with fine motor abilities and injury considerations as young as 5–7 years of age). Bowel program initiated at about 3 years of age, transitioning to independence and directing caregivers in late school age to adolescence (Massagli, 2000; Vogel et al., 2004).
2) Skin care
3) Autonomic dysreflexia (if injury is at T6 or above)
4) Medications
5) Community reintegration strategies
6) Sexuality: Effects on sexual function in children are similar to those in adults with SCI (pregnancy, fertility, erectile dysfunction, and ejaculation dysfunction). Education with parents and child or adolescent is similar to that of children without SCI and is developmentally appropriate (Vogel et al., 2004).
7) Emotional support: Sense of hope is important throughout rehabilitation and at all ages (Lohne & Severinsson, 2004).

3. Burns
a. Definitions:
1) The loss of any of the 3 layers of skin by fires, scalds (including immersion or splashing by hot liquids, grease, and steam), contact (touching hot object or substance), chemical, electrical, or radiation burns (Weed & Berens, 2005).
2) Classification:
a) First degree: superficial
b) Second degree: partial thickness
c) Third degree: full thickness
d) Some centers include fourth degree—includes muscles and bone (Weed & Berens, 2005).
3) Classifications in children:
a) Mild or minor: 10% total body surface area (TBSA) partial-thickness and < 2% full-thickness unless eyes, ears, face, or perineum is involved
b) Moderate: 10%–20% TBSA regardless of depth and 2%–10% TBSA full thickness unless the eyes, ears, face, or perineum is involved
c) Major: >20% TBSA partial thickness, >10% TBSA full thickness, all burns involving face, eyes, ears, feet, and perineum, all burns that are electrical or involve inhalation injury, all burns with ancillary injury (e.g., fracture, tissue trauma) (Weed & Berens, 2005)
4) Further studies and informational demographics are tracked through research burn model system databases (Klein et al., 2007).
b. Assessment components:
1) Skin integrity: Consider photo journal.
2) Respiratory condition
3) Mobility and functional levels (e.g., WeeFIM™).
4) Pain: assessment scales such as comfort scale, Premature Infant Pain Profile for young children; older children may use scales such as Poker Chip Tool, 0–10, Faces, Visual Analogue Scale (Stoddard et al., 2002).
5) Nutrition
6) Self-image
7) Developmental level (using Battelle Developmental Inventory)
8) Family history and coping

9) Sleep (itching, splinting, and night terrors may be common)

c. Rehabilitation issues and interventions: Children are more likely than adults to develop hypertrophic scars and keloids as a result of vigorous healing, compliance may be challenged by uncomfortable and unsightly treatment modalities and extreme social pressure for acceptance by peers (Passaretti & Billmire, 2003).

1) Potential for infection (e.g., skin, respiratory, mild restrictive disease in thermal burns; exercise or activity improves pulmonary function) (Suman, Mlcak, & Herndon, 2002)

2) Burn locations most challenging to functional ability: axillary, neck, flexion areas, bottoms of feet.

3) Comfort level and pain management: pharmacological (narcotic, nonnarcotic, anti-itching and anti-anxiolytic formulations), cognitive behavioral therapy, relaxation training, hypnosis, reassurance, parental support, guided imagery, biofeedback, distraction, therapeutic touch, art, music, and play therapy (Stoddard et al., 2002)

4) Nutrition deficit related to hypermetabolic state for as long as 1 year after burn injury; enteral or parenteral nutrition for supplementation should be considered at a rate of 1.4 times resting energy expenditure in pediatric population (Gordon, Gottschlich, Helvig, Marvin, & Richard, 2004; Pereira, Murphy, & Herndon, 2005).

5) Pressure garments: Average length of wearing is 1–2 years after acute burn, while scarring is still in inflammatory stage (Passaretti & Billmire, 2003).

6) Restoration of self-image

7) Elimination pattern

8) Contracture management and surgeries for function or cosmesis: scar contraction, joint contractures, muscle shortening, and growth restriction in pediatrics; physical and occupational therapy, splinting, massage, pressure garments, and surgical evaluation during the child's growing years (Passaretti & Billmire, 2003; Vehmeyer-Heeman, Lommers, Van den Kerckhove, & Boeckx, 2005)

9) Risk for pressure ulcers related to immobility, significant edema, nutrition alterations, injuries or operative procedures, moisture imbalance, splinting, and pressure garments: Consider pressure-reducing mattress, frequent turning (more often than every 2 hours), nutrition support, skin emollients and protective moisture barriers, skin checks with splint and pressure garment removal (Gordon et al., 2004).

10) Risk for long bone fractures: increased incidence in children <3 years of age and with burns greater than 40% (potential contributory factors: hormonal changes after burn, depressed vitamin D status, inadequate protein intake, decreased weight-bearing activity, opposition to physical therapy) (Mayers, Gottschlich, Scanlon, & Warden, 2003)

11) Medication management: potential treatment of hypermetabolic state (in children with >40% burns) with insulin, anabolic steroids, catecholamine antagonists, anabolic and anticatabolic agents (Pereira et al., 2005; Przkora et al., 2006)

12) School reintegration: potential compliance resistance necessitating assistance from school therapists for ongoing therapeutic management or behavior management program (Pidcock, Fauerback, Ober, & Carney, 2003)

d. Patient education topics

1) Importance of prevention of complications, contractures, loss of function, and ongoing exercise and therapy

2) Care and use of pressure garments

3) Signs and symptoms of infection

4) Skin and wound care

5) Social reintegration strategies

6) School and community reintegration strategies, camp opportunities

7) Psychosocial and behavioral interventions

8) Personal care

9) Nutrition

10) Pain and itching management

11) Medications

12) Home environment and safety as indicated; prevention of further injury

4. Limb deficiency

a. Definition: The absence of one or more

limbs, caused by congenital conditions, trauma or accidents, tumors, or diseases. Congenital amputations in children are more common than acquired amputations (Morrissy, Giavedoni, & Coulter-O'Berry, 2006).

1) Congenital: may be spontaneous, genetic, related to prenatal exposure to virus or teratogens in 1st trimester (Kozin, 2004). May have high incidence of other associated congenital anomalies, including genitourinary defects, cardiac defects, and cleft palate (Eilert, 2007).
   a) Upper extremity: below-elbow transverse arrest (most common), humeral deficiency, longitudinal arrest, failure of differentiation (i.e., synostosis), constriction or amniotic band syndromes, cleft hand, phocomelia (distal portion of extremity appears to attach directly to body), amelia (missing limb) (Kozin, 2004; Morrissy et al., 2006)
   b) Lower extremity: fibular hemimelia (missing fibula; most common), tibial hemimelia, proximal femoral focal deficiency (PFFD) (Morrissy et al., 2006; Mosca, 2006)
   c) Digits: syndactyly (fused), adactylia (absent)
2) Acquired:
   a) Trauma: leading cause is lawnmower accidents, followed by motor vehicle, farm machinery, gunshot wounds, fire or other burns, amputations from triggered landmines (in war-torn countries) (Morrissy et al., 2006).
   b) Malignancies or tumors
   c) Diseases (e.g., meningococcemia: decreased tissue perfusion leading to amputation)
3) Amputation terminology:
   a) Trans: amputation across axis of long bone
   b) Disarticulation: amputation through joint
   c) Partial: amputation distal to the wrist or ankle joint
b. Assessment components:
   1) Developmental level
   2) Musculoskeletal system
   3) Mobility: ambulation and use of prosthesis
   4) Skin integrity or residual limb care
c. Rehabilitation issues:
   1) Developmental and independence level.
   2) Function of limb: Goal is for most functional support. Varying degrees of limb difference and function may occur with or without use of prosthesis (Shida-Tokeshi et al., 2005); cosmesis, function, and comfort contribute to prosthetic wear; team decision with limb deficiency clinic practitioners, patient, and family.
   3) Prosthetic management: Consult with physical or occupational therapist and prosthetist experienced in pediatric limb deficiencies (Gitter & Bosker, 2005); secure funding and long-term planning to allow for frequent refittings and new prostheses related to growth:
      a) Upper extremity: cosmetic, body powered, myoelectric, hybrid (with control cable system for function)
      b) Lower extremity: function, above knee, below knee, special types of feet for various functions (Morrissy et al., 2006; Mosca, 2006)
   4) Mobility: ambulation and prosthesis introduction at developmentally appropriate milestones, more likely to succeed and incorporate prosthesis into new tasks:
      a) Upper extremity: when child has developed sitting balance (approximately 6 months of age)
      b) Lower extremity: When child has had amputation before learning ambulation, introduce prosthesis as pulling to stand and beginning walking motions (approximately 9–14 months) (Eilert, 2007; Gitter & Bosker, 2005).
   5) Skin or residual limb management: Monitor for pressure areas, bony prominences, rashes from excessive moisture and heat (confinement in prosthesis), surgical incisions for newer amputations, stump care, skin breakdown at amputation terminal ends related to bony overgrowth at distal end of residual limb (Gitter & Bosker, 2005; Mosca, 2006).
   6) Pain management:

a) Most common causes and contributors of pain: postoperative surgical incision pain, anxiety, bony overgrowth (most common in children who have had amputation through a long bone, especially lower extremity)

b) Phantom pain: Few children experience this phenomenon, less likely if amputation occurred before age 4 years (Morrissy et al., 2006; Wilkins, McGrath, Finley, & Katz, 2004).

7) Self-esteem and self-concept:

a) Facilitate networking with other parents and children with limb deficiencies or differences, often available through limb deficiency specialized outpatient clinics.

b) Provide support network resource information (e.g., National Amputation Foundation, Inc.; American Amputee Foundation, Inc.; Amputee Coalition of America; International Child Amputee Network; limbDifferences.org, from http://www.questdiagnostics.com/kbase/shc/shc05.htm; Superhands Network).

c) Discussion with parents, teachers, and peers to facilitate communication about differences, reactions, and responses as developmentally appropriate and ready (Morrissy et al., 2006)

d) Adaptations for activities and sports: critical for emotional, physical, self-esteem, and social development

d. Patient education topics:

1) Use and care of equipment or prosthesis

2) Residual limb wrapping or "stump sock"

3) Skin care

4) Pain management

5) Community reintegration strategies

6) Resources and supports

7) Therapy and prosthetic centers

8) Safety and community education prevention

9) For congenital deficiencies, genetic counseling (for the parents or the child) (Morrissy et al., 2006)

10) Emotional and social support:

Review support systems to deal with family distress, shock and possible feelings of guilt (in trauma and congenital events) (Morrissy et al., 2006; Mosca, 2006).

B. Acquired Diseases: Cancer is the fourth leading cause of death in children, behind unintentional injuries, homicides, and suicides. Treatment modalities have improved such that 5-year survival rate is greater than 75% (better than in adults). Most common malignancies are acute lymphocytic leukemia (ALL), acute myeloid leukemia (AML), brain tumors (most common of solid tumors in children), lymphomas, neuroblastomas, bone tumors, retinoblastomas, hepatic tumors, and Langerhans cell histiocytosis (Maloney et al., 2007).

1. Brain tumors: rehabilitation needs during and after intervention

a. Behavioral and cognitive function impairments, short- and long-term memory problems, similar to acquired brain injury (Poggi et al., 2005; Vargo & Gerber, 2005)

b. Dysphagia, treatment similar to stroke (Wesling et al., 2003)

c. Weakness and often gait disturbance

d. Visual–perceptual impairment

e. Increased incidence of seizures

2. General cancer care and rehabilitation nursing: assessment and monitoring

a. Developmental level

b. Family assessment

c. Community resources

d. Functional ability related to disease progression

e. Complications: growth, endocrine, cardiopulmonary, renal, neuropsychological, secondary malignancies

f. Monitoring laboratory results for nadir (low point of white blood cell count and platelet count after chemotherapy) and need for protective precautions

3. Rehabilitation issues

a. Pain management

b. Independence level related to developmental level

c. Disease progression

d. Coping

e. Self-image (especially with chemotherapy effects, amputation, scarring, alopecia)

f. Fatigue

g. Integration of rehabilitation and cancer treatment and palliative care plan

h. Skin integrity, especially with radiation

4. Patient education topics

a. Use and care of equipment and assistive devices

b. Medication regimen

c. Pain management techniques

d. Energy conservation

e. Community reintegration strategies

C. Congenital Diseases and Birth Defects

1. Myelodysplasia or myelomeningocele (spina bifida):

a. Definition: A condition in which the neural tube fails to close during the first 3–4 weeks of fetal development, resulting in incomplete closure of the spinal column. The opening in the spine may be at any level, but thoracic and lumbar levels are most common. There are different types of spina bifida:

1) Myelomeningocele: the most severe form. The spinal cord and meninges protrude from the opening in the spine; they may be covered with a sac or open.

a) Hydrocephalus occurs in about 80% of cases.

b) Motor and sensory nerves below the level of the lesion are affected, resulting in paraplegia, neurogenic bowel and bladder, and lack of sensation.

2) Meningocele: meninges protrude from the open spine. Motor and sensory nerves below the level of the lesion may be affected.

3) Spina bifida occulta: an abnormal opening in the spinal column, without any nerve tissue protruding, and completely covered by skin.

a) There may be a patch of hair covering the site but no unusual appearance.

b) There usually is no disability (Kaufman, 2004; Spina Bifida Association of America [SBAA], 2007).

b. Cause and incidence:

1) The exact cause is unknown, but is thought to be multifactorial, involving genetics and environment.

2) Folic acid supplementation in women of childbearing age significantly reduces the risk of a neural tube defect.

3) Women who take valproic acid for seizures are more likely to have a child with a neural tube defect (Koren, Nava-Ocampo, Moretti, Sussman, & Nulman, 2006).

4) Occurrence is one in every 1,000 live births (SBAA, 2007).

c. Outcomes:

1) Cognitive functioning: Children with hydrocephalus are more likely to be affected, with problems ranging from learning disabilities to mental retardation.

a) Motivation is a significant problem and stems in part from executive function deficits.

b) Depression and anxiety are common but may also be signs of shunt malfunction or infection, so organic causes must be ruled out before treatment (Oddson, Clancy, & McGrath, 2006; SBAA, 2007).

2) Neurogenic bowel and bladder:

a) Timed voiding, clean intermittent catheterization, and continent stomas that may be catheterized are some management methods.

b) Urinary tract infections are common and may damage ureters and kidneys.

c) Bowel programs focus on preventing constipation and maintaining continence (Zickler & Richardson, 2004); use of antegrade continence enema (ACE) has contributed to increased continence in a flaccid bowel.

3) Shunting of hydrocephalus: Shunts may malfunction, become infected, or need revision for growth.

4) Sensory deficits: Sensation is partially or completely lost below the level of the lesion.

5) Mobility: Depending on the level of the lesion and the muscles enervated, bracing, crutches, walker, or wheelchair may be used. Children who are able to walk short distances with crutches and braces when they are small often move to wheelchair mobility in adolescence, when they are older and heavier (Verhoef et al., 2006).

6) Latex allergy is very common in people with spina bifida and may be mild or very severe.

7) Neurologic complications: Although these do not occur in every person, they may significantly affect function and long-term outcome:
   a) Tethered spinal cord: The spinal cord is "caught" and cannot move as the child grows.
   b) Symptomatic Chiari malformation: a brain malformation, associated with hydrocephalus, that becomes symptomatic in about one-third of children with spina bifida (SBAA, 2007).
8) Orthopedic problems:
   a) Hip dysplasia
   b) Clubfoot
   c) Scoliosis and kyphosis
d. Nursing assessment and interventions:
   1) Developmental and cognitive assessment
   2) Neurologic assessment:
      a) Presence of neurologic complications
      b) Signs of shunt malfunction
   3) Bladder and bowel function:
      a) Signs of urinary tract infection
      b) Constipation
      c) Child's readiness to begin self care (Zickler & Richardson, 2004).
   4) Skin integrity: prevention and management of pressure ulcers (Butler, 2006).
   5) Orthopedic concerns:
      a) Pre- and postoperative surgical repair
      b) Use of braces and mobility devices
   6) Latex allergies: prevention and treatment (Association of Perioperative Registered Nurses, 2004)
   7) Visual perceptual deficits.
   8) Cardiopulmonary function: may be compromised in children with high thoracic lesion levels or with symptomatic Chiari malformation
   9) Nutritional status: adequate growth and development, prevention of obesity
   10) Ability to perform activities of daily living (ADLs)
   11) Self-concept and self-esteem: participation in adaptive sports can be helpful (Leger, 2005).
   12) Family assessment: ability to care for child, stressors, support systems
e. Rehabilitation issues:

1) Promotion of development, attainment of milestones as much as possible
2) Self-care as appropriate for age, ability to perform ADLs
3) Independence level related to growth and developmental level
4) Promotion of mobility and upright position
5) Bowel and bladder management
6) Skin care
7) Special education
8) Community inclusion (Lomax-Bream, Barnes, Copeland, Taylor, & Landry, 2007)
f. Family and child education topics:
   1) Bladder and bowel program (Mason, Tobias, Lutkenhoff, Stoops, & Ferguson, 2004)
   2) Skin care and pressure relief techniques
   3) Use and care of equipment and orthoses
   4) Promotion of independence and ADLs at home and school (Greenley, Coakley, Holmbeck, Jandasek, & Wills, 2006)
   5) Transfers and ambulation (if appropriate to level of lesion)
   6) Service coordination and advocacy
2. Diseases related to muscular dystrophy: Most children with a progressive neuromuscular condition are cared for and followed in an outpatient setting. Inpatient rehabilitation services may be sought for postoperative endurance reconditioning or as a secondary condition unrelated to the reason for the rehabilitation admission (e.g., car accident). The rehabilitation nurse may be called on for consultation to acute care inpatient surgical services.
a. Types and definitions (Muscular Dystrophy Association, 2007)
   1) Duchenne muscular dystrophy. Occurrence in males caused by absence of dystrophin. Age of recognition: 2–6 years, progresses rapidly. Genetics: X-linked recessive. Most common.
      a) Medical and mobility issues: Wheelchair use often by age of 9, gross motor strength significantly affected, able to do some fine motor independent skills with setup. Most often warrants surgical intervention for heel

cord releases, scoliosis corrective spine surgery, respiratory support; cardiomyopathy is common (in late teenage years).

b) Lifespan: Depending on respiratory support interventions and cardiac, often into 20s or 30s. Without intervention: late teens, early 20s. Support network: http://www. parentprojectmd.org.

2) Becker muscular dystrophy: a condition similar to but less severe than Duchenne, caused by insufficient production of dystrophin. X-linked recessive.

a) Medical and mobility issues: often ambulatory through the teen years

b) May consider using wheelchair for long distances

3) Congenital muscular dystrophy: a group of genetic, degenerative diseases affecting voluntary muscles. Onset at or near birth. Progression and disability vary; often seen as generalized muscle weakness. Autosomal recessive.

4) Myotonic dystrophy: affects generations, progressively more involved with each generation. Generalized weakness, muscle wasting, myotonia, developmental disability in children. Caused by repeated section of DNA on chromosome 19. Autosomal dominant. Medical and mobility issues: Often ambulatory into late teens, wheelchair for long distances.

5) Limb girdle muscular dystrophy: mutation of different genes affecting proteins for muscle function. Presents as weakness and wasting of muscles around shoulders and hips. Can be autosomal dominant or autosomal recessive. May look similar in functional challenges to Duchenne, less severely progressive.

6) Facioscapulohumeral muscular dystrophy: missing area of chromosome 4, onset usually by age 20. Weakness of eye and mouth muscles, shoulders, upper arms, and lower legs. Autosomal dominant.

7) Spinal muscular atrophy. Definition: deficiency of motor neuron protein SMN on chromosome 5. Loss of motor neuron nerve cells in the spinal cord, resulting in loss of voluntary muscle control. All types are autosomal recessive (Muscular Dystrophy Association, 2007).

a) Type 1: Infantile (Werdnig–Hoffman), onset birth to 6 months. Rapid progression, often leading to death in first year of life.

b) Type 2: Intermediate, onset 6–18 months. Weakness in central core muscles: shoulders, hips, thighs, upper back, wheelchair dependent. At risk for respiratory compromise. Lifespan can be into childhood, teens, young adulthood.

c) Type 3: Juvenile (Kugelberg–Welander): onset after 18 months. Weakness similar to Type 2, with slower progression. Walking ability often maintained at least until adolescence. Lifespan usually not affected.

d) Support network: http://www. fsma.org

8) Charcot–Marie–Tooth (CMT) (Muscular Dystrophy Association, 2007): neurological damage to peripheral nerves. Caused by defects in axons or in genes for proteins found in myelin. Onset birth to adulthood. Different forms of CMT: autosomal dominant, autosomal recessive, and X-linked. Slowly progressive, often see muscle weakness, wasting, loss of sensation in periphery.

9) Friedreich's ataxia: genetic defect to frataxin protein, diminishing energy production in mitochondria, resulting in damage to peripheral nerves and cerebellum. Affects all ages as young as 2 years old. Most characterized by ataxia, loss of sensation, cardiac involvement, difficulty with speech and swallowing, diabetes. Support network: http://www.ataxia.org.

10) Leukodystrophy (National Institute of Neurological Disorders and Stroke, 2007): different types, genetic related, progressive degeneration of white matter of the brain from decreased growth and development of myelin sheath. Varies in prognosis, often quite debilitating, life-limiting.

b. Assessment components
1) Developmental level
2) Respiratory status
3) Cardiovascular
4) Scoliosis
5) Assistive, orthotic mobility devices
6) Medication history (esp. corticosteroid use)
7) Skin integrity
8) Nutrition and fluid intake
9) Seizures (in leukodystrophy)
10) Bladder and bowel function (retain sensation, decrease in motor control and decrease in motility as disease progresses)
11) Psychosocial
12) Home environment accessibility
13) Family history and genetics

c. Rehabilitation issues
1) Pulmonary management and support
2) Corticosteroid precautions (Moxley et al., 2005)
3) Maintenance of intact skin
4) Toileting
5) Assistance with ADLs dependent on severity and progression of condition
6) Seizure management (as applicable)
7) Maintain independence as much as possible
8) Accessibility of home environment

d. Patient education topics
1) Pulmonary and cardiovascular maintenance and precautions
2) Maintenance of skin integrity
3) Range of motion exercises
4) Use of assistive, orthotic, and mobility devices
5) Nutrition/fluid intake
6) Home environment modifications
7) Medication management
8) Mobility
9) Community integration strategies

3. Joint and orthopedic conditions:
a. Common types of disabling orthopedic conditions that may necessitate rehabilitation
1) Legg–Calvé–Perthes disease: a condition most common in males in which the femoral head develops avascular necrosis.
a) May occur at any age but usually between 3–9 years of age.
b) Cause is unknown, but various factors, such as attention deficit–hyperactivity disorder (ADHD), delayed skeletal age, metabolic

factors, and mechanical dysfunction may play a role in its development.
c) Treatment includes bed rest with periodic mobilization, abduction bracing, biphosphate medications, or surgery (McQuade & Houghton, 2005).
2) Osteogenesis imperfecta (OI): a metabolic bone and connective tissue disease that results in brittle bones; commonly associated with fractures that can occur with normal movement and care of the child with this condition. Fractures that are characteristic of this condition often are mistaken as child abuse (Paterson & McAllion, 2006).
a) Cause is a dominate genetic mutation.
b) There are many different types of OI, from very mild to lethal.
c) OI is present from conception, but depending on the severity, it may be diagnosed at birth or late in life.
d) About 50,000 people in the United States have OI.
e) In most types, more fractures occur in childhood, then become less frequent with age.
f) Treatment varies with severity. Special handling techniques for children more significantly affected reduce the number of fractures. Frequent surgery may be needed to repair bone deformities (Osteogenesis Imperfecta Foundation 2006; Rauch & Glorieux, 2006).
3) Leg length discrepancy: inequality of the leg lengths, usually greater than 2 centimeters, which may be the result of: congenital malformations of the fibula, infections, trauma affecting the epiphyses, or neurologic disorders such as poliomyelitis (Rose, Fuentes, Hanl, & Dizalo, 1999).
a) Discrepancies of 2–4 centimeters may be treated using lifts in the shoe.
b) Discrepancies of 4 centimeters or more usually are treated with leg-lengthening surgery, often using a device called the Ilizarov, which distracts the ends of the bone and soft tissues over a period of weeks (Ramakerl et al., 2000).

4) Juvenile rheumatoid arthritis: a chronic inflammation that involves the connective tissue, joints, and viscera, which begins before the age of 16.

5) Achondroplasia: a skeletal dysplasia causing short stature and bony deformities.
   a) The cause is genetic, occurring in 1 out of 30,000 live births.
   b) Developmental delays, kyphosis, flexion contractures of joints, bowed legs, other hip and spine problems and characteristic bowed forehead are associated with achondroplasia.
   c) Treatment includes physical therapies, bracing, and surgical treatment (Amirfayz & Gargan, 2005).

6) Arthrogryposis multiplex congenita: congenital joint contractures, decreased fetal movement in utero related to variety of reasons and conditions, most often associated with motor neuron involvement (amyoplasia). Limited function of upper and lower extremities and ADLs (Hall, 1997; Staheli, Hall, Jaffe, & Paholke, 1998).

b. Nursing assessment and interventions
   1) Developmental milestones and self-care ability
   2) Level of disability related to diagnosis
   3) Pain assessment and management preoperatively and postoperatively
   4) Preoperative and postoperative nursing care (Ireland, 2006)
   4) Mobility, use and care of equipment and assistive devices
   5) Ability to perform ADLs; self-care
   6) Family
      a) Medical history and genetics
      b) Coping and adaptive skills
      c) Ability to care for child
   7) Discharge planning, service coordination, and case management (Hewitt-Taylor, 2005; Ottenbacher et al., 2000)

c. Rehabilitation issues
   1) Promotion of maximum independence level based on the severity of diagnosis
   2) Mobility
   3) Joint protection
   4) ADL modification

5) Safety
6) Psychological implications (e.g., of prolonged bedrest, disability, painful procedures) (Ramakerl et al., 2000)
7) Community integration and school attendance (Rehm, 2002)

d. Family and child education topics
   1) Medication regimen
   2) ADLs
   3) Safety
   4) Mobility versus joint protection
   5) Pain management
   6) Use and care of equipment and assistive devices
   7) Community resources (Sullivan-Bolyai, Knafl, Sadler, & Gilliss, 2004)

4. Cerebral palsy (CP):
   a. Definition: a mild to severe condition that results from damage to the developing brain that produces a permanent but nonprogressive abnormality of muscle coordination, balance, and purposeful movement. CP is the most common childhood disability and usually is detected by the time the child is 3 years old. The terms used to describe CP relate to extremity involvement: monoplegia, diplegia, hemiplegia, quadriplegia.

   b. Types of CP:
      1) Spastic: hyperactive reflexes, increased muscle tone, muscle spasms, motor weakness, persistent reflexes
      2) Athetoid: abnormal involuntary movements, facial grimacing, dystonic movements, poor speech, distorted posturing
      3) Ataxia: hypotonia, floppy muscle tone, impaired balance and coordination, unsteady gait
      4) Mixed: combination of several types

   c. Assessment must be highly individualized and reflect the child's age, levels of involvement, and associated problems (Edwards, 2001).
      1) Developmental level
      2) Cognitive level
      3) Communication and speech
      4) Ability to perform ADLs
      5) Feeding pattern
      6) Toileting
      7) Muscle function
      8) Ambulation
      9) History of seizure disorders and other associated conditions
      10) Vision and hearing
      11) Skin integrity

12) Learning disability

d. Rehabilitation issues: Additional problems and symptoms may develop as the child progresses and grows (Edwards, 2001).
   1) Neurodevelopmental and sensory therapies
   2) Independent living skills
   3) Positioning and therapeutic handling (depending on severity)
   4) Feeding problems
   5) Communication
   6) Seizure management
   7) Spasticity management
   8) Motor control
   9) Assistive technology
   10) Social and sexual relationships
   11) Surgery and nonsurgical procedures: orthopedic procedures, intrathecal baclofen, dorsal rhizotomy, peripheral neurotomy (Steinbok, 2006)

e. Family and child education topics:
   1) Skin assessment and care
   2) Exercise and fitness programs
   3) Medications
   4) Spasticity management techniques
   5) Self-care
   6) Feeding and nutrition
   7) Bowel and bladder management
   8) Community integration strategies: school, leisure activities, transportation, independent living arrangements

D. Chronic Illnesses
   1. Bronchopulmonary dysplasia
      a. Definition: a range of conditions characterized by scarring or fibrosis of immature lung tissue that occur in premature infants. Also known as chronic lung disease of infancy, it can last throughout childhood and into adulthood. Contributing factors:
         1) Prematurity
         2) Mechanical ventilation and oxygen in response to severe respiratory distress syndrome caused by pneumonia, sepsis, meconium aspiration, or fluid overload
         3) Infection and inflammation
         4) Patent ductus arteriosus
         5) Possible genetic influences (Capper-Michel, 2004; Driscoll & Davis, 2007)
      b. Cause and incidence:
         1) Caused by exposure of the immature alveoli and microvasculature of the lungs to trauma from

mechanical ventilation, high oxygen concentrations, and respiratory distress itself. The resulting decrease in oxygenation affects the lungs, the heart, and the brain.
         2) Occurs most commonly in premature infants with a birth weight of less than 1,250 g and at less than 30 weeks' gestation.
         3) The occurrence can be reduced by use of glucocorticoid and surfactant treatment (Baveja & Christou, 2006).
         4) Incidence ranges from 17% to 57% because multiple factors influence its development (Driscoll & Davis, 2007).
      c. Commonly associated complications:
         1) Airway complications such as stenosis, granuloma, scarring, tracheomalacia, and frequent infections
         2) Growth retardation and poor weight gain; vitamin deficiencies
         3) Gastroesophageal reflux
         4) Cardiac conditions such as pulmonary hypertension and cor pulmonale
         5) Seizures
         6) Retinopathy of prematurity and other ophthalmic complications
         7) Frequent ear and sinus infections
         8) Renal calcification from long-term use of diuretics
         9) Inflammation and infection of stomas from tracheostomy and gastrostomy tubes (Capper-Michel, 2004)
         10) Developmental delays including cognitive disability, gross and fine motor deficits, speech and language problems, visual–motor integration disorders, ADHD, and behavioral problems (Anderson & Doyle, 2006; Hack et al., 2000)
         11) Long term outcomes may include all of the above, as well as pulmonary disease with risk of respiratory failure in adolescence and adulthood and long-lasting cardiac disorders (Doyle et al., 2006)
      d. Nursing assessment and interventions:
         1) Respiratory assessment: adequacy of ventilation, function of assistive technology, patency of tracheostomy and suctioning or replacement when necessary, early identification of infection and treatment, respiratory medications.

2) Developmental level in all domains; promote attainment of developmental milestones. Assess self-care skills and ADLs.

3) Cardiac assessment: pulse, blood pressure, symptoms of heart failure, cardiac medications.

4) Oral feeding if possible, maintenance of gastrostomy tube and tube feedings, promote good nutrition; evaluate for anemia and other deficiencies, monitor growth and gastroesophageal reflux, administer medications as appropriate (Hummel & Cronin, 2004).

5) Skin care: Assess stomas for irritation, granulomatous tissue, leakage.

6) Appropriate screenings: vision, hearing, dental, developmental.

7) Health promotion and prevention: immunizations, need for palivizumab (Synagis) to prevent respiratory syncytial virus (Capper-Michel, 2004).

8) Discharge planning (Hummel & Cronin, 2004).

9) Family stress and coping skills, ability to manage child's needs (Montagnino & Mauricio, 2004).

e. Rehabilitation issues:

1) Developmental interventions including physical therapy, occupational therapy, speech therapy, and recreational therapy; promotion of independence as appropriate for age (Anderson & Doyle, 2006)

2) Respiratory management with pulmonary specialists to ameliorate impact of long-term ventilation or tracheostomy on development; chest physiotherapy

3) Early intervention, special education, and school inclusion (Clements et al., 2006)

4) Behavioral issues (Ottenbacher et al., 2000)

f. Family and child education topics:

1) Management of technology in the home and community: troubleshooting the ventilator, suctioning and changing the tracheostomy, administering tube feedings, changing the gastrostomy tube

2) Medication management: administration, side effects

3) Prevention of complications and health maintenance

4) Promoting independence in self-care in the child (Rehm & Bradley, 2005)

5) Negotiating with caregivers in the home, service coordination, school liaison (Rehm, 2002)

6) Safety at home, at school, and in the community (Rehm, 2002)

7) Maintenance of family equilibrium, dealing with siblings

2. Technology dependence

a. Definition: Children who are technology dependent are defined as those who use "a medical device to compensate for the loss of a vital bodily function and substantial and ongoing nursing care to avert death or further disability" (Office of Technology Assessment, 1987, p. 3).

1) Examples include children with a tracheostomy or gastrostomy tube or who need home oxygen, mechanical ventilation, or other medical devices such as colostomies or intravenous fluid pumps.

2) Many children who are technology dependent use more than one device (e.g., gastrostomy tube and mechanical ventilation).

3) They need high-tech care from parents or caregivers who have been specially trained or from nurses (Wang & Barnard, 2004).

4) Up to 40% of children discharged from one urban pediatric hospital were technology dependent (Feudtner et al., 2005).

5) In one state, less than 1% of children birth through 19 years of age were found to be medically fragile and use technology; however, these children used almost 7% of the Medicaid dollars allocated for that age group (Buescher, Whitmire, Brunssen, & Kluttz-Hile, 2006).

6) Rehabilitation nurses may encounter children who are technology dependent in the inpatient unit, clinic, school, or home.

b. Nursing assessment of child:

1) Developmental level and cognitive level

2) Language skills and communication methods

3) Age-appropriate ability to perform ADLs and amount and type of assistance needed

4) Frequent physiologic assessment, particularly respiratory system, gastrointestinal system,

genitourinary system, skin integrity, musculoskeletal system

    5) Ability to eat or take nourishment; nutrition

    6) Toileting and bowel and bladder management; signs of urinary tract infection, constipation

    7) Ambulation or form of mobility

    8) Psychosocial issues (Charlton, 2004)

    9) Hospital discharge planning and assessment

      a) Equipment and supply assessment: appropriate for child, in good working order, sufficient supplies (e.g., suction catheters, gloves)

      b) Home assessment: accessibility, enrichment of the environment (e.g., books, toys). cleanliness, safety; presence of emergency backup plan for equipment or power failure, notification of emergency responders (e.g., child with a tracheostomy or using a ventilator), notification of public utility services (e.g., need for immediate attention to resumption of electrical service)

      c) School assessment: accessibility, plan for care while child is in school, equipment and supplies, individualized educational plan, appropriate caregiver training (e.g., school nurse, licensed practical nurse, or designated caregiver) (Earle, Rennick, Carnavale, & Davis, 2006; Hewitt-Taylor, 2005; Hummel & Cronin, 2004; Montagnino & Mauricio, 2004)

  c. Nursing assessment of family:

    1) Family stress and coping skills

    2) Ability to meet child's needs

    3) Family and caregiver skill assessment

    4) Financial stress

    5) Sibling stress

    6) Role confusion: parent role versus high-tech caregiver role

    7) Social isolation (Kirk, Glendinning, & Callery, 2005; Montagnino & Mauricio, 2004)

  d. Rehabilitation nursing interventions:

    1) Discharge planning.

    2) Promote return to home, school, community (Rehm, 2002).

    3) Promote independence as appropriate for the child's developmental level

and functional abilities.

    4) Ensure safety in the home, community, and school.

    5) Provide expert clinical nursing care as appropriate.

    6) Offer family support and referrals as needed.

    7) Share information on community resources.

  e. Family and child education topics:

    1) Operation and maintenance of assistive technology

    2) Clinical care of child

    3) Promotion of independence in self-care

    4) Community integration

    5) Training of community service providers (Reeves, Timmons, & Dampier, 2006)

  f. Family issues and concerns:

    1) Finances

    2) Availability of home nursing care, therapy, and medical services in the home community

    3) Accessible transportation for medical services and recreational activities

    4) Fatigue and burnout

    5) Balancing family and personal needs with child's needs

    6) Intrusiveness of technology and nursing care in the home (Montagnino & Mauricio, 2004; Rehm & Bradley, 2005).

III. Long-Term Planning: Community Services for Children and Youth with Disabilities

A. Philosophy of Inclusion

  1. Inclusion is a philosophical viewpoint that asserts that children with disabilities are an integral part of the community and should participate with their peers in typical activities such as school.

  2. Inclusion may occur in playgroups, school, recreation, social activities, and work.

  3. In the school setting, inclusion means that children with disabilities should receive educational services in a typical classroom, where other children without disabilities are schooled (Wisconsin Education Association Council, 2007).

B. School Programs

  1. The Individuals with Disabilities Education Act (IDEA Reauthorization 2004, final regulations published August 14, 2006) ensures that all children and youth ages

3–21 years receive a free, appropriate public education.

2. Education and special education services should be delivered in the least restrictive environment, as similar to settings for children without disabilities as possible.

3. Children who need special education are entitled to receive an individualized education plan that is reviewed yearly to best meet the child's educational needs.

4. Children with disabilities may also receive related services through the school (e.g., physical therapy, occupational therapy, speech therapy, nutrition, other health-related services), as mandated by IDEA, if those services are necessary for learning.

5. Child Find is a system each school district has in place to identify children who are eligible for special education services (U.S. Department of Education, 2007).

6. The No Child Left Behind legislation, passed in 2001, set high standards for the education of all children and requires accountability from schools in the areas of reading and math. Children are tested on a regular basis to determine whether their education meets standards. Children with disabilities that hinder learning may receive alternative testing or may be excluded from testing (Schrag, 2003).

C. Early Intervention
1. Part C of IDEA provides for early educational services for young children with or at risk for disabilities from birth to 3 years of age.

2. Eligible children and their families receive an individualized family service plan that plans interventions to eliminate or reduce the developmental delay or disability and offer family support.

3. Early intervention services may include speech and language, physical or occupational therapy, psychological services, service coordination, social work, vision screening, and medical services (U.S. Department of Education, 2007).

D. Other Legislation Affecting Children with Disabilities
1. Rehabilitation Act: provides for supportive services in school for children with physical disabilities who do not qualify for special education.

2. Title V of the Social Security Act was passed in 1935 and established the Maternal and Child Health Bureau to provide public health

services for mothers and children, as well as disabled children (U.S. Department of Health and Human Services, 2007).

3. The Children's Bureau was established in 1912 to promote child welfare. The Child Abuse Prevention and Treatment Act was passed in 1974 and reauthorized in 2003 (Child Welfare Information Gateway, 2007).

4. Americans with Disabilities Act of 1990. [Refer to Chapter 23.]

5. Vocational Rehabilitation Act.

E. Home Health Care
1. Children who are technology dependent as a result of prematurity, illness, or injury often need skilled care at home and at school.

2. Living at home is much better for the child's developmental, psychological, and social well-being than living in an institution (Neufield, Query, & Drummond, 2001).

3. Medicaid is the primary payer for home health care, with private health insurance covering only about 1% of costs. Medicaid's low reimbursement rate makes it difficult to locate qualified agencies to provide specialized pediatric care in the home (American Academy of Pediatrics Committee on Child Health Financing, Section on Home Care, 2006).

4. Although the assistance of home health is welcomed, the intrusiveness of strangers in the home on a daily basis may be stressful (Hewitt-Taylor, 2005).

5. Many families' insurance does not cover home health care, and families are forced to provide skilled nursing care without assistance, which may put extreme stress on them.
   a. In these cases, respite care, which gives families a break, can be very useful (Neufield et al., 2001).
   b. The Division of Developmental Disabilities in each state may have respite care funding available.

F. Health Promotion and Prevention
1. Children with disabilities need a "medical home" to coordinate specialty care and ensure well care (American Academy of Pediatrics, Council on Children with Disabilities, 2005).

2. Developmental screening (identification of children who need in-depth assessment related to developmental delays) is the responsibility of the primary healthcare provider (American Academy of Pediatrics, Committee on

Children with Disabilities, 2001).

3. All children need immunizations and health screening, and children with disabilities may need specific preventive activities such as prevention of secondary conditions (e.g., contractures in a child with CP) (Cooley & the American Academy of Pediatrics Committee on Children with Disabilities, 2004).

4. Health promotion for children with disabilities includes good nutrition, physical activity, friendships, and positive social interaction.

G. Transition to Adulthood and Independent Living Situations (Figure 16-1)

1. School to work transition services are provided by the school system, which links with vocational education (Betz, 2007).

2. Youth with disabilities must also transition health care from pediatric to adult providers.

   a. Many adult healthcare providers are unfamiliar with the health consequences of growing up with a pediatric disability.

   b. Pediatric providers are unfamiliar with adult health issues (American Academy of Pediatrics, American Academy of Family Physicians, American College of Physicians, & American Society of Internal Medicine, 2002).

3. Primary factors in successful transition and independent living models:

   a. Attitude and attributes of the youth and family

   b. Self-care skills

   c. Availability of resources in the community, such as independent living services, accessible transportation, knowledgeable health and education providers, and supported employment

   d. Ability of the youth to perform ADLs and self-care independently or direct others to do so

   e. Independent mobility

   f. Healthcare needs

   g. Living arrangements (e.g., where, with whom, community options, housekeeping skills)

   h. Housing (e.g., adaptations needed, ability to maintain a home)

   i. Recreation and leisure activities

   j. Social skills

   k. Cognitive abilities and communication skills

   l. Job skills

m. Financial management strategies

n. Legal issues (Adolescent Youth Transition Project, 2006)

H. Vocational Rehabilitation and Higher Education

1. State and local vocational rehabilitation offices work closely with schools in transition programs and local employers.

2. Youth with disabilities who have academic capabilities may go on to higher education.

   a. Many city and community colleges and universities are reaching out to young adults with disabilities.

   b. Vocational rehabilitation offices may provide assistive technology to aid youth in educational pursuits.

3. Although not all children have the potential to be working members of society, many are overlooked simply because of lack of information about potential options (Adolescent Youth Transition Project, 2006; Betz, 2007).

IV. Trends and Future Directions

A. Health Care

1. More sophisticated technology will be available to preserve and improve life, at increasing expense. Funding may become more challenging to access and more dependent on private insurance or substantial income.

2. There will be a greater emphasis on quality and safety, tracking the impact of nursing care on outcomes.

3. Emphasis on research and evidence-based practice will address new ideas and validate current practice.

4. The nursing shortage will increase the need for education in pediatrics and rehabilitation for nurses practicing with children and adolescents in a variety of settings.

5. Quality of life and end-of-life decision making incorporating rehabilitation and developmental principles will be important, as will more nursing research to identify better treatment options.

6. Collaborative, interdisciplinary service models will continue to evolve, with growth in nonhospital settings.

7. Incidence of orthopedic and sports-related injuries will increase.

8. Genetics and stem cell research will provide linkage of diseases to certain genes with potential for new treatment options.

Figure 16-1. Transition to Adult Care Developmental Activities to Encourage Independence

Please note: The following recommendations are based on the child's developmental age and ability.

Birth–3 Years Old
- Encourage your child to assist with activities.
- Allow your child enough time to complete tasks.
- Talk with your child about his or her condition and abilities.

3–5 Years Old
- Teach your child about his or her special healthcare needs.
- Encourage your child to participate in self-care.
- Help your child to interact socially in various settings.
- Assign household chores or responsibilities particular to him or her.

6–12 Years Old
- Continue to assess your child's knowledge of his or her disability and provide additional information.
- Continue to teach your child self-care skills while addressing his or her special needs.
- Encourage his or her attempts to participate in self-care.
- Encourage hobbies and time for play.
- Allow your child to relate his or her experiences about the disability.
- Allow your child to participate in decision making by offering choices.
- Continue to assign appropriate chores or household duties that affect the child and the entire family.
- Help your child to interact with healthcare providers (allow him or her to speak directly to the doctor, nurse, or therapist).
- Talk about career options, interests, and abilities related to career choices.
- Take your child to work with you.

13–18 Years Old
- Help your teenager to develop self-awareness by focusing on interests, talents, and abilities.
- Continue to support your teenager's attempts to identify career choices.
- Continue to assess your teenager's knowledge and perception of his or her disability while providing additional information as needed.
- Continue to assist and encourage your teenager's attempts to do self-care.
- Encourage your teenager to do volunteer work or find part-time employment.
- Continue to assign chores and discuss the importance of family responsibilities.
- Obtain information about your teenager's state vocational rehabilitation program and school transition program.
- Discuss a plan for adult living, including healthcare services.
- Apply for SSI and Medicaid, if appropriate, at age 18 if previously denied for financial reasons.
- Discuss adult healthcare financing with your teenager.
- Discuss sexuality with your teenager, including how his or her disability may affect future health, career options, marriage, and the ability to have children.
- Encourage your teenager to speak freely with healthcare providers.
- Begin to look for adult care providers while allowing your teenager to participate in the decision-making process.
- Help your teenager keep a record of appointments, medications, and medical history (surgeries, treatments, hospitalizations, and allergies).
- Allow your teenager to make his or her own appointment, call for medication refills and supplies.
- Teach your teenager how to have medical information sent.

19–21 Years Old
- Identify an adult healthcare provider with your young adult.
- Transfer medical record to the adult care provider.
- Assist the young adult with finalizing adult healthcare financing and insurance options.
- Assist your young adult to schedule an appointment with adult care provider while still under pediatric care to ensure that the transfer to adult care will be uninterrupted and complete.
- Remain as a resource, support system, and safety net for your young adult as he or she assumes the responsibility of self-care.

Reprinted with permission of Lippincott, Williams & Wilkins from *Orthopaedic Nursing*, Sept/Oct, Vol.23, No. 5, p.306.

B. Community

1. There will be less hospital-based care with shorter stays and more outpatient, community, and home-based care.

2. There will be a greater need for accommodations for children who are technology dependent in schools and in the community.

3. There will be an increased need for home care education and for training caregivers in various settings.

4. Foster parents will be more likely to accept medically fragile children if they have a good medical home.

5. Legislation and litigation will continue to be a means to provide services to the pediatric population at the state and federal levels.

V. Advanced Practice Nurses (APNs) in Pediatric Rehabilitation

A. Qualifications: The APN has acquired the knowledge and practice experience for specialization, expansion, and advancement of pediatric rehabilitation nursing practice.

B. Characteristics of Graduate Nursing Education:

1. Greater depth and breadth of knowledge

2. Ability to synthesize data to a greater degree

3. Complexity of skills and interventions developed

4. Autonomy of practice

C. Broad Range of Titles and Variety of Settings

D. Scope of Practice:

1. Level of autonomy of practice

2. Dominance of nurse-initiated treatment regimens

3. Complexity of situations or cases managed

4. Leadership provided in the interdisciplinary team

5. In-depth understanding of interacting pathophysiologic and psychosocial changes associated with chronicity and disability

E. Advanced Practice Roles:

1. Clinician

a. Facilitates the design and implementation of the individualized plan of care and the transition from hospital to home and community

b. Assesses health needs; develops diagnoses; plans, implements, and manages care; and evaluates outcomes of care

2. Educator

a. Provides health education for professionals and consumers about the needs of children with disabilities and their families

b. Bases teaching methods on developmental level, functional ability, learning needs and abilities, and sociocultural factors

3. Leader and consultant

a. Serves as a model for child, adolescent, and family advocacy through direct intervention

b. Promotes community and government knowledge of pediatric rehabilitation issues and works to influence policy-making bodies to improve care

c. Involves stakeholders in the decision-making process and considers factors related to safety, effectiveness, cost, and impact on practice

d. Provides consultation to influence the plan of care, enhances the practice of team members, and affects resource use

4. Researcher

a. Participates in research and quality improvement projects and is responsible for providing evidence-based care

b. Critically evaluates current practice and uses scientific findings to improve patient care outcomes

c. Identifies research questions and disseminates relevant research findings to various constituencies

References

Adolescent Youth Transition Project. (2006, June). Working together for successful transition. *Washington State adolescent transition resource notebook.* Publication no. 970-110, Retrieved June 22, 2007 from http://depts.washington.edu/healthtr/notebook/default.html.

Agency for Health Care Policy and Research. (1999). *Rehabilitation for traumatic brain injury in children and adolescents. Summary, evidence report/technology assessment (number 2, supplement).* Rockville, MD: Agency for Health Care Policy and Research. Retrieved June 22, 2007 from http://www.ahrq.gov/clinic/epcsums/tbisum2.htm.

American Academy of Pediatrics. (2007). *What is a medical home?* Retrieved February 8, 2007, from http://www.medicalhomeinfo.org

American Academy of Pediatrics, American Academy of Family Physicians, American College of Physicians, & American Society of Internal Medicine. (2002). A consensus statement on health care transitions for young adults with special health care needs. *Pediatrics, 110*(6), 1304–1307.

American Academy of Pediatrics, Committee on Child Health Financing, Section on Home Care. (2006). Financing of pediatric home health care. *Pediatrics, 118*(2), 834–838.

American Academy of Pediatrics, Committee on Children with Disabilities. (2001). Developmental surveillance and screening in infants and young children. *Pediatrics, 108*(1), 192–197.

American Academy of Pediatrics, Council on Children with Disabilities. (2005). Care coordination in the medical home: Integrating health and related systems of care for children with special health care needs. *Pediatrics, 116*(5), 1238–1244.

Amirfayz, R., & Gargan, M. (2005). Achondroplasia. *Current Orthopaedics, 19*(6), 467–470.

Anderson, P.J., & Doyle F.W. (2006). Neurodevelopmental outcome of bronchopulmonary dysplasia. *Seminars in Perinatology, 30*(4), 227–232.

Association of Perioperative Registered Nurses. (2004). AORN latex guideline. *AORN Journal, 79*(3), 653–672.

Association of Rehabilitation Nurses (ARN). (2007). *Pediatric rehabilitation nursing role description* [Brochure]. Skokie, IL: Author.

Baveja, R., & Christou, H. (2006). Pharmacological strategies in the prevention and management of bronchopulmonary dysplasia. *Seminars in Perinatology, 30*(4), 209–218.

Betz, C.L. (2007). Facilitating the transition of adolescents with developmental disabilities. Nursing practice issues and care. *Journal of Pediatric Nursing, 22*(2), 103–115.

Blissit, P.A. (2006). Care of the critically ill patient with penetrating head injury. *Critical Care Nursing Clinics of North America, 18*(3), 321–332.

Brand, M. (2006). Focus on the physical series: Part 1: Recognizing neonatal spinal cord injury. *Advances in Neonatal Care, 6*(1), 15–24.

Buescher, P.A., Whitmire, J.T., Brunssen, S., & Kluttz-Hile, C.E. (2006). Children who are medically fragile in North Carolina: Using Medicaid data to estimate prevalence and medical care costs in 2004. *Maternal and Child Health Journal, 10*(5), 461–466.

Butler, C.T. (2006). Pediatric skin care: Guidelines for assessment, prevention and treatment. *Pediatric Nursing, 32*(5). 112-116.

Capper-Michel, B. (2004). Bronchopulmonary dysplasia. In P.J. Allen & J.A. Vessey (Eds.), *Primary care of the child with a chronic condition* (4th ed., pp. 282–298). St. Louis: Mosby.

Charlton, B. (2004). Pediatric assessment tool: A self instructional guide. *Journal of Radiology Nursing, 23*(3), 78–83.

Child Welfare Information Gateway. (2007). *About CAPTA: A legislative history.* Retrieved June 22, 2007 from http://www.childwelfare.gov/pubs/factsheets/about.cfm.

Chung, C.Y., Chen, C.L., Cheng, P.T., See, L.C., Tang, S.F., & Wong, A.M. (2006). Critical score of Glasgow Coma Scale for pediatric traumatic brain injury. *Pediatric Neurology, 34*(5), 379–387.

Clements, K.M., Barfield, W.D., Kotelchuck, M., Lee, K.G., & Wilbur, N. (2006). Birth characteristics associated with early intervention referral, evaluation for eligibility, and program eligibility in the first year of life. *Maternal and Child Health Journal, 19*(5), 433–441.

Cooley, C., & the American Academy of Pediatrics Committee on Children with Disabilities. (2004). Providing a primary care medical home for children and youth with cerebral palsy. *Pediatrics, 114*(4), 1106–1113.

Dawodu, S.T. (2007). *Traumatic brain injury: Definition, pathophysiology, epidemiology.* Retrieved June 22, 2007 from http://www.emedicine.com/PMR/topic212.htm.

Doyle, L.W., Faber, B., Callanan, C., Freezer, N., Ford, G.W., & Davis, N.M. (2006). Bronchopulmonary dysplasia in very low birth weight subjects and lung function in late adolescence. *Pediatrics, 118*(1), 108–113.

Driscoll, W., & Davis, J. (2007). *Bronchopulmonary dysplasia.* Retrieved June 22, 2007 from http://www.emedicine.com/PED/topic289.htm.

Earle, R.J., Rennick, J.E., Carnavale, F.A., & Davis, G.M. (2006). "It's okay, it helps me to breathe": The experience of home ventilation from a child's perspective. *Journal of Child Health Care, 10*(4), 270–282.

Edwards, P. (2001). Pediatric rehabilitation nursing. In J. Derstine & S. Hargrove (Eds.), *Comprehensive rehabilitation nursing* (pp. 545–570). Philadelphia: W.B. Saunders.

Eilert, R. (2007). Orthopedics: Disturbances of prenatal origin—Congenital amputations & limb deficiencies. In W.W. Hay, M. Levin, J.M. Sondheimer, & R.R. Deterding (Eds.), *Current diagnosis & treatment in pediatrics* (18th ed., pp. 787–805). New York: McGraw-Hill.

Feudtner, C., Villareale, N.L., Morray, B., Sharp, V., Hays, R.M., & Neff, J.M. (2005). *Technology-dependency among patients discharged from a children's hospital: A retrospective cohort study.* BMC Pediatrics, 5(1), 8.

Gitter, A., & Bosker, G. (2005). Upper and lower extremity prosthetics. In J.A. DeLisa, G.B.M. Gans, N.E. Walsh, W.L. Bockenek, &W.R. Frontera, et al. (Eds.), *Physical medicine & rehabilitation: Principles and practice* (4th ed.). Philadelphia: Lippincott, Williams & Wilkins.

Giza, C.C., Mink, R.B., & Madikians, A. (2007). Pediatric traumatic brain injury: Not just little adults. *Current Opinion in Critical Care, 13*(2), 143–152.

Gordon, M., Gottschlich, M., Helvig, E., Marvin, J., & Richard, R. (2004). Review of evidence-based practice for the prevention of pressure sores in burn patients. *Journal of Burn Care Rehabilitation, 25,* 388–410.

Greenley, R.N., Coakley, R.M., Holmbeck, G.N., Jandasek, B., & Wills, K. (2006). Condition-related knowledge among children with spina bifida: Longitudinal changes and predictors. *Journal of Pediatric Psychology, 31*(8), 828–839.

Hack, M., Wilson-Costello, D., Friedman, H., Taylor, G.H., Schluchter, M., & Fanaroff, A.A. (2000). Neurodevelopment and predictors of outcomes of children with birth weights of less than 1000 grams: 1992–1995. *Archives Pediatrics and Adolescent Medicine, 154*(7), 725–731.

Hackbarth, R.M., Rzeszutko, K.M., Sturm, G., Donders, J., Kuldanek, A.S., & Sanfilippo, D.J. (2002). Survival and functional outcome in pediatric traumatic brain injury: A retrospective and analysis of predictive factors. *Critical Care Medicine, 30*(7), 1630–1635.

Hall, J.G. (1997). Arthrogryposis multiplex congenital: Etiology, genetics, classification, diagnostic approach, and general aspects. *Journal of Pediatric Orthopedics, Part B, 6*(3), 159–166.

Hewitt-Taylor, J. (2005). Caring for children with complex and continuing health needs. *Nursing Standard, 19*(42), 41–47.

Hummel, J., & Cronin, J. (2004). Home care of the high risk infant. *Advances in Neonatal Care, 4*(6), 354–364.

Ireland, D. (2006). Unique concerns of the pediatric surgical patient: Pre-, intra-, and post-operatively. *Nursing Clinics of North America, 41*(2), 265–298.

Kaufman, B.A. (2004). Neural tube defects. *Pediatric Clinics of North America, 51*(2), 389–419.

Kirk, S., Glendinning, C., & Callery, P. (2005). Parent or nurse? The experience of being a parent of a technology-dependent child. *Journal of Advanced Nursing, 51*(5), 456–464.

Klein, M., Lezotte, D., Fauerbach, J., Herndon, D., Kowalske, K., Carrougher, G., et al. (2007). The National Institute on Disability and Rehabilitation Research burn model system database: A tool for the multicenter study of the outcome of burn injury. *Journal of Burn Care Research, 28,* 84–96.

Koren, G., Nava-Ocampo, A.A., Moretti, M.E., Sussman, R., & Nulman, I. (2006). Major malformations with valproic acid. *Canadian Family Physician, 52,* 441–442, 444, 447.

Kozin, S. (2004). Classification of limb anomalies in congenital disorders: Classification and diagnosis. In R.A. Berger & A.C. Weiss (Eds.), *Hand surgery* (pp. 1405–1423). Philadelphia: Lippincott Williams & Wilkins.

Launay, F., Leet, A., & Sponseller, P. (2005). Pediatric spinal cord injury without radiologic abnormality: A meta-analysis. *Clinical Orthopedics and Related Research, 433,* 166–170.

Leger, R. (2005). Severity of illness, functional status, and HRQOL in youth with spina bifida. *Rehabilitation Nursing, 30*(5), 180–187.

Lohne, V., & Severinsson, E. (2004). Hope after the first months after acute spinal cord injury. *Journal of Advanced Nursing, 47*(3), 279–286.

Lomax-Bream, L.E., Barnes, M., Copeland, K., Taylor, H.B., & Landry, S.H. (2007). The impact of spina bifida on development across the first 3 years. *Developmental Neuropsychology, 31*(1), 1–20.

Maloney, K., Greffe, B., Foreman, N., Porter, C., Graham, D., Sawczyn, K., et al. (2007). Neoplastic disease and brain tumors. In A. Hay, W. William, A. Levin, J. Myron, J. Sondheiver, et al., *Diagnosis & treatment in pediatrics* (18th ed., pp. 885–916). New York: McGraw-Hill.

Martin, B., Dykes, E., & Lecky, F. (2004). Patterns and risks in spinal trauma. *Archives of Diseases in Childhood, 89*(9), 860–865.

Mason, D., Tobias, N., Lutkenhoff, M., Stoops, M., & Ferguson, D. (2004). The APNs guide to pediatric constipation management. *The Nurse Practitioner: American Journal of Primary Health Care, 29*(7), 13–15, 19–23.

Massagli, T. (2000). Medical and rehabilitation issues in care of children with spinal cord injury. *Physical Medicine and Rehabilitation of North America, 11*(1), 169–182.

Mayers, T., Gottschlich, M., Scanlon, J., & Warden, G. (2003). Four-year review of burns as an etiologic factor in the development of long bone fractures in pediatric patients. *Journal of Burn Care Rehabilitation, 24,* 279–284.

McQuade, M., & Houghton, K. (2005). Use of bisphosphonates in a case of Perthes disease. *Orthopaedic Nursing, 24*(6), 393–398.

Montagnino, B.A., & Mauricio, R.V. (2004). The child with tracheostomy and a gastrostomy tube: Parental stress and coping in the home. *Pediatric Nursing, 30*(5), 373–401.

Morgan, A., Ward, E., Murdoch, B., Kennedy, B., & Murison, R. (2003). Incidence, characteristics, and predictive factors for dysphagia after pediatric traumatic brain injury. *Journal of Head Trauma Rehabilitation, 18*(3), 239–251.

Morrissy, R., Giavedoni, B., & Coulter-O'Berry, C. (2006). The child with a limb deficiency. In R.T. Morrissy & S.L. Weinstein (Eds.), *Lovell & Winter's pediatric orthopaedics* (6th ed., pp. 1330–1444). Philadelphia: Lippincott Williams & Wilkins.

Mosca, V. (2006). Lower limb: Lower limb deficiencies. In L.T. Staheli, *Practice of pediatric orthopedics* (2nd ed., pp. 101–103). Philadelphia: Lippincott Williams & Wilkins.

Moxley, R., Ashwal, S., Pandya, S., Connolly, A., Florence, J., Mathews, K., et al. (2005). Practice parameter: Corticosteroid treatment of Duchenne dystrophy. *Neurology, 64,* 13–20.

Muscular Dystrophy Association (MDA). (2007). *Diseases.* Retrieved March 6, 2007, from http://www.mda.org/disease

National Center for Injury Prevention and Control (NCIPC). (2006). *Traumatic brain injury.* Retrieved June 20, 2007, from http://www.cdc.gov/ncipc/tbi/TBI.htm

National Dissemination Center for Children with Disabilities (NICHCY). (2006, May). *Traumatic brain injury, fact sheet 18, Susan's story.* Retrieved June 22, 2007 from http://www.nichcy.org/pubs/factshe/fs18txt.htm.

National Institute of Neurological Disorders and Stroke. (2007). *NINDS leukodystrophy information page.* Retrieved March 6, 2007, from http://www.ninds.nih.gov/disorders/leukodystrophy/leukodystrophy.htm

Neufield, S.M., Query, B., & Drummond, J.E. (2001). Respite care users who have children with chronic conditions: Are they getting a break? *Journal of Pediatric Nursing, 16*(4), 234–244.

Oddson, B.E., Clancy, C.A., & McGrath, P.J. (2006). The role of pain in reduced quality of life and depressive symptomology in children with spina bifida. *Clinical Journal of Pain, 22*(9), 784–789.

Office of Technology Assessment. (1987). *Technology-dependent children: Hospital v. home care—A technical memorandum* (report no. OTA-TM-H-38). Washington, DC: U.S. Government Printing Office.

Osteogenesis Imperfecta Foundation (OIF). (2006). *Osteogenesis imperfecta: A guide for medical professionals, individuals and families affected by OI.* Retrieved June 22, 2007 from http://www.oif.org.

Ottenbacher, K.J., Msall, M.E., Lyon, N., Duffy, L.C., Ziviani, J., Grander, C.V., et al. (2000). Functional assessment and care of children with neurodevelopmental disabilities. *American Journal of Physical Medicine and Rehabilitation, 79*(2), 114–123.

Passaretti, D., & Billmire, D. (2003). Management of pediatric burns. *The Journal of Craniofacial Surgery, 14*(5), 713–718.

Paterson, C.R., & McAllion, S.J. (2006). Classical osteogenesis imperfecta and allegations of nonaccidental injury. *Clinical Orthopaedics and Related Research, 452,* 260–264.

Pereira, C., Murphy, K., & Herndon, D. (2005). Altering metabolism. *Journal of Burn Care Rehabilitation, 26,* 194–199.

Pidcock, F., Fauerbach, J., Ober, M., & Carney, J. (2003). The rehabilitation/school matrix: A model for accommodating the noncompliant child with severe burns. *Journal of Burn Care Rehabilitation, 24,* 342–346.

Poggi, G., Liscio, M., Galbiati, S., Adduci, A., Massimino, M., Gandola, L., et al. (2005). Brain tumors in children and adolescents: Cognitive and psychological disorders at different ages. *Psycho-Oncology, 14*(5), 388–395.

Przkora, R., Barrow, R., Jeschke, M., Suman, O., Celis, M., Sanford, A., et al. (2006). Body composition changes with time in pediatric burn patients. *The Journal of Trauma Injury, Infections and Critical Care, 60,* 968–971.

Ramakerl, R.R., Lagro, S.W., van Roermund, A.B. & Sinnemal, G. (2000). The psychological and social functioning of 14 children and 12 adolescents after Ilizarov leg lengthening *Acta Orthopaedica Scandinavica, 71*(1), 55–59.

Rauch, F., & Glorieux, F.H. (2006). Treatment of children with osteogenesis imperfecta. *Current Osteoporosis Reports, 4*(4), 159–164.

Reeves, E., Timmons, D., & Dampier, S. (2006). Parents' experiences of negotiating care for the technology dependent child. *Journal of Child Health Care, 10*(3), 228–239.

Rehm, R. (2002). Creating a context of safety and achievement at school for children who are medically fragile/technology dependent. *Advances in Nursing Science, 24*(3), 71–84.

Rehm, R.S., & Bradley, J.F. (2005). Normalization in families who are raising a child who is medically fragile, technology dependent and developmentally delayed. *Qualitative Health Research, 5*(6), 807–820.

Rice, S.A., Blackman, J.A., Braun, S., Linn, R.T., Granger, C.V., & Wagner, D.P. (2005). Rehabilitation of children with traumatic brain injury: Descriptive analysis of a nationwide sample using the WeeFIM. *Archives of Physical Medicine and Rehabilitation, 86*(4), 834–836.

Rose, R., Fuentes, A., Hanel, B.J., & Dzialo, C.H. (1999). Pediatric leg length discrepancy: Causes and treatments. *Orthopedic Nursing, 18*(2), 21–31.

Schrag, J. (2003, Spring). NCLB and its implications for students with disabilities. *The Special Edge, 16*(2). Retrieved June 22, 2007 from http://www.calstat.org/publications/pdfs/edge_spring_03.pdf.

Shida-Tokeshi, J., Bagley, A., Molitor, F., Tomhave, W., Liberatore, J., Brasington, K., et al. (2005). Predictors of continued prosthetic wear in children with upper extremity prostheses. *Journal of Prosthetics and Orthotics, 17,* 119–124.

Spina Bifida Association of America (SBAA). (2007). Retrieved June 23, 2007, from http://www.sbaa.org/site/c.liKWL7PLLrF/b.2642343/k.8D2D/Fact_Sheets.htm

Staheli, L., Hall, J., Jaffe, K., & Paholke, D. (Eds.). (1998). *Arthrogryposis: A text atlas.* New York: Cambridge University Press.

Steinbok, P. (2006). Selection of treatment modalities in children with spastic cerebral palsy. *Neurosurgical Focus, 12*(2), e4.

Stoddard, F., Sheridan, R., Saxe, G., King, B.S., King, B.H., Chedekel, D., et al. (2002). Treatment of pain in acutely burned children. *Journal Burn Care Rehabilitation, 23,* 135–156.

Sullivan-Bolyai, S., Knafl, K.A., Sadler, L., & Gilliss, C.L. (2004). Great expectations: A position description for parents as caregivers: Part II. *Pediatric Nursing, 30*(1), 52–56.

Suman, O., Mlcak, R., & Herndon, D. (2002). Effect of exercise training on pulmonary function in children with thermal injury. *Journal Burn Care Rehabilitation, 23,* 288–293.

Swift, E.E., Taylor, H.G., Kaugars, A.S., Drotar, D., Yeates, K.O., Wade, S.L., et al. (2003). Sibling relationships and behavior after pediatric traumatic brain injury. *Journal of Developmental and Behavioral Pediatrics, 24*(1), 24–31.

Tomlin, P., Clarke, M., Robinson, G., & Roach, J. (2002). Rehabilitation in severe head injury in children: Outcome and provision of care. *Developmental Medicine & Child Neurology, 44*(12), 828–837.

U.S. Department of Education. (2007). Individuals with Disabilities Education Act (IDEA). Retrieved June 29, 2007, from http://idea.ed.gov/explore/home

U.S. Department of Health and Human Services. (2007). *Maternal and Child Health Bureau.* Retrieved June 22, 2007 from http://mchb.hrsa.gov/about/default.htm.

Vargo, M., & Gerber, L. (2005). Rehabilitation for patients with cancer diagnosis. In J.A. DeLisa, B.M. Gans, N.E. Walsh, W.L. Bockenek, W.R. Fontera, S.R. Geiringer, et al. (Eds.), *Physical medicine & rehabilitation: Principles and practice* (4th ed., pp. 1771–1794). Philadelphia: Lippincott Williams & Wilkins.

Vehmeyer-Heeman, M., Lommers, B., Van den Kerckhove, E., & Boeckx, W. (2005). Axillary burns: Extended grafting and early splinting prevents contractures. *Journal of Burn Care Rehabilitation, 26,* 539–542.

Verhoef, M., Barf, H., Post, M., van Asbeck, F., Gooskens, A., Rob, H., et al. (2006). Functional independence among young adults with spina bifida in relation to hydrocephalus and level of lesion. *Developmental Medicine & Child Neurology, 48*(2), 114–119.

Vinck, A., Maassen, B., Mullaart, R., & Rotteveel, J. (2006). Arnold–Chiari II malformation and cognitive functioning in spina bifida. *Journal of Neurology, Neurosurgery & Psychiatry, 77*(9), 1083–1086.

Vogel, L., Hickey, K., Klaas, S., & Anderson, C. (2004). Unique issues in pediatric spinal cord injury. *Orthopedic Nursing, 23*(5), 300–308.

Wade, S.L., Taylor, H.G., Drotar, D., Stancin, T., Yeates, K.O., & Minich, N.M. (2004). Interpersonal stressors and resources as predictors of parental adaptation following pediatric traumatic injury. *Journal of Consulting and Clinical Psychology, 72*(5), 776–784.

Wang, K.W.K., & Barnard, A. (2004). Technology-dependent children and their families: A review. *Journal of Advanced Nursing, 45*(1), 36–46.

Weed, R., & Berens, D. (2005). Basics of burn injury: Implication for case management and life care planning. *Lippincott's Case Management, 10*(1), 22–29.

Wesling, M., Brady, S., Jensen, M., Nickell, M., Statkus, D., & Escobar, N. (2003). Dysphagia outcomes in patients with brain tumors undergoing inpatient rehabilitation. *Dysphagia, 18*(3), 203–210.

Wilkins, K., McGrath, P., Finley, G., & Katz, J. (2004). Prospective diary of nonpainful and painful phantom sensations in a preselected sample of child and adolescent amputees reporting phantom limbs. *Clinical Journal of Pain, 20,* 293–301.

Wisconsin Education Association Council. (2007). *Special education inclusion.* Retrieved from http://www.weac.org/resource/june96/speced.htm.

Zickler, C.F., & Richardson, V. (2004). Achieving continence in children with neurogenic bowel and bladder. *Journal of Pediatric Health Care, 18*(6), 276–283.

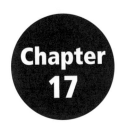

Chapter 17

Gerontological Rehabilitation Nursing

Kristen L. Mauk, PhD RN CRRN-A APRN BC • Cheryl Lehman, PhD RN CRRN-A BC

The rapid growth in the older adult population will have a major impact on the healthcare delivery system. In 1990, people older than 65 years accounted for 12.7% of the U.S. population, or 38 million people (Fowles, 1994). By 2025, the number of people over 65 years of age living in the United States is predicted to be nearly 20% (Munnell, 2004), and the oldest old—or frail older adults—will be the fastest-growing age group in the country. As a person's age increases, so does the likelihood of chronic illness and functional limitations. In light of these statistics, rehabilitation nurses must be prepared to meet the demands of an aging society. This can be accomplished only through special knowledge and training in the areas of gerontology and rehabilitation.

I. Theories of Aging

A. Biological

   1. Genes or biological clock: Each person has a genetic program that helps predetermine life expectancy.

   2. Wear and tear: The length of life is inversely related to the rate of living (i.e., the more wear and tear placed on the body, the faster one ages).

   3. Lipofuscin and connective tissue: This lipoprotein byproduct of metabolism increases with age, resulting in visible signs of aging.

   4. Free radicals: Unstable molecules damage cells, causing injury and signs of aging. Examples include tobacco smoke, herbicides and pesticides, radiation, and ozone.

   5. Stress: Aging is related to or influenced by life stress.

   6. Orgel: Errors in protein synthesis occur with aging, causing genes to mutate.

   7. Autoimmune or immunological: The body perceives old, irregular cells as hostile agents and begins to attack itself; the immune system becomes less effective with age.

   8. Nutritional: Length of life and age-related changes can be either positively or negatively influenced by nutritional intake.

   9. Environmental: Pollutants in one's surroundings, such as air and noise pollution, or radiation, adversely affect health and cause signs of aging.

B. Psychological

   1. Human needs (Maslow, 1954)

     a. Hierarchy of five basic needs that motivate human behavior:

       1) Physiologic

       2) Safety and security

       3) Love and belonging

       4) Self-esteem

       5) Self-actualization

     b. Failure in self-growth may lead to feelings of failure and depression (Lange & Grossman, 2006).

   2. Individualism (Jung, 1960)

     a. Lifespan view of development versus need attainment.

     b. Older adults engage in an inner search to evaluate their lives.

     c. Successful aging includes accepting the past and coping positively with changes.

   3. Lifespan development paradigm (Buhler, 1933)

     a. Life occurs in stages.

     b. Life satisfaction is related to goal achievement.

     c. Successful adaptation to changes in life may include reevaluation of the older person's beliefs relative to societal expectations.

   4. Selective optimization with compensation (Baltes, 1987)

     a. Emerged from Buhler's work

     b. Successful aging comes from learning to cope with losses of aging through choices.

     c. Selective optimization with compensation suggests that as people age they make choices of activities and roles that provide the most satisfaction, and this in turn facilitates successful aging (Baltes & Baltes, 1990).

C. Sociological

1. Activity theory: Older adults should remain active, occupied, and contributing to society to age positively and avoid the negative effects of advanced age (Havighurst, Neugarten, & Tobin, 1963).

   a. Research has shown a direct relationship between life satisfaction and activity in older adults (Lemon, Bengston, & Peterson, 1972).

   b. Informal activities such as gathering with friends, having hobbies, and engaging in group activities provided more life satisfaction than solitary activities. and meaningful activities has also been correlated with successful aging and life satisfaction (Harlow & Cantor, 1996, Schroots, 1996; Vaillant).

2. Disengagement: Society and older adults mutually withdraw from one another as one ages; disengagement is thought to maintain social equilibrium (Cumming & Henry, 1961).

   a. This theory has been and continues to be challenged by numerous studies that support activity theory.

   b. The Harvard Aging Study, which followed three cohorts of over 800 people each for more than 50 years, provides evidence that happiness in later life is more related to individual lifestyle choices than genetics, wealth, race, or other largely uncontrollable factors (Vaillant, 2002), raising questions about the validity of disengagement theory.

3. Continuity: Older adults continue with the same personality and behavior patterns that they developed throughout their lives (Havighurst, Neugarten, & Tobin, 1968). Four personality types of older adults:

   a. Integrated: well adjusted, actively engaged

   b. Armored-defended: continue activities and roles from middle age

   c. Passive-dependent: disinterested or dependent on others

   d. Unintegrated: fails to cope successfully with aging

4. Gerotranscendence: Older adults move toward oneness with the universe by maintaining close relationships, accepting impending death, and remaining connected with those of other generations (Tornstam, 1994).

   a. Three main elements:
      1) The cosmic level
      2) The self
      3) Social and individual relations

   b. A study investigating whether staff could recognize signs of gerotranscendence revealed that an interpretive framework for use in settings such as a nursing home would be of assistance in acceptance of these behaviors as a normal part of aging (Wadensten & Carlsson, 2001).

II. Review of Normal Aging

A. Cardiac and Circulatory System

1. Decreased cardiac output

2. Valvular changes that may result stenosis (Pugh & Wei, 2001) or heart murmurs

3. Decreased ability to adapt to increased demands

4. Age-associated changes across time may vary between individuals (Plahuta & Hamrick-King, 2006).

5. Increased incidence of varicose veins

6. Increased thickness of heart and arterial walls (Ferrari et al., 2003)

7. Increased systolic blood pressure (Plahuta & Hamrick-King, 2006)

B. Respiratory System

1. Decreased elasticity of the lungs

2. Impaired gas exchange over time caused by loss of elasticity and decreased surface area of alveoli

3. Increased carbon dioxide retention caused by a less efficient system

4. Less useful oxygen with each breath

5. Reduced vital capacity but no change in total lung capacity (Krauss Whitbourne, 2002)

6. Decreased blood oxygen level

C. Musculoskeletal System

1. Decreased muscle mass (sarcopenia) (Roubenoff, 2001) and related loss of muscle strength (Ivey et al., 2000)

2. Changes in range of motion in joints

3. Decreased overall height caused by compression of vertebrae over time

4. Decreased bone density, leading to increased risk for fractures

5. Decreased cartilage surface of joints, leading to possible limitations in range of motion

D. Genitourinary System

1. In women
    a. Decreased estrogen with perimenopause and menopause.
    b. Ovaries atrophy, vagina shortens and narrows, uterus decreases in size, and supporting ligaments weaken (Digiovanna, 2000).
    c. Decreased vaginal lubrication, often leading to pain during sexual intercourse
    d. Stress incontinence (common but treatable)
    e. Other types of incontinence (common but not a normal part of aging)
2. In men
    a. Testes decrease in size and weight, penis shows fibrous changes in erectile tissues by age 55 or 60 (Digiovanna, 2000).
    b. No significant changes in sexual libido or previous patterns of behavior
    c. Longer refractory times during phases of sexual intercourse
    d. Less complete erections and less frequent orgasms
    e. Enlarged prostate, resulting in poor urinary stream
3. In both men and women
    a. Decreased bladder capacity caused by bladder shrinkage and change in capacity and contractility (Digiovanna, 2000)
    b. Increase in urinary frequency and nocturia

E. Neurological System
    1. Brain decreases in size and weight.
    2. Loss of 10% of functioning neurons over lifespan in both genders, but neuron loss may be less than previously thought (Peters, 2002)
    3. Cognition:
        a. Some memory loss is common but should be distinguished from abnormalities such as those that occur with Alzheimer's disease.
        b. Intelligence and ability to learn are not affected.
    4. Proprioception (awareness of body position in space) may decrease with age, which can result in less coordination and balance, which could lead to falls.
    5. Slower voluntary reflexes
    6. Deep tendon reflexes still responsive
    7. More difficulty responding to multiple stimuli

8. Decreased kinesthetic sense
9. Complaints of feeling tired (even if staying in bed longer) caused by sleep pattern changes such as a decrease in stage IV, rapid eye movement sleep
10. Decreased dopamine levels, which may contribute to Parkinsonian features such as abnormal gait
11. Spinal cord cells begin to decline around age 60 (Beers & Berkow, n.d.) and spine may narrow, causing pressure on spinal cord that over time can cause changes in sensation.

F. Sensory System
    1. Vision
        a. Presbyopia: farsightedness or trouble focusing on near objects, caused by age-related changes in the shape of the eye that begin around age 40 (Digiovanna, 1994).
        b. Decreased peripheral vision
        c. Most common age-related eye diseases are cataracts (extremely common but highly treatable with surgery and intraocular lens implants), glaucoma, macular degeneration, and diabetic retinopathy (Jackson & Owsley, 2003).
        d. Decreased tear production, which leads to increased susceptibility to infections
        e. Changes in depth perception
    2. Hearing
        a. Presbycusis: decrease in hearing acuity, especially the ability to detect high-frequency tones and ability to discern speech (Rees, Duckert, & Carey, 1999)
        b. Impacted wax
        c. Need for hearing aids, which may amplify extraneous noises
    3. Smell: general decrease in acuity (Seiberling & Conley, 2004)
    4. Taste: atrophied taste buds, slight decrease in taste around age 60, and more exaggerated past age 70 (Seiberling & Conley, 2004)
    5. Touch: decreased ability to distinguish sensations and textures (Digiovanna, 2000)
    6. Pain
        a. Increased tolerance for pain
        b. General decreased sensitivity to light touch
        c. Increased pain threshold

G. Endocrine System
    1. Changes in sex hormones
    2. Decreased efficiency of the entire system

3. Changes in thyroid hormone production and glucose tolerance, which may warrant treatment (e.g., thyroid changes may lower the metabolic rate)

H. Hematological System
   1. Anemia common in 8%–44% of older adults (Nilsson-Ehle, Jagenburg, Landahl, & Svanborg, 2000), particularly iron deficiency and pernicious types
   2. Hypoalbuminemia
      a. Serum albumin has been shown to be a predictor of geriatric rehabilitation outcomes (Aptaker, Roth, Reichhardt, Duerden, & Levy, 1994).
      b. Albumin of less than 3.5 g/dl may place a person at risk for poor outcomes, including pressure ulcers (Aptaker et al., 1994).

I. Immune System
   1. Generally less efficient; immunosenescence is the aging of the immune system.
   2. Less effective T cells
   3. Possibly less resistant to infections
   4. Possible absence of typical symptoms of illness (e.g., elevated temperature with pneumonia)

J. Integumentary System
   1. Skin (Plahuta & Hamrick-King, 2006)
      a. Becomes more wrinkled, thinner
      b. Loses elasticity
      c. Is dry, which may lead to itching
      d. Has greater potential for tears and bruising
      e. Decreased number of sweat glands, which may lead to impaired thermoregulation
   2. Hair
      a. Pigment loss, resulting in what appears as gray or white hair
      b. Development of facial hair (in women)
      c. Thinning, balding (in men)
   3. Nails: more brittle, changes in color and texture
   4. Fat: distributed more on the trunk and less on the arms and legs

K. Gastrointestinal System (Plahuta & Hamrick-King, 2006)
   1. Slowed absorption in intestines
   2. Decreased digestive enzymes
   3. Decreased saliva production
   4. Decreased esophageal and intestinal peristalsis

5. Constipation
6. Weaker gag reflex or delayed swallowing, which can increase the risk of aspiration

L. Renal System
   1. Kidneys shrink, with potential loss of up to half of the functioning nephrons (Minaker, 2004).
   2. Decreased glomerular filtration rate, related in part to changes in blood flow (Digiovanna, 2000)
   3. Less effective filtration of wastes, which may allow medications to stay in the body longer and increase the risk of side effects

III. Aging and Disability: Acquiring a Disability at an Advanced Age

There are two distinct ways in which disability can affect older adults: Acquiring a disability at an advanced age and aging with an early-onset disability. The effects of age and aging can differ in each case.

A. Factors Affecting Rehabilitation Potential
   1. Age:
      a. Scivoletto, Morganti, Ditunno, Ditunno, and Molinari (2003) found that adults over 50 with new spinal cord injury (SCI) have less favorable outcomes than younger people with the same injuries in regard to walking and bladder and bowel independence and tend to have more associated medical problems.
      b. Bagg, Pombo, and Hopman (2002) reported that the Functional Independence Measure (FIM™) score at admission is a better predictor than FIM™ score at discharge in older adults with stroke and recommended that age not be a factor in the decision to admit a patient to rehabilitation.
      c. Yu (2005) found that age of 80 or older and admission function affected functional gains and rehabilitation efficiency in an outpatient rehabilitation program.
   2. Frailty:
      a. One definition of frailty is unintentional weight loss, exhaustion, low energy expenditure, slow walking speed, and weakness in the older adult (Fried, Ferrucci, Darer, Williamson, & Anderson, 2004).
      b. Another research-based definition of frailty is an accumulation of deficits, which include symptoms, signs, diseases, and disabilities. The more deficits, the

more frail (Rockwood, Mitniski, Song, Steen, & Skoog, 2006).

   c. Overall, frailty is the outcome of declines at the molecular, cellular, and physiologic system levels (Bandeen-Roche et al., 2006).

   d. Frail older adults are at higher risk for morbidity, disability, and mortality.

3. Effects of normal aging:

   a. Exercise tolerance: Pulmonary, cardiac, and muscle effects of aging affect exercise tolerance

   b. Strength

   c. Balance

   d. Mobility

4. Effects of chronic diseases:

   a. Diabetes:
      1) Glucose control
      2) Peripheral neuropathy
      3) Gastroparesis
      4) Vision
      5) Skin
      6) Vascular disease
      7) Amputation

   b. Heart disease:
      1) Exercise tolerance
      2) Ejection fraction
      3) Fluid balance
      4) Angina
      5) Edema

   c. Vascular disease:
      1) Wounds
      2) Amputation
      3) Pain
      4) Mobility
      5) Exercise tolerance

   d. Lung disease:
      1) Exercise tolerance
      2) Oxygenation

   e. Parkinson's disease:
      1) Cognition
      2) Mobility
      3) Balance
      4) Tremors

   f. Dementia:
      1) Ability to learn
      2) Memory
      3) Behavior

   g. Depression:
      1) Ability to learn
      2) Cognitive status
      3) Motivation

   h. Anemia:
      1) Exercise tolerance

      2) Healing
      3) Postural hypotension

   i. HIV and AIDS:
      1) Exercise tolerance
      2) Healing
      3) Nutritional status

   j. Cancer:
      1) Pain
      2) Exercise tolerance
      3) Mobility

   k. Patrick et al. (2001) found that the severity of medical comorbidity was a significant predictor of rehabilitation efficiency (gains in functional independence divided by length of stay) in older adults with various disabilities.

   l. Yu (2005) reported that the number of medical comorbidities and age affected length of stay in an outpatient rehabilitation program for older adults.

5. Baseline functional status: Yu (2005) found that age of 80 or more and admission function affected functional gains and rehabilitation efficiency in an outpatient rehabilitation program.

6. Baseline cognitive status:

   a. Ability to learn

   b. Memory

   c. Motivation

   d. Mast, MacNeill, and Lichtenberg (1999) reported that 34.7% of stroke patients and 27.8% of lower extremity fracture patients in their study met the criteria for dementia. Also, 33.3% of stroke patients and 25.1% of lower extremity fracture patients scored as depressed on the Geriatric Depression Scale. They noted that older stroke and lower extremity fracture patients need treatment not only of the reason for admission to rehabilitation but also of geriatric-specific problems such as depression, dementia, and multiple comorbidities.

7. Polypharmacy:

   a. Defined as using 2 or more medicines to treat the same condition, using 2 or more drugs from the same chemical class, or using 2 or more drugs with similar actions to treat different conditions (Brager & Sloand, 2005). Also defined as the prescription, administration, or use of more medications than are clinically indicated in a given patient (Charles & Lehman, 2006).

b. The risks of polypharmacy include increased likelihood of drug–drug or drug–disease interactions, adverse drug events, and patient nonadherence to medication plan (Charles & Lehman, 2006).

c. Home health nurses in one study reported that up to 21% of older adults did not understand their medications on discharge from hospital, that 78% took 5 or more drugs, that 11% had limited cognitive ability, and that 9% had medications ordered by more than one provider (Ellenbecker, Frazier, & Verney, 2004).

d. Ostwald, Wasserman, and Davis (2006) reported that stroke survivors in their study were discharged home with an average of 11.3 medications from 5 different drug classifications. The number of medications prescribed was correlated with the number of stroke-related comorbidities. Receipt of medication from several different drug categories was also correlated with having more stroke-related comorbidities and more complications. The authors of this study reported that the average monthly cost for a stroke survivor taking 10 commonly prescribed poststroke medications was $724.29 per month.

8. Social supports:
   a. Family or significant others
   b. Sources of income:
      1) Social Security
      2) Pension
   c. Funding for health care:
      1) Medicare
      2) Medicaid
      3) Private insurance
   d. Housing:
      1) Members of household
      2) Physical layout of home environment
   e. Transportation:
      1) Medical visits
      2) Grocery store
   f. Beaupre et al. (2005) demonstrated that functional status in a population aged 65 and older was lower in hip fracture patients with poor social supports than in those with good social supports. Subjects with poor social supports were also more likely to be living in an institution 6 months after discharge from rehabilitation than those with better social support.
   g. The Duke EPESE study (Mendes De Leon, Gold, Glass, Kaplan, & George, 2001) revealed that the larger the social network and the more interaction with that network, the less disability was present in study subjects (age 65 and older). Social interactions with friends were associated with lower disability, but interaction with children or relatives was not related to disability. The receipt of instrumental support was correlated with disability: The higher the support, the more disability.

9. Commonly acquired disability in older adults:
   a. Stroke
      1) Stroke is a leading cause of long-term disability in the United States.
      2) Onset is secondary to cardiovascular disease, high blood pressure, diabetes, smoking, high cholesterol, obesity, and family history.
      3) On average, one person in the United States has a stroke every 45 seconds.
      4) 88% of stroke deaths occur in people aged 65 and over.
      5) More women than men die of stroke each year because of their longer life expectancy.
      6) 88% of strokes are ischemic, 9% intracranial hemorrhage, 3% subarachnoid hemorrhage.
      7) In 2002, 71% of people discharged from short-stay hospitals with a primary diagnosis of stroke were older than 65 (American Heart Association [AHA]/American Stroke Association, 2006; AHA, 2004).
   b. Head injury
      1) Falls are the second leading cause of traumatic brain injury (TBI) and the leading cause of TBI hospitalizations in people aged 65 and older.
      2) These injuries often result in death or impairment for older adults.
      3) TBIs in older adults account for 80,000 emergency room visits per year, 75% of which result in hospitalization.
      4) 51% of TBIs in older adults are caused by falls, 9% by motor vehicle accidents.
      5) Older age negatively influences outcome after TBI.
      6) Older women are more likely to be hospitalized after injury than older men.
      7) The rate of TBI in the general

population is 60.6 per 100,000 people; after age 65, it increases to 155.9 per 100,000.

      8) Overall, in 2002 the U.S. incidence rate of hospitalization after fall with TBI was 29.6 per 100,000 population; in people aged 65–74, it increased to 58.6 per 100,000, and in those 75 years and older it was 203.9 per 100,000.

      9) Older age is recognized as an independent predictor for worse outcomes from TBI (Centers for Disease Control [CDC], 2003; Thompson, McCormick, & Kagan, 2006).

  c. Falls with fracture

      1) Secondary to muscle weakness, balance, osteoporosis, sensory loss.

      2) One-third of falls in older adults are caused by environmental hazards in home (see Figure 17-1).

      3) 3%–5% of falls in U.S. older adults result in fracture, with 360,000–480,000 fall-related fractures per year in the United States.

      4) Hip fractures cause the most deaths and disability in older adults.

      5) Up to 25% of community-dwelling older adults experiencing hip fracture from falls remain institutionalized after 1 year (CDC, 2006a).

  d. Deconditioning: Often a result of the enforced immobility of acute hospitalization superimposed on the normal changes of aging

B. Geriatric Syndromes That Can Affect Rehabilitation

  1. Delirium

    a. Defined as acute onset of confusion; fluctuates during the course of the day; short attention span, impaired memory, and usually an identifiable and treatable cause

    b. Multiple causative factors

    c. Delirium has been found to predict poor outcomes in orthopedic surgery patients (Duppils & Wikblad, 2004; Segatore & Adams, 2001).

    d. Nurses often do not recognize the symptoms of delirium (Inouye, Foreman, Mion, Katz, & Cooney, 2001).

  2. Falls

    a. More than one-third of older adults fall each year.

    b. Multiple causative factors

    c. Falls are a leading cause of death and disability among older adults and the most common cause of nonfatal injuries.

    d. Of those who fall, 20%–30% sustain moderate to severe injuries that reduce independence and mobility.

    e. For people 75 and older, those who fall are 4–5 times more likely to be admitted to a long-term care facility for a year or longer.

    f. Falls are a leading cause of TBI and fractures in older adults (CDC, 2006a).

  3. Dizziness

    a. Multiple causative factors

    b. Tinetti, Williams, and Gill (2000) reported that 24% of people 72 years and older reported dizziness, 74% of these reported several triggering factors, and 56% of the dizzy subjects reported differing sensations. Associated factors included anxiety, depression, impaired hearing, polypharmacy, postural hypotension, impaired balance, and past myocardial infarction. The risk of dizziness increased with each added characteristic.

  4. Incontinence

    a. Multiple causative factors

    b. Risk factors include immobility, decreased fluid intake, cognitive impairment, medications, constipation, environmental barriers, urinary tract infections, diabetes, and stroke.

    c. Consequences include falls, depression, pressure ulcers, and social isolation (Geronurseonline, 2005d).

Figure 17-1. Potential Environmental Risk Factors for Falls

- Flooring, such as throw rugs, high-pile carpeting, or slippery or wet tile
- Outdoor walkways that are wet or have leaves, snow, or ice on them
- Small children and pets
- Stairs and steps (especially those without handrails and those not clearly marked)
- Clutter in walkways and around the bedroom and bathroom areas
- Lack of handrails in the bathroom
- Adaptive equipment such as rolling walkers, canes, or splints
- Poor lighting in rooms or walkways
- Lack of a system to call for help (e.g., whistle, bell)
- Long cords such as those for phones or supplemental oxygen tanks
- Poor arrangement of living space, which requires a person to reach or move in ways that upset balance

5. Pressure ulcers
   a. Multiple causative factors
   b. Caused by immobility, moisture, poor nutrition, and pressure
6. Malnutrition
   a. Multiple causative factors
   b. Major risk factor for complications and delayed recovery
   c. Often caused by disease or functional impairments
   d. Natural progression of end-stage dementia; supplemental, invasive feeding in demented patients is an ethical concern.
   e. Includes both obese and underweight people
   f. Malnutrition increases risk of complications and death.
   g. 40%–60% of older hospitalized adults have been found to be malnourished (Institute of Medicine, 2000).
7. Dehydration
   a. Multiple causative factors
   b. Decreased thirst, reduced total body water in proportion to weight, body composition changes, impaired renal conservation of water, decreased effectiveness of vasopressin, multiple comorbidities
   c. Risk factors for dehydration include age greater than 85, decreased mobility, decreased ability to perform activities of daily living (ADLs), more than 4 chronic conditions, more than 4 medications, poor oral intake, communication difficulties, fever, few opportunities to drink.
   d. Atypical presentation in older adults: confusion, falls, change in level of consciousness, weakness, fatigue (Geronurseonline, 2005b)
8. Functional loss
   a. 22% of people 85 and older need assistance with personal care.
   b. 20%–40% of older adults experience functional decline during hospitalization.
   c. Risk factors include acute illness, exacerbation of chronic illness, injuries, medications, depression, malnutrition, decreased mobility, restraints.
   d. Complications include loss of independence, falls, incontinence, malnutrition, depression, decreased socialization, increased risk for

institutionalization (Geronurseonline, 2005a).
9. Polypharmacy
   a. 25%–40% of all prescriptions in the United States are written for older adults.
   b. 5%–15% of all hospitalizations are medication related.
   c. 40%–50% of all over-the-counter medications are consumed by older adults.
   d. 106,000 fatal adverse drug events occur annually in the United States.
   e. Community-dwelling adults average 4–6 medications daily.
   f. Symptoms of problems with medications include mental status changes, weight loss, dehydration, agitation, anorexia, urinary retention, and decline in functional status (Geronurseonline, 2005c).

C. Rehabilitation Nursing Interventions to Promote Successful Aging (see Figure 17-2)
   1. Primary prevention
      a. Young age groups without disability: prevention of chronic disease through promotion of healthy lifestyles
         1) Nutrition
         2) Exercise
         3) Weight management
         4) Smoking prevention or cessation
         5) Safety awareness
      b. Older adults with or without disability: prevention of new chronic disease or disability through promotion of healthy lifestyles
         1) Nutrition
         2) Exercise
         3) Weight management
         4) Smoking prevention or cessation
         5) Safety awareness
            a) Home environment
            b) Home safety evaluation
         6) Medication management
            a) Polypharmacy
            b) Psychoactive medications
         7) Driving skills
         8) Fall prevention
         9) Vision correction
         10) Hearing correction
         11) Seatbelts
         12) Limited alcohol intake
         13) Social supports
   2. Secondary prevention for all age groups, with and without disability
      a. Cancer screening

b. Smoking cessation

c. Pneumonia vaccine

d. Flu vaccine

3. Tertiary prevention in older adults without disability

a. Chronic disease management

b. Educating the older adult about
   1) The disease process
   2) How to prevent disease progression
   3) Recognition of complications and what to do
   4) Treatment compliance

4. Societal level

a. Redesign of cars

b. Redesign of roadways

c. License renewal restrictions

IV. Aging and Disability: Aging with an Early-Onset Disability

A. Longevity: People with early-onset disability are living longer. An estimated 12 million people are currently living into middle and late life with an early-onset disability.

1. Antibiotics and other medication advances

Figure 17-2. Suggestions for Teaching Older Adults

Visual

Use bright, direct lighting unless contraindicated because of visual disturbances (such as recent cataract surgery).

Do not stand by a window; avoid glare.

When using visual aids, use large, well-spaced letters (black on white is best).

Keep clients close to the speaker, or if in a large room, be certain that the audience can see and hear the speaker.

For individual teaching, make sure that the client's glasses are clean.

Auditory

Limit distractions: Eliminate extraneous noise, close doors, turn off television or radio, limit interruptions.

Face the audience; speak directly to the individual in a one-to-one setting..

Never cover your mouth when speaking (many older adults rely on lip reading to compensate for hearing deficits).

Speak slowly and clearly If appropriate, wear bright lipstick to help elderly people who lip read.

Before proceeding, ask whether the client can hear you.

Use assistive devices as needed (make certain that hearing aids and microphones are turned on and that batteries are working) .

General Teaching and Learning Suggestions

Keep teaching sessions short and to the point.

Design handouts to be simple and clear.

Relate the relevance of the topic to adult experiences within the group.

Use the principles of adult learning when planning an educational session.

Pace the presentation to reflect the unique needs and understanding of the group or individual.

Avoid the temptation to overload with too much information.

Remember that adults need a motivation to learn.

Provide immediate feedback to questions and comments.

Give an overview of the material to be covered and explain its relevance.

Keep information simple and specific; avoid technical jargon.

Use a variety of teaching modalities such as videotapes, hands-on experiences, samples of products, group discussion, overheads, pamphlets, handouts.

Emphasize the client's learning responsibility.

Be enthusiastic about the subject; if the teacher isn't, the learner will not be.

Summarize important points.

Teach a procedure close to the time it will take place.

When teaching skills, allow time for practice, return demonstrations, questions, and review sessions.

Stick to the essentials needed to maintain life and prevent complications but be prepared to address additional questions.

Keep the environment conducive to learning; for group sessions, the room temperature should be comfortable for the majority, potentially noxious stimuli (such as cigarette smoke) should be avoided, seats must be easily accessible.

Use a large enough room to accommodate those with wheelchairs, walkers, and other assistive devices, make certain exits are not blocked, have additional nursing personnel available should needs arise (such as toileting).

Be thoroughly familiar with resources available in the community and the individual facility.

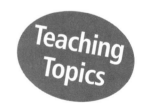

Reprinted with permission of W.B. Saunders Company from Easton, K.L. (1999). *Gerontological rehabilitation nursing* (p. 176). Philadelphia: W.B. Saunders.

---

2. Advances in technology

3. Improvements in public health

4. Improved medical care (Kemp & Mosqueda, 2004)

B. Aging as an Uncharted Course:
1. Atypical aging seems to be the norm. Unanticipated changes occur in midlife (Kemp & Mosqueda, 2004).

2. Higher rates of medical and functional problems 20–25 years earlier than those without disability:
   a. Often occurs in those who have been most active
   b. Changes occur in the amount of assistance needed (Kailes, 2002; Kemp & Mosqueda, 2004).

3. This population has 3–4 times the number of secondary health problems as age-matched peers (Kailes, 2002).

4. Accelerated aging is aging related to the disability itself at the cellular or organ level (Kailes, 2002).

5. *Wear and tear* refers to increased stress on body from living with disability over time (Kailes, 2002).

6. Depends on era of onset: People disabled 30, 40, or 50 years ago received rehabilitation in a different era. Many factors have changed over time. People disabled today may not have the same outcomes in 20, 30, or 40 years (Kailes, 2002).

7. Latent illness: An impairment such as polio or cerebral palsy (CP) can start a cascade of events that cause illnesses in later life (Kailes, 2002).

8. Contributing factors:
   a. Environment:
      1) Accessibility
      2) Modifications in home and the community
   b. Nonaccommodating environments may increase stress on the body (Kailes, 2002).
   c. Equipment: Manual equipment may increase stress on joints and limbs over time.
   d. Medications: Long term use of medications may affect the aging and health of body systems.
   e. Sedentary lifestyles increase the risk over time for cardiovascular disease and disuse syndromes.
   f. Preventive service use: Many people with

disabilities do not maintain preventive services over lifetime (e.g., vaccinations, cancer screening) because of a lack of knowledge, funding, or available and accessible services.

C. Unexpected Medical, Functional, and Psychosocial Problems (Kailes, 2002):
1. Loss of strength, endurance, and range of motion
2. Pain
3. Employment difficulties
4. Decreased quality of life
5. Family stress

D. Late Life Syndrome: Disability-specific changes with aging are common, superimposed on normal changes of aging.
1. Polio:
   a. Postpoliomyelitis syndrome (PPS):
      1) 440,000 people are at risk for PPS; 25%–60% of these survivors may develop PPS.
      2) Signs and symptoms appear 30–40 years after original onset of polio.
      3) Exact cause is unknown, thought to be degeneration of overworked nerve terminals in motor units that remain after initial illness.
      4) Slow, stepwise, unpredictable course.
      5) Decreased strength, fatigue:
         a) In muscles previously affected by polio and in muscles not previously affected by polio
         b) Muscle atrophy occurs in some cases.
         c) PPS fatigue affects more than 1.63 million American polio survivors (Bruno, Cohen, Galski, & Frick, n.d.).
      6) Decreased respiratory efficiency: pneumonia
      7) Dysphagia: aspiration pneumonia
      8) Joint pain
      9) Muscle pain, cramping
      10) Decreased function
      11) Depression
   b. Severity of PPS is predicted by severity of initial residual disability after polio (Klingbiel, Baer, & Wilson, 2004; NINDS, 2006b).
2. Cerebral palsy:
   a. 65%–90% of children with CP live into adulthood.
   b. Organ systems (heart, lungs) age prematurely.

c. Postimpairment syndrome includes pain, weakness, and fatigue.

d. Decline in functional status:
   1) Walking
   2) Self-care

e. Increased falls

f. Contractures, especially lower extremities in nonambulators

g. Progressive deformity

h. Kyphoscoliosis:
   1) Pneumonia, right-sided heart failure, hypoxemia, decreased vital capacity
   2) Problems with positioning, seating

i. Increased bowel and bladder dysfunction:
   1) Urinary tract infections
   2) Incontinence

j. Osteoporosis, osteopenia, and fractures

k. Oral motor and dental disorders:
   1) Increased difficulty chewing, eating, and swallowing
   2) Increased risk of aspiration, malnutrition, and dental decay
   3) More common in those with dyskinesias or spastic CP

l. Arthritis: association between presence of pain in weight-bearing joints and a cessation of ambulation around age 45

m. Spasticity

n. Pain:
   1) Often related to musculoskeletal dysfunction, degenerative arthritis, and overuse syndromes
   2) Common sites include hip, knee, ankle, and lumbar and cervical spine.

o. Spinal stenosis (Klingbiel et al., 2004; NINDS, 2006a)

p. Life expectancy lower for those with severe impairment and poor mobility (De Vivo, 2004).

q. Strauss, Ojdana, Shavelle, and Rosenbloom (2004) found a marked decline in ambulation with aging for those with CP who were mobile when they became adults; greater need for assistance with ADLs as age increased; greater need for residence in nursing facilities; and poorer survival among those who lost mobility. People with the most severe disability did not live to age 60.

3. Spina bifida:
   a. Overuse syndrome
      1) Wheelchair users: shoulders, wrists, hands; carpal tunnel syndrome; rotator cuff injuries
      2) Ambulators: hip and knee pain
   b. Shunt malfunction
   c. Tethered cord syndrome
   d. Knee pain
   e. Osteoporosis: increased risk for fractures
   f. Kyphosis and scoliosis
   g. Charcot joints
   h. Skin changes: pressure ulcers
   i. Increased incidence and severity of latex allergy
   j. Obesity
   k. Renal system changes
      1) Renal damage leading to renal failure
      2) Bladder cancer associated with neurogenic bladder
      3) Changes in bladder control
   l. Increased risk of latex allergies (Klingbiel et al., 2004)

4. Down's syndrome:
   a. 50% of infants who survive to age 1 can be expected to live past 50 years of age.
   b. Show signs of aging 20–30 years ahead of others in general population:
      1) Accelerated deterioration after stressful event
      2) Depression
      3) Hypothyroidism
      4) Hearing and visual impairment
      5) Vascular disease
      6) Graying hair
      7) Glucose intolerance and degenerative bone disease
      8) High rates of cancer
      9) Cognitive losses
   c. Early-onset dementia:
      1) Typically around age 40–50, as many as 75% of people with Down's syndrome exhibit signs of Alzheimer's-type dementia.
      2) Atypical signs and symptoms:
         a) Seizures
         b) Changes in ADL ability
   d. Accelerated rate of functional losses after age 45:
      1) Need the same health promotion programs at an earlier age as nondisabled people aged 50–80 (Chen, 2006; Merck Manuals Online Medical Library, 2003)
      2) Menopause may occur 5-–6 years earlier than in the general population (Holland & Benton, 2004).
   e. Quality of life (Brown, Taylor, & Matthews, 2001):

1) The majority report being happy.
2) Privacy is important.
3) Reminiscence may be helpful.
4) Tidiness and cleanliness of surroundings are valued.

5. Spinal cord injury:
   a. Three post-SCI phases identified:
      1) Acute restoration phase (first 2 years after SCI): Maximal function regained within limitations of SCI.
      2) Maintenance phase:
         a) Stable level of function over time
         b) Stable time varies
      3) Decline phase:
         a) Degenerative effects of SCI
         b) Aging
         c) Aging caregivers
   b. Functional decline begins 10–20 years after injury:
      1) Depends on genetics, lifestyle, age at time of injury, current age, level of injury, weight, health history, comorbidities, available social support.
      2) Children with SCI may have 20 years of stable functioning after injury, whereas adults over 50 may have just 5–7 years before decline begins.
   c. Overuse syndrome:
      1) Pain:
         a) Incidence of pain found to increase from 41% 1 year after injury to about 80% more than 5 years after injury.
         b) More than 70% of people with SCI report upper extremity pain.
         c) Nearly two-thirds of people with SCI have compressive neuropathies in the upper extremities.
      2) Most common overuse syndromes are degenerative joint disease, rotator cuff tears, rotator cuff tendonitis, subacromial bursitis, and capsulitis.
   d. Osteoporosis and fractures:
      1) 6% of people with SCI have a lower extremity fracture, most commonly femur.
      2) As many as 10% of these fractures result in nonunion.
   e. Scoliosis:
      1) Nearly 97% of pediatric patients with SCI develop scoliosis.
      2) Nearly 50% of adults with SCI develop scoliosis.
   f. Cardiovascular function:
      1) Incidence of cardiovascular disease is more than 200% higher than expected for noninjured population.
      2) Hypertension is twice as common in paraplegics as in general population.
   g. Gastrointestinal tract: Complications increase with age.
   h. Genitourinary tract: Incidence of bladder cancer increases from 0.2% in the first 10 years after injury to 9% after 30 years.
   i. Skin:
      1) Susceptibility to pressure ulcers increases with age.
      2) Sitting tolerance may decrease with age.
      3) Incidence of pressure ulcers increases with age.
   j. Decreased immunity:
      1) Urinary tract infections
      2) Pneumonia
   k. Decreased pulmonary function
   l. Insulin resistance
   m. Hardware breakdown: spinal rods
   n. Social isolation (Menter, 1998; Winkler, 2006)

6. TBI: A recent study of 286 survivors of moderate to severe TBI revealed the following chronic health conditions an average of 14.2 years after injury:
   a. Nervousness and tension
   b. Arthritis
   c. Sleep disturbances
   d. Vision changes
   e. Hearing changes
   f. Allergies
   g. Seizures
   h. Breathing problems (Colantonio, Ratcliff, Chase, & Vernich, 2004)

7. Multiple sclerosis (MS):
   a. People over 65 have greater disability.
   b. Disease course and length of time after diagnosis are stronger predictors of current status than current age and other demographics (DeVivo, 2004).
   c. Finlayson, Van Denend, and Hudson (2004) found that women aging with MS perceived that they had less freedom and needed more assistance than peers without MS. They shared concerns about unmet needs in the areas of personal care, housework, support groups, assistive technology, travel, and socialization.

E. Rehabilitation Nursing Interventions to Promote Successful Aging in Those with Early-Onset Disability:
  1. Primary prevention
    a. Young age groups
      1) Prevention of chronic disease through promotion of healthy lifestyles
        a) Nutrition
        b) Exercise
        c) Weight management
        d) Smoking prevention or cessation
        e) Safety awareness
      2) Early education about potential problems of aging and how to prevent them
        a) In rehabilitation setting
        b) In maintenance (stable) phase of disability
    b. Older adults
      1) Prevention of new chronic disease or disability through promotion of healthy lifestyles
        a) Nutrition
        b) Exercise
        c) Weight management
        d) Smoking prevention or cessation
        e) Safety awareness
        f) Medication management
          (1) Polypharmacy
          (2) Psychoactive medications
        g) Driving skills
        h) Fall prevention
        i) Vision correction
        j) Hearing correction
        k) Seatbelts
        l) Limited alcohol intake
        m) Social supports
      2) Lifelong education about, surveillance for, and prevention of combined problems of aging and disability
  2. Ongoing secondary prevention for all age groups with disability
    a. Cancer screening
    b. Smoking cessation
    c. Pneumonia vaccine
    d. Flu vaccine

V. **Psychosocial Issues**
  A. Grief and Loss
    1. Life changes with
      a. Retirement
      b. Death of a spo
      c. Possible decli chronic illnes
      d. Menopause
      e. Possible change in economic status
      f. Possible social isolation
      g. Possible change in living arrangements
    2. Role changes with age
      a. Widowhood
      b. Caregiver role reversal (i.e., the person who has provided care becomes the person who is being cared for)
  B. Stress and Coping
    1. The ability to deal well with stress and adopt positive coping mechanisms is associated with successful aging (Vaillant, 2002).
    2. Assess coping strategies in relation to the amount of stress the person is experiencing and promote the use of positive coping strategies:
      a. Increased social support
      b. Activity and exercise
      c. Faith, hope, and spirituality
      d. Involvement in leisure activities one enjoys
  C. Depression and Anxiety
    1. Depression
      a. It is estimated that 2 million older adults experience depression in some form (National Institute of Mental Health [NIMH], 2006).
      b. Risk factors:
        1) Incontinence
        2) History of substance abuse
        3) Social isolation
        4) Chronic pain or illness
        5) Being a caregiver
        6) Living alone
        7) Functional disability
        8) Poor social support
      c. Signs and symptoms:
        1) Insomnia
        2) Memory impairment
        3) Feelings of worthlessness or powerlessness
        4) Fatigue
        5) Vague physical complaints

d. Results of depression (Cowley, Diebold, Gross, & Hardin-Fanning, 2006):
   1) Decreased quality of life
   2) Associated anxiety
   3) Higher mortality rates from other conditions
   4) Higher risk for cancer
   5) Poorer outcomes after surgery
   6) Higher rate of suicide
e. Nursing interventions (Butcher & McGonigal-Kenney, 2005):
   1) Psychotherapy or counseling.
   2) Medications, especially tricyclic antidepressants, selective serotonin reuptake inhibitors, antipsychotics (monoamine oxidase inhibitors used less because of side effects).
   3) Encourage participation in social activities.
   4) Promote a healthy lifestyle including proper nutrition, good sleeping habits, and a daily routine.
   5) Enhance coping strategies.
   6) Connect to community resources.
   7) Enhance social support systems.
   8) Inspire hope.
   9) Be alert to suicidal ideations.

2. Anxiety
   a. Should be treated in conjunction with depression for best outcomes.
   b. Most older adults with major depression also have anxiety.
   c. Not well understood or studied in older adults.
   d. Selective serotonin reuptake inhibitors (used to treat depression) are medications of choice (Anxiety Disorders Association of America, 2006).
   e. Also treated with cognitive behavioral therapy.
   f. Nursing interventions similar to those for depression; in addition, person should develop a good trusting relationship with the primary healthcare provider.

D. Life Review and Reminiscence
   1. Older adults may be undertaking an end-of-life review.
   2. They may experience anticipatory grieving.
   3. Erikson's development stage for older age: Ego integrity versus despair suggests that older adults need to feel that their life has purpose and meaning. [Refer to Chapter 15 for more information on developmental stages.]

   4. Rehabilitation nurses can use reminiscence therapy to help older adults remember and recall positive memories that can be shared and discussed (Kart & Kinney, 2001).

E. Suicide
   1. Older white men are at highest risk for suicide.
   2. Older men tend to use more lethal means of suicide (e.g., firearms, hanging), whereas older women use less lethal means such as pills.
   3. Suicide is associated with alcoholism, diagnosis of a terminal disease, depression, presence of a chronic disease, being unmarried and living alone, having few support systems, drug abuse, bereavement, intractable pain, and social isolation; depression is the most notable associated condition.
   4. In 2000, 18% of suicide deaths were in older adults (NIMH, 2006).
   5. Up to 75% of those committing suicide visited their primary care physician within a month beforehand (NIMH, 2006).
   6. The risk can be lessened by strengthening social supports, treating depression, increasing involvement in social activities, and taking definitive action when suicidal ideations are expressed (Kart & Kinney, 2001).

F. Rehabilitation of Clients Who Are Terminally Ill
   1. Nurses should explore their own feelings about the rehabilitation of those who are at the end of life.
   2. There are many potential examples of situations that involve rehabilitating older adults with terminal illnesses:
      a. Late-stage cancer, including melanoma
      b. Rapidly growing, inoperable tumors
      c. End-stage renal disease
      d. Last stages of AIDS
      e. Other incurable diseases
   3. Explore with patient and family the goals of rehabilitation therapy:
      a. Increased quality of life
      b. Increase independence enough to go home to die rather than remaining in facility
   4. Discuss purposes of palliative care and hospice.

VI. General Aging Issues

A. Preventive Services for Older Adults:

1. Primary
   a. Activities for health promotion and disease prevention
   b. Immunizations to prevent illness; those recommended by the CDC for adults over age 65 and those at high risk include the following (CDC, 2006b):
      1) Annual flu vaccine
      2) Pneumococcal vaccine once after age 65 and one-time revaccination for those over age 75
      3) Tetanus and diphtheria vaccine every 10 years

2. Secondary
   a. Follow recommendations of Healthy People 2010 (http://www.healthypeople. gov/).
   b. Screenings for those at risk
   c. Screenings recommended by the U.S. Preventive Services Task Force with sufficient evidence to support (Nelson, 2006):
      1) Tobacco use
      2) Depression
      3) Hyperlipidemia
      4) Hypertension
      5) Osteoporosis for women older than 65
      6) Vision and hearing for older adults
      7) Mammography every 1–2 years for women
      8) Colorectal cancer screening by fecal occult blood test or sigmoidoscopy

3. Tertiary
   a. Rehabilitation of chronic health alterations as discussed throughout this core curriculum
   b. Focus on prevention of complications and maintenance of function

B. End of Life:

1. Hospice
   a. More than 75% of hospice patients die at home (National Hospice and Palliative Care Organization, 2004).
   b. Hospice care provides support for people in last phase of terminal illness.
   c. For people with less than 6 months to live, per physician
   d. Promotes the concept "live until you die"
   e. Hospice recognizes dying as a normal part of living.
   f. Focuses on maintaining quality of life until death
   g. Grief and bereavement support for patient and family
   h. Pain management is a priority.

2. Palliative care
   a. Comfort based, not curative
   b. Patients can receive treatment for conditions and still receive palliative care; pursuing treatment does not exclude patients from palliative care.
   c. Interdisciplinary team based
   d. Rehabilitation nurses can assist patient in the process of dying well because there is potential for self-growth even in the dying process (Byock, 1997).

3. Nursing interventions
   a. Advance directives
      1) Living will
         a) Is used in cases of terminal illness
         b) Makes the client's wishes known in advance when death is imminent, as certified by a physician
      2) Declaration document of life-prolonging procedures
         a) Describes steps to take to prolong life
         b) Is determined by the client
      3) Durable power of attorney for health care
         a) Allows another person to make decisions on behalf of the client
         b) Can encompass health, financial, property, and other issues
      4) Healthcare representative: allows a healthcare professional to make decisions at the client's behest regarding health-related issues
      5) Five wishes (My Health Directive, 2006; http://www.myhealthdirective. com)
         a) Not legally recognized in all states
         b) In the states where this is recognized, people may complete the forms, available online, without the use of an attorney.
         c) Cost effective and easy to use
         d) A nontraditional type of advanced directive that answers these five items according to a person's wishes:
            (1) Who makes healthcare decisions when the person is unable
            (2) What kind of medical

treatment is wanted or not wanted

    (3) Comfort measures the person wants

    (4) How people should treat the person

    (5) What he or she wants loved ones to know

  6) Allow natural death (Meyer, 2001; Warring & Krieger-Blake, 2006): more descriptive and positive than a do-not-resuscitate order

  b. Intervening with common problems at the end of life

    1) Dyspnea:

      a) Opioid therapy such as morphine can reduce shortness of breath.

      b) Elevate head of the bed 30–45 degrees.

      c) Provide a fan to move air in the room.

      d) Cool, humidified air

      e) Control oral secretions.

    2) Anxiety can be worsened by fear of suffering; antianxiety agents such as lorazepam given orally, sublingually, or rectally can help (McKinnis, 2002).

    3) Constipation:

      a) Immobility, lack of exercise, decreased fluids, and pain medications contribute to constipation.

      b) Use stool softener and stimulant combination.

    4) Nausea and vomiting:

      a) Treatment depends on the cause.

      b) A combination of medications may be indicated.

      c) Prepare foods away from patient's room.

    5) Poor appetite:

      a) Eat for pleasure as desired.

      b) There is a natural withdrawal of desire for food at end of life.

      c) Artificial hydration may prolong suffering and increase edema through fluid overload (End of Life Nursing Education Consortium, 2004).

      d) Provide meticulous mouth care as fluid intake decreases.

    6) Pain:

      a) Typically undertreated in older adults.

      b) Identify and treat the type of pain.

      c) Fear of addiction should not be a factor.

      d) Cancer pain treatment generally follows 3-step ladder (World Health Organization, 1990) of nonsteroidal anti-inflammatory drugs, opioids, and analgesic adjuvants in combinations.

  c. Educating families about what to expect at end of life

    1) Signs of impending death (Marrone, 1997):

      a) Decreased urine output

      b) Changes in breathing patterns

      c) Increasing periods of unresponsiveness

      d) Mottling of extremities

      e) Changes in vital signs

    2) Ask about specific cultural or spiritual practices at end of life and death.

  d. Ethical and moral dilemmas

    1) Withholding treatment: not beginning treatment (advance directives make the client's wishes explicit)

    2) Withdrawing treatment: removing life-sustaining interventions after they have been implemented (e.g., disconnecting a ventilator from a person who is unable to breathe independently, discontinuing nutritional interventions for a person who cannot otherwise eat or drink independently)

    3) Assisted suicide

      a) Defined as helping a person to terminate his or her own life

      b) Illegal in most states

      c) Legal in Oregon for a terminally ill patient to be prescribed a lethal dose of medication by the physician; must be taken by the patient

    4) Euthanasia

      a) Purposefully hastening the death of another person.

      b) An outside person may play a more active role in hastening the death of another with the purpose of ending his or her suffering.

C. Use of Physical and Chemical Restraints:

  1. About 15% of nursing homes residents are restrained for some portion of the day (Beers & Berkow, n.d.):

    a. Falls

    b. Confusion

c. Death

d. Pressure ulcers

e. Pneumonia

f. Urinary tract infections

3. The use of physical restraints must be justified and documented.

4. Physical restraints should be used only when the person is a danger to himself or herself or others.

5. Chemical restraints are inappropriate except in the most extreme circumstances for client safety.

6. Good alternatives to restraints exist and should be explored (Cowley et al., 2006):

   a. Companions or close supervision

   b. Modifying the environment

   c. Reality orientation

   d. Activities for diversion

   e. Increasing physical activities

7. Restraint use can increase the likelihood of injury in many instances.

8. A physician order is required for restraint use and must include documentation of the medical condition necessitating restraint, the type of restraint, the length of time for use, and guidelines for release and repositioning (according to OBRA 1987 guidelines). (Cowley et al., 2006)

D. Abuse or Mistreatment of Older Adults: May take many forms, including neglect or financial, passive or active physical, and sexual abuse:

1. Elder abuse is difficult to obtain statistics on and difficult to research (National Center on Elder Abuse, 2006).

   a. Often not reported or underreported by victims

   b. As many as 5 million victims of financial abuse.

   c. 2%–10% of older adults may be victims of abuse

   d. Between 1 and 2 million Americans may have been victimized in some way by those they depended on.

2. Characteristics of abusers:

   a. May have been victims of abuse themselves

   b. May be men or women

   c. May be family members or caregivers

   d. May have social and emotional problems or a history of psychological problems

   e. May abuse drugs or alcohol

   f. May have a high level of stress or frustration, minimal coping abilities, and lack of knowledge

3. Characteristics of victims (DeCalmer & Glendenning, 1993; Pritchard, 1995, 1996): Many rehabilitation clients are at risk because of the following factors:

   a. Are socially isolated

   b. Are elderly

   c. Are in poor health

   d. Are widowed

   e. Have significant physical limitations

   f. Can be men or women (although women are victims more often)

   g. Are dependent on others

   h. Have a history of family violence

4. Possible signs and symptoms of abuse or mistreatment:

   a. Poor physical hygiene

   b. Dehydration or malnutrition

   c. Multiple bruises of different colors (indicating different stages of healing)

   d. A withdrawn, cowering, fearful, anxious, depressed, or hopeless demeanor

   e. Presence of burns, skin tears, broken bones, or severe rashes that, when explained, do not fit the injury or trauma

5. Nursing interventions (see Figure 17-3):

   a. Perform a complete history and physical assessment.

   b. Make certain the explanation fits the injury, realizing that rehabilitating older adults may experience falls as they increase their level of independence.

   c. Be alert to possible signs and symptoms of abuse or neglect.

   d. Interview the suspected abuser and the victim separately.

   e. Consult with available resources as needed (e.g., psychologist, social worker).

   f. Report any suspected case of abuse. This can be done anonymously to an office of Adult Protective Services.

   g. Do not alienate the suspected perpetrator.

   h. Take necessary steps to protect the client.

E. Polypharmacy:

1. Polypharmacy is defined as the use of multiple medications (often inappropriately).

   a. Older adults commonly take many medications, which can increase the risk of adverse reactions for many reasons:

1) Drugs are excreted more slowly by the kidneys.
2) Absorption in the intestines is slower.
3) Metabolism slows with age.

b. Older adults consume 34% of prescription medications and about 40% of nonprescription medications (American Society of Consultant Pharmacists, 2000).

c. The aforementioned factors cause the drugs to remain present in the body for a longer time.

d. Adverse drug reactions may occur at any time, or at a later time than expected with younger adults.

e. Older adults may use over-the-counter medications or herbal therapies that they do not consider "drugs" but that also may interact with other medications.

f. Incidence of polypharmacy is thought to increase with age.

g. Those over 85 are at higher risk because they typically take more medications.

h. Polypharmacy is associated with:
1) Number and severity of illnesses
2) Hospitalization
3) Number of physicians seen
4) Number of pharmacies used
5) Increased patient age

i. In long-term care facilities, psychotherapeutics often misused.

j. Interventions to avoid polypharmacy have not been well researched or documented.

2. Nursing interventions:

a. Avoid unnecessary polypharmacy:
1) Teach clients and families to use

primary care provider to coordinate care.
2) Obtain list of all physicians and pharmacies used.
3) Check for duplication of medications.
4) Encourage use of one pharmacy.
5) Be sure all physicians are informed of all medications prescribed by other physicians.

b. Avoid negative effects of polypharmacy:
1) Obtain a comprehensive medication history.
2) Monitor blood urea nitrogen, creatinine, and creatinine clearance to check kidney function.
3) Consider the possibility of adverse drug reaction when new symptoms appear (Cowley et al., 2006).
4) Use or consider use of nonpharmacologic treatment when possible.
5) Simplify the medication regimen.
6) Educate family and clients to be informed consumers.

c. Family and client education regarding decreasing medication errors:
1) Include the client and the family or caregiver.
2) Follow the principles of teaching and learning with family members and with the client.
3) Allow time for demonstration and return demonstration.
4) Teach more than one family member whenever possible.
5) Use medication boxes to assist with organization of medications and promote independence of client when appropriate.
6). Use large and simple medication lists that are readily accessible.
7) Use pictures of medications on the list to assist with recognition.
8) Be sure that the client and family understand the purpose of the medication, time to be taken, amount, and route.

d. Use of medication boxes:
1) Organizes the client's medications
2) Provides a system for management to decrease the risk of making medication errors at home
3) Allows family members to help monitor or set up the client's medications

F. Caregiver Issues

Figure 17-3. Nursing Indications for the Prevention of Elder Abuse

- Establish a trusting relationship with the elderly person.
- Be able to refer families to resources available in the community.
- Strengthen social supports.
- Encourage regular respite for the caregiver.
- Identify caregivers who are at the highest risk of being abusers and target interventions to prevent stress from caregiver burden.
- Be aware of risk factors and contributing factors.
- Perform thorough physical assessments and carefully document findings, including the client's appearance, nutritional state, skin condition, mental attitude and awareness, need for aids to enhance sensory perception.
- If abuse is suspected, interview the caregiver and other possible informants to confirm or refute suspicions.
- Know the laws governing the reporting of abuse.

Reprinted with permission from Easton, K.L. (1999). *Gerontological rehabilitation nursing* (p. 336). Philadelphia: W.B. Saunders.

1. Aging caregivers
   a. Many caregivers of older adults are older themselves.
   b. When the caregiver's health is poor, caregiver stress is likely to be higher; older caregivers are more likely to have more chronic illnesses by virtue of their age.
   c. Caregiving may also fill a need for the caregiver (Krieger-Blake, 2006).
2. Caregiver stress
   a. Defined as the emotional burden of caregiving.
   b. The burden of caring can lead to depression, anxiety, difficulty coping, and problems with physical health of the caregiver.
   c. Women are more prone to this problem.
   d. Signs of caregiver stress (U.S. Department of Health and Human Services, 2006):
      1) Sleeping problems
      2) Weight loss or gain
      3) Fatigue
      4) Irritability
      5) Withdrawal
      6) Headaches, stomach upset, or frequent vague physical symptoms
   e. Interventions for caregiver stress:
      1) Obtain respite care as needed.
      2) Get assistance in the home.
      3) Take care of one's own health through diet, daily exercise, and relaxation.
      4) Use community resources (e.g., National Family Caregiver Support Program).
      5) Use faith-based resources if possible.

G. Postrehabilitation Care
   1. Settings for care
      a. Long-term care facilities
         1) Provide a variety of levels of care
         2) May range from independent living through nursing home or skilled care
         3) Costs vary widely but depend largely on geographic location and nature of services needed
      b. Independent living
         1) Senior living apartment
         2) Private home
         3) Apartment within a long-term care facility
      c. Assisted living
         1) Freestanding facilities

         2) Within a long-term care facility
         3) Group or foster homes
         4) Other community-based homes
         5) Adult day care services (for daytime only, not 24-hour supervision)
      d. Home health care
         1) Services vary according to agency.
         2) Many agencies provide companion services that include light housekeeping and meal preparation or assistance with ADLs.
         3) If further in-home therapy or nursing services are needed, investigate the exact nature of services that each agency will render and how expenses are billed.
   2. Assisting patients and families with postrehabilitation placement
      a. Address cultural influences.
      b. Realize that people with some cultural backgrounds consider placement in a nursing home to be unacceptable and that other resources must be explored.
      c. Explore cultural norms and influences with the family and client.
   3. Helping to select a facility
      a. Know the options available in the community.
      b. Obtain information through industry organizations such as the American Health Care Association.
      c. Access facilities' survey histories from the Centers for Medicare and Medicaid Services (formerly Health Care Financing Administration) or from state health departments.
   4. Assisting family members with placement decisions
      a. Provide the family with viable options and lists of community resources.
      b. Use mutual goal-setting techniques.
      c. Consult with the client's case manager or social worker for specific information on area facilities.
      d. Refer the family to information checklists available in the facility or through agencies such as the American Association of Retired Persons or the United Way.

H. Funding: Public programs for long-term care needs:
   1. See Chapter 4 for discussion of funding and insurance.

2. Medicare Parts A and B (Beam & O'Hare, 2003):
   a. A social insurance program for people age 65 and over and certain younger people with disabilities.
   b. Part A:
      1) Hospital insurance
      2) Funds hospital care, skilled nursing facility, hospice, and home health care
   c. Part B:
      1) Medical insurance
      2) Fees for physicians, surgeons, other healthcare providers
      3) Medical equipment rental
      4) Medical procedures, labs, diagnostics, X-rays, radiations, certain screenings
      5) Monthly premium is paid.
   d. Medicare does not provide for custodial care unless skilled nursing or rehabilitation is also needed.

3. Medicare Part D (Medicare, 2006):
   a. Available for anyone with Medicare.
   b. Income does not matter.
   c. A prescription drug plan through the federal government.
   d. Private companies issue plans through Medicare.
   e. Many different plans in each state.
   f. Many different categories from which plans must offer at least two prescription drugs in each category, but plans do not cover all drugs.
   g. Nurses can educate older adults to choose the best plan for them.
   h. A monthly premium is paid for the drug plan.
   i. Most plans have an annual deductible before Medicare pays.
   j. Costs to the person range from paying 100% out of pocket for those with low annual drug costs to 5% for those with high costs (e.g., more than $5,100, although this varies by plan).
   k. Financial assistance is available for those with low income; this is called "extra help."
   l. There is no cost containment for these drugs.

4. Medicaid (Beam & O'Hare, 2003). Medicaid laws change frequently, so these are general guidelines:
   a. State run program
   b. Largest source of medical care payments for low-income people
   c. Largest payer for nursing home services.
   d. About 30 states offer optional personal care services for people to remain in the home.
   e. Individual income must be less than a designated dollar amount to qualify.
   f. Applicants must pass an asset limitation test (i.e., assets must be spent down).

5. Veteran's Benefits (Beam & O'Hare, 2003):
   a. A potential source of long-term care benefits from a government source.
   b. Veterans who satisfy a means test that looks at income and assets may be eligible.
   c. Care is generally provided in Veterans Administration facilities.
   d. Basic health benefits of the Veterans Administration:
      1) Prevention and screenings
      2) Primary health care
      3) Diagnosis and treatment
      4) Surgery
      5) Mental health and substance abuse treatment
      6) Urgent care
      7) Medications
      8) Hospice and palliative care
      9) Limited other services such as certain nursing homes and adult day care in some programs

6. Long-term care insurance:
   a. For cost coverage outside a hospital.
   b. May cover any or all of the following services (Beam & O'Hare, 2003):
      1) Nursing home
      2) Assisted living
      3) Hospice
      4) Home health
      5) Adult day care
      6) Respite
      7) Caregiver training
      8) Home health coordinators
   c. Premiums (at age 65) range from $1,000 to $2,650/year.
   d. Premiums increase with age.
   e. Benefits include peace of mind, more choices, preservation of assets (Mauk & Mauk, 2006).
   f. Nurses should always ask whether patients have this type of coverage.

VII. Role of the Advanced Practice Nurse (APN)

A. Clinician:
1. According to the American Nurses Credentialing Center (ANCC, 2005), gerontological clinical nurse specialists:
   a. Provide, direct, and influence care of older adults and their families
   b. Work in a variety of settings
   c. Have in-depth knowledge of aging
   d. Have intervention skills focused on health promotion and management of health alterations
   e. Provide comprehensive gerontological services
   f. Engage in practice, research, theory use, collaboration, consultation, and administration
2. Gerontological nurse practitioners (ANCC, 2005):
   a. Are experts in healthcare provision to older adults
   b. Work in a variety of settings, particularly primary care
   c. Practice independently and collaboratively with other healthcare professionals
   d. Maximize patients' functional abilities
   e. Promote, maintain, and restore health
   f. Prevent or minimize disabilities
   g. Promote death with dignity
   h. Engage in case management, education, consultation, research, administration, and advocacy for older adults

B. Educator: The APN in the educator role may work in a variety of settings related to gerontological rehabilitation nursing.
1. Settings
   a. Rehabilitation unit in acute care hospital
   b. Freestanding rehabilitation facility
   c. Primary care practice in collaboration with physicians
   d. Outpatient clinic
   e. Academic setting or joint appointment collaborative agreement
   f. Private practice as consultant or seminar leader
2. Target audience
   a. Patients and families
   b. Interdisciplinary staff
   c. Physicians or other APNs
   d. Rehabilitation nurses
      1) Locally
      2) Regionally or nationally as an educational consultant
   e. Nursing students or other students in an academic setting

C. Leader:
1. As a leader, the gerontological rehabilitation nurse may be involved in a variety of organizations relating to both specialties or in organizations dedicated to the advancement of the nursing profession through research:
   a. Association of Rehabilitation Nurses
   b. American Gerontological Society (interdisciplinary)
   c. Association for Geriatrics in Higher Education (interdisciplinary)
   d. National Gerontological Nursing Association
   e. John A. Hartford Institute for Geriatric Nursing (devoted to education of nurses in excellent care of older adults)
   f. Sigma Theta Tau (international nursing honor society)
2. As a leader, the gerontological rehabilitation nurse in an advanced practice role may engage in the following activities:
   a. Membership in interdisciplinary care teams
   b. Developing standards of care for the specialty and professions
   c. Developing clinical guidelines
   d. Writing and advocating for certain healthcare policies
   e. Educating and mentoring colleagues in gerontological rehabilitation nursing
   f. Participating in research related to gerontological rehabilitation
   g. Membership in professional organizations

D. Consultant:
1. Legal
   a. Expert opinion
   b. Expert testimony or expert witness
   c. Type of cases may commonly include the following:
      1) Elder abuse or neglect
      2) Wrongful death
      3) Malpractice
      4) Other cases related to practice below the appropriate standard of care
   d. Employment as a regular part of a law office

---

2. Educational
   a. Through rehabilitation facilities giving presentations in various locations
   b. Self-employed
   c. Working for others to develop online courses for continuing education, academic credit, or instructional materials for purchase
3. Clinical
   a. May be combined with other types of consulting, including legal and educational
   b. The expert clinician may be highly sought after as an educator in a variety of settings.
   c. May develop subspecialty in other areas such as wound care or incontinence related to older adults with disabilities
4. Other
   a. Life care planning
   b. Advocacy
   c. Guardianship

E. Researcher:
   1. Evidence-based practice related to APNs in palliative care or hospice:
      a. Current trends suggest that APNs may play a significant role in the delivery of palliative care services to people at the end of life.
      b. Educational programs for APNs should incorporate components of palliative and hospice care.
      c. APNs caring for the dying patient and his or her family should have a broad knowledge base related to the dying process and strategies to provide comfort to patients and families.
   2. Clinical question: Is there a special role for APNs in care of patients receiving palliative care at end of life?
   3. Appraisal of evidence:
      a. One level I article with good evidence (Skilbeck & Payne, 2003)
      b. National guidelines: level I with good evidence (Clinical Practice Guidelines for Quality Palliative Care, 2004). Although the practice guidelines are not specific to APNs, there is a strong recommendation to have an interdisciplinary team of advanced clinicians.
      c. One level IV article with good evidence (Froggatt & Hoult, 2002)
      d. Two level VI articles with good evidence (Volker, Kahn, & Penticuff, 2004a, 2004b)
      e. Three level VII sources in textbooks and article with good evidence (Matzo & Sherman, 2001; Ferrell & Coyle, 2001; Pitorak, 2003)
   4. Recommendation for best rehabilitation nursing practice:
      a. The evidence generally demonstrates good support for APNs to play a significant role in palliative care at the end of life.
      b. The evidence suggests that there are educational and direct care deficits in some settings for palliative or end-of-life care, including residential care and nursing homes, that can be directly addressed through APN interventions.
      c. APNs can be instrumental in establishing links to health systems and resources.
      d. APNs can provide a unique level of emotional support to patients and families through their expertise and effective communication skills.
      e. APNs use advanced clinical skills to assess dying patients, provide comfort, and communicate essential information to the family.
      f. More research is needed to explore strategies used by APNs to provide high-quality care to those at the end of life.
   5. As researcher, the APN may also participate in the following activities:
      a. Clinical expert on an interdisciplinary team
      b. Link to clinical setting for collaborative research with academics.
      c. Advocate for using evidence-based practice in long-term care and rehabilitation facilities.
      d. For those prepared at the doctoral level:
         1) Design and conduct original research.
         2) Contribute to the development of nursing theory in gerontological rehabilitation.
         3) Obtain funding for research in the field.
         4) Publish findings to be used by others.
         5) Disseminate findings through presentations at conferences.

References

American Heart Association. (2004). *Statistical fact sheet: Populations*. Retrieved November 3, 2006, from: http://www.americanheart.org/downloadable/heart/1136584495498OlderAm06.pdf

American Heart Association/American Stroke Association. (2006). *Heart disease and stroke: 2006 update*. Dallas, TX: American Heart Association.

American Nurses Credentialing Center. (2005). *Gerontological nurse: Application for ANCC*. Retrieved November 11, 2006, from http://www.nursingworld.org/ancc

American Society of Consultant Pharmacists. (2000). Senior care pharmacy: The statistics. *Consultant Pharmacist, 15,* 310.

Anxiety Disorders Association of America (ADAA). (2006). *Anxiety in the elderly*. Retrieved November 9, 2006, from http://www.adaa.org/GettingHelp/AnxietyDisorders/Elderly.asp

Aptaker, R.L., Roth, E.J., Reichhardt, G., Duerden, M.E., & Levy, C.E. (1994). Serum albumin level as a predictor of geriatric stroke rehabilitation outcome. *Archives of Physical Medicine and Rehabilitation, 75*(1), 80–84.

Bagg, S., Pombo, A.P., & Hopman, W. (2002). Effect of age on functional outcomes after stroke rehabilitation. *Stroke, 33,* 179–185.

Baltes, P.B. (1987). Theoretical propositions of life-span developmental psychology: On the dynamics between growth and decline. *Developmental Psychology, 23,* 611–626.

Baltes, P. B., & Baltes, M.M. (1990). Psychological perspectives on successful aging: The model of selective optimization with compensation. In P.B. Baltes & M.M. Baltes (Eds.), *Successful aging: Perspectives from the behavioral sciences* (pp. 1–34). New York: Cambridge University Press.

Bandeen-Roche, K., Xue, Q.-L., Ferrucci, L., Walston, J., Guralnik, J.M., Chaves, P., et al. (2006). Phenotype of frailty: Characterization in the Women's Health and Aging Studies. *The Journals of Gerontology Series A: Biological Sciences and Medical Sciences, 61,* 262–266.

Beam, B.T., & O'Hare, T.P. (2003). *Meeting the financial need of long-term care*. Bryn Mawr, PA: The American College.

Beaupre, L.A., Cinats, J.G., Senthilselvan, A., Scharfenberger, A., Johnston, D.W., & Saunders, L.D. (2005). Does standardized rehabilitation and discharge planning improve functional recovery in elderly patients with hip fracture? *Archives of Physical Medicine and Rehabilitation, 86,* 2231–2239.

Beers, M. & Berkow, R. (Eds.). (n. d.). *The Merck Manual of Geriatrics*, internet edition. Merck & Company, Inc. and Medical Services USMEDSA, USHH. Retrieved January 20, 2005, from http://www.merck.com/mrkshared/mm_geriatrics/home.jsp

Brager, R., & Sloand, E. (2005). The spectrum of polypharmacy. *The Nurse Practitioner, 30,* 44–50.

Brown, R., Taylor, J., & Matthews, B. (2001). Quality of life: Ageing and Down syndrome. *Down Syndrome Research and Practices, 6*(3), 111–116.

Bruno, R.L., Cohen, J.M., Galski, T., & Frick, N.M. (n.d.). *The neuroanatomy of post-polio fatigue*. Retrieved October 28, 2006, from http://www.ott.zynet.co.uk/polio/lincolnshire/library.html

Buhler, C. (1933). *Der menschliche Lebenslauf als psychologisches Problem* [Human life as a psychological problem]. Oxford, England: Hirzel.

Butcher, H.K., & McGonigal-Kenney, M. (2005). Depression and dispiritedness in later life. *American Journal of Nursing, 105*(12), 52–61.

Byock, I. (1997). *Dying well*. New York: Free Press.

Centers for Disease Control (CDC). (2003). Public health and aging: Non-fatal fall-related traumatic brain injury among older adults: California 1996–1999. *MMWR Weekly, 52,* 276–278.

Centers for Disease Control (CDC). (2006a). *Falls and hip fractures among older adults*. Retrieved November 3, 2006, from http://www.cdc.gov/ncipc/factsheets/falls.htm

Centers for Disease Control (CDC). (2006b). MMWR quick guide. Recommended adult immunization schedule: United States—October 2006–September 2007. *MMWR, 55*(40), 1–4.

Charles, C.V., & Lehman, C.A. (2006). Medications and laboratory values. In K. Mauk (Ed.), *Gerontological nursing: Competencies for care* (pp. 293–320). Sudbury, MA: Jones and Bartlett.

Chen, H. (2006). *Down syndrome*. Retrieved November 6, 2006, from http://www.emedicine.com/ped/topic615.htm

Clinical practice guidelines for quality palliative care. (2004). Brooklyn, NY: National Consensus Project for Quality Palliative Care.

Colantonio, A., Ratcliff, G., Chase, S., & Vernich, L. (2004). Aging with traumatic brain injury: Long-term health conditions. *International Journal of Rehabilitation Research, 27*(3), 209–214.

Cowley, J., Diebold, C., Gross, J.C., & Hardin-Fanning, F. (2006). Management of common problems. In K. Mauk (Ed.), *Gerontological nursing: Competencies for care* (pp. 475–560). Sudbury, MA: Jones and Bartlett.

Cumming, E., & Henry, W. (1961). *Growing old*. New York: Basic Books.

DeCalmer, P., & Glendenning, F. (Eds.). (1993). *The mistreatment of the elderly people*. London: Sage.

DeVivo, M.J. (2004). Aging with a neurodisability: Morbidity and life expectancy issues. *NeuroRehabilitation, 19,* 1–2.

Digiovanna, A. G. (2000). *Human aging: Biological perspectives* (3rd Ed.). Boston: McGraw-Hill.

Duppils, G. & Wikblad, K. (2004). Cognitive function and health related quality of life after delirium. *Orthopedic Nursing, 23,* 195–203.

Easton, K.L. (1999). *Gerontological rehabilitation nursing*. Philadelphia: W.B. Saunders.

Ellenbecker, C.H., Frazier, S.C., & Verney, S. (2004). Nurses' observations and experiences of problems and adverse effects of medication management in home care. *Geriatric Nursing, 25*(3), 164–170.

End of Life Nursing Education Consortium (ELNEC). (2004). *ELNEC curriculum*. Robert Woods Johnson Foundation and City of Hope.

Ferrari, A., Radaelli, A., & Centola, M. (2003). Invited review: Aging and the cardiovascular system. *Journal of Applied Physiology, 95*(6), 2591-2597.

Ferrell, B.R., & Coyle, N. (2001). *Textbook of palliative nursing*. New York: Oxford University Press.

Finlayson, M., Van Denend, T., & Hudson, E. (2004). Aging with multiple sclerosis. *Journal of Neuroscience Nursing, 26,* 245–248.

Fowles, D.G. (1994). *A profile of older Americans*. Washington, DC: American Association of Retired Persons and Administration on Aging, U.S. Department of Health and Human Services.

Fried, L.P., Ferrucci, L., Darer, J., Williamson, J.D., & Anderson, G. (2004). Untangling the concepts of disability, frailty, and comorbidity: Implications for improved targeting and care. *The Journals of Gerontology. Series A, Biological Sciences and Medical Sciences, 59A,* 255–263.

Froggatt, K.A., & Hoult, L. (2002). Developing palliative care practice in nursing and residential care homes: The role of the clinical nurse specialist. *Journal of Clinical Nursing, 11,* 802–808.

Geronurseonline.org. (2005a). *Function*. Retrieved November 3, 2006, from http://www.geronurseonline.org/index.cfm?section_id=41&geriatric_topic_id=21&sub_section_id=163&page_id=288&tab=2

Geronurseonline.org. (2005b). *Hydration management*. Retrieved November 3, 2006, from http://www.geronurseonline.org/index.cfm?section_id=39&sub_section_id=110&geriatric_topic_id=19&page_id=267&tab=2

Geronurseonline.org. (2005c). *Medication*. Retrieved November 3, 2006, from http://www.geronurseonline.org/index.cfm?section_id=25&geriatric_topic_id=5&sub_section_id=37&page_id=59&tab=2

Geronurseonline.org. (2005d). *Urinary incontinence*. Retrieved November 3, 2006, from http://www.geronurseonline.org/index.cfm?section_id=28&geriatric_topic_id=8&sub_section_id=46&page_id=89&tab=2

Harlow, R.E., & Cantor, N. (1996). Still participating after all these years: A study of life task participation in later life. *Journal of Personality and Social Psychology, 71,* 1235-1249.

Havighurst, R.J., Neugarent, B.L., & Tobin, S.S. (1968). Disengagement and patterns of aging. In B. L. Neugarten (Ed.), *Middle age and aging*, pp. 67–71. Chicago: University Press.

Havighurst, R.J., Neugarent, B.L., & Tobin, S.S. (1963). Disengagement, personality and life satisfaction in the later years. In P. Hansen (Ed.), *Age with a future*, pp. 419–425. Copenhagen: Munksgoasrd.

Holland, T., & Benton, M. (2004). *Ageing and its consequences for people with Down's syndrome: A guide for parents and carers.* Retrieved November 6, 2006, from http://www.downs-syndrome.org.uk/pdfs/ageing%20&%20consequences.pdf

Inouye, S.K., Foreman, M.D., Mion, L.C., Katz, K.H., & Cooney, L.M. (2001). Nurses' recognition of delirium and its symptoms: Comparison of nurse and researcher ratings. *Archives of Internal Medicine, 161*(20), 2467–2473.

Institute of Medicine. (2000). Overview: Nutritional health in the older person. In *The role of nutrition in maintaining health in the nation's elderly: Evaluating coverage of nutrition services for the Medicare population.* Retrieved November 6, 2006, from http://fermat.nap.edu/books/0309068460/html/46.html

Ivey, F., Tracy, B., Lemmer, J., NessAiver, M., Metter, E., Fozard, J., et al. (2000). Effects of strength training and detraining on muscle quality: Age and gender comparisons. *Journals of Gerontology: Biological Sciences, 55A*(3), B152–B157.

Jackson, G., & Owsley, C. (2003). Visual dysfunction, neurodegenerative diseases, and aging. *Neurology Clinics of North America, 21,* 709–728.

Jung, C. G. (1960). *The structure and dynamics of the psyche. Collected works.* (Vol. VIII). Oxford, England: Pantheon.

Kailes, J.I. (2002). *Aging with disability.* Retrieved November 7, 2006, from http://www.jik.com/awdrtcawd.html

Kart, G.S., & Kinney, J.M. (2001). *The realities of aging.* Boston: Allyn & Bacon.

Kemp, B.J., & Mosqueda, L. (2004). Introduction. In *Aging with a disability: What the clinician needs to know.* Baltimore: Johns Hopkins University Press.

Klingbiel, H., Baer, H.R., & Wilson. P.E. (2004). Aging with a disability. *Archives of Physical Medicine and Rehabilitation, 85*(93), S68–S73.

Krauss Whitbourne, S. (2002). *The aging individual: Physical and psychological perspectives* (2nd ed.). New York: Springer.

Krieger-Blake, L.S. (2006). Changes that affect independence in later life. In K. Mauk (Ed.), *Gerontological nursing: Competencies for care* (pp. 321–354). Sudbury, MA: Jones and Bartlett.

Lange, J., & Grossman, S. (2006). Theories of aging. In K. L. Mauk's (Ed.) *Gerontological Nursing: Competencies for Care,* pp. 57 – 84. Sudbury, MA: Jones and Bartlett Publishers.

Lemon, B.W., Bengston, V.L., & Peterson, J.A. (1972). An exploration of the activity theory of aging: Activity types and life satisfaction among in-movers to a retirement community. *Journal of Gerontology, 27,* 511-523.

Marrone, R. (1997). *Death, mourning & caring.* Philadelphia: Wadsworth.

Maslow, A.H. (1954). *Motivation and personality.* New York: Harper & Row.

Mast, B.T., MacNeill, S.E., & Lichtenberg, P.A. (1999). Geropsychological problems in medical rehabilitation: Dementia and depression among stroke and lower extremity fracture patients. *The Journals of Gerontology: Biological Sciences and Medical Sciences, 54,* M607–M612.

Matzo, M.L., & Sherman, D.W. (2001). *Palliative care nursing: Quality care to the end of life.* New York: Springer.

Mauk, J.M., & Mauk, K.L. (2006). Future trends in gerontological nursing. In K. Mauk (Ed.), *Gerontological nursing: Competencies for care* (pp. 815–828). Sudbury, MA: Jones and Bartlett.

McKinnis, E.A. (2002). Dyspnea and other respiratory symptoms. In B.M. Kingbrunner, J.J. Weinreb, & J.S. Pliczer (Eds.), *Twenty common problems in end-of-life care* (pp. 147–162). New York: McGraw-Hill.

Medicare. (2006). *Medicare prescription drug coverage.* Retrieved November 7, 2006, from http://www.medicare.gov/pdp-basic-information.asp

Mendes De Leon, C.F., Gold, D.T., Glass, T.A., Kaplan, L., & George, L.K. (2001). Disability as a function of social networks and support in elderly African Americans and whites. *The Journals of Gerontology: Psychological Sciences and Social Sciences, 56,* S179–S190.

Menter, R. (1998). *Aging with spinal cord injury.* Retrieved November 7, 2006, from http://www.thecni.org/reviews/09-1-p16-menter.htm

Merck Manuals Online Medical Library. (2003). *Aging body.* Retrieved November 6, 2006, from http://www.merck.com/mmhe/sec01/ch003/ch003a.html

Meyer, C. (2001). *Allow natural death: An alternative to DNR?* Retrieved November 4, 2005, from http://www.hospicepatients.org/and.html

Minaker, K. (2004). Common clinical sequelae of aging. In L. Goldman & D. Ausiello (Eds.), *Cecil Textbook of Medicine,* (22nd ed.). Philadelphia: W.B. Saunders. Retrieved January 10, 2005, http://home.mdconsult.com/das/book/45511299-2/view/1231

Munnell, A.H. (2004). Population aging: It's not just the baby boom. An issue in brief. *Center for Retirement Research at Boston College, 16,* 1–7.

My Health Directive. (2006). *Five wishes and storage.* Retrieved November 7, 2006, from http://www.myhealthdirective.com/page_server/FiveWishes/Five%20Wishes.html

National Center on Elder Abuse. (2006). *Elder abuse prevalence and incidence. Fact sheet.* Washington, DC: Author.

National Hospice and Palliative Care Organization. (2004). *Keys to quality care.* Retrieved November 4, 2005, from http://www.nhpco.org

National Institute of Mental Health (NIMH). (2006). *Depression and suicide facts.* Retrieved November 9, 2006, from http://www.nimh.nih.gov/publicat/elderlydepsuicide.cfm

National Institutes of Neurological Disorders and Stroke (NINDS). (2006a). *Cerebral palsy: Hope through research.* Retrieved November 6, 2006, from http://www.ninds.nih.gov/disorders/cerebral_palsy/detail_cerebral_palsy.htm

National Institutes of Neurological Disorders and Stroke (NINDS). (2006b). *Post-polio syndrome fact sheet.* Retrieved November 6, 2006, from http://www.ninds.nih.gov/disorders/post_polio/detail_post_polio.htm

Nelson, J.M. (2006). Identifying and preventing common risk factors in the elderly. In K. Mauk (Ed.), *Gerontological nursing: Competencies for care* (pp. 357–388). Sudbury, MA: Jones and Bartlett.

Nilsson-Ehle, H., Jagenburg, R., Landahl, S., & Svanborg, A. (2000). Blood haemoglobin declines in the elderly: Implications for reference intervals from age 70 to 88. *European Journal of Haematology, 65*(5), 297–305.

Ostwald, S., Wasserman, J., & Davis, S. (2006). Medications, comorbidities and complications in stroke survivors: The CAReS study. *Rehabilitation Nursing, 31,* 10–14.

Patrick, L., Knoefel, F., Gaskowsk, P., & Rexrath, D. (2001). Medical comorbidity and rehabilitation efficiency in geriatric patients. *Journal of the American Geriatrics Society, 49,* 1471–1477.

Peters, A. (2002). The effects of normal aging on myelin and nerve fibers: A review. *Journal of Neurocytology, 31,* 581–593.

Pitorak, E.F. (2003). Care at the time of death. *American Journal of Nursing, 103*(7), 42–52.

Plahuta, J.M., & Hamrick-King, J. (2006). Review of the aging of physiological systems. In K. Mauk (Ed.), *Gerontological nursing: Competencies for care* (pp. 143–264). Sudbury, MA: Jones and Bartlett.

Pritchard, J. (1995). *The abuse of older people: A training manual for detection and prevention.* London: Jessica Kingsley Publishers.

Pritchard, J. (1996). Darkness visible: Elder abuse. *Nursing Times, 92*(42), 26–31.

Pugh, K., & Wei, J. (2001). Clinical implications of physiological changes in the aging heart. *Drugs & Aging, 18*(4), 263–276.

Rees, T., Duckert, L., & Carey, J. (1999). Auditory and vestibular dysfunction. In W. Hazzard, J. Blass, W. Ettinger Jr., J. Halter, & J. Ouslander (Eds.), *Principles of geriatric medicine and gerontology* (4th ed., pp. 617–632). New York: McGraw-Hill.

Rockwood, K., Mitniski, A., Song, X., Steen, B., & Skoog, I. (2006). Long-term risks of death and institutionalization of elderly people in relation to deficit accumulation at age 70. *Journal of the American Geriatrics Society, 54,* 975–979.

Roubenoff, R. (2001). Origins and clinical relevance of sarcopenia. *Canadian Journal of Applied Physiology, 26*(1), 78–89.

Schroots, J. J. F. (1996). Theoretical developments in the psychology of aging. *Gerontologist, 36,* 742-748.

Scivoletto, G., Morganti, B., Ditunno, P., Ditunno, J.F., & Molinari, M. (2003). Effects of age on spinal cord lesion patients' rehabilitation. *Spinal Cord, 41,* 457–464.

Segatore, M., & Adams, D. (2001). Managing dilirium and agitation in elderly hospitalized orthopaedic patients: Part 1: Theoretical aspects. *Orthopaedic Nursing, 20* 31–46.

Seiberling, K. & Conley, D. (2004). Aging and olfactory and taste function. *Otolaryngologic Clinics of North America, 37*(6), 1209-1228.

Skilbeck, J., & Payne, S. (2003). Emotional support and the role of clinical nurse specialists in palliative care. *Journal of Advanced Nursing, 43*(5), 521–530.

Strauss, D., Ojdana, K., Shavelle, R., & Rosenbloom, L. (2004). Decline in function and life expectancy of older persons with cerebral palsy. *Neurorehabilitation, 19,* 69–78.

Thompson, H.J., McCormick, W.C., & Kagan, S.H. (2006). Traumatic brain in jury in older adults: Epidemiology, outcomes and future implications. *Journal of the American Geriatrics Society, 54,* 1590–1595.

Tinetti, M.E., Williams, C.S., & Gill, T.M. (2000). Dizziness among older adults: A possible geriatric syndrome. *Annals of Internal Medicine, 132,* 337–344.

Tornstam, L. (1994). Gerotranscendence: A theoretical and empirical exploration. In L.E. Thomas & S.A. Eisenhandler (Eds.), *Aging and the religious dimension* (pp. 203-226). Westport, CT: Greenwood.

U.S. Department of Health and Human Services. (2006). *Caregiver stress.* Retrieved November 9, 2006, from http://www.womenshealth.gov/faq/caregiver.htm

Vaillant, G. (2002). *Aging well.* Boston: Little, Brown.

Volker, D.L., Kahn, D., & Penticuff, J.H. (2004a). Patient control and end-of-life care Part I: The advanced practice nurse perspective. *Oncology Nursing Forum, 31*(5), 945–953.

Volker, D.L., Kahn, D., & Penticuff, J.H. (2004b). Patient control and end-of-life care Part II: The patient perspective. *Oncology Nursing Forum, 31*(5), 954–960.

Wadensten, B., & Carlsson, M. (2001). A qualitative study of nursing staff members' interpretations of signs of gerotranscendence. *Journal of Advanced Nursing, 36,* 635–642.

Warring, P.A., & Krieger-Blake, L.S. (2006). End-of-life care. In K. Mauk (Ed.), *Gerontological nursing: Competencies for care* (pp. 779–814). Sudbury, MA: Jones and Bartlett.

Winkler, T. (2006). *Spinal cord injury and aging.* Retrieved November 7, 2006, from http://www.emedicine.com/pmr/topic185.htm

World Health Organization (WHO). (1990). *Cancer pain relief and palliative care.* Geneva: World Health Organization.

Yu, F. (2005). Factors affecting outpatient rehabilitation outcomes in elders. *Journal of Nursing Scholarship.* Retrieved November 1, 2006, from www.blackwellpublishing.com/journals/jns.

Section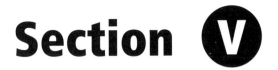

The Delivery and Evaluation of Rehabilitation Services

. . . .

Environment of Care and Service Delivery

Patricia A. Quigley, PhD MPH ARNP CRRN FAAN

Scientific and technological advances, the aging population, duration and quality of life, and cost-conscious healthcare systems have influenced the delivery of rehabilitation services, the environments in which rehabilitation services are provided, and the role of rehabilitation nurses in all healthcare settings. Additionally, models of care delivery have been redesigned to maximize continuity and coordination of client care in settings with diminishing lengths of stay and changes in skill mix. The delivery and evaluation of rehabilitation services warrant oversight by expert rehabilitation nurses who serve as client advocates to maximize client care services without jeopardizing quality of outcomes and client safety throughout the continuum of care.

This chapter compares rehabilitation environments throughout the continuum of care and demonstrates how the nursing and rehabilitation process is applied and integrated in the delivery of rehabilitation services. Rehabilitation nurses must become familiar with ethical principles, decision-making models, and alternatives to deal with the many challenges of healthcare reorganization and service redesign.

Rehabilitation should be practiced in all healthcare settings. Rehabilitation nursing should be an integral component of care delivery. The role of the rehabilitation nurse is to ensure that basic and advanced rehabilitation techniques are performed and that specialized rehabilitation care is provided in the appropriate setting based on the client's medical stability and tolerance for rehabilitation efforts.

I. Practice and Settings in Which Rehabilitation Occurs

A. Models of Nursing Care Practice and Delivery

1. Primary care nursing:
   a. One nurse is responsible for the total care of a client during the shift of care.
      1) Ensures that the client and other providers know who is accountable for the specific client's care
      2) Provides 24-hour accountability for the client's care
   b. For successful primary nursing, extensive communication and collaboration are needed with all members of the healthcare team, client, and family (Lyon, 1993).

2. Primary nurse for a shift of care:
   a. Financial constraints, the decreased availability of nurses, and the shift of acute nursing care to outpatient care settings (so that length of stay on medical and surgical units is less than 72 hours) have caused many acute care settings to adopt this model.
   b. One nurse is assigned as a primary nurse for a client for the shift rather than for the client's length of stay.

3. Case managers:
   a. Background
      1) Although case management has been practiced since the early 1900s, nurses have only recently accepted responsibility for this role (Case Management Society of America [CMSA], 2002).
      2) Case management is one of the most recent care delivery models for nurses to embrace (Beaty, 2005; McBride, 1992).
      3) This model of care delivery is comprehensive and client centered and allows continuous care across the continuum.
      4) Optimizes acute rehabilitation services (Carr, 2005)
   b. Roles of nurse case managers
      1) Licensed healthcare professionals providing patient assessment, treatment planning, healthcare facilitation, and patient advocacy according to the industry's standards (CMSA, http://www.cmsa.org)
      2) Coordinate care and service delivery, improve continuity of care, and monitor outcomes

3) Function as client advocates
4) Direct, coordinate, and supervise care
5) Improve financial outcomes and use continuous quality improvement and utilization review (Beaty, 2005; Johnson & Schubring, 1999; Tahan & Huber, 2006)
6) Rehabilitation includes case management (Haussler, 2006).

4. Nurse liaisons evaluate clients and help them gain access to services for the next level of medical care (e.g., at freestanding rehabilitation facilities).

5. Minimum Data Set (MDS) coordinators:
   a. Initiate and instruct the care team in completing MDS assessment forms and Resource Utilization Group codes
   b. Serve as a resource for team members about the prospective payment system (PPS) process in subacute and long-term care settings

6. Advanced practice nurses (e.g., clinical nurse specialists, advanced registered nurse practitioners):
   a. Provide clinical leadership and expertise as direct and indirect care providers
   b. Coordinate care and discharge planning rounds (Halm et al., 2003)

B. Aspects of Rehabilitation Nursing Care
   1. Prevent medical and functional complications (e.g., positioning, passive range of motion) and readmission
   2. Maintain function by engaging clients to participate in care (e.g., eating, bathing, dressing) within medically indicated restrictions and precautions
   3. Promote independence by engaging clients in increasing self-care actions and monitoring progress toward goal achievement
   4. Delegate and supervise aspects of rehabilitation and restorative care provided by licensed practical nurses, technicians, and unlicensed assistive personnel

C. Documentation: centers on medical management
   1. System review: Assess and manage physiological systems.
   2. System outcomes: Stabilize physiological status.
   3. Critical or clinical pathways: Use process standards as adjuncts to a client's plan of care that define when and by whom critical care interventions must be done.

D. Client and Family Education
   1. Medical management
   2. Self-care management
   3. Exercise and health promotion

E. Discharge Planning: focuses on the transition to the most appropriate level of care (Birmingham, 2004, p. 12)

F. Critical Care and Acute Care
   1. Description: Intensive medical and surgical care settings in hospitals; 25% of rehabilitation nurses practice in acute care facilities.
   2. Critical care:
      a. Clients are critically ill, with life-threatening illnesses or conditions.
         1) 1:1 or 1:2 nurse/client staffing ratio is appropriate.
         2) Clients need physiological assessment more frequently than every 4 hours.
      b. Clients cannot tolerate intensive rehabilitation.
      c. Care focuses on preventing complications to promote patient's ability to later participate in rehabilitation.
   3. Acute care: Clients need medical management by physicians or advanced practice nurses.
      a. Medically stable: Medical management is secondary to or concurrent with rehabilitation needs.
         1) Clients need ongoing medical management.
         2) Clients need 24-hour nursing care, 7 days per week.
      b. Ability to tolerate intensive rehabilitation:
         1) Clients need 1–3 hours of therapy per day.
         2) Clients need rehabilitation nursing and care.
   4. Settings:
      a. Episodic care settings (in hospitals and acute rehabilitation units) for acute illness
      b. Acute rehabilitation settings (the traditional setting for rehabilitation care)
      c. Rehabilitation units in general hospitals
      d. Freestanding rehabilitation centers
      e. Comprehensive integrated inpatient rehabilitation programs: "coordinated and integrated medical and rehabilitation service that is provided 24 hours per day and endorses the active participation and choice of the persons served throughout

the entire program" (Rehabilitation Accreditation Commission [CARF], 2006)

5. Models of nursing care delivery:
   a. Team nursing: task-oriented client care delivery
   b. Modified primary nursing: uses a primary nurse (RN) and associate nurses (RNs or licensed practice nurses)
   c. Interdisciplinary team care
      1) Team members share accountability to meet client and family rehabilitation needs.
      2) Shared goals cross discipline-specific boundaries.
      3) "Characterized by a variety of disciplines that participate in the assessment, planning, and/or implementation of a person's program: There must be close interactions and integration among the disciplines so that all members of the team interact to achieve team goals" (CARF, 1998, p. 310).
   d. Transdisciplinary team care: boundary-free plans of care that focus on client and family goals

6. Aspects of rehabilitation nursing care:
   a. Prevent complications
   b. Restore abilities
   c. Initiate rehabilitation services as soon as appropriate

7. Documentation:
   a. Some systems choose to focus on clinical pathways, combining aspects of critical pathways to focus on client needs or problems. Outcomes are achieved according to predetermined goals at predetermined intervals (Haley, 1995).
   b. Clinical pathways address the client's individualized needs and plan of care through teamwork by various team members.

8. Client and family education provides outcome-directed teaching and learning.

9. Discharge planning:
   a. "A major challenge faced today by nurses is the increased complexity of patients' discharge needs caused by decreased length of stay in the hospital" (Closson, Mattingly, Finne, & Larson, 1994, p. 287).
   b. The period immediately after rehabilitation is the most critical to clients; many gains may be lost within the first 3 months of discharge from an acute

rehabilitation program (Mor, Granger, & Sherwood, 1983), and discharge planning facilitates continued services (Lee, 2006).
   c. Interdisciplinary rounds facilitate successful discharge planning for patients and families (Halm et al., 2003).
   d. Follow-up interventions can help improve clients' functional outcomes and reduce healthcare use after discharge from rehabilitation.
      1) Deterioration was found to be related to the client's or caregiver's failure to understand or sustain the rehabilitation program (Moskowitz, Lightbody, & Frietag, 1972).
      2) Frequent follow-up after discharge (e.g., by telephone) may reduce healthcare use and improve functional outcomes (Evans et al., 1990).

G. Subacute and Postacute Care
   1. Descriptions:
      a. "Subacute care is a comprehensive, cost-effective inpatient level of care for patients who: have had an acute event resulting from injury, illness or exacerbation of a disease process; have a determined course of treatment; though stable, require diagnostics or invasive procedures, but not intensive procedures requiring an acute level of care" (National Association of Subacute/Post Acute Care [NASPAC], 2005, p. 1).
      b. A service area available since the mid-1980s for people who are not quite ready for intensive, acute rehabilitation therapy or need additional time transitioning to the community
      c. A care option that serves as an alternative to an acute care hospital admission or as an alternative to continued hospitalization. The client receives less acute nursing care and less intense rehabilitation (CARF, 1998) than in a freestanding or hospital-based setting.
      d. Uniform Data System for Medical Rehabilitation (UDSMR) data show that patients receiving care in subacute rehabilitation programs show measurable functional improvement and that a high percentage of patients are discharged to community-based settings (Deutsch, Fiedler, Iwanenko, Granger, & Russell, 2003).
      e. "Post-Acute Care (PAC) is a program introduced to improve the transition from hospital to the community. Post-Acute

Care facilities provide services to patients needing additional support to assist them to recuperate following discharge from an acute hospital" (NASPAC, 2005, p. 1).

2. Severity of clients' medical stability: varied acuity levels and problems:
   a. Medically complex but stable (e.g., cardiovascular clients with congestive heart failure, clients with septicemia or osteomyelitis):
      1) Need skilled nursing care
      2) Need medical monitoring and specialized care
      3) Need assistance with activities of daily living
   b. Medically unable to tolerate an intensive rehabilitation program (e.g., clients recovering from surgery, oncology clients, wound care clients):
      1) Need less than 1 hour of therapy daily
      2) Need at least 3 hours of therapy weekly
   c. Clients needing respiratory care:
      1) Need ventilator care or weaning
      2) Need nursing care
   d. Clients recuperating from surgery:
      1) Need skilled nursing care
      2) Need rehabilitation services
   e. Clients with chronic wounds need skilled nursing care.

3. Models of nursing care delivery:
   a. Team nursing: One RN is the designated team leader for staff members who provide care to a group of clients (this model was created to advance nursing care in functional nursing models).
   b. Functional nursing: Client care is divided by tasks.
   c. Case management: 1:1 care usually is provided by a live-in nurse (this form of nursing care was practiced in the early 20th century).
   d. Multidisciplinary team care: Discipline-specific care is directed to client needs but not integrated across disciplines or services; boundaries and turf issues exist between disciplines.

4. Aspects of rehabilitation nursing care:
   a. Prevent complications
   b. Maintain functional status and capabilities
   c. Restore self-care skills in functional activities of daily living

5. Client and family education provides outcome-directed teaching and learning.

H. Long-Term Care
   1. Description:
      a. Long-term acute care:
         1) Postacute hospital settings with an average length of stay of 25 days, according to the National Association of Long Term Hospitals, combining services for clients in need of intensive medical and extended skilled nursing care and rehabilitation and respiratory management.
         2) Highly specialized centers of care: Some acute rehabilitation facilities are licensed as long-term acute care facilities.
      b. Long-term care:
         1) Posthospital centers for clients who need extended skilled nursing care and attendant care because they are unable to live alone.
         2) Inpatient settings may provide long-term rehabilitation for clients with chronic disability:
            a) Skilled nursing facilities
            b) Residential facilities
            c) Transitional living centers
      c. Person-centered long-term care communities (PCLTCCs, or nursing homes): Person-centered long-term care communities (PCLTCCs) foster a culture that supports autonomy, diversity, and individual choice. Leadership, along with the community, cultivates relationships among residents, families/support systems, and personnel. In PCLTCCs, residents are the experts regarding life in their home. Residents participate in deciding about the rhythm of their day, the services provided to them, and the issues that are important to them in their home. Their families/support systems are welcomed. In partnership with residents and their families/support systems, personnel understand what services residents want, how the services should be delivered, and how they can help in their home (CARF, 2006).

   2. Severity of clients' medical stability:
      a. Medically stable clients have low potential for medical instability.
      b. Clients cannot tolerate intensive rehabilitation programs but have regular, direct individual contact with

rehabilitation physicians as determined by medical and rehabilitation needs.

c. Clients need routine rehabilitation nursing and have a low risk of needing high–medical acuity skilled nursing.

d. Clients receive a minimum of 1 hour of services 5 days per week from interdisciplinary team members.

e. Clients receive client and family education and training opportunities on an ongoing basis (CARF, 1998).

3. Models of nursing care delivery:

a. Functional nursing:
1) Nursing care is divided by labor (i.e., assembly-line nursing); this model dates back to the 1920s.
2) The division of labor determines the technical aspects of the job to be performed.
3) Each job is broken down to its simplest component to increase attention on quantity, not quality.
4) Nurses' aides provide care.

b. Partners in care: Cross-trained staff, which often includes teams of professional licensed nurses and technical support personnel, assist with specific tasks.

c. Nurses Improving Care to Health System Elders promotes innovative care across care settings in a comprehensive program that hospitals use to foster system-wide improvements in the care of older patients (Mezey et al., 2004).

4. Documentation:

a. Minimum Data Set–Post Acute Care (MDS-PAC) assessment:
1) Medicare's payment system for medical rehabilitation facilities, which took effect October 1, 2000, includes standard assessment data and disability and outcome data.
2) The MDS-PAC assessment will include as much of the Functional Independence Measure (FIM™) instrument as possible.

b. Clinical pathways:
1) Monitor client outcomes at predetermined intervals to provide a framework for interdisciplinary team members to plan, monitor, revise, and evaluate client responses to care throughout the rehabilitation process
2) Determine trend variances in outcomes for clinical cohorts (Quigley, Smith, & Strugar, 1998)

c. Nursing Intervention Classification (Moorehead, McCloskey, & Bulechek, 1993) and Nursing Outcomes Classification systems:
1) Designed to standardize nursing intervention and outcome terms and link them with the North American Nursing Diagnosis Association classification for nursing diagnoses
2) Contain 6 domains (physiological [basic], physiological [complex], behavioral, safety, family, health system), 26 classes, and more than 400 interventions that are also compatible with International Classification of Diseases codes and Diagnosis-Related Group classification systems
3) Have been tested for use in long-term care settings
4) Have a comprehensive coding structure for all nursing practice (Iowa Intervention Project, 1995)

d. Omaha Classification System (Martin & Scheet, 1992):
1) Serves as a guide for nursing practice and nursing documentation in home health care and nurse-managed care centers
2) Has three components
a) Problem Classification Scheme, which contains 44 actual or potential nursing diagnoses that affect the client or family
b) Problem Rating Scale for Outcomes, which was designed by community health nurses to help them systematically measure client changes and responses
c) The Intervention Scheme, which delineates four categories of interventions: health teaching, guidance, and counseling; treatments and procedures; case management; and surveillance

e. Outcome and Assessment Information Set (OASIS):
1) A standardized patient assessment instrument for adult home care patients that was developed by a research partnership between the federal government, the Robert Wood Johnson Foundation, and the home health industry over a 10-year period.
2) The goal was to develop an assessment and outcome dataset that would

provide the basis for outcome-based quality improvement in home health.

3) All home healthcare agencies that are reimbursed by the Medicare or Medicaid programs are required to participate in the OASIS data system, develop an outcome-based quality improvement system based on the OASIS data, and electronically submit their standardized data and assessment reports to their state system (Pentz & Wilson, 2001; State and Territory Injury Prevention Directors Association, 2006).

f. FIM™ instrument measures client outcomes in terms of functional status gains from admission to discharge throughout the continuum of care and is developed and updated by the UDSMR.

5. Client and family education promotes self-care actions to prevent complications, maintain functional status, and increase functional gains.

I. Community-Based Care

1. Description:

a. Care is based in the communities in which people with rehabilitation needs manage their care and daily activities independently, with assistance, or with supervision.

b. Clients and family members work as partners with healthcare providers to attain mutually established goals (Hoeman, 1996).

c. Rehabilitation is provided in community or residential settings.

d. According to CARF (1998, p. 296), when a residence is provided by the organization, it is "designed, constructed, furnished, and maintained in ways similar to others in the neighborhood consistent with the needs and preferences of the person served."

2. Types of community-based care:

a. Day treatment care or programs and adult day services provide supervised care and therapeutic recreational activities: A community-based group program designed to meet the needs of adults with impairments through individual plans of care. This type of structured, comprehensive, nonresidential program provides a variety of health, social, and related support services in a protective setting. By supporting families and caregivers, an adult day services program enables the persons served to live in the community. An adult day services program assesses the needs of the persons served and offers services to meet those needs. The persons served attend on a planned basis. The environment of care of an adult day services program is designed to maximize the functional levels of the persons served. Such a program encourages relationships and creates a culture that supports, involves, and validates the persons served. The environmental design considers the impairments and limitations of the persons served, promotes improvement and maintenance of their physical and mental health, supports their sense of control and self-determination, and provides them with a safe environment (CARF, 2006).

b. Independent living centers and congregate living facilities provide daily supervision and skilled nursing care.

c. Community reentry programs and assisted care living facilities [provide] coordinated, personalized 24-hour assistance and support (both scheduled and unscheduled) in a congregate residential setting. The choices, privacy, independence, and rights of the persons served are proactively protected and promoted as an essential part of assisted living's core values and mission. The assisted living environment is designed to enhance the functional levels of the persons served. Assisted living encourages, supports, involves, and validates the decision making of the persons served. The environmental design:
- Considers the abilities and limitations of persons served.
- Promotes improvement and maintenance of their physical health.
- Supports their sense of dignity, privacy, control, and self-determination.
- Facilitates family and community interaction.
- Provides persons served with a safe and accessible environment. (CARF, 2006)

d. Rural outreach programs

e. Home care and home healthcare services: Neal (1999) reported the results of a study examining the congruence between rehabilitation principles and home health nursing practice. Data from 30 home health nurses suggested congruence between rehabilitation and home health nursing principles (Neal-Boylan, 2006).

    f. Hospice services

    g. Nursing centers (e.g., Pine Street Inn, Boston): healthcare clinics run by nurses

    h. Outpatient clinics

    i. Senior citizen centers

    j. Continuing care retirement community: In recent years, many attractive options for retirement living have emerged. One popular option is the continuing care retirement community, or CCRC. This type of community is different from other housing and care options for older people because it offers a long-term contract that provides for housing, services and nursing care, usually all in one location. At the same time, CCRCs offer some distinct advantages, including physical and financial security, independence and access to health care, companionship of friends and neighbors of similar age and access to community facilities and privacy. The CCRC's emphasis on the individual, coupled with a supportive environment, allows you to continue to pursue your lifelong interests (CARF, 2006).

  3. Documentation:

    a. Home Healthcare Classification

      1) Generated from a study funded by the Health Care Financing Administration (now Centers for Medicare and Medicaid Services) to develop a method to assess and classify home health Medicare clients, predict resource needs, and measure outcomes (Bowles & Naylor, 1996)

      2) Bases cohort models on four types of provider visits for 30 days or for the episode of care (30–120 days or more)

      3) Includes measures of socioeconomic and functional status, medical diagnosis, surgical procedures, and nursing components of diagnoses, interventions, and discharge status (Saba, 1992)

    b. HomeFIM^SM instrument

      1) Designed to measure the functional status of people receiving home care rehabilitation services

      2) Provides documentation of functional gains for insurance effectiveness and efficiency for third-party payers

      3) Offers the critical link in the continuum of care between the comprehensive inpatient rehabilitation program, outpatient care, and home health services (Kedron, 1998)

  4. Client and family education provides information about continuous life planning.

II. Care Delivery Across the Lifespan

  A. Young Children

    1. Heery (1992) described pediatric rehabilitation as the process of restoring childhood.

    2. Interactions between parent and child are critical.

  B. Adolescents

    1. Critical development needs include independence, socialization, and sexuality education.

    2. The major focus is on helping the adolescent with a disability to adapt to educational settings.

  C. Adults

    1. Programs focus on the client's unique social, psychological, and vocational needs.

    2. Healthcare professionals should consider how working partners affect the care of family members.

  D. Older Adults

    1. Because of the increasing age of the population and the increasing number of older adults with disabilities, rehabilitation nurses must focus on this population.

    2. Healthcare professionals should consider how long-distance care affects the family.

  E. Old-Old Adults (over 85 years of age)

    1. This is the fastest-growing age group in the United States.

    2. Fall-related deaths are the primary cause of death.

III. Continuum of Care: Longitudinal Outcomes and Documentation

  A. Overview

    1. Clients, families, and other providers (e.g., visiting nurses associations) participate in mutual goal setting and monitoring goal achievement.

    2. Outcomes are setting-oriented and cumulative throughout the continuum of care.

    3. Long-term outcomes can be achieved only

after short-term, integrated outcomes are met.

    4. Outcomes must be monitored in relation to expected outcomes within a time frame and across settings.

    5. Family meetings are critical to reaching consensus about future hospitalizations, planning for healthcare needs, and insurance coverage.

B. Association of Rehabilitation Nurses (ARN) Standards

    1. Rehabilitation nurses provide services designed to prevent complications of physical disability, restore optimal functioning, and help the client adapt to an altered lifestyle (ARN, 1994).

    2. Rehabilitation nursing is practiced in rehabilitation settings, defined as any environment in which nurse–patient interactions are grounded in the philosophy and concepts of rehabilitation nursing practice (ARN, 1994).

C. Documentation

    1. Each environment of care has specific requirements for documentation defined by standards of nursing care and practice, accreditation bodies, third-party payers, and regulatory and institutional policies.

    2. Rehabilitation nurses must develop or select a standardized language for use with computerized, integrated team documentation systems that link to all points on the continuum of care (Cervizzi & Edwards, 1999).

    3. Documentation systems must promote high-quality, cost-effective client care, customer satisfaction, and outcomes.

D. Client and Family Education

    1. Educate families about 24-hour responsibilities and care needs

    2. Discuss issues of coordination of services and increased responsibility of care providers

    3. Provide access to support groups

E. Discharge Planning

    1. "Discharge preparation: Hospital-based activities to anticipate a safe, smooth transition from that setting" (Steele & Sterling, 1992, p. 80)

    2. "Discharge readiness: A multifaceted, multistaged concept that provides an estimate of a client's ability to leave an acute care facility" (Steele & Sterling, 1992, p. 80)

    3. Rehabilitation team meetings include the client and family and enable all participants to reach consensus about the ongoing needs and plans for rehabilitation throughout the continuum of care and a method to evaluate the effectiveness of that care.

IV. Changes in Health Care

A. In the Healthcare Environment

    1. Managed care and Medicare PPSs are affecting care delivery and client access to rehabilitation services.

    2. Rehabilitation services are moving to specialty centers, home care, and outpatient care.

B. In the Roles of Rehabilitation Nurses

    1. Managed care and Medicare PPSs rely on rehabilitation nurses' leadership as client advocates and care managers.

    2. Rehabilitation nurses must ensure that clients receive timely, high-quality, comprehensive, cost-effective care with appropriate providers in the appropriate setting.

    3. Rehabilitation nurses must practice within and across a variety of settings as case managers and clinical practitioners.

References

Association of Rehabilitation Nurses (ARN). (1994). *Standards and scope of rehabilitation nursing practice* (3rd ed.). Glenview, IL: Author.

Beaty, L. (2005). A primer for understanding diagnosis-related groups and inpatient hospital reimbursement with nursing implications. *Critical Care Nursing Quarterly, 28*(4), 360–369.

Birmingham, J. (2004). *Discharge planning guide: Tools for compliance.* Marblehead, MA: HCPro.

Bowles, K., & Naylor, M. (1996). Nursing intervention classification systems. *Image: The Journal of Nursing Scholarship, 28*(4), 303–308.

Carr, D.D. (2005). The case manager's role in optimizing acute rehabilitation services. *Lippincott's Case Management, 10*(4), 190–200.

Case Management Society of America (CMSA). (2002). *Standards of practice for case management, revised 2002.* Little Rock, AR: Author.

Cervizzi, K., & Edwards, P. (1999). Where is rehabilitation nursing documentation going? *Rehabilitation Nursing, 24*(3), 92.

Closson, B., Mattingly, L., Finne, K., & Larson, J. (1994). Telephone follow-up program evaluation: Application of Orem's self-care model. *Rehabilitation Nursing, 19*(5), 287–292.

Commission on Accreditation of Rehabilitation Facilities. (2006). Retrieved May 12, 2007 from www.carf.org.

Deutsch, A., Fiedler, R.C., Iwanenko, W., Granger, C.V., & Russell, C.F. (2003). The uniform data system for medical rehabilitation report: Patients discharged from subacute rehabilitation programs in 1999. *American Journal of Physical Medicine & Rehabilitation, 82*(9), 703–711.

Evans, R., Hendricks, R., Bishop, D., Lawrence-Umlau, D., Kirk, C., & Halar, E. (1990). Prospective payment for rehabilitation: Effects on hospital readmission, home care, and placement. *Archives of Physical Medicine and Rehabilitation, 71*, 291–294.

Haley, J.A. (1995). *Clinical pathways for in-patient rehabilitation programs.* Tampa, FL: Author.

Halm, M.A., Gagner, S., Goering, M., Sabo, J., Smith, M., & Zaccagnini, M. (2003). Interdisciplinary rounds: Impact on patients, families, and staff. *Clinical Nurse Specialist, 17*(3), 133–142.

Haussler, P. (2006, March–April). CDMS, CCM, ABDA rehabilitation as a model for case management. *Lippincott's Case Management, 11*(2), 115–117.

Heery, K. (1992). Restoring childhood through rehabilitation. *Rehabilitation Nursing, 17,* 193–195.

Hoeman, S. (Ed.). (1996). *Rehabilitation nursing: Process and application* (2nd ed.). St. Louis: Mosby.

Iowa Intervention Project. (1995). Validation and coding of the NIC taxonomy structure. IMAGE: The *Journal of Nursing Scholarship, 27*(1), 43–49.

Johnson, K., & Schubring, L. (1999). The evolution of a hospital based decentralized case management model. *Nursing Economics, 17*(1), 29–48.

Kedron, M. (1998). Introducing HomeFIM™ instrument. *The FIM™ SystemSM Update, 2*(3), 1.

Lee, J. (2006). An imperative to improve discharge planning: Predictors of physical function among residents of a Medicare skilled nursing facility. *Nursing Administration Quarterly: Ethics/Integrity and Trust, 30*(1), 38–47.

Lyon, J.C. (1993). Models of nursing care delivery and case management: Clarification of terms. *Nursing Economics, 11,* 163–169.

Martin, K., & Scheet, N. (1992). The Omaha system: *Application for community health nursing.* Philadelphia: W.B. Saunders.

McBride, S.M. (1992). Rehabilitation case managers: Ahead of their time. *Holistic Nursing Practice, 6,* 67–75.

Mezey, M., Kobayashi, M., Grossman, S., Firpo, A., Fulmer, T., & Mitty, E. (2004). Nurses Improving Care to Health System Elders (NICHE): Implementation of best practice models. *Journal of Nursing Administration, 34*(10), 451–457.

Moorehead, S., McCloskey, J., & Bulechek, G. (1993). Nursing Intervention Classifications: A comparison with the Omaha and the Home Healthcare Classification. *Journal of Nursing Administration, 23*(10), 23–29.

Mor, V., Granger, C., & Sherwood, C. (1983). Discharged rehabilitation patients: Impact of follow-up surveillance by a friendly visitor. *Archives of Physical Medicine and Rehabilitation, 64,* 346–353.

Moskowitz, E., Lightbody, F., & Frietag, N. (1972). Long-term follow-up of poststroke patients. *Archives of Physical Medicine and Rehabilitation, 59,* 167–172.

National Association of Subacute/Post Acute Care (NASPAC). (2005). FAQ. Retrieved May 7, 2007, from http://www.naspac.net/faq.asp

Neal, L. (1999). Research supporting the congruence between rehabilitation principles and home health nursing practice. *Rehabilitation Nursing, 24*(3), 115–121.

Neal-Boylan, L. (2006). The rehabilitation nurse specialist in home care. *Home Healthcare Nurse, 24*(7), 457–458.

Pentz, C., & Wilson, A. (2001). Ensuring the quality of OASIS data: One agency's plan. *Home Healthcare Nurse, 19*(1), 38–42.

Quigley, P., Smith, S., & Strugar, J. (1998). Successful experiences with clinical pathways in rehabilitation. *Journal of Rehabilitation, 64*(2), 29–32.

Rehabilitation Accreditation Commission (CARF). (1998). *Standards manual and interpretive guidelines for medical rehabilitation.* Tucson, AZ: Author. Retrieved October 19, 2006, from http://www.carf.org/Providers.aspx?content=content/Accreditation/Opportunities/AS/What.htm#Comprehensive

Saba, V. (1992). Home health care classification. *Caring, 11*(5), 58–60.

State and Territory Injury Prevention Directors Association (STIPDA). (2006). *Consensus recommendations for surveillance of falls and fall-related injuries.* Report of the Injury Surveillance Workgroup on Falls, ISW4.

Steele, N., & Sterling, Y. (1992). Application of the case study design: Nursing interventions for discharge readiness. *Clinical Nurse Specialist, 6*(2), 80–84.

Tahan, H., & Huber, D. (2006). The CCMC's national study of case manager job descriptions: An understanding of the activities, role relationships, knowledges, skills, and abilities. *Lippincott's Case Management, 11*(3), 127–144.

Suggested Resources

Bower, K. (1995). Case management designed for the care continuum. In K. Zander (Ed.), Managing outcomes through collaborative care: *The application of care mapping and case management* (pp. 20, 167). Chicago: American Hospital Publishing.

Clinton, B. (1992). The Clinton health care plan. *New England Journal of Medicine, 327*(11), 804–806.

Crummer, M., & Carter, V. (1993). Clinical pathways: The pivotal tool. *Journal of Cardiovascular Nursing, 7,* 30–37.

Erkel, E. (1993). The impact of case management in preventative services. *Journal of Nursing Administration, 23*(1), 27–32.

Hampton, D. (1993). Implementing a managed care framework through care maps. *Journal of Nursing Administration, 23,* 21–27.

Tahan, H. (1993). The nurse case manager in acute care settings: Job description and function. *Journal of Nursing Administration, 23*(10), 53–61.

Wood, R., Bailey, N., & Tilkemeier, D. (1992). Managed care, the missing link in quality improvement. *Journal of Nursing Care Quality, 6,* 55–65.

Chapter 19

Outcome Measurement and Performance Improvement

Terrie Black, MBA BSN RN BC CRRN

Accountability and validation of value have become essential components of the healthcare delivery process. Today, outcomes of care are emphasized as never before (Black, 1999). Outcomes focus on the effectiveness of care or the results of services delivered by a clinician or team of clinicians. Monitoring outcomes can help do the following:

- Track efficiency and effectiveness
- Identify trends
- Facilitate communication between the patient, family, treatment team, payers, referral source, and other stakeholders
- Assess follow-up measures to determine whether progress is continuing after discharge
- Identify areas for improvement
- Measure access to programs

Internal stakeholders interested in outcomes may include a rehabilitation program's case managers, administrator, board of directors, clinicians, and parties such as researchers and quality improvement practitioners who are interested in outcome data. Externally, stakeholders who often evaluate programs and services using outcome data include case managers, payers, referral sources, and direct consumers of healthcare services.

Outcomes can be benchmarked according to past trends within an organization or corporation, against national and regional standards or norms, and against best practice standards. Corporations can identify outcomes and use various sites or regions as bases for comparison. Rehabilitation outcomes can be measured and monitored to market an individual program or organization, meet accreditation standards, and identify areas for performance improvement (Wilkerson, 1997b). Data can also be used to improve rehabilitation nursing care and as the basis for outcome research. This chapter examines outcomes of care in rehabilitation, describes the tools used by rehabilitation clinicians to collect information about outcomes, and profiles the agencies that accredit rehabilitation programs.

I. Overview

A. Primary Accreditation Agencies for Rehabilitation Providers

1. The Joint Commission (JC), formerly the Joint Commission on Accreditation of Healthcare Organizations (JCAHO)

2. The Commission on Accreditation of Rehabilitation Facilities (CARF)

B. Benefits of Accreditation

1. Assists with the business, management, and quality strategies that organizations should have in place to meet consumer needs and maintain operations

2. Demonstrates to stakeholders that certain standards have been met, systems are in place to deliver high-quality services, results are as expected based on norms, and processes thought to be of expert consensus are followed

3. Assures consumers that an independent review process focuses on improving the quality of services

4. Provides organizations with a template for efficient and effective operations

5. Establishes a common level of program expectations and performance

6. Focuses on meeting the needs of people with disabilities and others who need rehabilitation

7. Offers a mechanism for purchasers, providers, and consumers to interact

8. Identifies organizations or programs that have met standards and reinforces and supports those organizations

9. Affects reimbursement (CARF, 1998)

II. Accrediting Agencies

A. The JC:

1. General:

   a. Mission: to continuously improve the safety and quality of care provided to the public through the provision of healthcare accreditation and related services that support performance improvement in healthcare organizations (JC, 2006).

   b. "Compliance": JC's term for referring to standards

   c. Organizational structure: governed by the Board of Commissioners

2. Historical perspective:

   a. 1910: Dr. Ernest Codman proposed a system of hospital standardization in which hospitals track every patient to determine whether treatment is effective.

   b. 1918: The American College of Surgeons began on-site inspections of hospitals.

   c. 1926: The first 18-page standard manual was published.

   d. 1950: More than 3,200 hospitals achieved approval under the new program; as a result, the standard of care gradually improved.

   e. 1951: The American College of Physicians, the American Hospital Association, the American Medical Association, and the Canadian Medical Association joined to create the Joint Commission on Accreditation of Hospitals, whose primary purpose was to provide voluntary accreditation.

   f. 1964: The Joint Commission on Accreditation of Hospitals began charging for surveys.

   g. 1966: Long-term care accreditation began.

   h. 1970: Nurses joined physicians in conducting surveys.

   i. 1982: The first public member began serving on the JCAHO Board of Commissioners.

   j. 1988: Accreditation for home care organizations began.

   k. 1989: Accreditation for managed care began.

   l. 1993:

      1) The number and nature of Type 1 recommendations against an organization became public information.

      2) JCAHO began making random, unannounced surveys of accredited organizations.

   m. 1996: The Home Care Accreditation Program became JCAHO's largest accreditation program based on number of accredited organizations.

   n. 1997:

      1) The ORYX initiative was launched to integrate outcomes and other performance measures into the accreditation process.

      2) JCAHO established cooperative agreements with CARF for freestanding rehabilitation hospitals and rehabilitation units in hospitals.

   o. 1998: JCAHO announced its intent to begin offering international accreditation services.

   p. 2002: Accredited hospitals began collecting data on standardized, or core, performance measures.

   q. 2004: The JC launched its new accreditation process, Shared Visions–New Pathways, on January 1.

3. Accreditation process:

   a. An organization submits an application to the JC.

   b. The survey date is given to the organization.

   c. An initial conference with the organization's leaders is held on the first day of the survey to finalize the survey schedule.

   d. The survey includes a tour of the facility, reviews of medical records and documentation, observation of staff, and interviews with patients and staff.

   e. The major focus is on direct input from care providers, with the surveyors providing education while measuring compliance with standards.

4. Accreditation decisions or outcomes:

   a. Accreditation with commendation

   b. Accreditation without Type I recommendations

   c. Accreditation with Type I recommendations

   d. Provisional accreditation

   e. Conditional accreditation

   f. Preliminary nonaccreditation

   g. Nonaccreditation

5. The ORYX initiative:

   a. Introduced in 1997

   b. Designed to help organizations strengthen their quality improvement efforts and to identify issues that warrant attention

c. Uses data from organizations to monitor performance between on-site survey visits

d. Supports the JC's mission and is a critical link between accreditation and patient care outcomes

e. Affects various rehabilitation settings, including hospitals, rehabilitation, long-term care, and home care (Dobrzykowski, 1997)

6. Benefits of JC accreditation and certification:

a. Strengthens community confidence in the quality and safety of care, treatment, and services

b. Provides a competitive edge in the marketplace

c. Improves risk management and risk reduction

d. Helps organize and strengthen patient safety effort

e. Provides education on good practices to improve business operations

f. Provides professional advice and counsel, thereby enhancing staff education

g. Enhances staff recruitment and development

h. Provides deeming authority for Medicare certification

i. Recognized by insurers and other third parties

j. May reduce liability insurance costs (JC, 2006)

7. Tracer methodology: Tracer methodology is an evaluation method in which surveyors select a patient, resident, or client and use that person's record as a roadmap to move through an organization to assess and evaluate the organization's compliance with selected standards and the organization's systems of providing care and services.

8. Unannounced surveys: The JC conducts unannounced surveys:

a. To help healthcare organizations focus on providing safe, high-quality care at all times, not just when preparing for survey

b. To affirm the expectation of continuous standards compliance both by the JC of its accredited organizations and by these organizations of themselves

c. To increase the credibility of the accreditation process by ensuring that surveyors observe organization performance under normal circumstances

d. To reduce the unnecessary costs healthcare organizations incur to prepare for surveys

e. To address public concerns that the JC receives an accurate impression of the quality and safety of care

9. Sentinel events: In support of its mission to continuously improve the safety and quality of health care provided to the public, the JC reviews organizations' activities in response to sentinel events in its accreditation process. A sentinel event is an unexpected occurrence involving death or serious physical or psychological injury or the risk thereof. Such events are called "sentinel" because they signal the need for immediate investigation and response.

B. CARF:

1. General

a. Mission: to promote the quality, value, and optimal outcomes of services through a consultative accreditation process that centers on enhancing the lives of the people served (CARF, 1998)

b. "Conformance": CARF's term referring to standards

c. Organizational structure

1) Six divisions

a) Medical Rehabilitation: accredits programs such as comprehensive integrated inpatient rehabilitation, brain injury, spinal cord injury systems of care, pain programs, outpatient, health enhancement, occupational rehabilitation, case management, and home- and community-based rehabilitation programs

b) Behavioral Health: accredits providers of behavioral health programs (e.g., alcohol and drugs, mental health, psychosocial rehabilitation, integrated behavioral health)

c) Employment and Community Services: accredits organizations that provide employment services, community services, and psychosocial rehabilitation programs

d) Aging Services: accredits programs that provide services to older adults and other adults in residential or community-based group settings

e) Child and Youth Services: accredits programs that provide child welfare, protection, and well-being services to children, youths, and their families

f) Opioid Treatment: accredits programs that provide rehabilitation and medical support for people addicted to opioid drugs

2) Board of Trustees: approves standards, awards accreditation, and oversees policies and financial matters (CARF, 1999)

2. Historical perspective

a. 1966: Founded as a nonprofit organization

b. 1973: Published a new program evaluation section of its standard manual for rehabilitation facilities

c. 1993: Accredited its first program in Canada

d. 1995: Enacted new standards for occupational rehabilitation and comprehensive pain management programs in the medical rehabilitation division

e. 1996: Accredited its first program in Sweden

f. 1997

1) Signed an agreement to accredit all Veterans Affairs rehabilitation programs over a 5-year period

2) Began to offer a combined survey process with JCAHO to freestanding rehabilitation hospitals

g. 1998: Rewrote standards to be unidimensional as a result of the Standards Conformance Rating Scale initiative.

h. 1998: Accredited medical rehabilitation programs that are part of a larger entity, are recognized by JCAHO, and do not have to undergo JCAHO surveys for larger organizations

i. 1999: Published standards for adult day services

j. 2000: Published standards for assisted living programs

k. 2001: Recognized by Substance Abuse & Mental Health Services Administration as an approved accrediting organization for opioid treatment programs

l. 2002: Incorporate CARF Canada

m. 2003: Acquired the Continuing Care Accreditation Commission

n. 2005: Published the *Child and Youth Standards Manual* and accredited its first program in South America

o. 2006: Published *Aging Services Standards Manual and Stroke Specialty Programs Standards*

3. Development and creation of standards

a. National Advisory Committees (NACs): Each year, NACs are formed to review existing standards and create new standards. This is usually the starting point in the development of new standards. In years when there are no NACs, CARF solicits informal feedback from surveyors, consumers, other purchasers, and interested stakeholders.

b. Field review: Proposed standards are sent to the rehabilitation field for review by national professional groups, third-party purchasers, consumers, surveyors, and advocacy groups. Feedback, suggestions, and requests are evaluated by CARF.

c. Vote by Board of Trustees: New or revised standards are approved by the board before they go into effect (CARF, 1999).

4. Accreditation process

a. Contact CARF office to verify which standard manual to use. Each standard manual year runs from July 1 to June 30.

b. Perform a self-study. A facility may opt to complete a self-study and evaluation before and in preparation for the survey. CARF publishes numerous resources to help organizations in this process.

c. Submit application at least 3 months before requested survey.

d. Schedule the survey date. Surveyors are selected based on their expertise and knowledge of the programs being surveyed. Generally, there is an administrative surveyor and at least 1 program surveyor for medical rehabilitation programs.

e. Have an orientation conference. This is done the first day of the survey to allow surveyors to give an overview of the survey process and the organization to describe itself to the survey team.

f. Have an exit conference. This provides immediate feedback to the organization about strengths, areas for improvement, suggestions, and any recommendations made by the survey team.

g. Surveyors' report is edited by CARF and sent to the Board of Trustees for accreditation decision.

h. Survey report with accreditation outcome is sent to the organization.

i. Organization submits a quality improvement plan that addresses any recommendations in the survey report.

j. Submit an annual conformance to quality report (CARF, 2006).

5. Key terminology related to CARF's survey process

a. Standard conformance rating scale:

1) 0 = Nonconformance: The program does not even partially conform to a standard.

2) 1 = Partial Conformance: The program or service has achieved some components of a standard or made progress toward conformance yet does not meet expectations for full conformance.

3) 2 = Conformance: The program or service fully meets the intent of a standard.

4) 3 = Exemplary Conformance: The program or service significantly exceeds the level of practice necessary to achieve conformance to a standard.

b. Consultation: Suggestions from the survey team for improving services in the organization based on experience in the rehabilitation field. Suggestions are not linked to conformance to the standards in that an organization is not required to implement or act on them (CARF, 2006).

6. Accreditation decisions, ultimately made by the Board of Trustees

a. 3-Year Accreditation: Demonstrates substantial conformance to the standards.

b. 1-Year Accreditation: Indicates that the organization is basically meeting the standards, but there are some significant areas of deficiency.

c. Provisional Accreditation: Indicates that an organization received a 1-Year Accreditation on its immediately preceding survey, and although the organization is basically meeting the standards, there continue to be significant problem areas. Upon resurvey, an organization that has a Provisional Accreditation must achieve a 3-Year Accreditation or it will be nonaccredited.

d. Nonaccreditation: Major deficits exist

in meeting standards, and concerns exist about whether the organization meets the needs of the people it serves.

e. Preliminary Accreditation is awarded to allow new programs to establish demonstrated use and implementation of the standards (CARF, 2006).

C. JC/CARF Integrated Survey: Integrated surveys apply only to the medical rehabilitation division.

1. Minimal integration: involves 2 survey teams, 2 standard manuals, 2 survey processes, 2 outcome decisions, and 1 survey timeframe

2. Moderate integration: began in February 1999 and involves 2 survey teams, 2 manuals, 2 outcome decisions, 1 survey process, and 1 survey timeframe

3. Full integration: anticipated to involve 1 survey process, 1 survey timeframe, 1 survey team, and 2 separate outcome decisions

D. National Council on Quality Assurance:

1. Oversees managed care companies

2. Uses the Health Employment Data Information Set as its dataset

III. Key Concepts in Rehabilitation

A. World Health Organization (2001) Model: International Classification of Functioning, Disability, and Health (ICF) is a classification of health and health-related domains that describe body functions and structures, activities, and participation. The domains are classified from body, individual, and societal perspectives. Because a person's functioning and disability occur in a context, ICF also includes a list of environmental factors.

B. Body Functions and Structures: An abnormality of body structure, appearance, and organ or system function resulting from any cause. Impairments occur at the organ level (e.g., dysphagia, hemiparesis)

C. Activities and Participation: The consequences of impairment in terms of a person's functional performance and activity; the nature and extent of function at the individual level. There may be activity disturbances at the level of the person (e.g., bathing, dressing, communication, walking, grooming). Participation: The disadvantages in work, family, and social roles experienced as a result of impairments; the nature and extent of a person's involvement in life and various activities. Participation reflects interaction with and adaptation to one's surroundings.

D. Environmental Factors: Barriers and facilitators

IV. Tools for Monitoring Rehabilitation Outcomes

A. Global Adult Scales (which measure motor, physical, and cognitive elements)

1. Functional Independence Measure (FIM™) instrument (see Figure 19-1)

   a. Looks at severity of disability and need for assistance (burden of care)

   b. Designed to promote a uniform language among the rehabilitation team and to describe the severity of disability

   c. Is included in the Uniform Data Set for Medical Rehabilitation (UDSMR), which includes demographic, diagnostic, financial, and functional information about rehabilitation patients. UDSMR maintains databases for acute rehabilitation, subacute and skilled nursing facilities, and long-term hospitals.

   d. Includes 18 items (13 motor, 5 cognitive)

   e. Involves a hierarchy of motor items that progress from eating (easiest) to using stairs (most difficult)

   f. Uses a 7-level scale in which 1 = *total assistance* (patient performs less than 25% of an activity) and 7 = *total independence* (patient performs an activity without an assistive device or a helper in a safe and timely manner)

   g. Is used internationally and considered to be the gold standard in assessing functional status

   h. Is easy to use by members of any discipline

   i. Provides the basis for predicting outcomes for various patient populations (Black, Soltis, & Bartlett, 1999)

   j. Is the foundation for establishing Function-Related Groups and Case Mix Groups (CMGs)

   k. Can be used to estimate the burden of care for activities of daily living (ADLs) (based on the FIM™ "Rule of Thumb Burden of Care" chart) (Deutsch, Braun, & Granger, 1997; UDSMR, 1996)

2. Inpatient Rehabilitation Facility Patient Assessment Instrument (see Figure 19-2)

   a. Is the data collection instrument for the Inpatient Rehabilitation Facility Prospective Payment System.

   b. Required by Centers for Medicare and Medicaid (CMS) to be completed for all Medicare Part A patients admitted to inpatient rehabilitation facilities

   c. Has the FIM™ instrument as a core component for rating patients (12 motor items, 5 cognitive items; tub and shower transfer is excluded in determining the CMG).

   d. Completed on admission and discharge; admission rating determines the CMG to which the patient is assigned.

   e. CMG then determines unadjusted federal prospective payment; additional facility adjusters include the wage index, rural vs. urban setting, and the low-income patient rate.

   f. Code 0 (*activity does not occur*) is used for admission only for items not occurring during the 3-day admission assessment timeframe.

3. Patient Evaluation and Conference System (see Figure 19-3)

   a. Comprehensive, lengthy interdisciplinary tool that examines 76 distinct functional areas

   b. Uses a 7-level scale in which 1 = *most dependent* and 7 = *independent*; 0 = a functional area that is not tested or unmeasurable

4. PULSES: Represents the initial letters of the categories it measures

   a. Physical condition

   b. Upper extremities

   c. Lower extremities

   d. Sensory components

   e. Excretory function

   f. Social and mental status

5. Functional Assessment Measure (Hall, 1997)

   a. Developed to serve as an adjunct to the FIM™ instrument to address some functional items that are essential to brain injury rehabilitation

   b. Measures 12 items, including cognitive, behavioral, communication, and community functioning

   c. Uses a 7-level scoring method similar to that of the FIM™ instrument

B. ADL Scales (which measure motor and physical elements) (Dittmar & Gresham, 1997) (see Figure 19-4)

1. Barthel Index:

   a. Uses a 0–100 scoring system (100 = *total independence*, 0 = *dependence*) that assesses 10 domains

   b. Is popular in European rehabilitation facilities

Figure 19-1. Functional Independence Measure (FIM™) Instrument

FIM™ Instrument

	7 Complete Independence (timely, safely) 6 Modified Independence (device)	**NO HELPER**
L E V E L S	**Modified Dependence** 5 Supervision (subject = 100%) 4 Minimal Assistance (subject = 75%+) 3 Moderate Assistance (subject = 50%+) **Complete Dependence** 2 Maximal Assistance (subject =25%+) 1 Total Assistance (subject = less than 25%)	**HELPER**

	ADMISSION	DISCHARGE	FOLLOW-UP
Self-Care A. Eating B. Grooming C. Bathing D. Dressing - Upper Body E. Dressing - Lower Body F. Toileting			
Sphincter Control G. Bladder Management H. Bowel Management			
Transfers I. Bed, Chair, Wheelchair J. Toilet K. Tub, Shower			
Locomotion L. Walk/Wheelchair M. Stairs	W Walk C Wheelchair B Both	W Walk C Wheelchair B Both	W Walk C Wheelchair B Both
Motor Subtotal Rating			
Communication N. Comprehension O. Expression	A Auditory V Visual B Both	A Auditory V Visual B Both	A Auditory V Visual B Both
Social Cognition P. Social Interaction Q. Problem Solving R. Memory			
Cognitive Subtotal Rating			
TOTAL FIM™ RATING			

NOTE: Leave no blanks. Enter 1 if patient is not testable due to risk.

Figure 19-2. Patient Assessment Instrument

DEPARTMENT OF HEALTH AND HUMAN SERVICES
CENTERS FOR MEDICARE & MEDICAID SERVICES

Form Approved
OMB No. 0938-0842

INPATIENT REHABILITATION FACILITY – PATIENT ASSESSMENT INSTRUMENT

Identification Information*

1. Facility Information
   A. Facility Name
   _____
   _____
   _____

   B. Facility Medicare
      Provider Number _____

2. Patient Medicare Number _____

3. Patient Medicaid Number _____

4. Patient First Name _____

5A. Patient Last Name _____

5B. Patient Identification Number _____

6. Birth Date _____/_____/_____
   MM / DD / YYYY

7. Social Security Number _____

8. Gender (1 - Male; 2 - Female)   _____

9. Race/Ethnicity (Check all that apply)
   American Indian or Alaska Native   A. _____
   Asian   B. _____
   Black or African American   C. _____
   Hispanic or Latino   D. _____
   Native Hawaiian or Other Pacific Islander   E. _____
   White   F. _____

10. Marital Status   _____
    (1 - Never Married; 2 - Married; 3 - Widowed;
    4 - Separated; 5 - Divorced)

11. Zip Code of Patient's Pre-Hospital Residence _____

Admission Information*

12. Admission Date _____/_____/_____
    MM / DD / YYYY

13. Assessment Reference Date _____/_____/_____
    MM / DD / YYYY

14. Admission Class   _____
    (1 - Initial Rehab; 2 - Evaluation; 3 - Readmission;
    4 - Unplanned Discharge; 5 - Continuing Rehabilitation)

15. Admit From   _____
    (01 - Home; 02 - Board & Care; 03 - Transitional Living;
    04 - Intermediate Care; 05 - Skilled Nursing Facility;
    06 - Acute Unit of Own Facility; 07 - Acute Unit of Another
    Facility; 08 - Chronic Hospital; 09 - Rehabilitation Facility;
    10 - Other; 12 - Alternate Level of Care Unit; 13 – Subacute
    Setting; 14 - Assisted Living Residence)

16. Pre-Hospital Living Setting   _____
    (Use codes from item 15 above)

17. Pre-Hospital Living With   _____
    (Code only if item 16 is 01 - Home;
    Code using 1 - Alone; 2 - Family/Relatives;
    3 - Friends; 4 - Attendant; 5 - Other)

18. Pre-Hospital Vocational Category   _____
    (1 - Employed; 2 - Sheltered; 3 - Student;
    4 - Homemaker; 5 - Not Working; 6 - Retired for
    Age; 7 - Retired for Disability)

19. Pre-Hospital Vocational Effort   _____
    (Code only if item 18 is coded 1 - 4; Code using
    1 - Full-time; 2 - Part-time; 3 - Adjusted Workload)

Payer Information*

20. Payment Source
    A. Primary Source   _____

    B. Secondary Source   _____

    (01 - Blue Cross; 02 - Medicare non-MCO;
    03 - Medicaid non-MCO; 04 - Commercial Insurance;
    05 - MCO HMO; 06 - Workers' Compensation;
    07 - Crippled Children's Services; 08 – Developmental
    Disabilities Services; 09 - State Vocational Rehabilitation;
    10 - Private Pay; 11 - Employee Courtesy;
    12 - Unreimbursed; 13 - CHAMPUS; 14 - Other;
    15 - None; 16 – No-Fault Auto Insurance;
    51 – Medicare MCO; 52 - Medicaid MCO)

Medical Information*

21. Impairment Group   _____   _____
                            Admission   Discharge
    Condition requiring admission to rehabilitation; code
    according to Appendix A, attached.

22. Etiologic Diagnosis   _____
    (Use an ICD-9-CM code to indicate the etiologic problem
    that led to the condition for which the patient is receiving
    rehabilitation)

23. Date of Onset of Impairment _____/_____/_____
                                MM / DD / YYYY

24. Comorbid Conditions; Use ICD-9-CM codes to enter up to
    ten medical conditions

    A. _____   B. _____

    C. _____   D. _____

    E. _____   F. _____

    G. _____   H. _____

    I. _____   J. _____

Medical Needs

25. Is patient comatose at admission?   _____
                                        0 - No, 1 - Yes

26. Is patient delirious at admission?   _____
                                        0 - No, 1 - Yes

27. Swallowing Status   _____   _____
                            Admission   Discharge

    3 - _Regular Food_: solids and liquids swallowed safely
        without supervision or modified food consistency
    2 - _Modified Food Consistency/ Supervision_: subject
        requires modified food consistency and/or needs
        supervision for safety
    1 - _Tube /Parenteral Feeding_: tube / parenteral feeding
        used wholly or partially as a means of sustenance

28. Clinical signs of dehydration   _____   _____
                                        Admission   Discharge

    (Code 0 – No; 1 – Yes) e.g., evidence of oliguria, dry
    skin, orthostatic hypotension, somnolence, agitation

*The FIM data set, measurement scale and impairment
codes incorporated or referenced herein are the property of
U B Foundation Activities, Inc. ©1993, 2001 U B Foundation
Activities, Inc. The FIM mark is owned by UBFA, Inc.

Figure 19-2. Patient Assessment Instrument *continued*

DEPARTMENT OF HEALTH AND HUMAN SERVICES
CENTERS FOR MEDICARE & MEDICAID SERVICES

INPATIENT REHABILITATION FACILITY – PATIENT ASSESSMENT INSTRUMENT

Function Modifiers*

Complete the following specific functional items prior to scoring the FIM™ Instrument:

		ADMISSION	DISCHARGE
29.	Bladder Level of Assistance (Score using FIM Levels 1 - 7)	☐	☐
30.	Bladder Frequency of Accidents (Score as below)	☐	☐

    7 - No accidents
    6 - No accidents; uses device such as a catheter
    5 - One accident in the past 7 days
    4 - Two accidents in the past 7 days
    3 - Three accidents in the past 7 days
    2 - Four accidents in the past 7 days
    1 - Five or more accidents in the past 7 days

Enter in Item 39G (Bladder) the lower (more dependent) score from Items 29 and 30 above.

		ADMISSION	DISCHARGE
31.	Bowel Level of Assistance (Score using FIM Levels 1 - 7)	☐	☐
32.	Bowel Frequency of Accidents (Score as below)	☐	☐

    7 - No accidents
    6 - No accidents; uses device such as an ostomy
    5 - One accident in the past 7 days
    4 - Two accidents in the past 7 days
    3 - Three accidents in the past 7 days
    2 - Four accidents in the past 7 days
    1 - Five or more accidents in the past 7 days

Enter in Item 39H (Bowel) the lower (more dependent) score of Items 31 and 32 above.

	ADMISSION	DISCHARGE
33. Tub Transfer	☐	☐
34. Shower Transfer	☐	☐

(Score Items 33 and 34 using FIM Levels 1 - 7; use 0 if activity does not occur) See training manual for scoring of Item 39K (Tub/Shower Transfer)

	ADMISSION	DISCHARGE
35. Distance Walked	☐	☐
36. Distance Traveled in Wheelchair	☐	☐

(Code items 35 and 36 using: 3 - 150 feet; 2 - 50 to 149 feet; 1 - Less than 50 feet; 0 – activity does not occur)

	ADMISSION	DISCHARGE
37. Walk	☐	☐
38. Wheelchair	☐	☐

(Score Items 37 and 38 using FIM Levels 1 - 7; 0 if activity does not occur) See training manual for scoring of Item 39L (Walk/Wheelchair)

*The FIM data set, measurement scale and impairment codes incorporated or referenced herein are the property of U B Foundation Activities, Inc. ©1993, 2001 U B Foundation Activities, Inc. The FIM mark is owned by UBFA, Inc.

39. FIM™ Instrument*

	ADMISSION	DISCHARGE	GOAL
SELF-CARE			
A. Eating	☐	☐	☐
B. Grooming	☐	☐	☐
C. Bathing	☐	☐	☐
D. Dressing - Upper	☐	☐	☐
E. Dressing - Lower	☐	☐	☐
F. Toileting	☐	☐	☐
SPHINCTER CONTROL			
G. Bladder	☐	☐	☐
H. Bowel	☐	☐	☐
TRANSFERS			
I. Bed, Chair, Whlchair	☐	☐	☐
J. Toilet	☐	☐	☐
K. Tub, Shower	☐	☐	☐

W - Walk
C - wheelChair
B - Both

LOCOMOTION	ADMISSION	DISCHARGE	GOAL
L. Walk/Wheelchair	☐ ☐	☐ ☐	☐
M. Stairs	☐	☐	☐

A - Auditory
V - Visual
B - Both

COMMUNICATION	ADMISSION	DISCHARGE	GOAL
N. Comprehension	☐ ☐	☐ ☐	☐
O. Expression	☐ ☐	☐ ☐	☐

V - Vocal
N - Nonvocal
B - Both

SOCIAL COGNITION	ADMISSION	DISCHARGE	GOAL
P. Social Interaction	☐	☐	☐
Q. Problem Solving	☐	☐	☐
R. Memory	☐	☐	☐

FIM LEVELS
No Helper
  7 Complete Independence (Timely, Safely)
  6 Modified Independence (Device)

Helper - Modified Dependence
  5 Supervision (Subject = 100%)
  4 Minimal Assistance (Subject = 75% or more)
  3 Moderate Assistance (Subject = 50% or more)

Helper - Complete Dependence
  2 Maximal Assistance (Subject = 25% or more)
  1 Total Assistance (Subject less than 25%)

  0 Activity does not occur; Use this code only at admission

Form CMS-10036 (01/06)

2

Figure 19-2. Patient Assessment Instrument

DEPARTMENT OF HEALTH AND HUMAN SERVICES
CENTERS FOR MEDICARE & MEDICAID SERVICES

INPATIENT REHABILITATION FACILITY – PATIENT ASSESSMENT INSTRUMENT

Discharge Information*

40. Discharge Date ____/____/____
MM / DD / YYYY

41. Patient discharged against medical advice? _____
(0 - No, 1 -Yes)

42. Program Interruption(s) _____
(0 - No; 1 - Yes)

43. Program Interruption Dates
(Code only if Item 42 is 1 - Yes)

A. 1st Interruption Date

[ ]
MM / DD / YYYY

B. 1st Return Date

[ ]
MM / DD / YYYY

C. 2nd Interruption Date

[ ]
MM / DD / YYYY

D. 2nd Return Date

[ ]
MM / DD / YYYY

E. 3rd Interruption Date

[ ]
MM / DD / YYYY

F. 3rd Return Date

[ ]
MM / DD / YYYY

44A. Discharge to Living Setting _____
(01 - Home; 02 - Board and Care; 03 - Transitional Living; 04 - Intermediate Care; 05 - Skilled Nursing Facility; 06 - Acute Unit of Own Facility; 07 - Acute Unit of Another Facility; 08 - Chronic Hospital; 09 - Rehabilitation Facility; 10 - Other; 11 - Died; 12 - Alternate Level of Care Unit; 13 - Subacute Setting; 14 - Assisted Living Residence)

44B. Was patient discharged with Home Health Services? _____
(0 - No; 1 - Yes)
(Code only if Item 44A is 01 - Home, 02 - Board and Care, 03 - Transitional Living, or 14 - Assisted Living Residence)

45. Discharge to Living With _____
(Code only if Item 44A is 01 - Home; Code using 1 - Alone; 2 - Family / Relatives; 3 - Friends; 4 - Attendant; 5 - Other

46. Diagnosis for Interruption or Death _____
(Code using ICD-9-CM code)

47. Complications during rehabilitation stay
(Use ICD-9-CM codes to specify up to six conditions that began with this rehabilitation stay)

A. _____   B. _____

C. _____   D. _____

E. _____   F. _____

Quality Indicators

RESPIRATORY STATUS
(Score items 48 to 50 as 0 - No; 1 - Yes)

	Admission	Discharge
48. Shortness of breath with exertion	_____	_____
49. Shortness of breath at rest	_____	_____
50. Weak cough and difficulty clearing airway secretions	_____	_____

* The FIM data set, measurement scale and impairment codes incorporated or referenced herein are the property of U B Foundation Activities, Inc. ©1993, 2001 U B Foundation Activities, Inc. The FIM mark is owned by UBFA, Inc.

Quality Indicators

PAIN

51. Rate the highest level of pain reported by the patient within the assessment period:
Admission: _____ Discharge: _____

(Score using the scale below; report whole numbers only)

```
0   1   2   3   4   5   6   7   8   9   10
|                   |                    |
No               Moderate              Worst
Pain               Pain           Possible Pain
```

Pressure Ulcers

52A. Highest current pressure ulcer stage
Admission _____   Discharge _____

(0 - No pressure ulcer; 1 - Any area of persistent skin redness (Stage 1); 2 - Partial loss of skin layers (Stage 2); 3 - Deep craters in the skin (Stage 3); 4 - Breaks in skin exposing muscle or bone (Stage 4); 5 - Not stageable (necrotic eschar predominant; no prior staging available)

52B. Number of current pressure ulcers
Admission _____   Discharge _____

PUSH Tool v. 3.0 ©

SELECT THE CURRENT LARGEST PRESSURE ULCER TO CODE THE FOLLOWING. Calculate three components (C through E) and code total score in F.

52C. Length multiplied by width (open wound surface area)
Admission _____   Discharge _____

(Score as   0 - 0 cm^2; 1 - < 0.3 cm^2; 2 - 0.3 to 0.6 cm^2; 3 - 0.7 to 1.0 cm^2 ; 4 - 1.1 to 2.0 cm^2; 5 - 2.1 to 3.0 cm^2; 6 - 3.1 to 4.0 cm^2; 7 - 4.1 to 8.0 cm^2; 8 - 8.1 to 12.0 cm^2; 9 - 12.1 to 24.0 cm^2; 10 - > 24 cm^2)

52D. Exudate amount
Admission _____   Discharge _____
0 - None; 1 - Light; 2 - Moderate; 3 - Heavy

52E. Tissue type
Admission _____   Discharge _____
0 - Closed/resurfaced: The wound is completely covered with epithelium (new skin); 1 - Epithelial tissue: For superficial ulcers, new pink or shiny tissue (skin) that grows in from the edges or as islands on the ulcer surface. 2 - Granulation tissue: Pink or beefy red tissue with a shiny, moist, granular appearance. 3- Slough: Yellow or white tissue that adheres to the ulcer bed in strings or thick clumps or is mucinous. 4 - Necrotic tissue (eschar): Black, brown, or tan tissue that adheres firmly to the wound bed or ulcer edges.

52F. TOTAL PUSH SCORE (Sum of above three items -- C, D and E)
Admission _____   Discharge _____

SAFETY	Admission	Discharge
53. Balance problem *(0 - No; 1 - Yes)* *e.g., dizziness, vertigo, or light-headedness*	_____	_____
54. Total number of falls during the rehabilitation stay		Discharge _____

The Specialty Practice of Rehabilitation Nursing: A Core Curriculum, 5th Ed.

Figure 19-3. Listing of Patient Evaluation and Conference System (PECS) Items and Item Groupings

I. **Rehabilitation Medicine (MED)**
1. Motor Loss
2. Spasticity/Involuntary Movement
3. Joint Limitations
4. Autonomic Disturbance
5. Sensory Deficiency
6. Perceptual & Cognitive Deficits
7. Associated Medical Problems
8. Postural Deviations

II. **Rehabilitation Nursing (NSG)**
1. Performance of Bowel Program
2. Performance of Urinary Program
3. Performance of Skin Care Program
4. Assumes Responsibility for Self-care
5. Performs Assigned Interdisciplinary Activities
6. Patient Education
7. Safety Awareness

III. **Physical Mobility (PHY)**
1. Performance of Transfers
2. Performance of Ambulation
3. Performance of Wheelchair Mobility
4. Ability to Handle Environmental Barriers (e.g., stairs, rugs, elevators)
5. Performance of Car Transfer
6. Driving Mobility
7. Assumes Responsibility for Mobility
8. Position Changes
9. Endurance
10. Balance

IV. **Activities of Daily Living (ADL)**
1. Performance in Feeding
2. Performance in Hygiene/Grooming
3. Performance in Dressing
4. Performance in Home Management
5. Performance of Mobility in the Home Environment (including utilization of environmental adaptations for communication)
6. Bathroom Transfers

V. **Communication (COM)**
1. Ability to Comprehend Spoken Language
2. Ability to Produce Language
3. Ability to Read
4. Ability to Produce Written Language
5. Ability to Hear
6. Ability to Comprehend and Use Gesture
7. Ability to Produce Speech
8. Ability to Swallow
12. Impairment in Thought (Verbal Linguistic) Processing (NP4)

VI. **Medications (DRG)**
1. Knowledge of Medications

VII. **Nutrition (NUT)**
1. Nutritional Status—Body Weight
2. Nutritional Status—Lab Values
3. Knowledge of Nutrition and/or Modified Diet
4. Skill with Nutrition & Diet (Adherence to Nutritional Plan)
5. Utilization of Nutrition & Diet (Nutritional Health)

VIII. **Assistive Devices (DEV)**
1. Knowledge of Assistive Mobility Devices

2. Skill with Assuming Operating Position of Assistive Mobility Devices
3. Utilization of Assistive Mobility Devices

IX. **Psychology (PSY)**
1. Distress/comfort
2. Helplessness/self-efficacy
3. Self-directed Learning Skills
4. Skill in Self-management of Behavior and Emotions
5. Skill in Interpersonal Relations
6. Ability to Participate in the Rehabilitation Program
7. Acceptance/understanding of Disability

X. **Neuropsychology (NP)**
1. Impairment of Short-term Memory
2. Impairment of Long-term Memory
3. Impairment in Attention-concentration Skills
4. Impairment in Verbal Linguistic Processing
5. Impairment in Visual Spatial Processing
6. Impairment in Basic Intellectual Skills
7. Orientation
8. Alertness/Coma State

XI. **Social Issues (SOC)**
1. Ability to Problem Solve and Utilize Resources
2. Family: Communication/Resources
3. Family: Understanding of Disability
4. Economic Resources
5. Ability to Live Independently
6. Living Arrangements

XII. **Vocational/Educational Activity (V/E)**
1. Active Participation in realistic Voc/Ed Planning
2. Realistic Perception of Work-related activity
3. Ability to Tolerate Planned Number of Hours of Voc/Ed
4. Vocational/Educational Placement
5. Physical Capacity for Work

XIII. **Therapeutic Recreation (REC)**
1. Participation in Group Activities
2. Participation in Community Activities
3. Interaction with Others
4. Participation and Satisfaction with Individual Leisure Activities
5. Active Participation in Sports

XIV. **Pain (PAI)**
1. Pain Behavior
2. Physical Activity
3. Social Interaction
4. Pacing
5. Sitting Tolerance
6. Standing Tolerance
7. Walking Tolerance
8. Use of Body Mechanics
9. Use of Relaxation Techniques
10. Performance of Medication Program

XVI. **Pastoral Care (PC)**
1. Awareness of Spiritual Dimensions of Illness/Disability
2. Knowledge of Spiritual Resources
3. Skill in Self-management of Spirituality
4. Utilization of Spiritual Resources

Reprinted with permission of Marianjoy Rehabilitation Hospital and Clinics and PECS, Inc., from Patient Evaluation and Conference System, Inc. (PECS). (Available from Marianjoy Rehabilitation Hospital and Clinics, PO Box 795, Wheaton, IL 60189)

2. Kenny Self-Care Evaluation:

   a. Examines 6 domains: transfers, bed activity, feeding, personal hygiene, dressing, and locomotion

   b. Uses a 5-level scale in which 0 = *completely dependent* and 4 = *independent*

3. Katz Index of Independence in Activities of Daily Living: uses letters (e.g., A = *independent*, G = *dependent*) to score various functional areas

4. Klein–Bell Activity of Daily Living Scale:

   a. Designed to assess the patient's current level of function

   b. Includes 170 items in 6 functional areas: dressing, elimination, mobility, eating, bathing and hygiene, and emergency telephone communication

5. Quadriplegia Index Function:

   a. Is specific to people with quadriplegia

   b. Involves the domains of transfers,

grooming, bathing, feeding, dressing, wheelchair mobility, bed activity, bladder program, bowel program, and understanding of personal care

   c. Uses a 5-level scale in which 4 = *independent* and 0 = *dependent*; 9 = *not applicable*

C. Instrumental Activities of Daily Living (IADLs) Scale (Dittmar & Gresham, 1997)

1. Encompasses activities that go beyond basic ADLs

2. Examples of IADLs include doing laundry, shopping, preparing meals, using a phone, and managing finances.

D. Scales That Measure the Effects of Primary and Secondary Handicaps

1. Community Integration Questionnaire, a 15-item tool that assesses home integration, social integration, and productive activity (Willer, Ottenbacher, & Coad, 1994)

2. Craig Handicap Assessment Reporting Technique (Hall, Dukers, Whiteneck, Brooks, & Krause, 1998)

   a. Designed to assess the reintegration of people with spinal cord injury

   b. Includes 27 items categorized into 5 dimensions (physical independence, mobility, occupation, social integration, and economic self-sufficiency)

   c. Has a maximum score of 100 for each dimension

E. Pediatric Tools

1. WeeFIM™ instrument (see Figure 19-5) (Braun, 1998)

   a. Designed for children aged 6 months to 7 years and older

   b. Derived from the FIM™ instrument.

   c. Can be used by members of any discipline

   d. Measures actual performance across various settings

   e. 0–3 Module (optional) of WeeFIM™ instrument is designed to measure precursors to function in children ages 0–3 years who have a variety of disabilities:

     1) 0–3 Module includes 3 domains: motor (16 items), cognitive (14 items), and behavioral (6 items).

     2) Intended to complement the WeeFIM™ instrument by measuring early functional performance and changes in performance over time

     3) Used across many settings,

Figure 19-4. Characteristics of Selected Activity of Daily Living (ADL) Scales

Scale	Items Included	Type of Scale	Evaluation
Katz Index of ADL	Bathing, dressing, toileting, transferring, continence, feeding; order of items reflects natural progression in loss and acquisition of function	Dichotomous rating of independence or dependence on each item; forms a six-level Guttman Scale	By professional raters
Kenny Self-Care Evaluation	Seventeen activities in six categories: bed activities, transfers, locomotion, personal hygiene, dressing, and feeding	Each activity rated on a four-point scale (0= complete dependence, 4= complete independence); an average score is created for each of six categories, allowing a possible total score of 24	By rehabilitation staff; scores constructed on the basis of observations
Barthel Index	Feeding, transferring, grooming, toileting, bathing, walking, or propelling a wheelchair; climbing stairs, bladder control, bowel control	Partial scores for performing ADLs with help, full score for independent performance; items weighted; full score of 100 signifies ability to do all tasks independently	By rehabilitation staff

Source consulted

Jacelon, C.S. (1986). The Barthel Index: A review of the literature. *Rehabilitation Nursing, 11*(4), 9–11.

including early intervention and preschool

2. Pediatric Evaluation of Disability Inventory (Haley, 1999)

   a. Provides an assessment of key functional areas in children between the ages of 6 months and 7 years

   b. Examines performance in 3 domains: self-care, mobility, and social

3. Home Observation for Measurement of the Environment (Molnar & Alexander, 1999)

   a. Consists of 45 items

   b. Identifies risk of developmental delay caused by lack of environmental support for a child in the home

   c. Assesses quality of child care

   d. Bases data collection on actual observation

F. Outpatient Tools

   1. LIFEware™ assessment tools (Granger, 1999)

      a. Designed for outpatient medical rehabilitation programs

      b. Examines physical function, pain, affective well-being, and cognitive functioning

      c. Customized for various patient populations

         1) Musculoskeletal (2 versions, 1 of which is abbreviated)

         2) Neurological

         3) Pulmonary

         4) Comprehensive

         5) Multiple sclerosis

Figure 19-5. WeeFIM™ Instrument

WeeFIM™ Instrument

L E V E L S	7 Complete Independence (timely, safely) 6 Modified Independence (device)	**NO HELPER**
	Modified Dependence 5 Supervision (subject = 100%) 4 Minimal Assistance (subject = 75%+) 3 Moderate Assistance (subject = 50%+) **Complete Dependence** 2 Maximal Assistance (subject = 25%+) 1 Total Assistance (subject = less than 25%)	**HELPER**

Self-Care   ASSESSMENT   GOAL
A. Eating
B. Grooming
C. Bathing
D. Dressing - Upper Body
E. Dressing - Lower Body
F. Toileting
G. Bladder
H. Bowel

Self-Care Total

Mobility
I. Chair, Wheelchair
J. Toilet
K. Tub, Shower
L. Walk, Wheelchair
M. Stairs

    W Walk
    C Wheelchair
    L Crawl
    B Combination

Mobility Total

MOTOR SUBTOTAL RATING

Cognition
N. Comprehension
O. Expression
P. Social Interaction
Q. Problem Solving
R. Memory

    A Auditory
    V Visual
    B Both
    V Vocal
    N Nonvocal
    B Both

Cognition Total

WEEFIM® TOTAL RATING

NOTE: Leave no blanks. Enter 1 if patient is not testable due to risk.

2. Focus on Therapeutic Outcomes (Dobrzykowski & Nance, 1997)
   a. Created in 1992 as an outcome measurement system for outpatient orthopedic rehabilitation
   b. Monitors the efficiency and effectiveness in the outpatient orthopedic population
3. Short Form 36, developed to assess a patient's well-being and perception of overall health (Ware & Sherbourne, 1992)

G. Home Environment Tools: Outcome and Assessment Information Set
   1. Mandated by the CMS for use in home care
   2. Has 100 questions covering 14 categories of care (e.g., ambulation, management of medication, psychological and emotional behavior, living arrangements)
   3. Involves data information being sent to state agencies
   4. Is a standardized measurement for monitoring outcomes of adults in the home setting

H. Other Tools
   1. Minimum Data Set (MDS) assessment [Refer to Chapter 4.]:
      a. Mandated by CMS for use in long-term care and subacute or postacute settings
      b. Serves as the data collection instrument for prospective payment systems
      c. Uses Resource Utilization Groups, Version III, a 53-group patient classification system in which periodic assessments are done
      d. Involves patient information being sent to the fiscal intermediaries for reimbursement and MDS information being sent to state survey and certification agencies (Medicare Payment Advisory Commission, 1999)
   2. Nursing home quality measures: The nursing home quality measures come from resident assessment data that nursing homes routinely collect on the residents at specified intervals during their stay. These measures assess the resident's physical and clinical conditions and abilities, preferences, and life care wishes. These assessment data have been converted to develop quality measures that give consumers another source of information about how well nursing homes are caring for their residents' physical and clinical needs. The quality measures have 4 intended purposes:

   a. To give information about the care at nursing homes to help people choose a nursing home for themselves or others
   b. To give information about the care at nursing homes where people already live
   c. To get people to talk to nursing home staff about the quality of care
   d. To give data to the nursing home to help them with their quality improvement efforts

V. Program Evaluation

A. Overview
   1. Performance indicators play a key role in the development of a successful outcome system.
   2. Performance indicators are quantitative values that can be collected by providers and reported to stakeholders.

B. General Considerations
   1. When assessing the efficiency, effectiveness, and other critical outcomes of rehabilitation, an organization must use a system that has demonstrated reliability and validity.
      a. Reliability: reproducibility of an instrument's findings
      b. Validity: ability of the tool to measure what it was designed or intended to measure
   2. Data collection instruments and systems used by rehabilitation programs should be valid and reliable.
   3. Development of a successful program evaluation and outcome system with an emphasis on rehabilitation nursing interventions should include specific critical design elements.
      a. Functional status: documents the rehabilitation gains of physical function
      b. Destination: determines whether discharge to the community or to the least restrictive environment has been achieved
      c. Efficiency: the extent to which a specific intervention, procedure, regimen, or service, when applied in routine circumstances, does what it is intended to do for a specific population (Last, 1995)
      d. Patient perception: satisfaction of the patient, family, and other stakeholders
      e. Effectiveness: the end results achieved in relation to the resources (e.g., money, time) expended (Last, 1995)
      f. Follow-up: determines whether progress

was made or maintained after discharge from a rehabilitation program

VI. Quality and Performance Improvement in Health Care

A. Overview

1. Definition of quality improvement: "a management process or approach to continuous study and improvement of the processes of providing health care services to meet the needs of individuals and others" (JCAHO, 1999)

2. Historical figures in the development of quality improvement

   a. Walter Shewhart (1920s): Created the quality cycle of Plan, Do, Check, Act.

   b. Armand Feigenbaum (1940s to present): Developed phrases "total quality control" and "cost of quality."

   c. W. Edwards Deming (1930s to present): Developed a 14-point plan that serves as the basis for total quality management. Although Deming's model originally was designed for manufacturing industries, the concepts and philosophy have been adopted by the healthcare industry.

   d. Joseph Juran (1950s): An engineer and attorney whose philosophy was to build on quality improvement, quality control, and quality planning (i.e., the quality trilogy). Juran's philosophy supports the frameworks of CARF and the JC.

   e. Philip Crosby (1960s to present): Identified zero defects as a performance standard with an emphasis on preventing errors.

B. Tools for Quality Improvement (Brassard & Ritter, 1994)

1. Brainstorming: Allows team members to create as many creative ideas and solutions as possible; all suggestions are recorded to be evaluated at a later time.

2. Cause-and-effect diagram (fishbone diagram): Allows team members to visually and graphically explore the relationship between the effects and possible causes of identified problems.

3. Affinity diagram: Gathers large amounts of data and helps organize the information into groupings based on the relationships between the items.

4. Check sheet: Allows team members to record and collect data from various sources so that patterns and trends may be identified.

5. Run chart: Used to visually display data and to identify any changes that occur.

6. Histogram: Displays the distribution of data and reveals the amount of variation within a process.

7. Scatter diagram: Used to study the possible cause-and-effect relationship between 2 variables.

8. Control chart: Used to monitor, control, and improve variances in performance by identifying the source; is similar to a run chart but with statistical upper and lower limits.

9. Flowchart: A pictorial representation of various steps of a process that allows team members to easily identify the flow of events.

10. Force field analysis: Identifies the forces in place that affect an issue or problem; ideally, it reinforces positives and eliminates negatives.

11. Pareto chart: A display of bar graphs that can help focus on and determine which problems to solve and in which order so that efforts are directed to the problems that have the greatest improvement potential.

C. Models for Performance Improvement

1. American Nurses Association (ANA) and Association of Rehabilitation Nurses (ARN) standards of care

   a. 1973: ANA established generic standards of nursing practice for determining the quality of nursing care.

   b. 1977: ANA published standards of rehabilitation nursing practice.

   c. 1986: ARN and ANA collaborated to revise the standards of rehabilitation nursing practice (McCourt, 1993).

   d. 2001: ARN published revised standards for rehabilitation nursing practice.

2. JC's Plan, Do, Check, Act approach

   a. Plan what you want to accomplish.

   b. Do what you planned to do.

   c. Check the results.

   d. Act on the information.

3. CARF's Quality and Accountability Initiative

   a. Goals: to increase the value of accreditation, conduct accreditation program research, and direct attention to outcome measurement and management

   b. Includes the 4-level Standards Conformance Rating Scale:

      1) 0 = Nonconformance (does not meet standard)

2) 1 = Partial Conformance (has substantial room for improvement)
3) 2 = Conformance (fully meets standard)
4) 3 = Exemplary Conformance (significantly exceeds expectation for conformance)

4. National Quality Forum (NQF)
   a. The NQF is a voluntary consensus standard-setting organization.
   b. Mission: The mission of the NQF is to improve the quality of American health care by setting national priorities and goals for performance improvement, endorsing national consensus standards for measuring and publicly reporting on performance, and promoting the attainment of national goals through education and outreach programs.

5. CMS
   a. The quality improvement organization (QIO) program consists of a national network of 53 QIOs responsible for each U.S. state, territory, and the District of Columbia.
   b. QIOs work with consumers, physicians, hospitals, and other caregivers to refine care delivery systems to make sure patients get the right care at the right time, particularly among underserved populations.
   c. The program safeguards the integrity of the Medicare trust fund by ensuring that payment is made only for medically necessary services and investigates beneficiary complaints about quality of care.

VII. The Future of Outcome Management

A. Increasing Importance of Outcomes
   1. Outcomes across the continuum will continue to have greater importance.
   2. Some systems (e.g., WeeFIM™, FIM™ instrument, LIFEware^SM) support measurement across the continuum of care.
   3. Computer adaptive testing
   4. The emphasis of satisfaction will move from provider to payer to patient or consumer (Jones & Evans, 1998).
      a. Satisfaction is evidenced by disclosure statements, which have a great influence in rehabilitation.
      b. Example: CARF's medical rehabilitation division maintains a public disclosure policy in which a person may request an organization's survey summary, and CARF provides the summary to the person at no charge. This meets the "need to know" element for various stakeholders (e.g., consumers).

B. Greater Accountability to Stakeholders
   1. Rehabilitation providers are experiencing an increase in accountability to demonstrate positive outcomes.
   2. Rehabilitation providers are increasingly expected to share information about programs and outcomes.

C. Increased Focus on Measuring and Monitoring Outcomes
   1. Measuring and monitoring outcomes and the quality and durability of outcomes will become an even larger component of rehabilitation nursing practice.
   2. Management of patients' needs across the continuum will be critical for successful chronic disease management.
   3. Rehabilitation nurses have the skills and knowledge to improve outcomes for patients.

References

Black, T.M. (1999). Outcomes: What's all the fuss about? *Rehabilitation Nursing, 24*(5), 188–189, 191.

Black, T.M., Soltis, T., & Bartlett, C. (1999). Using the Functional Independence Measure (FIM™) instrument to predict stroke rehabilitation outcomes. *Rehabilitation Nursing, 24*(3), 109–114, 121.

Brassard, M., & Ritter, D. (1994). *The Memory Jogger IITM: A pocket guide of tools for continuous improvement and effective planning.* Methuen, MA: Goal/QPC.

Braun, S. (1998). The Functional Independence Measure for children (WeeFIM^SM instrument): Gateway to the WeeFIM system. *Journal of Rehabilitation Outcomes Measurement, 2*(4), 63–68.

Deutsch, A., Braun, S., & Granger, C.V. (1997). The Functional Independence Measure (FIM™) instrument. *Journal of Rehabilitation Outcomes, 1*(2), 67–71.

Dittmar, S., & Gresham, G. (1997). Appendix A: Description and display of selected functional assessment and outcome measures in physical rehabilitation. In *Functional assessment and outcome measurement for the rehabilitation healthcare professional* (pp. 90–138). Gaithersburg, MD: Aspen.

Dobrzykowski, E. (1997). ORYX: The next evolution in accreditation. *Journal of Rehabilitation Outcomes, 1*(6), 22–23.

Dobrzykowski, E., & Nance, T. (1997). The Focus on Therapeutic Outcomes (FOTO) outpatient orthopedic rehabilitation database: Results of 1994–1996. *Journal of Rehabilitation Outcomes Measurement, 1*(1), 56–60.

Granger, C. (1999). The LIFEware System. *Journal of Rehabilitation Outcomes Measurement, 3*(2), 63–69.

Haley, S. (1999). The Pediatric Evaluation of Disability Inventory (PEDI). *Journal of Rehabilitation Outcomes, 1*(1), 61–69.

Hall, K. (1997). The Functional Assessment Measure (FAM). *Journal of Rehabilitation Outcomes Measurement, 1*(3), 63–65.

Hall, K., Dukers, M., Whiteneck, G., Brooks, C.A., & Krause, J. (1998). The Craig Handicap Assessment and Reporting Technique (CHART): Metric properties and scoring. *Journal of Rehabilitation Outcomes Measurement, 2*(5), 39–49.

Jacelon, C.S. (1986). The Barthel Index: A review of the literature. *Rehabilitation Nursing, 11*(4), 9–11.

The Joint Commission (JC). (2006). http://www.jointcommission.org. Oakbrook Terrace, IL: Author.

Joint Commission on Accreditation of Healthcare Organizations (JCAHO). (1999). *1999 accreditation manual for hospitals.* Oakbrook Terrace, IL: Author.

Jones, M., & Evans, R. (1998). Outcomes in a managed care environment. *Topics in Spinal Cord Injury Rehabilitation, 3*(4), 61–73.

Katz, S., Lord, A.B., Moskowitz, R.W., Jackson, B.A., & Jaffe, M.W. (1963). Studies of illness in the aged. The index of ADL: A standardized measure of biological and psychological function. *Journal of the American Medical Association, 185*, 914–919.

Last, J.M. (1995). *Dictionary of epidemiology* (3rd ed.). New York: Oxford University Press.

McCourt, A.E. (Ed.). (1993). *The specialty practice of rehabilitation nursing: A core curriculum* (3rd ed.). Skokie, IL: Rehabilitation Nursing Foundation of the Association of Rehabilitation Nurses.

Medicare Payment Advisory Commission (MedPac). (1999, March). Post acute care providers: Moving toward prospective payment. In *Report to Congress: Medicare payment policy* (pp. 81–98).

Molnar, G., & Alexander, M. (Eds.). (1999). *Psychological assessment in pediatric rehabilitation* (pp. 29–56). Philadelphia: Hanley and Belfus.

The Rehabilitation Commission (CARF). (1998). *Performance indicators for rehabilitation programs, version 1.1.* Tucson, AZ: Author.

The Rehabilitation Commission (CARF). (1999). *Standards manual for medical rehabilitation.* Tucson, AZ: Author.

The Rehabilitation Commission (CARF). (2006). *Standards manual for medical rehabilitation.* Tucson, AZ: Author.

Uniform Data System for Medical Rehabilitation (UDSMR). (1996). *Guide for the Uniform Data Set for Medical Rehabilitation.* Buffalo: State University of New York.

Ware, J.E., & Sherbourne, C.D. (1992). The MOS 36-item short health survey (SF-36): Conceptual framework and item selection. *Medical Care, 30*, 472–480.

Wilkerson, D. (1997b, August/September). Outcomes and accreditation. *Rehab Management,* pp. 112, 114–115, 124.

Willer, B., Ottenbacher, K., & Coad, M.L. (1994). The Community Integration Questionnaire. *American Journal of Physical Medicine and Rehabilitation, 73*(2), 103–111.

World Health Organization (WHO). (1980). *International classification of impairments, disabilities and handicaps.* Geneva: Author.

Suggested Resources

Hoeman, S. (Ed.). (1996). *Rehabilitation nursing: Process and application* (2nd ed.). St. Louis: Mosby.

Roberts, S., Wells, R., Brown, I., Bryant, J., Hutchinson, H.T., Kurushima, C., et al. (1999). The FRESNO: A pediatric functional outcome measurement system. *Journal of Rehabilitation Outcomes, 3*(1), 11–19.

WeeFIM™ Guide: Uniform Data System for Medical Rehabilitation. (2005). *The WeeFIM II system clinical guide, version 6.0.* Buffalo, NY: UDSMR.

Wilkerson, D. (1997a, Winter). On the language and classification of disablement and a new ICIDH. *American Congress of Rehabilitation Medicine Newsletter,* pp. 5–7.

World Health Organization (WHO). (2001). *International classification of functioning, disability and health (ICF).* Geneva: Author.

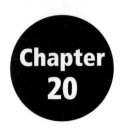

Chapter 20

Rehabilitation Nursing and Case Management

Donna Williams, MSN RN CRRN-A • Patricia L. McCollom, MS RN CRRN CDMS CCM CLCP

Case management is a model of care delivery that has been shown to be a key strategy and innovative approach to managing healthcare services and improving patient or client care. It is comprehensive, is patient or client centered, and promotes continuity of care across all settings. Our rapidly changing healthcare system demands financial and clinical outcomes within an appropriate timeframe and with appropriate use of resources. Case management provides a framework for planning, implementing, and evaluating care and is an effective process for dealing with the increasing complexity, fragmentation, and constraints of healthcare delivery.

Patients and clients of all ages are served by rehabilitation nurse case managers. In assigning a nurse case manager, consideration should be given to the client's age, the diagnosis, and the severity of the illness or injury because specialized knowledge may be an important factor in achieving goals.

The objectives of this chapter are to define case management, describe the role or model and functions of the nurse case manager and the scope of case management, and identify the processes that affect the quality and cost-effectiveness on healthcare services. The rehabilitation nurse is in a unique position to serve as a case manager because of his or her specialized knowledge and experience.

I. Historical Perspectives on Case Management

A. Early 1900s Social and Legislative Changes
   1. 1943: Vocational Rehabilitation Act
   2. 1945: Liberty Mutual nurses coordinate care.
   3. 1960: Workers' Compensation Rehabilitation Law
   4. Insurance Company of North America begins first private sector rehabilitation company.
   5. 1973: Rehabilitation Act, foundation for Americans with Disabilities Act (1990)

B. Insurance Industry
   1. 1970: Nurses and vocational rehabilitation counselors coordinate care and create long-term plans for people with disabilities.
   2. Entrepreneurs begin independent practice.
   3. 1993: Boston Consulting Group coins the term *disease management*, an approach to managing specific diseases and patient populations.

C. Facility-Based Case Management
   1. 1980s: Case management is developed in facilities to avoid duplication of services, evaluate care, and contain costs while improving the effectiveness of care (Cohen & Cesta, 2005).

   2. Roots in primary nursing.

D. Government Case Management Programs
   1. 1973: Title V of the Social Security Act and the Older Americans Act.
   2. 1985: Diagnosis-Related Groups propel case management into acute settings.
   3. Department of Veterans Affairs and TRICARE, health insurance for military dependents and retirees, use case management to optimize services and achieve high-quality care.

II. Definitions of Case Management

A. ARN: The process of assessing, planning, organizing, coordinating, implementing, monitoring, and evaluating the services and resources needed to respond to a person's healthcare needs (ARN, 2006).

B. Case Management Society of America (CMSA): A collaborative process of assessment, planning, facilitation, and advocacy for options and services that meet a person's health needs through communication and available resources to promote high-quality, cost-effective outcomes (CMSA, 2002).

C. American Nurses Association (ANA): A dynamic and systematic collaborative approach to provide and coordinate healthcare services to a defined population. It is a participative process to identify and facilitate options and services for meeting people's health needs while decreasing fragmentation and duplication of care and improving cost-effective clinical outcomes. The framework for nursing case management includes five essential functions: assessment, planning, implementation, evaluation, and interaction (ANCC, 2007).

D. Case Management Leadership Coalition (CMLC) consumer definition: Case managers work with people to get the health care and other community services they need when they need them and for the best value (CMLC, 2005).

III. Standards of Practice

A. ANA: *Standards of Practice* were updated in 2004 and articulate the who, what, when, where, and how of practice. *Code of Ethics for Nurses,* updated in 2004, establishes guidelines for carrying out nursing responsibilities in a manner consistent with quality in nursing care and the ethical obligations of the profession (see http://www.nursingworld.org).

B. CMSA: Standards were developed in 1995 and updated in 2002. Standards provide a parameter for knowledge, skill, behavior, and practice.

1. Provide a basis for evaluation of practice

2. Stimulate the development of the practice

3. Encourage research to validate the practice

C. ARN: Standards were developed in 1994 and updated in 2007. Rehabilitation nursing is viewed as a specialty practice guided by philosophy, theory, and research.

1. Scope of practice

2. Standards of care

3. Standards of professional performance

IV. Goals of Case Management

The goal of case management is the provision of high-quality, cost-effective healthcare services. The nurse case manager realizes this goal by organizing necessary healthcare services to promote outcomes for the client that include the highest possible level of independence and quality of life (ARN, 2006).

A. Improve Quality Through Appropriate and Timely Use of Services and Resources

1. Meets expected outcomes; promotes optimal functioning and independence in the least restrictive environment

2. Prevents complications

3. Improves coping with injury, illness, or disability

4. Helps patients or clients assume responsibility for directing their own care, being their own advocates, and making informed decisions

5. Facilitates successful return to work, school, and community

B. Facilitate Outcomes of Case Management

1. Coordinates care by ensuring access to healthcare services and monitoring all health care provided to the patient or client

2. Promotes collaborative practice through ongoing communication with the identified team in each setting on the continuum

3. Educates or promotes the education of patients or clients about their health status and prevention of complications or further disability. Emphasis is placed on self-management and responsibility for healthcare needs.

4. Advocates for the patient or client's optimal functioning and independence in the community by providing the tools necessary to achieve that level of functioning.

V. Models of Case Management

A. Setting: Case management services are provided in institutional, residential, outpatient, and community settings. These settings may include acute care facilities, rehabilitation facilities, outpatient facilities, skilled nursing facilities or nursing homes, residential facilities, day care agencies, private residences, or the workplace.

B. Employment: Case managers may be employees, contractors, or private practitioners.

1. Facility- or agency-based case manager: a case manager employed by a healthcare facility, government or private agency, or healthcare provider. This case manager is responsible for quality and cost-effectiveness of care delivery from admission to discharge.

2. Insurance-based case manager: a case manager employed by a third-party payer (e.g., an insurance company)

a. The case manager may be responsible for managing disease or incident-based injury or illness.

b. In workers' compensation the case manager is responsible for coordinating the care with a goal of return to work, and the file may close after return to work or at the time of settlement.

3. Employer-based case manager: a case manager retained by an employer to provide

case management services directly to employees.

    a. The case manager may be involved in industrial illness or injury.

    b. The case manager may be responsible for coordinating medical benefits provided by the employer and for promoting wellness.

4. Independent case manager: a private case manager whose services are retained by a third-party payer, facility, attorney, agency, or individual or family. Responsibilities may include all those of other case manager types, depending on the referral source.

VI. Role Functions and Processes

A. Patient Identification: Early identification of patients or clients who would benefit from case management is essential to successful achievement of outcomes and should occur at the onset of injury or diagnosis of chronic illness.

    1. Facility-based case managers, inpatient and outpatient, typically serve all admitted patients and initiate services upon admission.

    2. External case managers may receive referrals from insurance carriers, other third-party payers, attorneys, or physicians. Individual clients may also self-identify and self-refer. Case managers can help referral sources establish appropriate criteria.

B. Data Collection and Assessment:

    1. Obtains all necessary authorizations to contact the client and family for an initial interview and assessment

    2. Reviews and analyzes referral information in consultation with the client, health team members, employers, family, legal representatives, and claims and insurance personnel as indicated

    3. Reviews and assesses the client's personal and medical history, current status, diagnosis, prognosis, current treatment plan, and care provider's level of expertise. (For catastrophic injuries or illness, an on-site assessment of the client and anticipated or actual provider is highly recommended.)

    4. Assesses the client's learning needs related to the medical diagnosis and prognosis, treatment providers, treatment options, financial resources, psychosocial adjustment and coping mechanisms, and vocational rehabilitation needs and potential

    5. Assesses the family's knowledge base, health status, and expectations and the potential for or actuality of a family member acting as the primary caregiver if necessary

    6. Identifies the team members appropriate for each client

C. Data Analysis and Problem Identification:

    1. Identifies temporary or permanent alterations in function that have resulted from the injury or illness

    2. Identifies potential challenges or complications of physiological or psychosocial function

    3. Identifies potential difficulties in community reintegration where appropriate

    4. Identifies the learning needs of the client and significant others

    5. Considers vocational and history prognosis for reentering or entering the workforce when appropriate

D. Establishment of Goals and Plan of Care:

    1. Establishes realistic goals to achieve optimal outcomes for the client. This is done in collaboration with the client and family and with the interdisciplinary team, within available resources.

    2. Helps the client, the family, and team identify the variables that may influence the accomplishment of goals (see Figure 20-1)

    3. Develops a comprehensive plan that includes short- and long-term goals and preventive treatment measures. Identifies alternatives for the client's treatment when appropriate

    4. Establishes target dates for achievement of goals

E. Implementation and Coordination:

    1. Uses rehabilitation principles to promote optimal outcomes for the client

    2. Provides ongoing assessment of the client, family, and caregiver

    3. Coordinates access to accelerated or alternative care options when appropriate.

    4. Coordinates access to appropriate government and community programs and resources

    5. Coordinates and evaluates in a quality-conscious, cost-effective manner the client's and family's use of medical equipment, supplies, medications, and the full spectrum of services

    6. Provides instruction to the client and family based on identified learning needs.

    7. Coordinates referrals for instruction or counseling as is agreeable to the client and

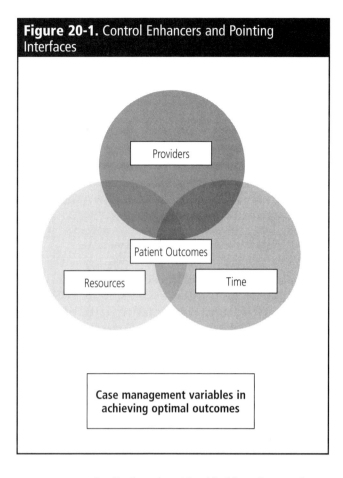

Figure 20-1. Control Enhancers and Pointing Interfaces

Providers

Patient Outcomes

Resources

Time

Case management variables in achieving optimal outcomes

family, based on identified learning needs.

8. Provides education, guidance, and recommendations to the payer about alternatives for care and services where appropriate.

9. Intervenes promptly when necessary to promote optimal functioning and prevention of complications.

10. Facilitates and collaborates with the healthcare team for timely discharge planning to an alternative level of care or return to the community when appropriate.

11. Coordinates the discharge plan with the healthcare team and providers.

12. Educates the client and family on care options and choices, allowing informed decisions, even when the decisions are suboptimal or different from the case manager's recommendations.

F. Monitoring:

1. Ongoing assessment to allow awareness of potential or real complications and need for plan revision

2 Adherence to plan

3. Achievement of benchmarks

G. Evaluation:

1. Goals and outcomes are monitored continuously.

2. Progress toward goals is evaluated and modified if necessary.

H. Quality Management: A method for ensuring that all the activities in the case management structure that are pursued to design, develop, and implement the service are effective and efficient with respect to the system and its performance.

I. Outcomes:

1. Outcome measurement provides professionals with feedback that helps them achieve goals. Key data in all sectors, including trends, history, clinical decisions, and identification of patterns allows review and alterations of or options for the treatment plan.

2. Categories of measurement of patient or client outcomes include physiological, psychosocial, functional, behavioral, knowledge, home functioning, family strain, safety, symptom control, quality of life, goal attainment, patient or client satisfaction, use of services, and nursing diagnosis resolution (Cohen & Cesta, 2005). These categories can be applied easily by case management practitioners to clarify and specify the results of intervention for individuals and groups.

J. Cost Management: The case manager's role in cost management depends on the setting, expected function, and situation. Case managers may recommend and arrange for purchase of services and supplies and negotiate and coordinate care and services, resulting in effective use of resources. This results in an opportunity for creativity and development of nontraditional options to meet individual client needs.

VII. Certification

A. CRRN®: First offered in 1984 by ARN. Requires 2 years of experience as a registered nurse in rehabilitation nursing.

B. CCM: First offered in 1993 by the Commission for Case Manager Certification. Requires licensure in professional healthcare and 2 years of experience in case management.

C. ANCC: First offered in 1998 by the American Nurses Credentialing Center. Focused on facility-based practice, the application criteria include licensure as a registered nurse with a minimum of 2 years' full-time work and 2,000 hours of practice.

VIII. Accreditation and Regulation

A. Joint Commission on Accreditation of Healthcare Organizations determined measures for meeting discharge planning criteria, including documentation of a formal plan of care with expected patient outcomes, in 1996. Case managers may be assigned responsibility for discharge planning.

B. Commission of Accreditation of Rehabilitation Facilities (CARF) developed standards for medical rehabilitation case management that were implemented July 1, 1999. CARF believes that case management is an integral part of rehabilitation care. Coordination, communication, and advocacy are primary themes in the CARF standards.

C. American Health Care Commission/Utilization Review Accreditation Commission developed a process in 1998 to accredit case management programs that promote innovation and best practice in the case management industry.

IX. Life Care Plans

A. Life care plans were introduced into rehabilitation and the legal literature in 1981 as part of a rehabilitation evaluation to project the impact of catastrophic injury on a person's future. A life care plan was distinguished from a discharge plan by its projection of costs of medical and associated care over a person's lifetime. The life care planner may be a case manager who prepares the dynamic plan. The case manager may also be involved in overseeing the implementation of the plan.

B. The International Academy of Life Care Planners (IALCP) defines a life care plan as a dynamic document based on published standards, a comprehensive assessment, data analysis, and research. It provides an organized, concise plan for current and future needs with associated costs for people who have sustained catastrophic injury or have chronic healthcare needs (IALCP, 2006).

1. Uses of life care plans
   a. Identification of costs for attorneys working on personal injury cases
   b. Identification of potential costs for insurance or reinsurance companies to specify damages resulting from injury
   c. A guide for families or clients for necessary healthcare and community resources
   d. A tool for clients of any age and their families to anticipate and self-monitor care
   e. A tool for expenditures from group

healthcare plans in catastrophic injury or illness

2. Descriptions of life care plans
   a. Consistent with the clinical needs of the client and should reflect risk factors that may affect available resources.
   b. Must include healthcare needs and quality of life needs.
   c. Comprehensive plans prepared by assessment of all medical records and other data that might affect the plan, interview or observation of the patient or client and care provider, and collaboration with treating professionals.
   d. Medicare set-asides: Regulated by the Centers for Medicare and Medicaid Services, a Medicare set-aside (MSA) is the required method to protect Medicare's interests in workers' compensation case settlements. The MSA allocates a portion of the settlement for future medical expenses that would otherwise be funded by Medicare.

X. Advanced Practice

A. Definition: ANA has recognized advanced practice as specialization, enhancement, expansion of practice and knowledge, and graduate-level education, although there is active dialogue among ANA and advanced practice nurses about the definition of the advanced practice nurse. ARN has recognized and certified advanced practice nurses in rehabilitation. Advanced practice nurses, certified and noncertified, have many responsibilities in the area of case management. It is recognized that advanced practice nurses conduct comprehensive assessments and function autonomously, showing expert skill in the diagnosis and treatment of complex responses to actual or potential health problems resulting from an altered functional ability and altered lifestyle secondary to a physical disability or chronic illness.

B. Advanced Practice Nurse Case Manager Functions:

1. Clinician: uses advanced assessment skills to determine healthcare needs, establish the plan of care, and monitor the progress and outcomes.

2. Educator: provides information about the plan of care to team members and information on the diagnosis and plan of care to the client.

3. Manager: manages, assigns, and delegates tasks to team members in a cost-effective

manner; organizes appropriate treatments.

4. Consultant: addresses factors affecting outcomes, ensures quality of care, acts as a resource.

5. Collaborates with physicians and other healthcare professionals using effective communication styles

6. Develops and coordinates the plan of care throughout the continuum of care

7. Researcher: redesigns plans of care based on outcomes and evidence-based practice and monitors the quality of each plan.

8. Fiscal responsibility: The advanced practice nurse should be familiar with pertinent financial, regulatory, and accreditation issues in whatever setting practice occurs.

XI. Issues

A. Multistate Licensure: Nurse licensure rules and regulations were formed when nursing was practiced primarily within the boundaries of one state and usually within a facility or agency. As access to health care, the mobility of the population, and coverage by insurance companies has changed, nurses may find themselves providing services to patients who travel across multiple state lines. Many state nursing licenses are not recognized by other states. The following are issues for multistate licensure.

1. There may be additional costs for licensure.

2. Nurses may be more vulnerable to lack of malpractice insurance. This may affect the employer as well.

3. As of January 2007, 20 state boards of nursing have joined together to form a Nurse Compact in which states mutually recognize nurse licenses from other states. Two additional states are pending implementation.

4. A CMSA position paper revised in 2005 addresses the problem and may be found at http://CMSA.org.

B. Education and Certification: The process of case management continues to develop as healthcare systems change, definitions are refined, job functions evolve, and the needs of the consumer and payer grow. Requirements for basic education and continued education will continue to change. Confusion about eligibility for the roles and certification must be addressed because there are trends toward increasing legislation, rules, and regulations in case management practice (Huber, 2006).

XII. Implications for Practice

A. Leadership

1. Case managers are in a prime leadership position. The case manager assumes responsibility for communication, collaboration, negotiation, and resolution of conflict between team members while identifying and coordinating the treatment plan. Conflict can arise from difficulty in fulfilling the plan because of economic, time, or other resource limitations or lack of patient or family understanding. In complex cases, multiple providers can be treating the client and may be unaware of the work of other providers. The case manager may be instrumental in identifying all current providers, establishing communication between them, and leading them through the process of coordinated care.

2. Review of leadership theory and processes may be useful to the nurse seeking more information.

B. Potential Ethical Conflicts in Case Management

1. Interdisciplinary teamwork involves collaboration, typically through team meetings. Members work together and share resources to arrive at a decision or position that balances ethical and cost concerns. Through this synergistic process, the team model provides support, expertise, and guidance that would not otherwise be available to individual professionals. Many managed care organizations are structured to allow this type of professional interaction.

2. Interdisciplinary teams present potential for ethical conflicts between members because they are:
   a. Holistic (addressing medical, social, and functional needs)
   b. Comprehensive in their analysis of cases
   c. Diverse in experience, cultural background, skills, and perspectives

3. Characteristics of case management that may present barriers to ethically appropriate care:
   a. Accountability for cost of care: When a physician or medical center is held financially accountable for the patients' costs of care, the patient–physician relationship may be significantly affected by attempts to contain costs at the expense of patient health and well-being. The case manager may feel pressure to prioritize financial goals above care outcome goals.

b. Proactive care planning: Professionals may compromise their loyalty and commitment to provide necessary care and individual autonomy.

c. Outpatient services: Such services, whether provided in the clinic or home, help to avoid more costly hospitalizations. Comprehensive assessments must be completed to ensure that care plan recommendations are practical and within the ability of the patient or client and family to perform. Conflict may arise if there is disagreement about ability to participate in a home or clinic setting.

d. Interventions suitable for the general population: Most managed care plans exclude inefficient or costly approaches or those that have not been shown in research studies to have sufficient efficacy. Therefore, treatments that may benefit patients with particular conditions are not covered by managed care organizations. Many payers are experimenting with various guidelines for treatment as they consider approval for plans of care.

4. Factors influencing the effectiveness of an interdisciplinary team:

a. One of the most basic barriers to the effectiveness of interdisciplinary team planning is related to autonomy and the goals and desires of the client and her or his family. When these goals and desires are at odds with those presumed by the team, recommendations are likely to bring little improvement.

b. Some cases are not suited for the team care approach. The overall effectiveness of a team may be compromised by the need to contain costs in specific cases that are unlikely to result in demonstrable improvement.

c. The means of measuring and demonstrating savings are inadequate when a team approach is used to plan for high-risk patients, particularly older adults. Further complicating this situation, it is very difficult to evaluate outcomes in older adults with debilitating conditions or comorbidities by using existing measures.

d. Because the team process is time consuming and costly, team members often are pressured to demonstrate that the approach meets the needs of patients in a cost-effective manner.

5. Maxims to promote organizational ethics:

a. Build on an organization's existing resources.

b. Understand that initially all ethics programs experience growing pains and may meet resistance.

c. Establish a high level of ethical behavior and accountability.

d. Encourage and support professionals' efforts toward spiritual growth.

6. Ethical concepts:

a. Elements of ethical competence

1) Commitment to patient or client well-being: Case managers must ensure that patient- or client-centered care and services are provided.

2) Responsibility and accountability: Through coordination activities, case managers monitor the effectiveness of the plan and can reinforce the accountability of others who are responsible for achieving specific goals or performing specific tasks within the plan.

3) Ability to act as an effective advocate: With access to and knowledge of the healthcare system, the case manager acts as an advocate for patients or clients within the system and in coordinating community-based services.

4) Ability to mediate ethical conflicts: Case managers are in a position to identify ethical conflicts and seek resolution through ethics consultations and other means.

5) Ability to recognize ethical dimensions of practice: Skill in identifying potential ethical dilemmas is derived from an ability to analyze situations from multiple perspectives.

6) Ability to critique the potential to influence a person's well-being: With the availability of new healthcare technologies, case managers must analyze the potential of various interventions (both positive and negative).

b. Ethical approaches

1) Generally, the principle-based approach consists of traditional principles of autonomy, beneficence, nonmaleficence, and justice. Ethical dilemmas arise when the case manager cannot uphold one or more of these principles.

2) The care-based approach is based on the professional–client relationship and focuses on the totality of the client's life. It attends to the client's needs and interests while attempting to resolve ethical conflicts by improving relationships between the client, professional, and family.

3) The shared decision-making model recognizes the importance of considering the expertise and opinion of both the patient or client and the professional when making a decision. Professionals give the patient or client the information, skills, data, and other support necessary to make an informed decision. The patient or client and the professional are active participants in the discussion leading to a decision. Each voices his or her thoughts and can consider the perspective of the other before making a decision.

4) Criteria to identify the appropriate ethical approach:

   a) The patient or client's ability to comprehend information that is relevant to the decision to be made.

   b) His or her ability to deliberate using a consistent set of values and goals.

   c) His or her ability to communicate preferences.

C. Legal Issues in Case Management Based on Changes in Healthcare Delivery

1. More knowledgeable patients and clients with increased access to information through technology such as the Internet

2. Clients' increased expectations from service providers because of their greater knowledge and access to health information

3. Case managers' greater exposure to lawsuits as they assume more responsibility for cost containment

4. Increased autonomy of case managers and other healthcare professionals in their practices

5. Increased caseloads of case management professionals as healthcare organizations downsize

D. Risk Factors in Case Management

1. Case managers are responsible for integrating care and services, advocating for patients or clients and their families, and acting as risk managers. Case managers may reduce the risk of litigation by performing their duties as defined by established standards and relevant scope of practice.

2. Case managers have a responsibility to communicate with the patient or client, the family, and the treatment team in a timely manner. This is particularly true when the condition of the patient or client changes significantly and warrants immediate attention. Case managers must ensure that the treatment plan remains accurate and relevant to the changing needs of the patient or client.

3. Case managers have a responsibility to integrate services. In doing so, case managers develop relationships with patients or clients, family, service providers, and others involved in the care and rehabilitation processes. Liability issues arise when the professional cannot integrate necessary care and services because of conflicting obligations (e.g., patient or client advocacy vs. contractual obligations to the employer).

4. Case management is a specialty practice with providers held to professional standards of practice. The elements of proof remain the same as in any professional malpractice case (e.g., duty, breach), but for a finding of malpractice, evidence must go beyond the reasonable man standard and establish that the professional did not meet the necessary standards of care.

5. The role and functions of case management according to relevant nurse practice acts, certification standards, standards of professional organizations, and other sources are well documented. The jury compares those standards with the actions of the professional and uses them as guides in the decision-making process in a court setting.

References

American Nurses Association (ANA). (2004). *Nursing: Scope and standards of practice.* Washington, DC: American Nursing Publishing.

Association of Rehabilitation Nurses (ARN). (2006). *The rehabilitation nurse case manager: Role description.* Glenview, IL: Author.

Case Management Society of America (CMSA). (2002). *Standards of practice for case managers.*

Cohen, E., & Cesta, T. (2005). *Nursing case management from essentials to advanced practice applications* (4th ed.). St. Louis: Elsevier.

Huber, D.L. (2006). *Leadership and nursing care management* (3rd ed.). Elsevier.

International Academy of Life Care Planners. (2006). *Standards of practice.* Glenview, IL: IALP.

Suggested Resources

ANA Nursing World: http://www.Nursingworld.org

Case Management Leadership Coalition: http://www.cmleaders.org

Case Management Society of America: http://CMSA.org

Commission on Accreditation of Rehabilitation Facilities: http://www.CARF.org

Rossi, P.A. (2003). *Case management in health care* (2nd ed.). Philadelphia: Elsevier Science.

The Joint Commission: http://Jointcommission.org

Weed, R.O. (1999). *Life care planning and case management handbook.* New York: CRC Press.

Section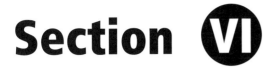

Rehabilitation Nursing Today

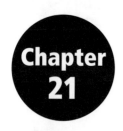

The Impact of Information Technology and Computer Applications on Rehabilitation Nursing

Kathleen A. Stevens, PhD RN CRRN

"The work of redefining human potential and creating a world of access to opportunity through technology has only just begun. It must continue until technology is a regular part of the lives of all individuals with disabilities who can benefit from it" (Alliance for Technology Access, 1996, p. ix).

Information technology and computer applications have developed and expanded beyond expectations. The electronic revolution has given birth to the information age and has changed health care dramatically. The ability to access and rapidly transfer information has created a digital knowledge revolution. Information technology is the use of computers and computer software to convert, store, protect, process, transmit, and retrieve information. According to the Institute of Medicine (IOM) report *Crossing the Quality Chasm*, information technology has the potential to promote health care that is "safe, effective, patient-centered, efficient and equitable" (IOM, 2001, p. 164). Technology has had a significant impact on the lives of people with disabilities as assistive technology improves access to services and the community.

In addition to improvements in technology, access to the World Wide Web and the Internet has created a global community. The Web allows everyone with a computer to access information and communicate with others without regard for location or times of day. People with disabilities can search the Web for medical information, treatment options, or research opportunities and communicate with others through virtual communities. Caregivers can access support groups around the clock to help them cope with caring for a family member. Information and support are no longer something we have to wait for; it's all available via the Internet.

Health care has changed as a result of new technology and access to the Internet. In 1992, nursing informatics was officially approved by the American Nurses Association (ANA) as a nursing specialty. Nursing informatics is the "specialty that integrates nursing science, computer science, and information science to manage and communicate data, information, and knowledge to support patients, nurses, and other providers in their decision making in all roles and settings. This support is accomplished through the use of information structures, information processes, and information technology" (ANA, 2001, p. 9). Rehabilitation nurses use nursing informatics in diagnosis, care, treatment, education, and research related to people with disabilities.

Health care can be more effective, efficient, and reliable because of computer technology and information systems. Information technology gives clinicians the opportunity to research best practices, share information, and locate vendors and clinical services that can improve the quality of care for people with disabilities. According to Schopp, Hales, Brown, and Quetsch, (2003, p. 163), "Rehabilitation informatics links the clinical expertise of health service providers with the technical expertise of information scientists to build new and innovative information technology applications to meet the needs of persons with neurological disabilities." Technology is also changing how rehabilitation services are delivered. Although assistive technology can play an important role in improving health and function and reducing barriers, personal factors and meanings associated with assistive technology play a decisive role in whether the person chooses to use the technology (Pape, Kim, & Weiner, 2002).

This chapter reviews the key concepts related to information technology used in health care and its relevance to rehabilitation nursing practice. Because of the amount of information available and the rapid changes in information technology, this chapter is only an introduction to resources available to rehabilitation nurses and people with disabilities. It is not a comprehensive study of the numerous areas of computer applications and information technology.

I. Precipitating Factors of Computerization in Rehabilitation

A. Health Care

1. Technology and consumer sophistication:
   a. More than 60% of Americans have Internet access.
   b. Studies report that 80% of Internet users, or approximately 93 million Americans, have searched the Internet for health information (Pew Internet and American Life Project, 2003).
   c. For patients and their families, Internet access is an inexpensive and an easy means of seeking knowledge, healthcare information, and support (Dickerson & Brennan, 2002).
   d. Healthcare information seeking is one of the most common reasons people use the Internet. Eight in 10 Internet users have looked for health information online. The greatest growth in online searching has occurred in information seeking about hospitals, doctors, experimental treatments, health insurance, medicines and supplies, fitness, and nutrition (Pew Internet and American Life Project, 2005).

2. Shorter hospital stays: Changes in payment systems and the risks associated with inpatient hospital care have resulted in shorter inpatient stays and shifted care to postacute settings.

3. Demand for postacute care:
   a. Since the 1970s, health care has shifted from acute hospital-based care to chronic care provided by postacute services in rehabilitation, long-term care, and home care.
   b. As the population ages, the demand for postacute care is expected to increase.
   c. As demand increases, access may be limited by the number and location of providers. Information technology may play a role in improving access and treatment.

4. Focus on outcomes, quality, and safety: Consumers using information technology and the Internet can access public records and hospital report cards published by individual states and agencies such as the Center for Medicare and Medicaid Services and the Joint Commission on quality outcomes for hospitals and long-term care facilities.

5. Staffing shortages: Rehabilitation therapies that use repetition to develop motor pathways and improve function often are labor intensive. There is growing interest in using technologies such as ceiling lifts and robotic devices to provide formerly labor-intensive care and treatment.

6. Changes in reimbursement and product costs:
   a. Reimbursement options are changing as a result of the Americans with Disabilities Act of 1990 and other legislation. Furthermore, computer hardware and software products that benefit people with disabilities are marketed to a larger commercial audience and are more reasonably priced and accessible.
   b. Consumers have greater knowledge about technological resources.

B. People with Disabilities

1. Programs that have affected growth of assistive technology:
   a. The Americans with Disabilities Act of 1990 mandated reasonable accommodation for people with disabilities, with particular attention to accommodations in communication and telecommunication.
   b. The Assistive Technology Act of 1998 provides funding to states to promote assistive technologies, help people purchase assistive technology services, and provide information to current and potential users of assistive technology.
   c. Rehabilitation Engineering Research Centers are funded by the National Institute of Disability and Rehabilitation Research to promote rehabilitation engineering research and development for innovative technologies and approaches to improve quality of life for people with disabilities.

2. Type and severity: As people with severe disabilities survive, more resources are being devoted to explore how technology can be used to promote physical health (e.g., portable mechanical ventilators, implanted intrathecal pumps, ventricular assistive devices) and improve quality of life (e.g., environmental control units).

3. Life expectancy: People with disabilities are living longer, and the need for assistive technology changes with age.

4. Changes in family structure and availability of caregivers: As the number of family caregivers shrinks and access to caregiver

services becomes more difficult, individuals and families are turning to technology to reduce caregiver workload (e.g., ceiling lifts in the home) or to provide caregiver support (e.g., Internet support groups).

    5. Access to technology:

        a. Products that previously were used solely by people with disabilities, such as voice-operated computer software and large-button phones, are now marketed to a wider range of consumers.

        b. Once what was special technology has become common.

II. Information and Computer Technology in Rehabilitation

  A. Consumer Access

    1. Despite gains in Internet access among the general population, the proportion of people with disabilities with home Internet access is less than the able-bodied population (Pew Internet and American Life Project, 2003; Schopp et al., 2003).

    2. People with disabilities who do have Internet access are active users and routinely search the Internet for health information. Health topics commonly searched:

        a. Specific diseases or conditions

        b. Specific medical treatments or procedures

        c. Diet, nutrition, vitamins

        d. Exercise and fitness

        e. Prescription and over-the-counter drugs

        f. Alternative treatments

        g. Clinical trials

    3. People with disabilities are also more likely to participate in online communications via bulletin boards or e-mail (Pew Internet and American Life Project, 2003).

        a. Common Web sites:

           1) Association of Cancer Online Resources: http://ACOR.org

           2) Spinal Cord Injury Information Network: http://www.Spinalcord.uab.edu

           3) Brain Injury Association of America: http://www.Biausa.org

        b. Referral to a support group is an important intervention and has been used by rehabilitation nurses to reduce social isolation associated with brain injury (Holley, 2007).

    4. Locating specialized care has become easier because consumers can access sites such as the Commission on Accreditation of Rehabilitation Facilities, Spinal Cord Injury Model Systems, National Spinal Cord Injury Association, and other national organizations on disability to locate centers with rehabilitation expertise when considering postacute care options.

  B. Delivery of Rehabilitation Services

    1. Imaging and diagnostic equipment advances have made diagnosis easier and increased our knowledge of neural function.

        a. Magnetic resonance imaging

        b. Positron emission tomography

        c. Functional magnetic resonance imaging

    2. Telemedicine is "the use of telecommunications to provide medical information and services" (Peredenia & Allen, 1995, p. 483).

        a. Common telemedicine uses

           1) Digital imaging data transfer, commonly used to transmit radiological images

           2) Interactive video

               a) May be used to conduct physical examinations of a patient from a remote site.

               b) Videoconferencing has been used to provide people in remote locations access to rehabilitation specialists for examination or consultation (Savard, Borstad, Tkachuck, Lauderdale, & Conroy, 2003).

        b. Telerehabilitation: Delivering rehabilitation services

           1) Telerehabilitation provides people in remote sites with access to rehabilitation services not available in their local community (Forducey et al., 2003).

           2) "Telerehabilitation is about the use of a more inclusive selection of tools and strategies to minimize barriers of distance and time for assessment and therapeutic interventions" (Winters & Winters, 2004, p. 205).

               a) Assessment:

                  (1) Collecting health histories: Koestler, Libby, Schofferman, and Redmond (2005) reported on a pilot study to assess the feasibility and consumer acceptance of using a Web-based touchscreen computer to collect history and clinical

information from patients with chronic low back pain.

  (2) Online personal health histories can be shared with healthcare providers and may be available through local hospital Web sites, physician offices, or, according to the American Health Information Management Association, a number of companies or Web services (e.g., http://myPHR.com).

  (3) Privacy is a major limitation and concern.

  b) Treatment: Teletherapy allows clinicians to deliver therapy services to remote sites via the Internet. A 2003 case study described how a physical therapist used teletherapy for patient with traumatic brain injury located 100 miles from rehabilitation center (Forducey et al., 2003).

  c) Educational interventions delivered by healthcare providers using videophone, telephone, and standard care protocols have been used to improve outcomes among patients with conditions such as multiple sclerosis, cancer, dementia, Alzheimer's disease, and arthritis in community settings (Dickerson, Boehmke, Ogle, & Brown, 2006; Egner, Phillips, Vora, & Wiggers, 2003; Glueckauf & Loomis, 2003; Tak & Hong, 2005).

  d) A Web-based system has been used to facilitate repetitive movement and give feedback as means of improving motor function for people with stroke (Reinkensmeyer, Pang, Nessler, & Painter, 2002).

3) Remote monitoring technologies allow clinicians to monitor:
  a) Vital signs (e.g., Digital Angel™)
  b) Weight
  c) Cardiac rhythms
  d) Blood glucose levels
  e) Physical activity levels (Slootmaker et al., 2005)
  f) Memory and location of people with brain injury (Schulze, 2004).

4) Support and education:

  a) The Internet has been used to provide education and support. Steiner and Pierce (2002) designed the Caring~Web, a Web-based in-home intervention to provide resources and support for caregivers of people with stroke during the first year after rehabilitation treatment.

  b) Dickerson et al. (2006) found that during cancer care, patients either directly or indirectly used the Internet to gather information and maintain a sense of hope through connections with others.

3. Educational therapeutic software.

C. Assistive Technology

  1. According to the 1998 Assistive Technology Act, an assistive technology device is "any item, piece of equipment, or product system, whether acquired commercially off the shelf, modified or customized, that is used to increase, maintain, or improve functional capabilities of individuals with disabilities" (Olson & DeRuyter, 2002, p. 4).

  2. Benefits associated with assistive technology:
     a. Allows people with chronic health needs to live in the community and still have access to medical equipment and monitoring essential for health and safety
     b. Increases level of independence and reduces dependence on caregivers
     c. Allows participation in community, vocational, leisure, or social activities that can enhance quality of life
     d. Allows people with disabilities to live independently

  3. Common resources for funding technology:
     a. Commercial insurance: If the technology is prescribed by a physician and a letter of medical necessity outlines use of the technology, some devices may be covered by individual policies.
     b. Medicare and Medicaid:
        1) May cover some mobility aids
        2) Will cover communication equipment
     c. Workers' compensation:
        1) Will cover most functional assistive devices
        2) May pay for modifications or equipment that is needed for return to work
     d. State Office of Rehabilitation Services

e. Veteran's Administration
f. Out-of-pocket payment
g. Alternative sources:
   1) Hospital charity care
   2) Lending libraries, either hospital based or associated with disability organizations
   3) Employers, if reasonable accommodation is needed for return to work

4. Principles of technology use:
   a. Assistive technology is a tool, not a solution.
   b. A person's perceptions of the device and how it may be used in their life are important. A person's level of psychosocial adaptation can be a significant factor in device use; for example, a person with a recent spinal cord injury who denies the permanence of the injury may not be interested in purchasing a customized van because he or she does not anticipate needing it, whereas a child with cerebral palsy may be quite excited about a new communication device that allows him or her to interact with peers at school.
   c. Professional consultation is an important factor to help match a device with the client's function and illness trajectory.
   d. Team input is essential (Olson & DeRuyter, 2002).
      1) Occupational therapists make recommendations on assistive technology and environmental controls to improve function.
      2) Speech–language pathologists evaluate communication and recommend augmentative communication devices.
      3) Rehabilitation engineers match, modify, or create technology to promote function or safety.
      4) Rehabilitation nurses evaluate a client's level of independence using equipment during daily activities.
   e. Any recommendation for a device should take into account training and repair and maintenance needs.
   f. Consumer involvement and choice are important considerations in selecting a device.
   g. Location and portability of the device:
      1) If the person is mobile, is the device sufficiently portable and functional in different environments? If it is not, this factor will limit use.
      2) If the device is not portable, will a comparable device and necessary software and accessibility be available in the school or work setting?
   h. More technology is not necessarily better; what matters most is matching the type of technology to the person.

5. Healthcare technology and self-monitoring:
   a. Chronic illness
      1) Heart disease
         a) Implanted defibrillators
         b) Home electrocardiographic monitoring
      2) Diabetes
         a) Blood sugar monitors
         b) Implanted insulin pumps
   b. Disability
      1) Arthritis: activity monitors
      2) Traumatic brain injury
         a) Global positioning system locators
         b) Emergency call systems
      3) Ventilator dependent: portable mechanical ventilators
      4) Spasticity: intrathecal baclofen pumps

6. Types:
   a. Low tech
      1) Devices that do not rely on computer or information technology, such as spelling boards or universal cuffs.
      2) Typically devices used for feeding, grooming, and dressing
   b. High tech: devices that rely on computer technology, switches, or external power sources, such as environmental control units or sip 'n' puff power wheelchairs

7. Assistive technology uses:
   a. Mobility:
      1) Manual wheelchair
      2) Battery-powered wheelchair
         a) Sip 'n' puff chairs
         b) Voice controls
   b. Self-care:
      1) Feeding
         a) Universal cuff, a simple cuff that allows people with minimal hand function to use a fork, toothbrush, or pencil to perform functional activities
         b) Mobile arm supports for people with limitations in shoulder movement necessary for feeding

2) Grooming: universal cuff
c. Communication:
1) Augmentative and alternative communication (AAC) systems are "an integrated group of components, including symbols, aids, strategies and techniques used by individuals to enhance communications" (Henderson & Doyle, 2002). (see Table 21-1).
2) Device types and features (E. Hitchcock, personal communication 2006):
a) Communication output
(1) Auditory digitized output: playback of message taped by user or another person
(2) Synthesized voice output: computer-generated voice
(3) Message display: graphical display on device
b) Written output: printer (internal to device or external)
c) Language features
(1) Item representation alphabet
(2) Whole word
(3) Photo or icon
(4) Object
d) Language storage and retrieval:
(1) Letter encoding
(2) Word prediction
(3) Icon encoding
e) Physical interface
(1) Direct selection: ability to push a single button to produce single result (e.g., pushing letter on keyboard)
(2) Encoded input (e.g., Morse code)
(3) Scanning
(4) Switches: can be used with any available motion to provide access or produce selected outcome (e.g., eyeblink switch used to activate device)
(a) Dual
(b) Multiswitch
(5) Directed (joystick)
(6) Speech or voice recognition
(a) Highly dependent on setup and user upgrades to maintain level of functionality.
(b) The most popular and accessible is Dragon Voice®. An advantage is speed; however, this device is the most cognitively demanding.

d. Sensory:
1) Vision
2) Hearing
a) Hearing aid
b) Cochlear implant
e. Safety:
1) Call systems
a) Hand bell
b) Motion-activated light or alarm
c) Intercom, from simple room-to-room intercom to sophisticated in-home wired system
d) Pocket pagers
e) Emergency call system and monitored phone service (e.g., Life Alert® or other medical alert system)
2) Monitors
a) Motion sensors
b) Medical alert system and phone link (e.g., Life Alert®)
c) Pagers or phones with global positioning system to track activity and location
3) Telephones
a) Amplified speakerphones
b) Big Keys® make dialing easier
c) Remote voice-activated dialing phones (e.g., RC 200 Speakerphone™)
f. Electronic aids to daily living are "devices that allow clients to control common household electronic items. A client who is unable to access a standard remote control can operate infrared devices through a number of different switch options that may be activated by head control or gross arm movement" (E. Hitchcock, personal communication).
1) Computer access
2) Keyboard options
a) Sticky keys available universally
b) BigKeys®
c) One-handed keyboards
3) Mouse options
a) Head movement–operated mouse
b) Eyegaze system
g. Education:
1) Electronic communication devices
2) Screen readers
h. Recreation and leisure:
1) Sit ski or sitting hockey sleds
2) Sports wheelchairs

Table 21-1. Key Issues for AAC Application Among Disability Groups

Diagnosis	Characteristic	AAC Intervention Strategy
Congenital		
Cerebral palsy	Developmental neuromotor involvement exists.	Oral motor training and speech therapy indicated for young children to develop word approximations.
	Type is characterized by motor impairment (e.g., spastic, athetoid).	Early intervention to train various motor sites should occur.
		Primary site (i.e., eye point) may be used for communication while switch and light beam are in training.
	Associated problems of developmental delay, seizure activity, visual and auditory perception, and acuity exist.	Use AAC to improve communication and enhance language development.
		Systems including devices change as skills improve and environmental demands change.
		Emphasize literacy skill development. May use prediction, Minspeak or dynamic display to increase speed of message transmission.
Autism	Social interaction skills are delayed or impaired.	Pragmatics need to be supplemented and trained.
		Voice output may help with pragmatics to decrease frustration.
Speech/oral apraxia	Receptive language may be age appropriate.	May use visual and spatial skills to advantage with an icon or words-based system.
	May be ambulatory with fine motor problems.	Portability is an issue.
	Verbal expression delays prevalent.	
	Structure and routine assists in training.	Teach use of AAC during routines. Can use a symbol-based calendar to anticipate new events.
		Consider use of simple signs or gestures. Use environmental and visual cues to structure and promote early communication.
		Use AAC to improve communication and language development.
	Receptive language may be age appropriate.	Use AAC to improve communication and language development.
	Fine motor problems may interfere with traditional sign language.	Teach gestural or modified manual sign language to the extent possible with motor planning.
	May see increased verbalizations as use of AAC lessons effort on communication.	Consider multiple portable components.
Cognitive limitations	Communication and language skills are delayed.	Use multimodal approach. Train in natural environment.
Acquired		
TBI	Majority of recovery occurs 6-9 months after injury.	Improve functional communication, teach family strategies, use flexible system, and use AAC to facilitate cognition and language recovery. Ensure user has insight and judgment before device purchase. Provide extensive trials before purchase. Educate family about the benefits of AAC; they may see AAC interfering with recovery of speech.
	Recovery of speech usually occurs within 12 months but may continue to improve several years postsurgery.	
	Cognitive, behavioral, and motor control problems occur.	
	Memory deficits an difficulties with new learning exist.	

(continued)

Table 21-1. Key Issues for AAC Application Among Disability Groups *(continued)*

Diagnosis	Characteristic	AAC Intervention Strategy
Acquired (cont.)		
CVA	Left CVA, nonfluent or Broca's are candidates.	Provide trials before purchasing.
	Language deficits primarily influence AAC use.	
	Majority of recovery is 6 months postonset, with gradual gains in speech and language processes several years postonset.	
	May be resistant to voice output.	Begin with manual components.
		May benefit from voice output in specific situations.
	Reading and spelling skills may be impaired.	Consider communication notebook with lists of names and blank paper for writing or drawing.
	May be able to recognize a written word.	May use voice output to practice verbalizing words or phrases.
	Visual cues (icons or words) may help word retrieval and verbal expression.	Teach to use a phone book, map, or catalog to retrieve information.
	Older populations want to talk about past events and experiences.	Use vocabulary to promote social closeness and sharing of information. Interview family about past history.
	Ability to use telephone is needed.	Voice output can be used for specific situations.
Brainstem	Recovery patterns are variable.	Establish alternative "yes" and "no" responses.
	May be called *locked-in syndrome*.	Eye-gaze boards may be used for interactions with nursing and caregivers.
	Visual perceptual and integration deficits may be present.	
	Generally, one reliable motor access site exists.	Integrate technologies.
Spinal cord injury	Level of injury influences intervention.	Speaking valves, voice amplifiers, and electro-larynges may be indicated.
	If complete injury, expect no spontaneous return.	Provide individual and family time to accept and cope with disability.
	Cognition and language usually intact.	Take time to explore various technologies.
	Patient may fatigue easily.	Monitor fatigue and task "loads."
Progressive		
ALS, or Lou Gehrig's disease	Different manifestations occur, generally rapid decline.	Provide flexible system.
		Intervene as mobility, motor control, or communication needs change.
	Usually no change in cognition occurs.	Use alphabet-based and text–based techniques.
	Patient may be resistant to further adaptations in technology as it indicates further loss of function.	Introduce new components as the need arises.
		Capitalize on residual skills.
		Maintain communication until death.
Multiple sclerosis	Manifestations differ; some symptoms are temporary.	Provide new components as symptoms arise.
	Progress is usually slower than ALS.	Use technologies for longer periods.
	Cognitive and visual perceptual deficits may be present.	Font size and complexity of visual display are important to monitor.
Parkinson's disease	Slow progression occurs.	Consider voice amplifiers.
	Hand tremors may influence motor access.	Manual systems and strategies may supplement speech (e.g., alphabet and initial letter cueing).
	Cognitive and language deficits may be present at end stages.	Icons may be useful.

Reprinted with permission of Mosby from Olson, D.A., & DeRuyter, F. (Eds.). (2002). *Clinicians guide to assistive technology* (pp. 128–129). St. Louis: Mosby.

TBI, traumatic brain injury; CVA, cerebrovascular accident; ALS, amyotrophic lateral sclerosis.

i. Vocational:
    1) Book holder with or without mechanical page turner
    2) Mouthstick
    3) Voice-activated computer
j. Transportation:
    1) Hand controls for automobile
    2) Wheelchair lift

D. Patient Education: Virtual libraries or databases such as the L.I.F.E. Center, hosted by the Rehabilitation Institute of Chicago or Spinalnetwork.org

E. Support and Long Term Care: Caring~Web, a Web-based in-home intervention for caregivers of people with stroke during the first year after rehabilitation treatment (Steiner & Pierce, 2002)

III. Benefits of Computer Technology for Nurses

A. Access to Education:

1. Internet access can increase educational opportunities and optimize use of time, money, educational staff, and other resources.

2. Nurses can take the time to participate in continuing education programs because of the increased availability of options.

3. Nurses can choose the most convenient time for a class, eliminating unnecessary rushing, fatigue, or concern about work. Being in control of time improves the efficacy of the educational offering.

4. All staff may receive education and still maintain adequate coverage on unit.

B. Networking: RehabNurse-L Listserve allows access to support groups and chat rooms. Dealing with high-stress jobs, sharing frustrations about new legislation, or using a particular assistive device are some areas that may be discussed in online chat groups (Thompson & Penprase, 2004).

C. Evidence Based Practice: The Internet provides nurses with access to information about evidence-based interventions.

1. National Library of Medicine via PubMed: http://www.ncbi.nlm.nih.gov/sites/entrez

2. National Guidelines Clearinghouse: http://www.guidelines.gov

3. Joanna Briggs Institute: http://www.joannabriggs.edu.au

D. Linking Interventions and Outcomes via Standardized Documentation:

1. Documentation systems using standardized languages allow researchers to study links between interventions and outcomes.

2. Common standardized languages used in nursing outcome research:

    a. Nursing Intervention Classification System

    b. Nursing Outcomes Classification (Moorehead, Johnson, & Maas, 2003)

    c. Minimum Data Set

    d. Home Health Outcomes (OASIS)

    e. Functional Independence Measure (FIM™ instrument; Keith, Granger, Hamilton, & Sherwin, 1987)

    f. WeeFIM™ Pediatric Functional Independence Measure (Msall et al., 1994)

3. Requests for information can be easily accessed in an accurate, timely manner.

4. Databases such as the National Database of Nursing Quality Indicators provide data on nursing outcomes and staffing effectiveness.

5. Financial accounting

6. Educational printouts or resources:

    a. Client education, a vital component of rehabilitative success, can be achieved through Web-based education programs reinforced by healthcare providers. Caregiver education, which is necessary for compliance and support of the rehabilitative client, can be facilitated through computer use.

    b. The quantity of education time can be distributed flexibly without a continuous or rigid schedule for one-on-one time. For example, a nurse can e-mail educational materials to family members who live across the country and discuss material or respond to questions via the Internet.

7. The family caregiver can supervise the client's practice sessions more accurately and needs less training to do so. For example, a Web camera allows family to view therapy sessions, or a digital recording of a procedure can be replayed at home.

IV. Rehabilitation and Clinical Research

A. Overview: Effective techniques and uses for technology to improve the lives of people with disabilities are being explored in research studies in medical rehabilitation. Health care is changing as a result of new technology, and every day these advances are expanding opportunities for people with disabilities. As technology evolves, the opportunities for people with disabilities will continue to grow.

B. Advancements Through New Technology:
1. Robotics:
   a. Kine-assis® is a new class of microprocessor-controlled devices that can help clinicians maintain patient safety during walking and balance exercises (Brown, 2004).
   b. Speech treatment.
   c. Use of robotic devices in sensorimotor training after stroke (Volpe, Krebs, & Hogan, 2003)
2. Neural engineering:
   a. Bionic Arm® (Kuiken et al., 2006) uses nerve transfers to improve control of upper arm prostheses, allowing the person to simultaneously operate multiple joints with more natural and intuitive control.
   b. BrainGate™ (Cyberkinetics Neurotechnology Systems, Inc.)
3. Health monitoring: Global positioning systems allow family members to track the location of people with cognitive deficits at risk for wandering.
4. Miniaturization and portability of devices.
5. Databases and outcome studies.
6. Nursing practice research: New paradigms arise with the advent of new technologies that can aid the advancement of rehabilitation nursing.
   a. Caring Web® (Pierce, Steiner, & Govoni, 2002)
   b. ComputerLink (Brennan, Moore, & Smyth, 1991)
   c. Developing tools to meet consumer needs
      1) Cultural sensitivity and language
      2) Accessibility
         a) Round-the-clock availability
         b) Nurses using the Web to evaluate patients or deliver education or support no longer need to be physically present with patients and families, so rehabilitation nurses are able to reach out to audiences beyond the inpatient rehabilitation unit.

References

Alliance for Technology Access. (1996). *Computer resources for people with disabilities: A guide to exploring today's assistive technology* (2nd ed.). Alameda, CA: Hunter House Publishing.

American Nurses Association (ANA). (2001). *Scope and standards of nursing informatics practice*. Washington, DC: American Nurses Publishing.

ASHA. (1991). Report on augmentative and alternative communication. *ASHA, 33*(Suppl. 5), 9–12.

Brennan, P.F., Moore, S.M., & Smyth, K. (1991). ComputerLink: Electronic support for the home caregiver. *Advances in Nursing Science, 13*(4), 14–27.

Brown, D.A. (2004, November). Creating a new balance. *Rehab Management.*

Cyberkinetics Neurotechnology Systems, Inc. (2005) *BrainGate™ clinical trials*. Retrieved April 8, 2007, from http://www.cyberkineticsinc.com/content/clinicaltrials/braingate_trials.jsp

Dickerson, S., Boehmke, M., Ogle, C., & Brown, J.K. (2006). Seeking and managing hope: Patients' experiences using the Internet for cancer care. *Oncology Nursing Forum, 33*(1), E8–E17.

Dickerson, S.S., & Brennan, P.F. (2002). The Internet as a catalyst for shifting power in provider–patient relationships. *Nursing Outlook, 50*(5), 195–203.

Egner, A., Phillips, V.L., Vora, R., & Wiggers, E. (2003). Depression, fatigue, and health-quality of life among people with advanced multiple sclerosis: Results from an exploratory telerehabilitation study. *NeuroRehabilitation, 18*, 125–133.

Forducey, P.G., Ruwe, W.D., Dawson, S.J., Scheideman-Miller, C., McDonald, N.B., & Hanita, M.R. (2003). Using telerehabilitation to promote TBI recovery and transfer of knowledge. *NeuroRehabilitation, 18*, 103–111.

Glueckauf, R.L., & Loomis, J.L. (2003). Alzheimer's caregiver support online: Lessons learned, initial findings and future directions. *NeuroRehabilitation, 18*, 135–146.

Henderson, J. & Doyle, M. (2002). Augmentative and alternative communication. In Olsen, D. and DeRuyter, F. *Clinicians guide to assistive technology*. St. Louis: Mosby.

Holley, U. (2007). Social isolation: A practical guide for nurses assisting clients with chronic illness. *Rehabilitation Nursing, 32*(2), 51–57.

Institute of Medicine. (2001). *Crossing the quality chasm: A new healthcare system for the 21st century*. Washington, DC: National Academy Press.

Keith, R.A., Granger, C.V., Hamilton, B.B., & Sherwin, F.S. (1987). The Functional Independence Measure: A new tool for rehabilitation. *Advances in Clinical Rehabilitation, 1*, 6–18.

Koestler, M.E., Libby, E., Schofferman, J., & Redmond, T. (2005). Web-based touch-screen computer assessment of chronic low back pain. *Computers, Informatics and Nursing, 23*(5), 275–284.

Kuiken, T.A., Miller, L.A., Lipschutz, A.B., Lock, B.A., Stubblefield, K., Marasco, P.D., et al. (2006). Targeted reinnervation for enhanced prosthetic arm function in a woman with a proximal amputation: A case study. *Lancet, 369*(9959), 371–380.

Msall, M.E., DiGaudio, K., Rogers, B.T., LaForest, S., Catanzaro, N.L., Campbell, J., et al. (1994). The Functional Independence Measure for Children (WeeFIM™). Conceptual basis and pilot use in children with developmental disabilities. *Clinical Pediatrics, 33*(7), 421–430.

Moorehead, S., Johnson, M., & Maas, M. (2003). *Nursing Outcomes Classification, NOC*. St. Louis: Mosby.

Olson, D.A., & DeRuyter, F. (Eds.). (2002). *Clinician's guide to assistive technology*. St. Louis: Mosby.

Pape, T., Kim, J., & Weiner, B. (2002). The shaping of individual meanings assigned to assistive technology: A review of personal factors. *Disability and Rehabilitation, 24*, 5–20.

Peredenia, X., & Allen, X. (1995). Telemedicine technology and clinical applications. *JAMA, 273*, 483–488.

Pew Internet and American Life Project. (2003). *Internet health resources: Health searches and email have become more commonplace, but there is room for improvement in searches and overall Internet access*. Retrieved November 17, 2005, from http://www.pewinternet.org/pdfs/PIP_Health_report_July_2003.pdf

Pew Internet and American Life Project. (2005). *Health information online*. Retrieved November 17, 2005, from http://www.pewinternet.org/pdfs/PIP_Health_report_May_2005.pdf

Pierce, L.L., Steiner, V., & Govoni, A.L. (2002). In-home support for caregivers of survivors of stroke: A feasibility study. *Computers, Informatics, Nursing, 20*, 157–164.

Reinkensmeyer, D.J., Pang, C.T., Nessler, J.A., & Painter, C.C. (2002). Web-based telerehabilitation for the upper extremity after stroke. *IREE Transactions on Neural Systems and Rehabilitation Engineering, 10*, 102–108.

Savard, L., Borstad, A., Tkachuck, J., Lauderdale, D., & Conroy, B. (2003). Telerehabilitation consultations for clients with neurological diagnoses: Cases from rural Minnesota and American Samoa. *NeuroRehabilitation, 18*, 93–102.

Schopp, L.H. Hales, J.W., Brown, G.D., & Quetsch, J.L. (2003). A rationale and training agenda for rehabilitation informatics: Roadmap for an emerging discipline. *NeuroRehabilitation, 18*, 159–170.

Schulze, H. (2004). MEMOS: A mobile extensible memory aid system. *Telemedicine Journal & e-Health, 10*(2), 233–242.

Slootmaker, S., Chin, A., Paw, M., Schuit, A.J., Seidelle, J.C., & van Mechelen, W. (2005). Promoting physical activity using an activity monitor and tailored Web-based advice: Design of a randomized control trial. *BMC Public Health, 8*, 134.

Steiner, V., & Pierce, L. (2002). Building a web of support for caregivers of persons with stroke. *Topics in Stroke Rehabilitation, 9*, 102–111.

Tak, S.H., & Hong, S.H. (2005). Use of the Internet for health information by older adults with arthritis. *Orthopaedic Nursing, 24*, 134–138.

Thompson, T.L., & Penprase, B. (2004). RehabNurse-L: An analysis of the rehabilitation nursing Listserv experience. *Rehabilitation Nursing, 29*, 56–61.

Volpe, B.T., Krebs, H.I., & Hogan, N. (2003). Robot-aided sensorimotor training in stroke rehabilitation. *Advances in Neurology, 92*, 429–433.

Winters, J.M., & Winters, J.M. (2004). A telehomecare model for optimizing rehabilitation outcomes. *Telemedicine Journal and e-Health, 10*, 200–212.

Chapter 22

Research and Evidence-Based Practice

Elaine Tilka Miller, DNS RN CRRN FAHA FAAN • Carole Ann Bach, PhD RN CRRN

The rehabilitation nurse is responsible for using best practices when caring for clients and fostering the advancement of rehabilitation nursing knowledge. Evidence-based practice (EBP) and research problems often emerge from nursing practice issues. Therefore, rehabilitation nurses should have a thorough understanding of and appreciation for the importance of the research process and the resultant knowledge that forms the foundation for EBP and high-quality patient care.

Each day, rehabilitation nurses make numerous important clinical practice decisions. However, the process of conducting research, publishing the findings, critiquing and synthesizing the current knowledge, and applying it to practice is time-consuming. Research shows that very few nurses use research findings when making clinical practice decisions. For example, it may take up to 17 years for research findings to be translated into nursing practice (Balas & Boren, 2002; Institute of Medicine, 2001). With the explosion of knowledge and the rapid changes that are taking place in health care today, it is imperative that research evidence be translated more quickly into clinical practice. According to Melnyk and Fineout-Overholt (2005), EBP is a way of getting information about the most up-to-date practice into the hands of clinicians. Furthermore, the research suggests that practitioners who use best practices in their clinical practice experience less burnout and higher job satisfaction than those whose practice is based on tradition (Melnyk & Fineout-Overholt, 2005).

Another major force guiding this blending of the research process with EBP is the Association of Rehabilitation Nursing (ARN) research agenda (Jacelon, Pierce, & Buhrer, 2007), which identifies the following four high-priority research areas:

"1. Nursing and nursing-led interdisciplinary intervention to promote function in people of all ages and disability and/or chronic health problems

2. Experience of disability and/or chronic health problems for individuals and families across the lifespan

3. Rehabilitation in the changing healthcare system

4. The rehabilitation nursing profession" (p. 29).

To provide leadership and guidance to staff who are participating in research, using research findings in their practice, and promoting ARN's research agenda, rehabilitation nurses need a thorough grounding in the fundamentals of the research process and EBP that together form the foundation for rehabilitation nursing practice. To assist in developing this knowledge and skill, this chapter differentiates research from EBP, describes the importance of EBP to the advancement of rehabilitation nursing, identifies basic sources of research and EBP problems, describes ways to evaluate these problems, distinguishes levels of evidence, identifies ways of locating and then evaluating the literature, and concludes with specific examples of key elements to the application of EBP in rehabilitation nursing practice.

I. Difference Between Research and EBP

Although sometimes used interchangeably, *research* and *EBP* are distinctly different in terms of definitions and associated processes. It is important to recognize that research creates the foundation for EBP.

A. Nursing Research: This is the "systematic inquiry designed to develop knowledge about issues of importance to the nursing profession, including nursing practice, education, administration, and informatics" (Polit & Beck, 2004, p. 3). The research process is orderly and planned, investigates a specific problem, ends with an outcome in the form of results and recommendations, and contributes to our understanding of the phenomena in question (e.g., pain, anxiety).

1. Major contributions of nursing research to rehabilitation nursing:

a. Builds professionalism that defines the parameters of rehabilitation nursing

b. Provides accountability (e.g., establishes standards of care, addresses cost containment issues)

c. Validates the social relevance of nursing and promotes the efficacy of nursing in the changing healthcare arena

d. Expands the knowledge related to rehabilitation nursing (e.g., education, consultation, administration, theory, the basis for nursing decision making, evaluation of expected outcomes)

2. Paradigms of nursing research: The researcher's worldview (professional perspective) has a tremendous impact on

what is investigated, how the research question is stated, and what methods are selected to generate the knowledge. Two paradigms, worldviews, or frameworks have had an immense impact on nursing and other disciplines: the empirical paradigm and the naturalistic paradigm.

    a. The empirical paradigm, or quantitative perspective, purports that there is an objective, ordered, and nonrandom reality.

    b. The naturalistic paradigm, or qualitative perspective, holds that reality is subjective, mentally constructed by those participating in the research, and variable.

    c. Neither viewpoint is better than the other; however, the orientation that the researcher selects determines how the research is conducted.

3. Purposes of nursing research (Burns & Grove, 2005):

    a. Description: depicts the characteristics of individuals, groups, situations, and health states

    b. Exploration: investigates the dimensions of a phenomenon and helps to develop and refine research hypotheses

    c. Explanation: attempts to understand the underpinnings of phenomena and their interrelationships

    d. Prediction and control: forecasts how combinations of variables will operate in different circumstances involving different individuals

4. Limitations of research:

    a. General limitations such as inevitable study flaws (e.g., in design, sampling techniques, measurement of variables)

    b. Moral and ethical constraints, such as those related to informed consent, risks and benefits, freedom from harm or exploitation, the right to privacy, and fair treatment

    c. Complexity of human beings

    d. Measurement and data collection difficulties, such as concerns about the ability to adequately capture the phenomenon that is the focus of the research via quantitative or qualitative methods

    e. Obstacles to having complete control in the research situation, such as extraneous variables and the dynamic nature of the study phenomena (Burns & Grove, 2005)

B. EBP: EBP is a problem-solving approach to clinical practice that integrates:

    1. A systematic search and critical appraisal of the most relevant evidence to answer an important clinical question

    2. One's own clinical experience

    3. Patient values and preferences (Melnyk & Fineout-Overholt, 2005). In addition, patient situations are not static, diagnoses may be imprecise, the pathophysiology may be unclear, and patient responses to interventions may vary. EBP indicates that evidence is used to either support current practice or guide changes in practice. However, EBP is broader than research-based practice because the evidence is collected from research and from other sources such as expert opinions and incorporates clinical expertise along with patient preferences (Pravikoff & Donaldson, 2001). EBP is the result of obtaining comprehensive information pertaining to a specific topic, critically evaluating the evidence, and synthesizing the evidence in order to make conclusions about the state of the knowledge about a topic (Polit & Beck, 2004). Also, clinical judgment demands a precise and critical examination of the most current science and application of this evidence only when it is relevant to a particular patient's condition. Two aspects must be present when one uses evidence or current science to make a clinical decision (Melnyk & Fineout-Overholt, 2005):

    a. Validity (level and rigor) of the evidence.

    b. Applicability to the specific situation. Research evidence does not always have a linear relationship to practice. Patient characteristics, study circumstances, and measurement factors can dramatically affect the applicability of findings to another practice situation.

C. Terminology Related to Research and EBP: Other terms that are often confused with EBP are "best evidence" and "best practice." Research involving clinical trials generally is equated with best evidence, whereas best practice is practice that results in the best possible patient outcomes (Melnyk & Fineout-Overholt, 2005; Youngblut & Brooten, 2001).

    1. Clinical nursing research: "research designed to generate knowledge to guide nursing practice and to improve the health and quality of life of nurses' clients" (Polit & Beck, 2004, p. 3)

    2. Phenomena: observable facts or events that

reflect concepts (e.g., observation of a high prevalence of falls on a unit leads one to identify related concepts such as fatigue, vision changes, and environmental factors such as slippery floors)

3. Qualitative research: "the investigation of phenomena, typically in an in-depth and holistic fashion, through the collection of rich narrative materials using a flexible research design" (Polit & Beck, 2004, p. 729)

4. Quantitative research: "the investigation of phenomena using manipulation of numeric data with statistical analysis. Can be descriptive, predictive or causal" (Melnyk & Fineout-Overholt, 2005, p. 592).

5. Descriptive research: "research studies that have as their main objective the accurate portrayal of the characteristics of persons, situations, or groups, and/or the frequency with which certain phenomena occur" (Polit & Beck, 2004, p. 716)

6. Experimental research: "a study whose purpose is to test the effects of an intervention or treatment on selected outcomes. This is the strongest design for testing cause and effect relationships" (Melnyk & Fineout-Overholt, 2005, p. 587).

7. Randomized clinical trials: "a full experimental test of a new treatment, involving random assignment to treatment groups and, typically, a large and diverse sample [also known as a phase III clinical trial]" (Polit & Beck, 2004, p. 730)

8. Quasiexperimental research: "a type of experimental design that tests the effects of an intervention or treatment but lacks one or more characteristics of a true experiment (e.g., random assignment, a control or comparison group" (Melnyk & Fineout-Overholt, 2005, p. 593)

9. Evidence-based theory: "a theory that has been tested and supported through the accumulation of evidence from several studies" (Melnyk & Fineout-Overholt, 2005, p. 587)

10. Opinion leaders: "individuals who are typically highly knowledgeable and well respected in a system; as such, they are often able to influence change" (Melnyk & Fineout-Overholt, 2005, p. 591).

11. Research application: "the use of research knowledge, often based on a single study, in clinical practice" (Melnyk & Fineout-Overholt, 2005, p. 593)

II. Importance of EBP to Rehabilitation Nursing

Rehabilitation nurses function in a dynamic healthcare setting that demands constant decision making in complex circumstances. EBP promotes the use of the best current evidence in these important day-to-day patient care decisions. For nurses who function at the highest professional level and strive for the best patient outcomes, EBP is a cornerstone of practice. EBP has four components essential to the advancement of rehabilitation nursing practice (Law, 2002):

A. Awareness of the evidence that forms the foundation of rehabilitation nursing practice

B. Consultation with the patient to choose the care strategy that best fits the patient and his or her circumstances. Central to this behavior are excellent communication skills and the ability to educate and work with the patient and family to achieve a positive outcome.

C. Clinical judgment is essential in ascertaining the quality of the evidence and the applicability of the interventions to the particular patient and care situation.

D. Creativity and insight must be coupled with nursing skills to determine how the evidence fits and is implemented in specific practice situations.

III. Importance of Research and EBP Dissemination and Use in Rehabilitation Nursing Practice

The generation and refinement of nursing knowledge through research, whether quantitative or qualitative, is a complex process that is time-consuming and requires a special set of skills and resources. An important and equally time-intensive aspect of the research endeavor is disseminating this newly obtained knowledge to other professionals through publication or presentation. Even for very motivated and well-educated researchers, dissemination of research and use of it in practice pose a special set of challenges. However, researchers must publish and present their findings in nursing and other professional forums. Ideally, the results will be published in refereed journals such as *Rehabilitation Nursing* or other professional journals that are widely recognized nationally or internationally.

For EBP to exist, it is imperative that researchers consistently disseminate their findings, making the research-generated information available to practitioners for scrutiny and application in their practice settings. Unfortunately, the literature suggests that the time between generation and implementation of research findings can be very long. For instance, in the case of research evidence indicating that aspirin could reduce the likelihood of myocardial infarction and stroke, it took almost 17 years for the U.S. Food and Drug Administration to approve this preventive use (Marwick, 1997).

A. Barriers to Research and EBP Use (Grol & Wensing, 2004; Omery & Williams, 1999)

1. Research findings may not address pressing clinical problems.

2. Findings are not communicated in a form that practitioners can readily understand.

3. Practitioners do not feel confident in reading research reports and articles.

4. Practitioners do not know how to apply research findings to practice.

5. A variety of models exist that describe how research dissemination and use should occur:

   a. Rogers's (1995) theory of diffusion of innovations

   b. Havelock's (1973) linker systems, describing how innovation connects to the user

   c. Stetler's (1994) model of research use

B. Specific Ways Rehabilitation Nurses Can Participate in Research and EBP Dissemination and Use

   1. Communicate and use the findings of nursing research through publications (journals, newsletters), posters, paper presentations, nursing grand rounds, and e-mail of research abstracts.

   2. Read and critique research articles to determine strengths, limitations, and applicability to your practice situation.

   3. Start or participate in a journal club.

   4. Participate in a research team.

   5. Replicate a study already reported in the literature.

   6. Promote excitement and a research-friendly atmosphere that encourages use of research and EBP.

   7. Form nursing committees to discuss the current state of research and EBP related to a common patient problem and, if needed, ways to overcome barriers to use of current knowledge and practice guidelines.

IV. Sources of Research Problems and Evidence-Based Problems

A. Common Sources of Research Problems and Evidence-Based Problems

   1. Experiences in the rehabilitation setting

   2. Unanswered questions in the literature

   3. Theories or conceptual frameworks that stimulate quandaries

   4. Outside sources such as agencies, patients, families, or other healthcare professionals who express concerns related to quality of care

Once a problem has been identified that sparks the researcher's interest, the topic must be broken down into a list of questions that can be transformed into researchable problem statements. The difficulty for most researchers is that the questions or hypotheses (relationship statements of concepts) are too broad and not researchable. Therefore, developing precise questions is a vital step in the research process. In addition, after the problem is stated succinctly, it must be evaluated to determine whether the next step in terms of performing the research is appropriate.

B. Determining the Significance of the Problem and Its Relevance to Rehabilitation Nursing

   1. Based on the literature and other forms of available knowledge, determine whether this problem is worth investigating further.

   2. Determine whether the problem will expand or improve rehabilitation nursing practice.

C. Assessing the Researchability of the Problem

   1. Avoid value-laden questions and problems.

   2. Determine whether it is possible to obtain the data to examine the questions emerging from the problem, whether quantitatively or qualitatively framed.

   3. Determine the feasibility of the research by giving early consideration to factors such as time, place, space, and resource materials, which can help identify practical problems such as financial constraints, theoretical problems, control of extraneous variables, or ethical issues that influence the researcher's decision about conducting the study.

   4. Estimate the time needed to complete the project.

   5. Assess the availability of subjects (e.g., access and willingness of people to participate).

   6. Determine what sort of cooperation from others (e.g., institutions and agencies, permission of the study population or their guardians or parents) is needed.

   7. Determine what facilities and equipment are needed (e.g., availability of office or interview space, computers, printers).

   8. Estimate financial resources, including funding from a variety of public or private international, national, regional, and local sources.

   9. Assess the experience of the researchers, including knowledge about and experience in executing all aspects of the investigation.

   10. Address ethical considerations related to working with human subjects, including informed consent, freedom from harm,

privacy, anonymity, confidentiality, and voluntary participation:

a. The principal investigator is responsible for ensuring that human rights are not violated.

b. All people involved in the research, such as the data collectors, have the same ethical responsibilities as the principal investigator.

V. Quantitative and Qualitative Research Designs That Build the Knowledge of EBP

Quantitative and qualitative research and mixed methods that incorporate both approaches create the scientific knowledge to expand and refine practice and form the foundation of EBP. This section is a brief overview of major distinctions between the two research paradigms and key elements to consider when examining the quality of the evidence generated and its generalizability or transferability to your practice situation. Even excellent research that is well designed but targeted at a different patient population may not be transferable to your practice setting. During scrutiny of all reported research studies, nurses must evaluate both the strengths and limitations of the study or studies pertaining to a topic of interest. This critique is a pivotal aspect of EBP, along with consideration of the clinician's expertise and the patient's preferences and values.

A. Quantitative Research Designs (Burns & Grove, 2005; Creswell, 2002; Polit & Beck, 2004): Table 22-1 describes the most common quantitative research designs.

B. Evaluating Quantitative Studies:

1. Quantitative research reports can be evaluated on several criteria (Polit & Beck, 2004; Rempher & Silkman, 2007):

a. Problem statement, research question, and study purpose
    1) Is the problem statement identified and clear?
    2) Are key study concepts identified?
    3) Does the posed research question fill a void in nursing knowledge or a theory or model?
    4) Does the research problem clearly flow from the stated research purpose?
    5) Are the who, what, where, when, and why clearly presented in the research question?
    6) Do the research problem and question flow coherently from the stated purpose of the study?
    7) Does the purpose statement indicate the study population and the dependent and independent variables?

8) Is the research hypothesis measurable and justifiable?

b. Literature review and conceptual or theoretical framework
    1) Does the literature give the reader an orientation to what is already known about the topic?
    2) Is the literature current, and does it include classic studies on the topic? The majority of the reported studies should be less than 5 years old. In addition, current literature should be related to the historical research.
    3) How does the current literature address knowledge gaps or reflect an improvement in how data are collected or consideration of other variables not studied in the past that could affect study outcomes?
    4) Is the significance of the problem being studied thoroughly explained?
    5) Is it clear what must be done to fill the void in current literature?
    6) If the researcher has provided a conceptual model or theory to guide the study design and data interpretation, does it coherently fit the problem and question under investigation?
    7) Are the research variables thoroughly defined?

c. Sample selection, methods, and design
    1) Is it clear what method was used to select the sample?
    2) Was the process of subject recruitment described?
    3) Is it clear what the inclusion and exclusion criteria were for subject selection?
    4) Is the sample size appropriate and representative of the population of interest?
    5) Is the research design the most rigorous design to address the hypothesis or research questions?
    6) Did the researcher provide a rationale for the choice of design?
    7) Is the sample size appropriate to address the hypothesis or research question?
    8) Was a power analysis used to determine the sample size, and does it appear justified?
    9) Does the data collection procedure avoid bias?
    10) If there was an intervention, was enough detail given to replicate the study?

Table 22-1. Types of Quantitative Research Designs

Type of Design	Description	Strengths	Limitations	Examples
Experimental research	A type of research that predicts and controls phenomena, examining causality: At least one variable is manipulated. Control exists over the experimental situation. Subjects are selected randomly.	The most effective way to test hypotheses The most powerful and best-controlled research	Not all variables can be manipulated. Manipulation can create ethical problems. Artificiality is problematic. Generalizability can be limited.	Pretest–posttest design Solomon four-group design Factorial design Repeated-measures design
Quasiexperimental research	One independent variable is manipulated. Lacks at least one of the other two properties that characterize a true experiment.	Practical Feasible Generalizable	Control is lacking, so other hypotheses may exist.	Nonequivalent control group (no randomization) Time series One-group, pretest–posttest design
Nonexperimental research	Researcher collects data without introducing any treatment or changes.			Ex post facto Descriptive research Retrospective and prospective studies Survey research Evaluation research Need assessments Meta-analysis Delphi survey Methodological research Content analysis study

11) Are the appropriate statistical procedures used to address the hypotheses?

12) Is a rationale provided for the use of the selected statistical tests?

  d. Human rights protection

    1) Was information included that addressed the protection of human subjects?

    2) Was a human subject review of some kind conducted?

    3) Is it clear that the study benefits outweighed the potential participant risk?

  e. Results, discussion, and limitations

    1) Is it clear how the statistical findings relate to the research questions or hypotheses and to the conceptual or theoretical framework?

    2) Were tables used to organize large amounts of data?

    3) Were limitations to the study discussed?

    4) Were important results discussed?

    5) Were the data interpretations consistent with the reported results?

    6) Did the researcher describe the implications to practice and future research?

2. Approaches to critiquing research literature vary. A more simplistic approach to evaluating quantitative research studies includes the following 3 questions, identified by O'Rourke and Booth (2000):

  a. Are the study results valid? This refers to whether the results of the study were obtained from rigorous methods and not compromised by bias, anything that would distort the findings, confounding variables, or some unknown variable not investigated (Melnyk & Fineout-Overholt, 2005).

  b. Are the results of the study reliable? This pertains to whether "the effects have sufficient influence on practice, clinically and statistically (i.e., the results can be counted on to make a difference when clinicians apply them to their practices)" (Melnyk & Fineout-Overholt, 2005, p. 83).

  c. Will the results help locally? Are the problems dealt with in the study sufficiently comparable to my setting to extrapolate the findings (O'Rourke & Booth, 2000)?

C. Characteristics of Qualitative Research Studies:

1. Are descriptive or theory building, can be used to develop hypotheses, and can be used to study phenomena about which little is known

2. Consist of a design that emerges from the data (i.e., questions may change, or the focus may be refined during data collection). See Tables 22-2, 22-3, and 22-4 for design specifics and differences depending on the qualitative approach selected.

3. Have a purposive sample: Participants are selected because they have some characteristic in common.

4. Allow collection of data to occur in the natural or field setting: Data are collected in the participant's home or natural context.

5. Involve the researcher closely with the participants:

    a. The researcher is immersed in the data.

    b. The researcher's goal is an in-depth understanding of the phenomena under study.

6. Entail holistic data collection (e.g., interviews, observation, focus groups, observation of participants)

7. Use inductive data analysis, which proceeds from the specific to the general

8. Use a narrative approach to reporting research outcomes: Lengthy, rich descriptions of the data are reported.

D. Evaluating Qualitative Research Reports (Polit & Beck, 2004; Rempher & Silkman, 2007): The focus of this section is a general narrative

Type	Description
Table 22-2. Types of Qualitative Research	
Grounded theory	Develops theories and theoretical propositions that are based on real-world observations; focuses on process
Ethnography	Focuses on the culture of the people being studied
Phenomenology	Considers the lived experience of the people being studied
Historical research	Explores the past and applies findings to present and future
Case studies	In-depth studies on one particular case
Field studies	Examine people and how they function in real life

literature approach that can be performed by nurses at all practice levels. It is not representative of a systematic review, integrative review, or meta-analysis but identifies key questions to assess the overall quality of a quantitative and qualitative study.

1. Problem statement, research question, and study purpose

    a. Is the problem statement identified and clear?

    b. Are key study concepts identified?

    c. Does the posed research question fill a void in nursing knowledge or a theory or model?

    d. Does the research problem clearly flow from the stated research purpose?

    e. Are the who, what, where, when, and why clearly presented in the research question?

    f. Do the research problem and question

Table 22-3. Methodological Considerations Involving Qualitative Research

Methodological Considerations	Item	Description
Sample size and selection		Depends on the type of qualitative design selected.
		Subjects are added until no new information is available (saturation).
Data organization and reduction	Preliminary activities	Listen to tapes to make sure transcription is accurate.
		Make several copies of transcript.
		Add comments about transcript (e.g., observations, tone of voice, feelings of researcher).
Data organization and reduction	Development of categories and codes	Convert data into smaller, more manageable units.
		Look for patterns in transcripts.
		Organize transcripts.
		Label materials.
		Develop definitions for each category of materials.
		Look for relationships between the materials.
Data organization and reduction	Analytic procedures	Summarize conclusions of the materials.
		Share the information at conferences or in journals.

Table 22-4. Trustworthiness of Qualitative Research

Establishing Trustworthiness of Qualitative Research	Description
Credibility	The research is authentic, truthful, believable; similar to internal validity.
Transferability	The research is generalizable, fits the data; similar to external validity.
Confirmability	Bias was minimized; another researcher could logically follow the process and procedures used; similar to objectivity.
Dependability	Results are consistent over time; methods were sound; similar to reliability.

flow coherently from the stated purpose of the study?

   g. Does the purpose statement indicate the study population and the dependent and independent variables?

   h. Is the research hypothesis measurable and justifiable?

2. Literature review and conceptual or theoretical framework

   a. Does the literature give the reader an orientation to what is already known about the topic?

   b. Is the literature current (with a majority of studies in the last 5 years), and does it include classic studies on the topic? Also, is current literature related to the historical research?

   c. How does the current literature address knowledge gaps or reflect an improvement in how data are collected or consideration of other variables not studied in the past that could affect the study outcomes?

   d. Is the significance of the problem being studied thoroughly explained?

   e. Is it clear what must be done to fill the void in current literature?

   f. If the researcher has provided a conceptual model or theory to guide the study design and data interpretation, does it coherently fit the problem and question under investigation?

   g. Are the research variables clearly defined?

3. Sample selection, methods, and design

   a. Is it clear what method was used to select the sample?

   b. Was the process of subject recruitment described?

   c. Is it clear what the inclusion and exclusion criteria were for subject selection?

   d. Is the sample size appropriate and representative of the population of interest?

   e. Is the research design the most rigorous design to address the hypothesis or research questions?

   f. Did the researcher provide a rationale for the choice of design?

   g. Does the selected qualitative research design fit with the type of qualitative research being performed?

   h. Does the sample size correspond to the type of qualitative research performed?

   i. Does the data analysis approach fit with the type of qualitative research performed?

   j. Has data quality been assessed according to the tradition of the qualitative research used?

4. Human rights protection

   a. Was information included that addressed the protection of human subjects?

   b. Was a human subject review of some kind conducted?

   c. Is it clear that the study benefits outweighed the potential participant risk?

5. Results, discussion, and limitations

   a. Are the findings clearly presented, and do they reflect the data gathered?

   b. Is it clear how the analysis of the qualitative data was performed, and is it consistent with the type of qualitative research performed?

   c. Is it clear how data were assessed, and was the assessment performed appropriately?

   d. Do the results relate back to the research questions or hypotheses?

   e. Do the results relate back to the literature or theoretical framework used?

   f. Were the limitations of the research discussed?

   g. Were the important results discussed?

   h. Were the data interpretations consistent with the reported results?

   i. Did the researcher describe the implications of the research findings to practice and future research?

VI. Levels of Evidence

The evidence on which EBP is based must be the result of sound, well-conducted studies using the appropriate design (whether quantitative or qualitative) that provides high-quality data to answer the research questions or hypotheses. It is imperative for the nurse to be able to critically evaluate research when performing a literature review on a specific topic.

A. Levels of Evidence: In the literature, there are a variety of descriptions of how to label levels of evidence. In this chapter, the levels of evidence described by Melnyk and Fineout-Overholt (2005, p. 10) are used:

"Level I: Evidence from a systematic review or meta-analysis of all relevant randomized controlled trials (RCTs), or evidence-based clinical practice guidelines based on systematic reviews of RCTs.

Level II: Evidence obtained from at least one well-designed randomized clinical trial.

Level III: Evidence obtained from well-designed controlled trials without randomization.

Level IV: Evidence from well-designed case control and cohort studies.

Level V: Evidence from systematic reviews of descriptive and qualitative studies.

Level VI: Evidence from a single descriptive or qualitative study.

Level VII: Evidence from the opinion of authorities and/or reports of expert committees."

B. Melnyk's 5 Critical Steps to EBP:

1. Ask the burning clinical questions (PICO components):
   a. P: patient population of interest
   b. I: intervention of interest
   c. C: comparison of interest
   d. O: outcome of interest

2. Collect the most relevant and best evidence: "Critically appraise the evidence. Integrate all evidence with one's clinical expertise, patient preferences, and values in making a practice decision or change. Evaluate the practice decision or change" (Melnyk & Fineout-Overholt, 2005, p. 9).

3. Critically appraise the evidence:
   a. What were the study results?
   b. Are the study results valid (sound scientific methods used)?
   c. Will the study findings facilitate care?

4. Integrate the evidence: Can the study evidence be incorporated into the clinician's practice, given the clinician's expertise, the clinical resources available, and the patient's preferences?

5. Evaluate the effectiveness of the evidence-based interventions for a particular patient or care situation.

VII. Locating the Evidence

There are many resources nurses can use when searching for evidence on a topic. More information is becoming available online, and it is important to evaluate the evidence online as thoroughly as evidence in print.

A. Searching the Evidence:

1. Melnyk and Fineout-Overholt (2005) identified the following essential steps for a search strategy:
   a. Step 1: Formulate a well-built clinical question without jargon or ambiguity.
   b. Step 2: Determine the type of database that is appropriate for the question.
   c. Step 3: Determine the type of study design that would best answer the question.
   d. Step 4: Enter a subject heading and or text word search, guided by the PICO components of the question.
   e. Step 5: Begin combining searches to find relevant evidence.
   f. Step 6: Further restrict combined searches for study design, methods, indicators of clinical meaningfulness, or other appropriate, available limits. Consider limiting the search to English language and human subjects, depending on the question and the searcher.
   g. Step 7: Apply a priori inclusion and exclusion criteria to studies gathered in the search to find the best available evidence (Melnyk & Fineout-Overholt, 2005, p. 51).

2. Online journals are accessible 24 hours a day and can include articles that are longer than those published in print journals. Their goal is to expedite dissemination so the information can get to the reader quickly. They must be subjected to the same critique as research reports in print journals (Pravikoff & Donaldson, 2001).
   a. The CINAHL index of nursing literature "contains studies in nursing, allied health, and biomedicine" (Melnyk & Fineout-Overholt, 2005, p. 41). The CINAHL database is available at http://www.cinahl.com.
   b. Cochrane Central Register of Controlled

Trials is "a bibliography of controlled trials identified by contributors to the Cochrane Collaboration and others" (Melnyk & Fineout-Overholt, 2005, p. 585).

3. Cochrane Database of Methodology Reviews "contains full text of systematic reviews of empirical methodological studies prepared by the Cochrane Empirical Methodological Studies Methods Group" (Melnyk & Fineout-Overholt, 2005, p. 585).

4. Cochrane Database of Systematic Reviews "contains reviews that are highly structured and systematic with evidence included or excluded on the basis of explicit quality criteria, to minimize bias" (Melnyk & Fineout-Overholt, 2005, p. 585).

   a. Cochrane Methodology Register: "a bibliography of articles and books on the science of research synthesis" (Melnyk & Fineout-Overholt, 2005, p. 585).

   b. Clinical Practice Guidelines: "systematically developed statements to assist clinicians and patients in making decisions about care; ideally the guidelines consist of a systematic review of the literature, in conjunction with consensus of a group of expert decision-makers, including administrators, policy-makers, clinicians, and consumers who consider the evidence and make recommendations" (Melnyk & Fineout-Overholt, 2005, p. 585).

   c. MEDLINE: "studies in medicine, nursing, dentistry, psychiatry, veterinary, and allied health. It is produced by the National Library of Medicine and is available free of charge through the PubMed search engine" (Melnyk & Fineout-Overholt, 2005 p. 43), available at http://www.ncbi.nlm.nih.gov/sites/entrez.

   d. The National Guideline Clearinghouse houses summaries of clinical practice guidelines and information on their development. A condensed version of the guideline and a link to the full clinical practice guideline are available at http://www.guideline.gov (Melnyk & Fineout-Overholt, 2005, p. 43).

   e. PsycINFO: "This database of scholarly literature in behavioral sciences and mental health contains more than 1 million citations. Professionals in psychology and related fields such as psychiatry, education, neuroscience, nursing, and other healthcare disciplines can find relevant evidence in this data base to answer specific clinical questions" (Melnyk & Fineout-Overholt, 2005, p. 45). Their Web site is http://www.apa.org/psycinfo/about/.

B. Outcomes of the Search: One of the most difficult decisions for the researcher to make is to decide when enough literature is enough.

   1. Use the most current literature for the search. Begin with the most recent 5 years.

   2. Incorporate the classic literature related to a topic. If you see a researcher's name in all the studies you read, and many studies refer to the seminal work by a certain author, then it is important to include that author in the literature you are using. For example, anyone working on the concept of locus of control would have to include Rotter, who conducted the seminal work on locus of control in 1966. If you did not refer to that body of knowledge, then your review would be incomplete.

VIII. **Assessing the Evidence for EBP**

A. Four Types of Literature Reviews:

   1. Narrative review:

      a. "A review that includes published papers that support an author's point of view; serves as a general background discussion for a particular issue" (Melnyk & Fineout-Overholt, 2005, p. 115)

      b. Not systematic in its approach to identifying articles and papers

   2. Integrative review:

      a. "A review of research that amasses comprehensive information on a topic, weighs pieces of evidence, and integrates information to draw conclusions about the state of knowledge" (Polit & Beck, 2004, p. 721)

      b. Does not have a summary statistic because the sample sizes cannot be summarized because of the heterogeneity of studies and their samples (Melnyk & Fineout-Overholt, 2005)

   3. Systematic review: "a summary of evidence typically conducted by an expert or expert panel on a particular topic, that uses a rigorous process (to minimize bias) for identifying, appraising, and synthesizing studies to answer a specific clinical question and draw conclusions about the data gathered" (Melnyk & Fineout-Overholt, 2005, p. 594).

4. Meta-analysis: "a statistical approach to synthesizing the results of a number of studies that produces a larger sample size and thus greater power to determine the true magnitude of an effect" (Melnyk & Fineout-Overholt, 2005, p. 115). A meta-analysis provides a single effect measure of all of the summarized study results (Melnyk & Fineout-Overholt, 2005).

In the 1980s and 1990s many articles and theories were written about EBP. Several centers throughout the country have focused on the promotion of EBP. For the purposes of this chapter, we use Melnyk's method for discussing EBP (Melnyk & Fineout-Overholt, 2005).

B. Systematic Reviews: These "provide summaries of the results of evidence-based healthcare, which can be made available to clinicians, policy decision makers, and patients" (Law, 2002, p. 110). A systematic review compiles many studies and relates them to a specific research question. It is the "most rigorous approach to minimization of bias" (Melnyk & Fineout-Overholt, 2005, p. 115).

1. Phases:
   a. Phase 1: deciding what clinical question to propose.
   b. Phase 2: determining how the validity of the studies will be assessed.
   c. Phase 3: research related to proposed question.
   d. Phase 4: assessment of studies.
   e. Phase 5: validity of studies is examined.
   f. Phase 6: data extraction.
   g. Phase 7: overview of studies and synthesis of results.
   h. Phases 8–10 include a peer review (Melnyk & Fineout-Overholt, 2005, p. 116).

2. Example of a systematic review in the literature: The citation for this systematic review is Pearson et al. (2006). What follows is a description of how the various phases of this approach pertain to Pearson's article, which represents a review of a topic with many facets. All phases are applicable to any systematic review.
   a. Phase 1: deciding what clinical question to propose:

   Question: What is the best available evidence on the effect of team characteristics, processes, structure, and composition in the context of collaborative practice among nursing teams to create a healthy work environment?
   b. Phase 2: determining how the validity of the studies will be assessed:

Search strategy was to find published and unpublished studies in the English language. Inclusion and exclusion criteria were described in terms of type of studies (qualitative and quantitative), type of participants, type of interventions (nursing staff outcomes, patient outcomes, organizational and system outcomes).

c. Phase 3: research related to proposed question. A 3-step search approach was used:
   1) Initial limited search of Medline and CINAHL databases to identify search terms followed by an analysis of text words contained in the title and abstract to describe the article.
   2) More extensive search using all the identified keywords and index terms:
      a) Search of the reference list led to the identification of more studies.
      b) The final databases searched included CINAHL (1982–2005), Medline, other nonindexed citations and OVID, Cochrane Library, Database of Abstracts of Reviews of Effectiveness, PsycINFO, Embase, Sociological Abstracts, Econ Lit, ABI/Inform, Education Resources Information Center (ERIC) and PubMed.

d. Phase 4: assessment of studies. Studies that met the inclusion criteria were identified and grouped into the following categories: experimental studies, descriptive, descriptive–correlational, interpretive and clinical research, cost minimization studies, and textual and opinion papers. All results were assessed by two independent reviewers for methodological quality, and the review was completed by the System for the Unified Management of the Review and Assessment of Information (SUMARI) package.

e. Phase 5: validity of studies is examined. The 2 independent reviewers determined that the examined studies fit the identified inclusion and exclusion criteria.

f. Phase 6: data extraction. Results of the methodological assessment indicated quantitative and qualitative data. The quantitative data were extracted using a work based on the Cochrane Collaboration and Canter for Reviews and Dissemination (Pearson et al., 2006, pp. 154–157), and qualitative data were extracted using the SUMARI package (Pearson et al., 2006, pp. 158–159).

g. Phase 7: overview of studies and synthesis of results of studies. Data were synthesized quantitatively and qualitatively involving several instruments and software packages that were clearly described (Pearson et al., 2006, pp. 121–122).

h. Phases 8–10 include a peer review involving 2 independent reviewers.

3. Checklist for appraising the evidence (Melnyk & Fineout-Overholt, 2005):

a. Does the review address a research question that is clear?

b. Are the inclusion and exclusion criteria for subjects plainly stated?

c. Are the interventions in the studies similar?

d. Are the outcome measures similar between the studies reviewed?

e. Is it reasonable to combine the studies to synthesize the designs and results?

f. What measures of exposure or occurrence are reported in each study?

g. Are the magnitude and precision of the effects (outcomes) reported?

h. Are study participants in the respective studies similar to your patients?

i. Are all important outcomes of the studies reported?

j. Would you consider a change in your practice based on the results presented in the systematic review? Why or why not?

4. Additional resources and examples:

a. Forbes (2003)

b. Peacock and Forbes (2003)

C. Meta-Analysis: A meta-analysis is the "statistical method used to obtain a single-effect measure of the summarized results of all studies included in a review" (Melnyk & Fineout-Overholt, 2005, p. 119). A meta-analysis is an analysis of several analyses and therefore contributes to building evidence. Although a meta-analysis provides a simple and precise estimate of the benefit and harm of the studies examined, it should be used with caution. In addition, sources of bias and differences may exist between the various clinical research trials, and the conclusions recommended as describing the "average" or "typical" patient may actually be unhelpful in clinical practice (Law, 2002, p. 120). The following example of a meta-analysis is from Hodgkinson, Koch, Nay, and Kim (2006).

1. Purpose: To present the best available evidence for strategies to prevent or reduce the frequency of mediation errors associated with prescribing, dispensing and administering medications in older adults (65 and older) who are in acute, subacute, and residential settings

2. Search strategy: PubMed, Embase, Current Contents, Cochrane Library

3. Selection criteria: Systematic reviews, RCTs, other research methods such as non-random controlled trials, longitudinal studies, cohort/case-control studies, descriptive studies evaluating strategies to reduce medication errors

4. Data collection and analysis: Tabulated relative risks, odds ratios, mean differences, and associated 95% confidence intervals calculated from comparative studies. All other information provided in a summary format.

5. Results of the meta-analysis: Most common medication errors occurred in hospitals and were medication ordering errors, dispensing, administration, and medication recording errors. Contributing factors associated with these hospital errors are largely unreported. In the community, there were also improper drugs ordered, administration errors, and incorrectly ordered doses.

6. The evidence from this meta-analysis revealed common medication errors, but the assumption cannot be made that this always happens.

D. Limitations of Systematic and Meta-Analyses Pertaining to the Assessment Process and Outcomes:

1. A disadvantage to systematic reviews is that the information cannot be generalized. A systematic review is so detailed that it can be applied only to the specific clinical question that was proposed.

2. A meta-analysis may be detrimental when the studies are too different to combine in a statistically meaningful way (Melnyk & Fineout-Overholt, 2005).

IX. Using the Evidence: Translating Research into Practice

Although EBP will advance the quality of care for patients and the practice of rehabilitation nursing, the use of EBP has lagged far behind expectations. Unfortunately, on average it takes 17 years for new knowledge generated by RCTs, the highest level of evidence, to be incorporated into clinical practice, and even then its application is highly irregular (Balas & Boren, 2000; Institute of Medicine, 2001). Additional research involving countries such as the United States and the Netherlands indicates that in all practice settings at least 30% of patients do not receive care according to current scientific evidence, and another 20% or more of the provided care is not needed or is potentially harmful to patients (Grol & Grimshaw, 2003). New strategies and models must be developed and implemented to increase the speed with which scientific evidence is instituted in clinical settings. In addition, rehabilitation nurses and researchers need to remain aware of ARN's research agenda (Jacelon et al., 2007), which identifies focus areas to be developed in our specialty.

A. Translating Research into Practice and Policy: Cosponsored by the Agency of Healthcare Research and Quality and the National Cancer Institute, TRIPP (2006) was formed to close the gap between knowledge and practice (between what we know and what we do) and to ensure continued improvement of health care. TRIPP's overriding purpose is to facilitate the translation of research findings into sustainable improvements in health outcomes, quality, effectiveness, efficiency, and cost effectiveness of care.

B. Approach: Although there is not uniform consensus on how to translate evidence into clinical practice, the following steps capture the essence of a suggested approach:

1. Assess the need for change in practice.
2. Link the problem with interventions and outcomes.
3. Synthesize the best evidence.
4. Design a change in practice.
5. Implement and evaluate practice.
6. Integrate and maintain the practice change.

C. Development of EBP in Rehabilitation Nursing:

1. Within rehabilitation nursing, EBP has been identified as critical to present and future practice. This commitment to EBP is reflected in ARN's publications and practice standards. Although great strides in knowledge have occurred, many areas of EBP in rehabilitation nursing are in their infancy. Specific gaps identified on the ARN Web site were "nursing and nursing-led interdisciplinary interventions to promote function in people of all ages with disability and/or chronic health problems, experience of disability and/or chronic health problems for individuals and families across the lifespan, rehabilitation in the changing healthcare system, the rehabilitation nursing profession."

2. Rehabilitation nurses must become EBP practitioners. Whether they are expert rehabilitation nurses or new nurses in this specialty area, all should strive to identify and evaluate current scientific information that can affect practice. Also, EBP practitioners need to foster adoption and sustainability of EBP and educate other nurses and health professionals about its value. A key component of successful EBP outcomes is the recognition and initiation of interventions at the individual and organizational level that begin to consider the interaction between the individual, social context, organizational, and economic factors that affect EBP.

X. Key Factors Affecting Implementation and Adoption of EBP (Grol & Wensing, 2004; Law, 2002; Melnyk & Fineout-Overholt, 2005)

A. Individual Context

1. Cognitive: thinking, decoding, benefits and risks
2. Educational: learning needs and styles
3. Attitudes: social norms, self-efficacy, perceived behavioral control, beliefs
4. Motivation: stages with varied features and barriers

B. Social Context

1. Social learning: incentives, feedback, reinforcement, observed behavior of others
2. Social network and influence: value and culture of network, opinions of key people
3. Patient influence: perceived patient expectations and behaviors
4. Leadership: style, commitment of leader, and type of power

C. Organization and Economic Context

1. Innovativeness of the organization: specialization, professionalism, functional differentiation
2. Quality management: culture, leadership, processes within the organization, customer focus

3. Complexity: interaction between parts and complex behavioral patterns between various levels of the organization

4. Organizational learning: capacity and continuous organizational development and learning supported and implemented

5. Economic: incentives, rewards, reimbursement

D. Examples of Prominent EBP Clinical Outcomes: What follows is a description of common clinical outcomes that promote the use and sustainability of EBP at the individual, institutional, and national level. It must be emphasized that evidence is dynamic and continues to expand, leading to revisions in rehabilitation practice and care standards.

1. Clinical practice guidelines (CPGs) are "systematically developed statements that assist practitioner and patient decisions about appropriate health care for specific clinical circumstances" (Law, 2002, p. 196). They may be based on "expert opinion/consensus and/or evidence-based practice as identified by research" (Law, 2002, p. 196). An example of a clinical practice guideline is the "Guideline for Radiography of the Ankle and Foot (Ottawa Ankle Rule)" (Law, 2002, p. 198).

2. Algorithms are "written guidelines to stepwise evaluation and management strategies that require observations to be made, decisions to be considered, actions to be taken, and basically CPGs arranged in a decision-tree format" (Law, 2002, p. 201). A good example of algorithms would be found in the Inpatient Rehabilitation Facility Patient Assessment Instrument manual and scoring of the Functional Independence Measure™ instrument.

3. A clinical pathway is "a cause and effect grid or framework, which identifies expected measurable patient/client outcomes (or behaviors) against a timeline for a specific case-type or group" (Law, 2002, p. 203). Interventions commonly included in a clinical pathway are consultations and referral; assessments and observations; tests, treatments, measurements, and diagnostics; nutrition, medications, activity, and mobility; safety, patient/client, and family education/teaching; and discharge planning and follow-up.

4. Healthcare policies and laws are derived from evidence. Legislators cannot propose legislation without having the necessary substantiation, based on various sources of evidence (Melnyk & Fineout-Overholt, 2005). According to Melnyk and Fineout-Overholt (2005), the level of evidence required for health policy and lawmaking is Level VII: expert opinions of researchers and clinicians.

References

Balas, E.A., & Boren, S.A. (2002). Managing clinical knowledge for health care improvement. In *Yearbook of medical informatics*. Bethesda, MD: National Library of Medicine.

Burns, N., & Grove, S.K. (2005). *The practice of nursing research conduct, critique, & utilization*. Philadelphia: W.B. Saunders.

Creswell, J.W. (2002). *Research design: Qualitative, quantitative and mixed method approaches* (2nd ed.). Thousand Oaks, CA: Sage.

Forbes, D.A. (2003). An example of the use of systematic reviews. *Western Journal of Nursing Research, 25*(2), 179–192.

Grol, R. & Grimshaw, J. (2003). From the evidence to best practice effective implementation of change in patient's care. *Lancet, 362*, 1225–1230.

Grol, R. & Wensing, M, (2004). What drives changes? Barriers to and incentives for achieving evidence-based practice. *Medical Journal of Australia, 180.* 557–560.

Havelock, R.G. (1973). *The change agent's guide to innovation in education*. Englewood Cliffs, NJ: Educational Technology in Education.

Hodgkinson, B., Koch, S., Nay, R., & Kim, N. (2006). Strategies to reduce medication errors with reference to older adults. *International Journal of Evidence-Based Healthcare, 4*(1), 2–41.

Institute of Medicine. (2001). *Crossing the quality chasm.* Washington, DC: National Academies Press.

Jacelon, C.S., Pierce, L.L., & Buhrer, R. (2007). Revision of the rehabilitation nursing research agenda. *Rehabilitation Nursing, 32*(1), 23–30.

Law, M. (2002). *Evidence-based rehabilitation: A guide to practice*. Thorofare, NJ: SLACK Incorporated.

Marwick, C. (1997). Aspirin's role in prevention now official. *Journal of the American Medical Association, 277*(9), 701–702.

Melnyk, B.M., & Fineout-Overholt, E. (2005). *Evidence-based practice in nursing & healthcare: A guide to best practice.* Philadelphia: Lippincott Williams & Wilkins.

Omery, A., & Williams, R.P. (1999). An appraisal of research utilization across the United States. *Journal of Nursing Administration, 29*(12), 50–56.

O'Rourke, A., & Booth, A. (2000). *Unit 4: Critical appraisal and using the literature.* Research Training Programme Literature Reviews and Critical Appraisal Module. School of Health and Related Research, University of Sheffield. Retrieved January 21, 2007, from http://www.shef.ac.uk/~scharr/ir/units/

Peacock, S., & Forbes, D. (2003). Interventions for caregivers of person with dementia: Systematic review. *Focus on Gerontology, 35*(4), 89–107.

Pearson, A., Porritt, A., Doran, D., Vincent, L., Craig, D., Tucker, D., et al. (2006). A comprehensive systematic review of the evidence on the structure, process, characteristics and composition of a nursing team that fosters a healthy work environment. *International Journal of Evidence Based Healthcare, 4*, 118–159.

Polit, D.F., & Beck, C.T. (2004). *Nursing research: Principles and methods* (7th ed.). Philadelphia: Lippincott Williams & Wilkins.

Pravikoff, D.S., & Donaldson, N.E. (2001). Online journals: Access and support for evidence-based practice. *AACN Clinical Issues, 12*(4), 586–596.

Rempher, K.J., & Silkman, C. (2007). How to appraise quantitative research articles. *American Nurse Today, 2*(1), 26–28.

Rogers, E.M. (1995). *Diffusion of innovations* (4th ed.). New York: Free Press.

Stetler, C.B. (1994). Refinement of the Stetler/Marram model of application of research findings to practice. *Nursing Outlook, 42*(1), 15–25.

Translating Research into Practice and Policy (TRIPP). (2006). Retrieved October 30, 2006, from http://www.epc3.net/TRIPP06/conference/index.html

Youngblut, J.M., & Brooten, D. (2001). Evidence-based nursing practice: Why is it important. *AACN Clinical Issues, 12*(4), 468–476.

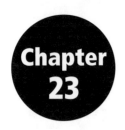

Changes in American Health Care and the Implications for Rehabilitation Nurses

Teresa L. Cervantez Thompson, PhD RN CRRN-A

Rehabilitation has moved from its era of research and development to one of scrutiny. In prior years reimbursement was a given and model systems and programs of research in major rehabilitation settings were common and well funded. Those days are gone. Today, 75% rules, intensity of service, and other insurance requirements result in rehabilitation nurses being very aware of rules and regulations as part of their care. At times, that is what nurses may feel drives their interventions or lack thereof. This chapter describes the major drivers of change, which include regulation and reimbursement. In addition, the focus of care is changing from a reactive approach to care to one that is preventive and proactive. The consumer is seeking out both alternative and traditional care, which changes the basic parameters of what is taken into consideration in assessment and intervention. The rehabilitation nurse is in an environment that is in continuous flux. Change theory is no longer a staged process with a beginning and an end. Instead, it is continuous, dynamic, and chaotic. This complex environment, fueled by the explosion of knowledge and communication, requires openness, passion, and resilience to ensure the best care for people with disabilities and chronic illnesses.

I. **Major Milestones in a Changing Environment**

  A. Legislated Acts

    1. The Americans with Disabilities Act (ADA) of 1990 (U.S. Department of Justice, 2006a)

      a. Title I

        1) Prohibits private employers, state and local governments, employment agencies, and labor unions from discriminating against qualified people with disabilities in job application procedures, hiring, firing, advancement, compensation, job training, and other terms, conditions, and privileges of employment

        2) Describes the traits of a person with a disability

          a) A physical or mental impairment that substantially limits one or more major life activities

          b) A record of such an impairment

          c) Regarded as having such an impairment

      b. Title II

        1) Provides comprehensive civil rights for qualified people with disabilities

        2) Addresses public entities and requires that all activities, services, and programs of public entities be covered by the ADA, including activities of state legislatures and courts, town meetings, police and fire departments, motor vehicle licensing, and employment

        3) Directly influences access, program integration, communication, construction, and alterations

      c. Title III

        1) Addresses the public sector

        2) Defines the private entities that must meet ADA requirements

      d. Title IV: telecommunication

      e. Title V: miscellaneous provisions to cover legal fees and to prohibit coercion and retaliation

      f. The impact of the ADA

        1) Allows people with disabilities to have equal opportunities, accessibility, and accommodations in employment, transportation, and public access

        2) Has spawned litigation and clarification to further define its actual implementation and application (U.S. Department of Justice, 2006b)

3) Has reinforced the advocate role of rehabilitation nurses based on their knowledge of the ADA as they inform patients, encourage ADA enforcement, and obtain resources

2. Rehabilitation Acts (U.S. Department of Justice, 2006a): foundation for federal funding and contract requirements
   a. Section 501: affirmative action and nondiscrimination in employment in federal agencies
   b. Section 503: affirmative action and nondiscrimination in federal contracts and subcontracts
   c. Section 504: affirmative action and nondiscrimination in programs that receive federal funding
   d. Section 508: requires that electronic and information technology used by the federal government be accessible

B. Changes in Rehabilitation Reimbursement
   1. Initial impact of diagnosis-related groups
      a. In the mid-1980s, there was an increase in rehabilitation acute units.
      b. In the early 1990s, the overall census in all inpatient settings decreased.
      c. In the 1990s, competition for rehabilitation patients began and the growth of acute rehabilitation subsided.
      d. Internal and external case management of all patients has increased.
      e. Home health care initially increased and later came under prospective payment systems, capping payment.
   2. Balanced Budget Act of 1997 (Esser, 1998)
      a. Called for Medicare spending cuts that affected rehabilitation (Esser, 1998)
      b. Required a prospective payment system (PPS)
      c. Required the use of Resource Utilization Groups (RUGs) as the basis for rehabilitation PPSs: RUGs-III are based on the Minimum Data Set assessment's Resident Assessment Instrument and Resident Assessment Protocols, which must be done for each patient. RUGs group patients into four major categories (Knapp, 1999; Nathenson, 1999).
      d. 75% rule (Centers for Medicare and Medicaid Services [CMS], 2007a):
         1) Initiated in 1984
         2) Established 10 diagnostic categories for admission to rehabilitation
         3) CMS increased to 13 diagnoses in

2003.
         4) Began enforcement in 2004 with initial compliance at 50%, with graded increase to 75% of all admissions by 2008 (Cournan, 2006; Zigmod, 2006)
         5) Impact is the denial of admissions or payment for services of those not meeting the diagnostic criteria.
         6) Lobbying efforts to expand the diagnostic categories persist.
      e. Capped Medicare Part B payments (CMS, 2007b):
         1) Rehabilitation therapy for postacute delivery has an annual financial limitation (cap).
         2) Combined outpatient physical therapy and speech–language pathology services share the same cap ($1,780 in 2007).
         3) Occupational therapy has a $1,780 cap per year.
         4) Treatment must be medically necessary.
         5) 20% of the Medicare-approved amount is the client's responsibility.
         6) No cap applies if therapy is provided at a hospital outpatient therapy department.
         7) Medicare-certified beds in skilled nursing facilities also have the same cap amounts.
   3. Impact on rehabilitation (Cournan, 2006)
      a. Decreased access for people with disabilities that do not fit within the defined categories
      b. Increased scrutiny of admission by payers
      c. Limited outpatient services
      d. Addition of nursing roles for admission and PPS coordinators to ensure compliance and reimbursement
      e. Decrease in census of inpatient rehabilitation settings

C. Focus on Outcomes
   1. Outcomes, especially as they relate to function, are the most common measures across all levels of rehabilitation programs.
   2. The Inpatient Rehabilitation Facility Patient Assessment Instrument, used to document for rehabilitation admission and reimbursement, is based on functional outcome data.
   3. Outcomes are used to communicate with consumers of rehabilitation services to describe the following:

a. Comparison

b. Contracting

c. Selection of a rehabilitation setting

d. Marketing and competition for the rehabilitation patient

D. Recognition of a Transcultural Environment

1. Acknowledges rapidly changing demographics and increased awareness of cultural expectations

2. Promotes cultural competence (Andrews & Boyle, 2003; Leininger & McFarland, 2002)

   a. Includes cultural self-awareness of values and beliefs

   b. Conscious awareness of the individual, family, and community context

   c. Confronts prejudices, biases, judgments, and generalizations

3. Promotes culturally sensitive care, which provides for the preservation and maintenance, accommodation and negotiation, and repatterning and restructuring of care to meet patients' cultural and healthcare needs (Leininger, 1997)

4. Blends well with rehabilitation nursing philosophy, which is based on a holistic approach to the patient and ensures equal opportunity to care

E. Major Shifts in the Delivery, Environment, and Expectations of Health Care (Issel & Anderson, 1996)

1. Customer orientation: This shift involved moving from viewing the person as the customer to viewing the population as the customer.

2. Wellness orientation: With the movement to a focus on patient populations, the emphasis became health promotion, which redefined the health services that were provided and prioritized.

3. Cost versus revenue: The emphasis is on managed care and capitation, and the responsibility lies with the provider to control costs.

4. Approach to care: This shift involved moving from a departmental or an individual professional approach to an integrated, interdependent approach to care.

5. Shift for patients: Patients are now viewed as consumers of cost and quality, which allows them to identify the types and cost of services needed to maintain wellness.

6. Continuity of information: Information is now brought to the patient across time and discipline boundaries.

F. Disease State Management

1. Disease state management is "a comprehensive, integrated approach to care and reimbursement based on a disease's natural course" (Todd & Nash, 1997, p. 4).

2. Disease management is population focused.

3. The managed care model of crib-to-grave enrollment motivates healthcare professionals to perform disease management. The use of services is disproportionate for patients with complicated medical problems.

4. Best practice guidelines to standardize approaches to care are expanding across healthcare settings.

5. Healthy People 2010 seeks to improve systems for personal and public health. (U.S. Department of Health and Human Services, n.d.):

   a. By increasing quality and years of healthy life

   b. By eliminating health disparities

   c. By promoting healthy behaviors

   d. By preventing and reducing diseases and disorders

   e. By promoting healthy communities

G. Alternative and Complementary Therapies

1. The use of alternative and complementary therapies has increased. These therapies often are incorporated into what is perceived as mainstream care.

2. In 2002, 36% of adults reported using alternative medicine; with the addition of megavitamin therapy and prayer, this figure rises to 62% (National Institute of Health National Center for Complementary and Alternative Medicine [NIH NCCAM], 2007b).

3. The NCCAM was established in the National Institutes of Health in 1998 (Marwick, 1998).

4. NCCAM identified four domains of complementary and alternative medicine (NIH NCCAM, 2007a):

   a. Mind–body medicine: focuses on enhancing the mind's capacity to affect the body.

   b. Biologically based therapies are natural and biologically based practices, interventions, and products.

   c. Manipulative and body-based systems

involve manipulation or movement of the body.

    d. Energy medicine includes biofield therapies and bioelectromagnetic-based therapies.

5. NCCAM recognizes whole medical systems: complete systems of theory and practice that may have developed in non-Western or Western cultures.

6. There are many types of alternative and complementary therapies, many of which have been linked to rehabilitation (Carlson & Krahn, 2006; Miller, 2005).

    a. Research has been reported in the areas of geriatrics (Gaylord & Grotty, 2002), chronic pain (McEachrane-Gross, Liebschutz, & Berlowitz, 2006), multiple sclerosis (Campbell et al., 2006; Stuifbergen & Harrison, 2003), neurogenic communication disorders (Laures & Shisler, 2004), and stroke.

    b. Modalities of tai chi (Bottomley, 2004), energy healing, ginkgo biloba, music therapy, prayer and meditation (Schoenberger, Matheis, Shiflett, & Cotter, 2002), and acupuncture have been reported in clinical trials, research reports, and surveys of rehabilitation practitioners.

7. Rehabilitation nurses should be aware of the cultural meanings of health and wellness and various alternatives that patients may use. The mainstream use of complementary and alternative medicine can affect the effects of medications, the value of various interventions, and the incorporation of these practices into what is perceived as the standard rehabilitation program. This information should be gathered during the patient assessment. Incorporation of techniques requires additional education and review of the science and related research.

II. Change in an Ever-Changing Time

A. Descriptions of Change:

1. Previously known situation, process, or adaptation that is now new or altered.

2. Clear delineation of beginning and end.

3. Today change is seen in terms of complexity, or chaos theory. Change is endless (Porter-O'Grady & Malloch, 2003).

B. Lewin's Change Theory (historic approach):

1. Social scientist Kurt Lewin (1947) is credited as the original theorist of change theory;

much of his work was done in the 1940s.

2. Change theory concepts:

    a. Behavior is a function of both personality and the environment, and the interaction between the two is dynamic.

    b. There are 3 stages of change:

      1) Unfreezing: movement from a steady state to a state that is unsteady and amenable to change

        a) Discomfort with the present situation is induced or emerges.

        b) Status quo is questioned.

        c) Change relationship is established.

      2) Movement to a higher level of behavior

        a) Problem is assessed and diagnosed.

        b) Options and alternatives are identified.

        c) Goals are established.

        d) Action is taken.

        e) Evaluation is made.

      3) Refreezing: integration and stabilization of new learning

        a) New responses are integrated into lifestyle and relationships.

        b) Change is complete.

C. Profound Change: This phrase is used to describe organizational change that combines inner shifts in people's values, aspirations, and behaviors with outer shifts in processes, strategies, practices, and systems (Senge et al., 1999). Nothing can change without personal transformation.

1. The beginning and end of change are no longer clearly defined. Profound change builds on ongoing data gathering and adaptation (Porter-O'Grady & Malloch, 2003).

2. Change often is multidimensional and entails a more fluid approach.

3. Senge (1994) described the learning organization as an approach to transition that is needed today. Learning organizations are those that seek to create their own future. Senge's model includes five disciplines:

    a. Mental models: the personal biases and assumptions we use to make decisions that drive our behavior

    b. Personal mastery: clarifying what is important and striving to see reality more clearly

    c. Shared vision: building a common sense of purpose and commitment by developing shared images of the future we seek to create

    d. Team learning: reflecting on action as a team and transforming collective thinking skills so that the team can develop intelligence and ability greater than the sum of individual members' talents

    e. Systems thinking: the language of relationships that shape the behavior of the systems in which we exist

  4. Senge et al. (1999) noted that companies that fail to sustain significant change end up facing crises.

    a. Organizations (and professionals) must change their basic ways of thinking to initiate and sustain change.

    b. There must be a commitment to change rather than a simple compliance with change.

  5. External forces for change include technology, customers, competitors, market structure, and the social and political environment.

  6 Internal realities of change depend on how the environment adapts.

  7. "The timeless concern is whether these internal changes—in practices, views, and strategies—will keep pace with the external change" (Senge et al., 1999, p. 14).

D. Rehabilitation Nurse as a Change Agent in Today's Healthcare Environment:

  1. Change is a central concern for nursing, healthcare, and society.

    a. "Change in the rehabilitation setting can involve change in knowledge, attitude, behavior, or group organization or functioning" (Chin, Finocchiaro, & Rosebrough, 1998, p. 71).

    b. As a change agent, the rehabilitation nurse proactively helps the patient or is involved in the change process in the organization.

    c. Change parallels the nursing process:
      1) Identify the problem to be addressed.
      2) Define the changes needed.
      3) Identify the purpose of the change.
      4) Gather and use the elements needed to accomplish the change.
      5) Implement actions to accomplish the change.
      6) Evaluate the change.

    d. Change is continuous, and the nursing process is not linear but is continually evolving, necessitating continuous reassessment.

  2. The current demands of health care create an environment of profound change.

  3. Rehabilitation nurses must have knowledge of change barriers, identify internal and external barriers to openness to change, and make a commitment to change.

    a. Internal demands
      1) Reorganization
      2) Redesign
      3) Reengineering
      4) Continuous quality improvement
      5) Redeployment

    b. External demands
      1) New knowledge
      2) Competition
      3) Regulations

  4. Rehabilitation nurses must understand the external forces driving change:

    a. Venue of care

    b. Expanded knowledge

    c. Upgrade of clinical knowledge and skills

    d. Fiscal accountability

  5. Rehabilitation nurses must recognize their own attitudes or personality traits related to change. They must know the role that best describes their own positions and learn how to work with people who fall into the other groups.

  6. Rogers (1995) described 6 types of behavioral groups:

    a. Innovators: adventuresome

    b. Early adopters: respected leaders in the organization

    c. Early majority: deliberate

    d. Late majority: skeptical

    e. Laggards: hang on to traditional ways and ideas

    f. Rejecters

  7. Major hurdles to change-ready thinking (Kriegel & Brandt, 1996):

    a. Fear

    b. Fatigue

    c. Comfort

  8. Reasons for taking a proactive approach to change and seeking out opportunities for change:

    a. To improve the quality of care

    b. To improve the cost-effectiveness of care delivery

    c. To make the adaptations needed to maintain change

  9. Resilience in facing change:

a. Attitudes and traits that are characteristic of change-resilient people (Conner, 1996; Giordono, 1997; Jacelon, 1997):
   1) Positive thinking
   2) Sense of being in control
   3) Resourcefulness
   4) Focus
   5) Self-discipline
   6) Flexibility
   7) Organization
   8) Proactive behavior
b. Resilience is needed to manage uncertainty (Porter-O'Grady & Malloch, 2003).
c. Traits that pose barriers to resilience to change (Giordono, 1997):
   1) Cynicism
   2) Distancing
   3) Avoidance

III. Conclusions

Rehabilitation nurses are driven to change both internally (as providers of care) and externally (as a part of healthcare organizations). Rehabilitation nurses who are aware of the various changes in health care and are open to new strategies are able to stay at the forefront of the complex changes that surround them. Rehabilitation nurses can develop a passion for change and seek to create a new reality for rehabilitation care (Porter-O'Grady, 2003).

References

Andrews, M.M., & Boyle, J.S. (2003). *Transcultural concepts in nursing care* (4th ed.). Philadelphia: Lippincott Williams & Wilkins.

Bottomley, J.M. (2004). Tai chi: Choreography of body and mind. In C.M. Davis (Ed.), *Complementary therapies in rehabilitation: Evidence for efficacy in therapy, prevention, and wellness* (2nd ed.). Thorofare, NJ: SLACK, Inc.

Campbell, D.G., Turner, A.P., Williams, R.M., Hatzakis, M., et al. (2006). Complementary and alternative medicine use in veterans with multiple sclerosis: Prevalence and demographic associations. *Journal of Rehabilitation Research and Development, 43*(1), 99.

Carlson, M., & Krahn, G. (2006). Use of complementary and alternative medicine practitioners by people with physical disabilities: Estimates from a national US survey. *Disability & Rehabilitation, 28*(5), 505–513.

Centers for Medicare and Medicaid Services (CMS). (2007a). *Inpatient rehabilitation facility prospective payment system (IRF PPS) final rule for fiscal year (FY) 2007.* http://www.cms.hhs.gov/inpatientrehabfacpps/downloads/cms_1540f.pdf

Centers for Medicare and Medicaid Services (CMS). (2007b). *Patient rehabilitation facility prospective payment system: Payment system fact sheet series.* Retrieved April 2, 2007, from http://www.cms.hhs.gov/MLNProducts/downloads/IRFPPSFactSheet0307.pdf

Chin, P.A., Finocchiaro, D.N., & Rosebrough, A. (1998). *Rehabilitation nursing practice.* New York: McGraw-Hill.

Conner, D.R. (1996). How can you survive continuous change? *Medical Economics, 73*(8), 109–114.

Cournan, M.C. (2006). The 75% rule: What rehabilitation nurses need to know. *ARN Network, 23*(5), 11.

Esser, C. (1998). Sorting out the Balanced Budget Act of 1997. *ARN Network, 14*(3), 1–2.

Gaylord, S., & Grotty, N. (2002). Enhancing function with complementary therapies in geriatric rehabilitation. *Topics in Geriatric Rehabilitation, 18*(2), 63–79.

Giordono, B.P. (1997). Resilience: A survival tool for the nineties. *AORN Journal, 65*(6), 1032–1034.

Issel, L.M., & Anderson, R.A. (1996). Take charge: Managing six transformations in health care delivery. *Nursing Economics, 14*(2), 78–85.

Jacelon, C.S. (1997). The trait and process of resilience. *Journal of Advanced Nursing, 25*, 123–139.

Knapp, M.T. (1999). Nurse's basic guide to understanding the Medicare PPS. *Nursing Management, 30*(5), 14–15.

Kriegel, R., & Brandt, D. (1996). *Sacred cows make the best burgers: Developing change-ready people and organizations.* New York: Warner Books.

Laures, J.S., & Shisler, R. (2004). Complementary and alternative medical approaches to treating adult neurogenic communication disorders: A review. *Disability and Rehabilitation, 26*(6), 315–325.

Leininger, M. (1997). Overview of the theory of culture care with the ethnonursing research method. *Transcultural Nursing, 8*(2), 32–52.

Leininger, M., & McFarland, M.R. (2002). *Transcultural nursing: Concepts, research and practice.* New York: McGraw-Hill.

Lewin, K. (1947). Frontiers in group dynamics: Concepts, methods, and reality in social science. *Human Relations, 5*(1), 5–42.

Marwick, C. (1998). Alterations are ahead at the OAM. *Medical News and Perspectives, 280*(18), 1553–1554.

McEachrane-Gross, F.P., Liebschutz, J.M., & Berlowitz, D. (2006). Use of selected complementary and alternative medicine (CAM) treatments in veterans with cancer or chronic pain: A cross-sectional survey. *BMC Complementary and Alternative Medicine 6*(34). Available: http://www.biomedcentral.com/1472-6882/6/34

Miller, E. (2005). Merging rehabilitation nursing with complementary and alternative therapies. *Rehabilitation Nursing, 30*(5), 170, 172.

Nathenson, P. (Ed.). (1999). *Integrating rehabilitation and restorative nursing concepts into the MDS.* Glenview, IL: Association of Rehabilitation Nurses.

National Institute of Health National Center for Complementary and Alternative Medicine (NIH NCCAM). (2007a). *Get the facts: Complementary and alternative medicine.* Retrieved March 30, 2007, from http://nccam.nih.gov/health/whatiscam/

National Institute of Health National Center for Complementary and Alternative Medicine (NIH NCCAM). (2007b). *The use of complementary and alternative medicine in the United States.* Retrieved March 30, 2007, from http://nccam.nih.gov/news/camsurvey_fs1.htm

Porter-O'Grady, T. (2003). Of hubris and hope: Transforming nursing for a new age. *Nursing Economic\$, 21*(2), 59–64.

Porter-O'Grady, T., & Malloch, K. (2003). *Quantum leadership: A textbook of new leadership.* Boston: Jones and Bartlett.

Rogers, E. (1995). *Diffusion of innovation* (4th ed.). New York: Free Press.

Schoenberger, N.E., Matheis, R.J., Shiflett, S.C., & Cotter, A.C. (2002). Opinions and practices of medical rehabilitation professionals regarding prayer and meditation. *The Journal of Alternative and Complementary Medicine, 8*(1), 59–69.

Senge, P. (1994). *The fifth discipline fieldbook.* New York: Currency Doubleday.

Senge, P., Kleiner, A., Roberts, C., Ross, R., Roth, G., & Smith, B. (1999). *The dance of change.* New York: Currency Doubleday.

Stuifbergen, A.K., & Harrison, T.C. (2003). Complementary and alternative therapy use in persons with multiple sclerosis. *Rehabilitation Nursing, 28*(5), 141–147, 158.

Todd, W., & Nash, D. (Eds.). (1997). *Disease management: A systems approach to improving patient outcomes.* Chicago: American Hospital Association.

U.S. Department of Health and Human Services. (n.d.). Healthy People 2010 homepage. Retrieved October 25, 2006, from http://www.healthypeople.gov/

U.S. Department of Justice. (2006a). ADA home page. Retrieved October 25, 2006, from http://www.usdoj.gov/crt/ada/adahom1.htm

U.S. Department of Justice. (2006b). *A guide to disability rights laws.* U.S. Department of Justice. Civil Rights Division, Disability Rights Section. Retrieved October 25, 2006, from http://www.usdoj.gov/crt/ada/cguide.htm

Zigmod, J. (2006). Adjusting to new rules. *Modern Healthcare, 36*(22), 24–26, 28.

Suggested Resources

Andrews, M.M. (1998). A model for cultural change. *Nursing Management, 29*(10), 62, 63, 66.

Bartol, G., & Richardson, L. (1998). Using literature to create cultural competence. Image: *Journal of Nursing Scholarship, 30*(1), 75–79.

Fadiman, A. (1997). *The spirit catches you and you fall down.* New York: Noonday.

Flowers, C.R., Edwards, D., & Pusch, B. (1996). Rehabilitation cultural diversity initiative: A regional survey of cultural diversity within CILs. *The Journal of Rehabilitation, 62*(3), 22–29.

Jonas, W.B., & Levin, J.S. (Eds.). (1999). *Essentials of complementary and alternative medicine.* Philadelphia: Lippincott Williams & Wilkins.

Kerfoot, K. (1999). Creating a forgetting organization. *Nursing Economics, 17*(1), 64–65.

King, W.R. (1997). Organizational transformation. *Information Systems Management, 14,* 63–65.

Kirkham, S.R. (1998). Nurses' descriptions of caring for culturally diverse clients. *Clinical Nursing Research, 7*(2), 125–146.

KMRREC. (2000). *RehabTrials.Org.* Retrieved October 25, 2006, from http://www.rehabtrials.org/

Leskowitz, E. (2006). *Complementary and alternative medicine in rehabilitation.* Philadelphia: Churchill Livingstone/Elsevier.

Morey, S.S. (1998). NIH issues consensus statement on acupuncture. *American Family Physician, 57*(10), 2545–2546.

National Institutes of Health. (n.d.). *Clinical trials.* Retrieved October 25, 2006, from http://www.clinicaltrials.gov/ct

Sampson, W. (1999). The braid of the "alternative medicine" movement. *Scientific Review of Alternative Medicine, 2*(2), 4–11.

Samdup, D.Z., Smith, R.G., & Song, S. (2006). Use of complementary and alternative medicine in children with chronic medical conditions: Research survey. *American Journal of Physical Medicine & Rehabilitation, 85*(10), 842–846.

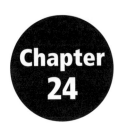

Chapter 24

Rehabilitation Nursing: Past, Present, and Future

Patricia A. Edwards, EdD RN CNAA

The history of rehabilitation nursing is inextricably linked to the history of medicine, nursing, and rehabilitation. The timelines in this chapter provide a historical overview of rehabilitation and the major events, people, and factors that shaped the healthcare specialty known as rehabilitation nursing.

The initial change in attitude toward people with disabilities came with an interest in crippled children, particularly those affected by the outbreak of polio at the turn of the 20th century. In the first decade of the 20th century, society began to focus on the needs of people with disabilities by providing a therapeutic environment for the treatment of specific disabilities and by beginning to address these people's educational and vocational needs. Many changes were stimulated as a result of society entering or recovering from war, enjoying the creativity and prosperity of peacetime, and attempting to treat and cure disease and its sequelae. In the second half of the 20th century, people with physical disabilities, composing a minority of approximately 45 million people in America, began to receive national support for their right to lead normal, high-quality lives despite their physical disabilities.

Rehabilitation was first practiced by nurses in the convalescent and sanitarium units of the early 1900s. The specialty practice of rehabilitation nursing began in the 1940s as World War II veterans returned home with spinal cord injuries and the aftermath of the polio epidemic left many people with disabilities. Both groups of patients needed hospitalization over long periods of time.

The change, growth, creativity, and technological advances that characterized the 20th century have challenged rehabilitation nurses to expand their knowledge base and practice across the continuum of care. At the beginning of the 21st century the challenges to rehabilitation nurses include the changing roles, especially at the advanced practice level, the nursing shortage and recruitment problems, changes in practice and care settings, and the healthcare crisis (access, equity, and reimbursement). This chapter concludes with a number of possibilities for the future practice of rehabilitation nursing in the 21st century from rehabilitation nursing leaders and experts in other nursing arenas.

I. Past: A Historical Overview of Rehabilitation

A. Rehabilitation from Ancient Egypt Through the 18th Century

1. From ancient to modern times, humankind has been adapting and coping with physical disability.

2. More than 5,000 years ago, an Egyptian physician recorded an assessment of a client.

3. 2380 BC: Earliest record of crutches, discovered in hieroglyphics on an Egyptian tomb.

4. Pre-Christian era: Many biblical references concerned the crippled, lame, blind, and afflicted.

5. 400–300 BC: Hippocrates, the father of medicine, recorded the use of artificial limbs as an attempt to replace amputated limbs and the basic principle that "exercise strengthens and inactivity wastes."

6. 200–100 BC: Galen, a Greek physician and writer, described the muscles and bones of the body.

7. 30 AD: Celsius advocated the use of exercise after a fracture had healed to prevent the loss of function.

8. 1601: The Poor Relief Act, the first show of responsibility and concern for people with disabilities, was passed in England.

9. 1633: Vincent dePaul founded institutions for crippled children in France.

10. 1750: John Hunter, a British physician, focused on the importance of the relationship between the client's will, range of motion, and muscle reeducation.

11. 1798: Philippe Pinel began practicing psychiatric rehabilitation and occupational and recreational therapies as treatment methods in England (McCourt, 1993).

B. Rehabilitation in the 19th Century

1. 1829: The Perkins Institute, the first sheltered workshop for people with disabilities in the United States, was founded by Samuel Gridley Howe. The goal was to train blind people so they could work in the community.

2. 1854: Florence Nightingale organized professional nursing in England.

3. 1873: The first U.S. school of nursing was founded in New York at Bellevue Hospital.

4. 1877: Clara Barton established the American Red Cross.

5. 1889–1893: Interest in crippled children grew. The Cleveland Rehabilitation Center began offering services for children, and the first U.S. schools for children with physical disabilities were established (see Figure 24-1).

6. Advances in science and medicine increased the potential for the survival and physical restoration of people with disabilities.

7. End of the 19th century: Public health departments were established in major cities.

C. Rehabilitation in the 20th Century

1. 1900–1919:

   a. Society began to focus on the needs of people with disabilities:

      1) By providing a therapeutic environment for the treatment of specific disabilities

      2) By addressing educational and vocational needs

   b. Certain people promoted occupational and vocational training:

      1) Susan Tracy, a nurse, teacher, and author who pioneered the discipline of occupational therapy

      2) Eleanor Slagle, a social worker

      3) George Barton, an architect recovering from tuberculosis

   c. The Home for Crippled Children was established in Pittsburgh in 1902 to care for children with disabilities.

   d. Electrotherapy was used as a therapeutic modality, and physical therapy modalities were instituted at Massachusetts General Hospital.

   e. The need for licensure and definition of the specialty of rehabilitation was identified.

   f. The Institute for Crippled and Disabled (est. 1917) and the Curative Workshop of Milwaukee (est. 1919) were pioneering ventures in the area of rehabilitation.

   g. World War I had a great impact on physical medicine.

      1) The federal division of specialty hospitals and physical reconstruction at Massachusetts General Hospital was developed in 1917 to treat wounded soldiers and others needing rehabilitation.

      2) Education and vocational rehabilitation was provided through the American Red Cross Institute for Disabled Men.

      3) The first spinal centers incorporated concepts of functional reeducation.

      4) The U.S. Veterans' Administration (VA) was created.

2. 1920–1943:

   a. 1920:

      1) The Vocational Rehabilitation law provided for federal control of vocational rehabilitation.

      2) The first Rehabilitation Act passed by Congress set in motion a focus on the emerging specialty of rehabilitation.

   b. 1921: The Division of Physical Reconstruction and the Federal Board for Vocational Education were established.

Figure 24-1. Early Pediatric Rehabilitation Facilities in the United States

1883	The Hospital for Sick Children, Washington, DC
1889	The Cleveland Rehabilitation Center, Cleveland, OH
1892	The Children's Country Home, Westfield, NJ, and The Blythedale Children's Hospital, Valhalia, NY
1893	The Boston Institute School for Crippled and Deformed Children
1895	Health Hill Hospital in Cleveland
1902	The Home for Crippled Children (now The Rehabilitation Institute), Pittsburgh, PA
1919	The Curative Workshop of Milwaukee
1922	Happy Hills Convalescent Center (now Mt. Washington Pediatric Hospital), Baltimore, MD
1930	Elizabethtown Hospital and Rehabilitation Center (now University Hospital Rehabilitation Center for Children and Adults), Elizabethtown, PA
1937	Children's Rehabilitation Institute (now the Kennedy Institute), Baltimore, MD
1940	Alfred I. DuPont Institute, Wilmington, DE (as a hospital for crippled children)
1949	Kennedy Memorial Hospital (now Franciscan Children's Hospital and Rehabilitation Center), Boston, MA
1950	Children's Orthopedic Hospital (now Cardinal Hill Rehabilitation Hospital), Lexington, KY

Source consulted

Edwards, P.A. (1992). The evolution of rehabilitation facilities for children. *Rehabilitation Nursing, 17*, 191-192.

c. Associations for physical and occupational therapists were developed. These organizations began to determine the role, placement, and governance of therapies, which became focus points of the emerging specialty of rehabilitation.

d. 1935: The Social Security Act defined rehabilitation as a process that helped a person with a disability become capable of engaging in a remunerative occupation. The government began providing rehabilitation services beyond the needs of the military and outside hospital walls.

e. 1938: The American Academy of Physical Medicine and Rehabilitation was founded to set standards and requirements for the practice of rehabilitation medicine.

f. 1938–1941: In 1938, Dr. Frank Krusen established the hallmarks of physical medicine as controlling disease, relieving suffering, and shortening the period of disability. In 1941, Krusen wrote *Physical Medicine*, the first comprehensive book about treatment methods.

g. 1943:
  1) The Sister Kenny Institute was established. Sister Kenny, a nurse, used muscular manipulation, which led to the theory of muscle reeducation. Her techniques pioneered the discipline of physical therapy, and her success with treatment of polio patients boosted the medical specialty of physiatry (McCourt, 1993).
  2) The Vocational Rehabilitation Act was enacted.
    a) Made funds available for professional training and research
    b) Broadened the scope of rehabilitation
    c) Provided a catalyst for the growth of the practice

h. World War II played a tremendous role in the further development of rehabilitation programs:
  1) Dr. Howard A. Rusk dramatically demonstrated the possibilities of rehabilitation when he showed how it could improve the lives of men who had been hospitalized since World War I.
  2) New methods of handling shock and treating infection, along with increasingly sophisticated trauma

care, meant more people would survive.

3. 1944–1960:
  a. The number of industrial-related injuries increased, as did motor vehicle–related accidents and injuries.
  b. 1945:
    1) Liberty Mutual hired the first rehabilitation nurse in the insurance industry, thus recognizing the importance of nurses in a rehabilitation role.
    2) The American Paraplegia Association was founded.
    3) World War II was the primary impetus for the clinical nurse specialist (CNS) role. Hildegard Peplau made the first reference to the CNS role in the psychiatric context.
  c. 1946:
    1) Rehabilitation programs began in U.S. VA hospitals.
    2) The term *physiatrist* began to be used to describe a physician with specialized training in rehabilitation medicine.
  d. 1947: Dr. Rusk established the first medical rehabilitation services in a U.S. civilian hospital.
  e. Late 1940s: The first board certification exams in physiatry were conducted.
  f. 1951: Alice Morrissey, BS RN, wrote the first textbook (*Rehabilitation Nursing*) in the field of rehabilitation nursing:
    1) Principal contributions of nurses in rehabilitative care identified by Morrissey:
      a) Basic bedside nursing
      b) Clinical teaching and rehabilitation nursing service management
      c) An emphasis on the importance of nutrition and activities of daily living
    2) Principal message of Morrissey's textbook: "Each sick person is regarded not as a patient with a disease but as a person with a future."
  g. 1956–1969: Lena Plaisted, MS RN, founded the first graduate rehabilitation nursing program at Boston University in 1956. Plaisted wrote *The Clinical Specialist in Rehabilitation*, the first publication to describe this role, in 1969.
  h. In the 1950s: Barbara Madden, MA

RN, contributed significantly to the development of nursing programs for acute and postpolio patients and helped establish regional respiratory centers.

    i. Important strides were made in technology, and greater emphasis was placed on the needs of those with disabilities and on rehabilitation.

    j. The realm of rehabilitation was expanded to include treatment for people with stroke, cardiac conditions, arthritis, orthopedic injuries, and brain injuries.

    k. Mary Ann Mikulic was one of the first rehabilitation nursing clinical specialists appointed by the VA.

4. 1960–1989:

    a. These 3 decades marked a period of increased recognition of the specialty practice of rehabilitation nursing. As one nurse said, "When starting my rehabilitation career in the '60s, I was frustrated that no one else in other specialty areas seemed to understand what we did in rehabilitation. My mentor acknowledged my frustration and said, 'Barbara, our day will come.' The day did come when I found others calling me about patient education, measuring outcomes, and discharge planning. Nurses in critical care wanted to know about autonomic hyperreflexia and how to talk to patients about sexuality. Finally I felt that what we did and what we knew were acknowledged and appreciated" (B. Warner, personal communication, July 7, 1999).

    b. The Korean and Vietnam wars influenced continued progress in rehabilitation, in part through the ability to treat wounded people more effectively on the battlefield and the availability of improved transport to medical treatment services, which led to a decrease in mortality rate (McCourt, 1993).

    c. Increased medical technology, institution-based trauma care, and paramedics led to an increased survival rate from injury and focused on the further need for rehabilitation programs and services (McCourt, 1993).

    d. The scope of rehabilitation broadened to include and meet needs of the following groups:

        1) People with chronic diseases
        2) An aging population
        3) People reentering the workforce after traumatic injury or disease

    e. 1962: Medicare legislation stimulated an increased demand for rehabilitation, and more rehabilitation nurses were hired by insurance companies (McCourt, 1993).

    f. 1965:

        1) The Workers' Compensation and Rehabilitation law passed, placing an emphasis on the workplace.
        2) The American Nurses Association published *Guidelines for the Practice of Nursing on the Rehabilitation Team: An Answer to a Growing Need.*
        3) The nurse practitioner role was originated by Loretta Ford, PhD RN, and Henry Silver, MD, in response to the inequities in the accessibility to health care, exacerbated by a physician shortage.

    g. 1966: The Commission on Accreditation of Rehabilitation Facilities was established to provide a consultative accrediting process in the rehabilitation industry. (Its current name is the Rehabilitation Accreditation Commission.)

    h. 1967: Amendments were passed to the Vocational Rehabilitation Act that focused on improving workforce reentry for people with disabilities.

    i. Early 1970s: Regional health care became a focal point in rehabilitation services.

    j. 1973: The Rehabilitation Act was passed, demonstrating increased public awareness of the needs of people with disabilities. The act included guidelines for nondiscrimination in employment and promoted community access by reducing or eliminating physical barriers.

    k. 1974: The Association of Rehabilitation Nurses (ARN) was established under the leadership of Susan Novak. In 1975, 4 chapters, representing the states of California, Illinois, and New York, were chartered. Dagny Engle was the first executive director.

    l. 1975: *ARN Journal* was developed, with Dagny Engle serving as the first editor. The introduction of the journal was a professional milestone for ARN and its members (see Table 24-1). In 1981, the journal's name was changed to *Rehabilitation Nursing,* and it became a refereed journal.

    m. 1976:

        1) ARN was recognized by the nursing profession as a specialty

organization, and the Rehabilitation Nursing Institute (RNI) was established.

   2) ARN developed and published the standards and scope of rehabilitation nursing practice.

n. 1978: Independent living programs helped change societal views of the dependency of people with catastrophic injuries (McCourt, 1993).

o. 1980: Publication of *Rehabilitation Nursing and Related Readings*, a useful resource compiled by Rita Boucher and Sharon Dittmar.

p. 1981: The International Year of the Disabled Person:

   1) The needs of people with disabilities became more prominent as a social issue.

   2) The 1st edition of ARN's core curriculum for rehabilitation nursing was published under the title *Rehabilitation Nursing: Concepts and Practice—A Core Curriculum.* The editor-in-chief was Shannon Sayles.

   3) A credentialing committee was created, with Jessie Drew as chair, to develop a plan for certification; this became the Rehabilitation Nursing Certification Board.

   4) The continuing education application review subcommittee was established.

   5) The first distinguished service award was presented to Sue Novak.

   6) The seminar "Application of Rehabilitation Concepts to Nursing Practice" was developed to prepare nurses for certification.

q. 1984:

   1) ARN developed a formal definition,

philosophy, and conceptual framework of rehabilitation nursing and the association.

   2) The first certification examination for the Certified Rehabilitation Registered Nurse (CRRN) credential was held, and 965 nurses sat for the exam.

r. 1986:

   1) RNI changed its name to the Rehabilitation Nursing Foundation (RNF), which more clearly represented the entity's goals and purpose to the outside world.

   2) ARN revised and updated the standards and scope of rehabilitation nursing practice.

   3) Membership campaign "Each One Reach One" was initiated.

   4) The *Rehabilitation Nursing* journal had a new look under the editorial leadership of Glee Walquist.

s. 1987:

   1) ARN revised its core curriculum, with Christina Mumma as the editor, and identified the following areas as future challenges (see Table 24-2):

      a) Insurance issues

      b) Increased impact and influence of rehabilitation

         (1) Increased knowledge and education

         (2) Medicine, drugs, and technological advances

         (3) Decreased social isolation and involvement

         (4) Continued independent living movement

         (5) Increased awareness of cost-effectiveness of rehabilitation

         (6) Clearly defined and available levels of rehabilitation care

   2) ARN formally implemented Special Interest Councils (currently called Special Interest Groups [SIGs]) in 9 areas: administrators; CNSs; educators and researchers; gerontology; home health care; pain; pediatrics; rehabilitation nurse consultants, insurance, and private practice; and staff nurses.

   3) The Nurse-in-Washington program began.

   4) Basic rehabilitation nursing course called "Rehabilitation Nursing: Directions for Practice" was

Table 24-1. *ARN Journal* Editors

1975–1977: Dagny Engle

1977–1980: Mary Ann Mikulic

1980–1985: Barbara McHugh

1985–1987: Glee Walquist

1987: Susan Novak

1988–1998: Belinda Puetz

1998–2003: Susan Dean-Baar

2003–present: Elaine Miller

Table 24-2. Comparison of Future Challenges in ARN's Core Curricula

Rehabilitation Nursing: Concepts and Practice (2nd ed., 1987)	The Specialty Practice of Rehabilitation Nursing: A Core Curriculum (3rd ed., 1993)	The Specialty Practice of Rehabilitation Nursing: A Core Curriculum (4th ed., 2000)
Insurance issues	Managed care	Healthcare crisis: Access, equity, reimbursement
Increased impact and influence of rehabilitation	Cost containment	Changing role of rehabilitation nurses at both the basic and advanced practice levels
Increased knowledge and education	Increased demand for rehabilitation nursing	Roles include case manager and expert rehabilitation clinical nurse specialist
Increased awareness of cost-effectiveness of rehabilitation	Increased need for services	Nursing shortage and recruitment and education issues
Clearly defined and available levels of rehabilitative care	Increased recruitment and further education of nurses	Value of rehabilitation across the continuum of care
	Increased insistence on certification	Changes in practice and care settings: Hospital is more acute and rehabilitation units are changing; more clients are cared for in the home and community
	Greater awareness of rehabilitation and its benefit to individuals and society	
	Alteration in practice settings	

developed.

t. 1989: RNF funded its first research grant, and the first job analysis was done.

u. Rehabilitation techniques became more widely used in a variety of settings:
   1) Nursing homes
   2) Extended care facilities
   3) Inpatient rehabilitation units
   4) Home care programs
   5) Outpatient programs
   6) Private practice

5. 1990s: a decade of healthcare reform and rehabilitation nursing initiatives:
   a. Healthcare reform
      1) The 1990s were marked by increasing survival and life expectancy rates, which consequently increased the need for rehabilitation services.
      2) 1990: The Americans with Disabilities Act increased accessibility options and opportunities for people with disabilities in community, employment, education, and healthcare arenas.
      3) Geriatric rehabilitation demanded greater attention, with an increased need for rehabilitation nurses and an increased emphasis on restorative care and prevention of disability.
      4) The decline in deaths from traumatic injuries and previously life-threatening diseases increased the need for rehabilitation nurses:
         a) In critical and acute care settings
         b) As case managers for complex, multifaceted problems
      5) The intensity of care increased at all points in the continuum, and care delivery expanded to outpatient and home care.
      6) Early interventions and intense technological treatment increased.
      7) Lifelong care planning issues arose because people began living longer with chronic illness and disease.
      8) New roles, including case management, emerged for nurses.
      9) Rehabilitation nurses influenced the standards set for rehabilitation facilities and participated in quality improvement and program evaluation activities.
   b. Rehabilitation nursing initiatives by ARN
      1) 1990: The first role description for case managers was written by an ARN SIG, with many other role descriptions to follow.
      2) 1992–1996: ARN published the journal *Rehabilitation Nursing Research*.
      3) ARN initiated research to determine interventions and outcomes of specific nursing diagnoses.
      4) 1993: ARN published the 3rd edition of its core curriculum with a new title, *The Specialty Practice of Rehabilitation Nursing: A Core Curriculum*, with Ann McCourt as editor. It included the areas of future challenges listed in Table 24-2.
   c. Meeting the increased demands and challenges for rehabilitation nurses
      1) Increased need for services
      2) Altered practice settings
      3) Greater demand for patient and family education
      4) Increased recruitment problems and need for further education of nurses

5) Increased insistence on CRRN certification
6) Expansion of professional activities into consultation and research
7) Ensuring a unified voice for the specialty

d. Dealing with the implications of healthcare reform and the need for greater awareness of rehabilitation and its benefits to individuals and society
1) Managed care
2) Cost containment
3) Legislative involvement and client activity
4) Advanced technology
5) Ethical issues

6. 1994:
a. ARN updated the standards and scope of rehabilitation practice.
b. ARN published *Basic Competencies for Rehabilitation Nursing Practice.*

7. 1995: ARN published *21 Rehabilitation Nursing Diagnoses: A Guide to Interventions and Outcomes.*

8. 1996: ARN published the scope and standards of advanced clinical practice in rehabilitation nursing; Anne Cordes replaced Dagny Engle as executive director.

9. 1997:
a. ARN published *Advanced Practice Nursing in Rehabilitation: A Core Curriculum.*
b. The Certified Rehabilitation Registered Nurse–Advanced (CRRN-A) credential was introduced, and the first exam was held.

10. 1998: ARN published *Rehabilitation Nursing in the Home Health Setting.*

11. 1999:
a. ARN published *Integrating Rehabilitation and Restorative Nursing Concepts into the MDS.*
b. ARN published *Restorative Nursing: A Training Manual for Nursing Assistants.*
c. The *Rehabilitation Nursing* journal, with Susan Dean-Baar as editor, took on a new look with the redesign of the cover and layout and two new columns: "Current Issues" and "Perspectives."

II. Present: The Beginning of the 21st Century

A. The Practice of Rehabilitation Nursing at the Beginning of the 21st Century

1. Rehabilitation nursing continues to be a prominent specialty in the new millennium, and increasing patient acuity is changing the basic scope of practice.

2. The value of rehabilitation nurses continues to increase as the healthcare system recognizes the impact of rehabilitation principles across the continuum of care. Nurses must be involved in efforts to raise public awareness of the value of rehabilitation nursing.

3. "Rehabilitation nurses today need to have more acute and critical care competence" (S. Burnett, personal communication, October 20, 2006).

4. Rehabilitation nurses continue to define their practice, conduct and use research in everyday work, ensure that rehabilitation nurses have adequate preparation, and support ARN so that it remains a strong voice for rehabilitation nurses in the healthcare community.

5. "Patients are more complex in their needs and require more technologically based, advanced treatment and services" (L. Pierce, personal communication, October 26, 2006).

6. Rehabilitation nurses with advanced degrees, including doctoral, act in many capacities:
a. As experts in research and evidence-based practice
b. As advocates and managers for large populations needing restorative care
c. As promoters of public policy for people with disabilities at the local and national levels

B. The Effect of Changing Demographics on the Demand for Rehabilitation Nurses and Practice Settings

1. As the population continues to age, the need for professional nurses who have the skills to treat chronic illnesses and their effects on function, quality of life, and access to care has grown significantly.

2. Rehabilitation nurses have seen a shift in the distribution of illness from acute to chronic and a shift in the kinds of injuries, especially in survivors of war.

3. Rehabilitation nurses, who are particularly suited to case management, market their approach and philosophy to a variety of employers, insurance companies, inpatient settings, physicians, and other community-based services.

4. The hospital is more acute, and the

rehabilitation unit (acute and subacute) has changed as more patients are cared for in their homes, retirement centers, and other living arrangements in the community. "Practice has expanded to schools, nurse managed clinics in the community, independent nursing practices and more rural and inner urban areas" (T. Patterson, personal communication, October 25, 2006).

5. "The expertise of case management and life care planning are roles that continue to grow" (T. Thompson, personal communication, October 25, 2006).

C. The Nursing Shortage and Recruitment Issues

1. A large number of nurses are reaching retirement age. This decrease in the workforce comes at a time when there is also declining enrollment in nursing schools and declining interest among young people in the nursing profession. Keeping nurses in the workforce into their retirement years at healthcare facilities and schools of nursing with flexible schedules and benefits will be essential.

2. "With an overabundance of therapy practitioners and a shortage of nursing practitioners, the challenge for rehabilitation nurses is to identify the value of what they do, demonstrate that it takes a registered nurse to do it, and help recruit the younger generation into the field" (K. Johnson, personal communication, July 12, 1999).

3. "Anything the rehabilitation healthcare organization can do to retain, motivate, and keep nurses safe and healthy will be key for the future; consider ergonomics and the environment and safe patient-handling equipment" (K. Cervizzi, personal communication, October 25, 2006).

D. The Healthcare Crisis: Access, Equity, and Reimbursement Issues

1. Cost and access to care continue to be big issues because of changes in reimbursement. "Inpatient rehabilitation facilities have become increasingly constrained in the type of patient they can accept for inpatient rehabilitation due to the changes in qualifying conditions found in the 75% rule and medical necessity criteria" (K. Cervizzi, personal communication, October 25, 2006). ARN has a published position statement on the 75% rule.

2. Health care continues to be at a crisis level, and the lack of funding and other resources has severely changed the landscape of the delivery system and allowed fiscal intermediaries to determine admission and length of stay.

3. Problems with environmental, financial, and geographic access to services and the availability of practitioners who understand the needs of patients who are older, chronically ill, and disabled are important issues.

4. "Reimbursement is tied to [the Inpatient Rehabilitation Facility Patient Assessment Instrument] and the RIC classification. Today's rehabilitation requires that there is someone who is dedicated to the documentation of need" (T. Thompson, personal communication, October 25, 2006).

5. "Attempts to limit the role of the [advanced practice registered nurse] and other care providers will affect access to those most in need: poor, rural areas, inner cities" (S. Burnett, personal communication, October 20, 2006).

E. Ethical Issues and Dilemmas

1. Nurses increasingly face the challenge of working with people who choose to end their own life and have considered their positions on laws dealing with patients' rights and choices.

2. Nurses have had to assess their own feelings and attitudes related to ethical issues and dilemmas such as cloning, organ transplantation, and assisted suicide.

F. Initiatives by ARN

1. 2000: ARN published the 4th edition of its core curriculum, with Patricia Edwards as editor. It included the areas of future challenges listed in Table 24-2.

2. 2002:
   a. A CRRN preparation CD-ROM was developed, with test questions based on the new content outline of the certification exam.
   b. A professional rehabilitation nursing course was implemented.

3. 2003:
   a. The Web site, http://rehabnurse.org, got a new look and a "Members Only" area.
   b. The Advanced Practice in Rehabilitation Nursing certification examination was discontinued.

4. 2005:
   a. A position statement on the rehabilitation nurse as case manager was developed.

It indicated that "rehabilitation nurses are the most qualified healthcare professionals to perform the case management function because they have the education, background and expertise needed to coordinate patients' healthcare services from the onset of injury or illness to safe return to work or assimilation into the community as productive members of society" (K. Cervizzi, personal communication, October 25, 2006).

    b. ARN created the Competencies Assessment Tool, with 12 basic rehabilitation nursing competency areas, to be used online.

    c. Anne Cordes stepped down from the executive director position after almost 10 years and was replaced by Karen Nason.

    d. A new rehabilitation nursing research agenda with 19 statements of research priorities was formulated, intended to drive rehabilitation nursing research for the next 10 years.

    e. The Rehabilitation Institute of Chicago became the first rehabilitation hospital to be awarded magnet status by the American Nurses Credentialing Center, recognizing excellence in nursing services. Craig Hospital became the second magnet rehabilitation hospital.

  5. 2006:

    a. *Evidence-Based Rehabilitation: Common Challenges and Interventions*, an updated version of *21 Rehabilitation Nursing Diagnoses*, was published.

    b. The Rehabilitation Nursing Certification Board (RNCB) celebrated its 25th anniversary. As of 2007, there are nearly 10,000 CRRNs. Certification in rehabilitation nursing shows employers, colleagues, patients, and the public that the nurse is committed to excellence in caring for people with physical disabilities and chronic illnesses. It indicates that she or he is an experienced rehabilitation or restorative nurse who has achieved a level of knowledge in this practice area and can lead to increased professional credibility, recognition of expertise, greater impact as a job candidate, and a heightened sense of personal achievement.

    c. As of 2007, there have been 32 presidents of ARN (see Table 24-3).

III. Future: Nurses' Perspectives on Health Care for the Next 10 Years

A. Integration of Information Technology into Rehabilitation Nursing Practice

  1. Advances in technology and telemedicine will link healthcare providers with patients across a greater distance (K. Cervizzi,

Table 24-3. ARN Presidents

1974–76: Susan Novak	1991–92: Aloma "Cookie" Gender
1976–77: Virginia Wright	1992–93: Kathleen Stevens
1977–78: Albinia Doll	1993–94: Karen Preston
1978–79: Barbara McHugh	1994–95: Susan Dean-Baar
1979–80: Rosemarian Berni	1995–96: Catherine Tracey
1980–81: Patricia Rizio	1996–97: Judy Hartmann
1981–82: Shannon Sayles	1997–98: Lois Schaetzle
1982–83: Carol Ann Imhoff	1998–99: Marilyn Ter Maat
1983–84: Diane Burgher	1999–00: Cynthia Jacelon
1984–85: Marilyn Pires	2000–01: Judy DiFilippo
1985–86: Renee Steele Rosomoff	2001–02: Donna Williams
1986–87: Phyllis Commeree	2002–03: Paul Nathanson
1987–88: Patricia McCollom	2003–04: Terrie Black
1988–89: Teresa Cervantez Thompson	2004–05: Joanne Ebert
1989–90: Beth Budny	2005–06: Stephanie Davis Burnett
1990–91: Malcolm Maloff	2006–07: Terri Patterson

personal communication, October 25, 2006).

2. Electronic medical records will continue to evolve, resulting in increased use of the computer for all documentation (K. Cervizzi, personal communication, October 25, 2006).

3. The information explosion in a high-technology world will continue to expand rehabilitation nursing research beyond national borders; an international collaborative research effort with colleagues across the globe is already occurring. With the World Wide Web connection, opportunities to design and carry out collaborative studies working "virtually" side by side have become a reality (L. Pierce, personal communication, October 25, 2006).

B. Emphasis on Research and Evidence-Based Practice

1. "Research is needed to address new ideas but also to validate old practices" (S. Burnett, personal communication, October 20, 2006).

2. ARN moved from a nursing diagnosis focus to evidence-based practice with its new publication *Evidence-Based Rehabilitation: Common Challenges and Interventions*.

3. "The emphasis on research will continue to grow and will require more data. Rehabilitation hospitals seeking magnet status will be looking at ways to increase their participation in this part of the process" (T. Thompson, personal communication, October 25, 2006).

C. Magnet Recognition Program for Nursing Excellence

1. "As more rehabilitation healthcare organizations seek magnet recognition, the desire for CRRN certification, continuing education programs, and advanced education will increase" (K. Cervizzi, personal communication, October 25, 2006).

2. The "Forces of Magnetism" may be used as guides to strengthen rehabilitation nursing services and programs.

3. The program may be cost prohibitive for some rehabilitation hospitals and long-term care facilities.

D. Recruitment and Education Issues

1. "The nursing shortage will continue to be an issue as baby boomers begin to retire. Ways must be found to continue to attract nurses into the field of rehabilitation across all practice settings" (M. Ter Maat, personal communication, October 25, 2006).

2. "Future efforts will be aimed at recruiting and retaining aging nurses with incentives and flexibility to motivate them to stay in the workforce well into their retirement years for leading, precepting, mentoring, education, and direct patient care" (K. Cervizzi, personal communication, October 25, 2006).

E. Issues Related to Quality of Life and End-of-Life Decision Making

1. "Rehabilitation nurses will continue to be involved with these issues and need to be able to support the patients' wishes and ensure that they have a comfortable and meaningful period of time while living with disability and experience a good death" (M. Ter Maat, personal communication, October 25, 2006).

2. "Pain management, alternative therapy, spirituality assessment, and bereavement counseling will have a greater emphasis in the aging population, with more nursing research to develop and implement better therapy options" (K. Cervizzi, personal communication, October 25, 2006).

3. Rehabilitation principles are of utmost importance to allow patients to live while dying and to help the family make this time productive and meaningful.

F. Changes in Practice and Care Settings

1. "Demand for home care and long-term care nurses will increase as the older adult population continues to increase" (M. Ter Maat, personal communication, October 25, 2006).

2. "Changing healthcare priorities that reflect ongoing concerns about spiraling healthcare costs, an emphasis on cost-effectiveness, and an outcome-oriented society will continue to change the landscape of rehabilitation nursing" (L. Pierce, personal communication, October 25, 2006).

G. Disaster Preparedness and Education

1. "Disaster education will become more important for rehabilitation nurses and patients in light of the changing world and the risk of natural and human-made disasters" (S. Burnett, personal communication, October 20, 2006).

2. "Many shelters are not wheelchair accessible, and many nurses are not trained in care for the disabled" (S. Burnett, personal communication, October 20, 2006).

3. "ARN will be defining its role in disaster preparedness and education" (T. Patterson,

personal communication, October 26, 2006).

H. Thoughts from Nursing Colleagues Outside Rehabilitation Nursing

1. Technology will transform the nursing profession:
   a. Create a global professional community
   b. Provide evidence at the point of service; patients will demand evidence-based nursing.
   c. Information technology use is a strategic imperative (R. Simpson, presentation at NYONE, October 15, 2006).

2. Mobility and portability will be the basis for any healthcare delivery model:
   a. There will be growth in nonhospital settings.
   b. "Technology will extend lives, and healing will take place in the home. Focus on making the transition to home" (T. Porter-O'Grady, *American Nurse Today*, October 2006).

3. Evidence-based practice helps nurses get "a handle on what we do that is valuable—what difference it makes. Can we do it again and can we do it even better the next time?" (T. Porter-O'Grady, *American Nurse Today*, October 2006).

4. Increasing emphases on quality and safety are trends that have benefited nursing:
   a. The National Database of Nursing Quality Indicators tracks nursing impact on patient care outcomes.
   b. Nurses may see more pay for performance: "Nurses must be involved in establishing payment criteria" (L. Aiken, *American Nurse Today*, October 2006).

5. High times for high tech:
   a. Linking diseases to genes and stem cell research will have an impact.
   b. Computer-assisted surgery is becoming more common.

6. Nursing workforce issues:
   a. The demand for nursing is rising with only slow increases in supply: "We're experiencing the calm before the storm" (P. Buerhaus, *American Nurse Today*, October 2006).
   b. "Aging nurses need to take the burden out of care; technology can help (L. Burnes Bolton, *American Nurse Today*, October 2006)."
   c. Use of foreign nurses is increasing.
   d. The physician shortage is increasing the demand for nurse practitioners.
   e. Push for staffing ratios and legislation on public reporting
   f. "The faculty shortage will worsen; schools are looking for options. Advanced practice nurses will partner in the education of students, and schools will develop certificate programs to develop faculty" (J. Lancaster, *American Nurse Today*, October 2006).
   g. Educational delivery and teaching methods will change through the use of distance learning, curriculum restructuring, and simulations.

7. Surviving in the new world:
   a. Be open to change.
   b. Emphasize the need for continual learning; recognize "need to have a mental model in which I have access to the most current data and information possible" (T. Porter-O'Grady, *American Nurse Today*, October 25, 2006).
   c. See "opportunities for significant reforms in our health care"; learn political skills to influence others and understand the healthcare business (R. Patton, *American Nurse Today*, October 2006).
   d. Move forward together! Nursing will continue to evolve, but the basics of human caring must remain. Nursing leadership must remain strong, and leaders must model change and mentor future nurse leaders.

References

McCourt, A.E. (Ed.). (1993). *The specialty practice of rehabilitation nursing: A core curriculum* (3rd ed.). Skokie, IL: The Rehabilitation Nursing Foundation of the Association of Rehabilitation Nurses.

Suggested Resources

Allan, W. (1958). *Rehabilitation: A community challenge*. New York: Wiley.

Association of Rehabilitation Nurses (ARN) 20th Anniversary Task Force. (1994). *Celebrating 20 years of magic*. Skokie, IL: ARN.

Bitter, J. (1979). *Introduction to rehabilitation*. St. Louis: Mosby.

Mumma, C. (Ed.). (1987). *Rehabilitation nursing: Concepts and practice* (2nd ed.). Evanston, IL: Rehabilitation Nursing Foundation.

Novak, S., & McCourt, A. (1994, September). *History in the making*. Session presented at the ARN 20th Anniversary Educational Conference, Orlando, FL.

Acknowledgments

Thanks go to Stephanie Burnett, Karen Cervizzi, Cynthia Jacelon, Kelly Johnson, Terri Patterson, Linda Pierce, Marilyn Ter Maat, Teresa Thompson, Cathy Tracey, and Barbara Warner for sharing their insights on the future of rehabilitation nursing.

Case Studies

The case studies can be used in classroom teaching, review sessions for certification, and as an individual learning activity. As you read the cases and answer the questions, refer to related sections of the core curriculum for specific content.

Case Study: ALS

Kristen L. Mauk, PhD RN CRRN-A APRN BC • Cindy Gatens, MN RN CRRN-A

Dr. George is a 59-year-old grandfather of 5 who was recently diagnosed with ALS. At the time of diagnosis, Dr. George had an active practice in dentistry, and was married to his wife, Ann, for 35 years.

Dr. George sees a physiatrist for management of his condition. A rehabilitation nurse works with the physiatrist and often consults with Dr. George on routine office visits. At the last visit, Dr. George was beginning to have difficulty with speech and reports an increased loss of strength in both hands. Physical examination and diagnostic tests confirm progression of the ALS. Dr. George confides to the nurse that he does not wish to face the possibility of total loss of function and the burden of care that he realizes will fall upon his wife as his condition progressively worsens. He tells the nurse that he intends to live as long as he feels okay and then end his own life by taking pills that will result in him losing consciousness and never awakening. He has access to these medications in his dental practice. Dr. George has discussed this with his wife, and although she has moral objections and will not assist him, she supports his right to decide.

Questions for discussion:
1. What should the rehabilitation nurse's next course of action be?
2. What education does the family and patient need?
3. Are there special considerations that need to be paid to the wife?
4. How should the nurse deal with this situation?
5. Are there realistic goals that may be discussed with Dr. George?
6. What legal and moral issues are involved in this situation?
7. If Dr. George follows through on his plan to end his own life, at what point will he likely do this? And is there a point at which he will be unable to do this on his own?
8. What would you do if you were the rehabilitation nurse in this scenario?

Case Study: Amputation

Kristen L. Mauk, PhD RN CRRN-A APRN BC • Cindy Gatens, MN RN CRRN-A

Mr. Jones is a 65-year-old African American male with a history of diabetes. He lives at home with his wife of 45 years, one adult son, and two grandchildren who are teenagers.

Mr. Jones is 5' 10" and weighs 230 pounds. He retired from his job in the mills at the age of 62. His favorite activities are watching television and eating out. Mrs. Jones states that she tries to get him to "eat better," but he likes snacks and does not want to exercise. Mr. Jones' Hgb A1C is greater than 9, and he has had some problems with foot ulcers in the past.

About a month ago, Mr. Jones was seen in the office because he has tried to remove a callus on his left foot by filing it. The area became infected and showed necrosis upon examination. Mr. Jones stated that he didn't notice it because it "didn't hurt" until recently. Traditional treatment was unsuccessful, and Mr. Jones was scheduled for a foot amputation performed 10 days prior to admission to acute rehabilitation.

Mr. Jones is admitted to the unit where you are the APN. A prosthetic foot is being considered, but the physician fears a BKA might be in the future for Mr. Smith because of noncompliance in managing his diabetes, as well as his pre-existing PVD.

Questions for discussion:

1. What unique discharge needs are likely in Mr. Jones' case?
2. What teaching should be done, and what team member should do it?
3. What are some team goals for Mr. Jones?
4. Of the family members listed, how can the APN involve them in promoting best care for Mr. Jones?
5. What might be the long term effects of diabetes and PVD for this patient?
6. What are Mr. Jones risk factors for future amputation? And how could they be minimized?
7. How can the APN direct the team so that diabetic control is addressed?
8. What are the benefits and risks of a foot prosthesis for this patient?
9. What consults would you recommend for Mr. Jones while he is in inpatient rehabilitation?
10. If a follow up program after discharge is available, how would it be structured?

Case Study: Arthritis

Kristen L. Mauk, PhD RN CRRN-A APRN BC • Cindy Gatens, MN RN CRRN-A

Sally is a 60-year-old woman with a long-standing history of severe rheumatoid arthritis. Over a number of years, Sally has experienced limited range of motion and pain as the most significant results of her disease. She has undergone several joint replacements in order to combat the effects of her illness, including replacements of both knees, shoulders, and one hip.

Sally has two grown children and lives in a large trailer within an upscale community with her husband of 40 years. She describes their relationship as strong and loving, but states that her illness has taken a toll both emotionally and financially. Her children help when they can, but a majority of her social support comes from friends and church members.

There are 5 steps into Sally's trailer. Her home is clean and well organized. The shelves in the kitchen have been lowered to help her reach items, but she needs assistance from her husband at times. The floor concept is open. The rooms are all on one level. Sally does most of the cooking and home maintenance.

The rehabilitation nurse first meets Sally in an outpatient rehabilitation program that incorporates aquatic therapy. Sally is recovering from shoulder replacement. The rehabilitation nurse's job is to act as case manager for each of the clients seen in this outpatient facility. The rehabilitation nurse assesses Sally's many care needs and devises a long term plan to help Sally and her husband cope with the effects of her arthritis.

Questions for discussion:

1. What are Sally's greatest care needs at the present? In the future?
2. How important are the following in Sally's overall rehabilitation? Pain management, activity/exercise, social and emotional support, spousal support?
3. Are there additional support systems into which Sally and her family could be linked?
4. Consider the environment in which Sally lives. Are there any suggestions you might make?
5. Is aquatic therapy an appropriate exercise treatment for Sally? Why or Why not?
6. What medications would you expect to see Sally taking? What will you teach her and her husband about side-effects from these?
7. What implications do numerous joint replacement surgeries have for Sally?

Case Study: Brain Injury (BI)

Kristen L. Mauk, PhD RN CRRN-A APRN BC • Cindy Gatens, MN RN CRRN-A

Mike is 24-years-old and sustained a traumatic brain injury from an assault. He was assessed at a Rancho Level IV on admission to rehabilitation. After completing a four week stay on an inpatient rehabilitation unit, he was discharged to his parent's home.

Prior to his injury, he lived with his girlfriend and worked full time as a housepainter. She has remained supportive and involved in his recovery. Since she worked full time, she was unable to provide his care. Mike had no major physical disabilities, but was scheduled to attend outpatient therapy (psychology and speech) for ongoing cognitive rehabilitation 3 days per week. Mike would be under supervision of his mother who worked out of a home office. His father worked approximately 50 hours/week outside the home.

After being home for a week, Mike became restless and was found wandering through the neighborhood. His mother started locking doors in an attempt to manage Mike's wandering. This angered Mike and he threatened to leave. A few days later Mike had left his parent's home and could not be found. His mother spent several hours in panic searching for him. He was later found by police who suspected he was on drugs because of his cognitive deficits, confusion, and odd behavior.

Mike and his parents are back for a follow up visit. As an APN in the rehabilitation outpatient clinic you are to see Mike and his mother.

Questions for discussion:

1. Can you identify the gaps or barriers in the interdisciplinary team's inpatient discharge plan?
2. How do you prioritize issues that can be dealt with in the clinic setting?
3. How will you approach Mike, his family, and community services about safety issues?
4. Are there any medications that might help with Mike's presenting problems?
5. What are other options or resources that could facilitate better outcomes for Mike and his mother?
6. Would this visit be an appropriate time to talk with Mike's mother about Advanced Directives for Mike?

Case Study: GBS

Kristen L. Mauk, PhD RN CRRN-A APRN BC • Cindy Gatens, MN RN CRRN-A

Nellie was a 52-year-old rehabilitation nurse who experienced a respiratory infection with fever about 3 weeks after receiving a flu shot (without informed consent) from her place of employment. She went to the doctor with complaints of strange sensations such as feelings of numbness in her big toe and one arm.

She presented with a hacking cough and fever. Nellie's trip to the ER revealed a negative chest x-ray and no other abnormal labs. Nellie's reflexes were also normal. Doctors placed her on antibiotics. She was told she had bronchitis and pneumonia.

Nellie finally called a neurologist when she felt progressive paralysis in her bilateral lower limbs, feeling she had symptoms of GBS. The neurologist confirmed the diagnosis with a spinal tap that revealed white blood cells in the CSF and decreased deep tendon reflexes. Nellie was admitted to acute care where she underwent several plasmapherisis treatments over two weeks.

The medical treatment arrested the course of her disease, and she entered rehabilitation for two weeks of acute care. After discharge, Nellie could no longer work as a rehabilitation nurse due to the residual effects of her illness that included severe fatigue. Nellie also had some lower extremity weakness, memory impairment, facial droop, photosensitivity, and decreased tearing of both eyes. She took a job as a home health nurse to better manage her own schedule but was unable to continue work as a rehab nurse due to ongoing fatigue and weakness.

Questions for discussion:

1. Are Nellie's residual deficits common for patients post-GBS?
2. What are the implications for what happened to Nellie in relation to the flu shot she was given at her place of employment?
3. Does Nellie have cause for a lawsuit if informed consent was not obtained prior to the flu shot she was given?
4. Identify priority issues to discuss at Nellie's first follow-up appointment.
5. What are some potential options/resources to facilitate Nellie's return to work in a different type of nursing position?
6. How could Nellie's medical situation have been handled differently? What should have been done?

Case Study: Multiple Sclerosis

Kristen L. Mauk, PhD RN CRRN-A APRN BC • Cindy Gatens, MN RN CRRN-A

Joanna is a 29 year-old married, white female with 2 small children. Things have been going well for the family. They have put a down payment on a new house and Joanna has been promoted to nurse manager in the SICU at your facility. Joanna was recently diagnosed with MS.

Her symptoms, at first, were vague: feelings of numbness in her legs and hands. She had experienced these for several months until one day at work, she experienced a sudden onset of numbness and weakness in her legs. A stat CT scan showed the presence of plaques, and the neurologists made a tentative diagnosis of MS. Joanna was hospitalized on the acute unit for initial treatment (IV methylprednisolone) and observation.

Over the next few days, her symptoms include rapidly worsening gait and speech, in spite of treatment. She describes continual numbness in her legs, chest, and face. Her observed gait is very unstable and ataxic, yet she refuses to remain in bed. She insists that, as an ICU nurse, she is perfectly able to return home and self administer the IV medications. Joanna has been open with her staff and colleagues about her diagnosis. Even with her current functional limitations and uncertain outcome, Joanna has already decided on the date that she will return to work.

The neurologists consult you as the Rehabilitation APN for further assessment and intervention. The SICU also asks for your help with staff support—the SICU staff have been devastated by the news that their manager has MS.

Questions for discussion:

1. What is the role of the APN in this case, as a colleague and as a rehabilitation specialist?
2. What nursing interventions should take priority in this case?
3. What can you anticipate will be the outcome of this acute episode?
4. What safety issues can you identify, and how may they be addressed?
5. What workplace issues should be addressed?
6. What long term needs can you address at this stage in the course of Joanna's disease?
7. How can you best support the staff in the ICU?
8. What medications may be helpful for long-term management of Joanna's disease?

Index

American Nurses Association (ANA)
case management, 412–413, 422
health care reform, *72*
performance improvement models, 409
rehabilitation teams, 458
standards and ethics, 4, 9, 29, 413
American Nurses Credentialing Center (ANCC), 379, 413, 415
American Pain Society (APS), 260, 262, 267, 270
American Paraplegia Association, 457
American Red Cross, 456
American Red Cross Institute for Disabled Men, 456
American Society for Pain Management Nursing, 271, 272
American Society for Parenteral and Enteral Nutrition, 96
American Society for Reproductive Medicine (ASRM), 119
American Society of Consultant Pharmacists, 376
American Speech-Language-Hearing Association, 93
American Spinal Injury Association (ASIA), 65–66, 67–68, 69, 198
American Stroke Association (ASA), 157, 166, 179, 364
American Urological Association, 117
"The Americans with Disabilities Act: More rights for people with disabilities" (Watson), 49
Americans with Disabilities Act (ADA), 2, 22, 48, 49, 423, 448–449
Amirfayz, R., 348
Amputation, 227–230, 468
Amyotrophic lateral sclerosis (ALS), 429, 467
"An interdisciplinary approach to the rehabilitation of open-heart surgical patients" (Carbone), 248
"ANA hails Congress' support," 149, 150
Anarthria, 162
Anderson, C., 339
Anderson, G., 362
Anderson, K., 48, 127
Anderson, L.P., 224
Anderson, P.J., 349, 350
Anderson, R.A., 450
Andragogical Model of Adult Learning, 128
Andrews, M.M., 450
Annon, J.S., 117
Ansell, B., 190
Anterior cord syndrome, 68, 198
Anti-inflammatory agents, 222
Antidiuretic hormone (ADH), 60

Antiplatelet and anticoagulation drugs, 165
Antirheumatic drugs, 222
Antle, B.J., 144, 151
Antonino, S., 235
Anxiety Disorders Association of America, 372
Apathy, 131, 135–136
Apkarian, A.V., 260
Application of Rehabilitation Concepts to Nursing Practice (seminar), 459
Apraxia of speech, 162
Aptaker, R.L., 362
Arachnoid mater, 56
Arbesman, M., 75
Architectural Barriers Act (1968), 21
Ardell, D.B., 72
ARN Health Policy Committee, 49
ARN Journal, 458, 459
ARN Position Statement on Ethical Issues, 29–31
Arnett, F.C., 220
Arnold, J., 13
Arnold, R., 205–206
Arthritis
case studies, 469
Degenerative Joint Disease (DJD), 223–227
juvenile, 220, 221–223
overview, 218–219
rheumatoid, 219–223
Arthritis Foundation, 219–220, 223
Arthrogryposis multiplex congenita, 348
ASIA impairment scale, 69–70, 198–199
Assessment and moral principles, 30
Assessment Instrument of Problem-Focused Coping, 132
Assessment of Pain in Children, 264
Assisted care living facilities, 391
Assisted suicide, 374
Assistive technology, 44, 423, 425–430
Association of Cancer Online Resources, 424
Association of Perioperative Registered Nurses, 345
Association of Rehabilitation Nurses (ARN)
case management, 413
competencies assessment tool, 463
core curricula, 459, 460
goals and values of rehabilitation, 2, 5
guidelines for political action, 51
initiatives, 462–463
pain assessment and management, 260, 268, 271–272
pediatric nursing, 336

performance improvement models, 409
presidents, 463
rehabilitation teams, 458
research agenda, 433
standards and ethics, 29–31, 393, 413
Web site, 179
Asthma, 249, 250, 251, 252, 253
Atherosclerotic process lesions, 240
Attention (mental), 130
Augmentative and alternative communication (AAC) systems, 427, 428–429
Autism, 428
"Autoimmune and endocrine conditions" (Youngblood & Edwards), 220
Autonomic nervous system, 68, 69
Autonomy of patients, 30
Avant, K.C., 6

B

Bader, M.K., 69, 165, 166
Baer, H.R., 368
Bagg, S., 362
Baggerly, J., 183, 184
Bailey, C., 305
Balanced Budget Act of 1997, 48, 449
Balanced Budget Refinement Act of 1999, 48
Balas, E.A., 433, 445
Balfanz-Vertiz, K., 144
Balluz,L.S., 43
Baltes, M.M., 359
Baltes, P.B., 359
Bandeen-Roche, K., 363
Bandura, A., 72–73, 126, 128, 131, 134
Baptiste, A.S., 111
Barber, D., 261, 262
Barker, E.
life care planning, 40
multiple sclerosis, 286
neuroanatomy, 56–59, 61–64, 66–68
Parkinson's disease, 289–291
traumatic injuries, 183, 185, 191
Barnard, A., 350
Barnason, S., 268, 272
Barnes, M., 345
Barry, P.D., 145
Bartel Index, 169, 199, 400
"The Bartel Index: A review of the literature" (Jacelon), 406
Barthel, D.W., 169
Bartlett, C., 400
Barton, Clara, 456
Barton, George, 456

Deficit Reduction Act of 2005, 48
DeFriez, C.B., 261, 262, 263
Defrin, R., 267
Degraff, D., 23, 24
DeGroot, I., 133
DeJong, B.A., 23
Delirium and dizziness, 365
DeLisa, J.A., 3
Dellasega, C. A., 150
Dementia, 369. *See also* Alzheimer's Disease (AD)
Deming, W. Edwards, 409
Denial behavior, 134–135
Deontology, 27
Department of Defense (DOD), 185
DePaul, Vincent, 455
DePippo, K.L., 180, 181
Depression, 135
DeRuyter, F., 425–426
Derwinski-Robinson, B., 132
Deutsch, A., 388, 400
Deutsch, P.M., 147
Developmental stages, 124–125
Developmental theories and tasks
    advanced practice, 333–334
    family developmental and function theories, 331–333
    individual human developmental theories, 324–331
DeVinney, D.J., 148
DeVivo, M.J., 369, 370
Di-Lucente, L., 135
Diabetes Control and Complications Trial (study), 277–278
Diabetes mellitus (DM)
    acute problems, 282–283
    diabetes and glycemic control, 281–282
    diagnostic criteria, 277
    epidemiology and incidence, 276
    etiology, 276–277
    exercise therapy, 279
    HbA1c (glycosylated hemoglobin test), 277–278
    management options, 278–281
    medication therapy, 279–281
    nursing process, 283–284
    overview, 275
    pathophysiology, 277, 278
    risk factors, 277
    symptomatic manifestations, 278
    types, 275–276
Diagnosis. *See specific disease or condition*
Diamond, P., 135
Dickerson, S., 423, 425
Diebold, C., 95, 372
Diencephalon, 59–60

Diener, E., 147
Dietary needs, 92–93
Diffuse azonal injuries (DAI), 185
Digiovanna, A.G., 361, 362
Dines, A., 72
Dirksen, S.R., 56, 285–286, 287
Disability, defined, 3
Disability in America: Toward a National Agenda for Prevention, 46
Disability insurance, 44–45
Disability Rating Scale, 187
Disability statistics, 45–46
Disaster preparedness, 464–465
Discharge planning for stroke patients, 176
Disease state management, 450
Disinhibition, 138
Dittmar, Sharon, 400, 406, 459
Ditunno, J.F., 362
Ditunno, P., 201, 362
Division of Physical Reconstruction, 456
Dizalo, C.H., 347
Dobrzykowski, E., 397, 408
Dochterman, J., 75, 78, 79
Doenges, M., 75, 78, 83
Donaldson, N.E., 434, 441
Doolittle, N., 147
Down's syndrome, 369
Doyle, F.W., 349, 350
Doyle, M., 427
Dracup, K., 148
Drew, Jessie, 459
Driscoll, W., 349
Drucker, J., 329
Drugs and Aging, 119
Drummond, J.E., 352
Duchene, P.M., 27, 28, 29, 32
Duckert, L., 361
Duerden, M.E., 362
Duff, D., 190
Dufour, L., 192
Duke EPESE study, 364
Dukers, M., 406
Dumas, V., 75
Duncan, G., 286
Duodecium, 109
Duppils, G., 365
Dura mater, 56
Durable power of attorney, 31
Durand, I., 6
Durham, P., 190
Duvall, E., 331–332
Dykes, E., 339
Dysarthria, 162
Dysphasia, 161–162, 174, 180
Dziewulski, P., 300

E

Earle, R.J., 351
Easton, K., 149, 177, 180, 367
Economics
    barriers to care, 42–44
    financing the delivery of healthcare services, 35–40
    funding for assistive technology, 44
    income support programs, 44
    prevention of disability, 45–46
    reimbursement for healthcare services, 40–42
Edelman, C., 71, 72–73, 74
Edelstein, J., 230
Education amendments, 48
Education for All Handicapped Children Act, 2
Edwards, P.
    cerebral palsy, 348–349
    continuum of care, 393
    juvenile arthritis, 220, 221
    pediatric rehabilitation facilities, 456
    setting-centered care, 4, 44
    wellness, 72
Edwards, Patricia, 462
Egner, A., 425
Eilert, R., 342
Electrotherapy, 456
Eleftheriou, E., 185
Elfstrom, M.L., 148, 151
Ellenbecker, C.H., 364
Ellis, D., 190
Ellis, J.R., 27, 28, 29, 31–32
Elvers, J., 133
Embolic strokes, 158
Emotional liability, 137–138
Emphysema, 247, 249, 250–251
Empirical paradigm, 434
End of life issues, 373–374, 464. *See also* Palliative care
End of Life Nursing Education Consortium, 374
Engberg, S.J., 104
Engle, Dagny, 458, 461
Environment of care and service delivery
    across lifespan, 392
    changes in health care, 393
    continuum of care, 392–393
    practice and settings, 386–392
Epidemiology. *See specific disease or condition*
Epidural hematoma, 183
Epidural space (brain), 57
Epps, C.D., 272
Equipment, 175. *See also* Assistive technology

G

Galen, 455
Galinsky, D., 147
Galveston Orientation and Amnesia Test, 187
Gangrene, 227–228
Gardner, V.O., 219
Gargan, M., 348
Gate Control Theory, 262–263
Gatens, C., 195
Gautheron, V., 147
Gaylord, S., 451
Geis, G., 235
Gennarelli, T.A., 185
Genomics, 52
Genuth, S., 278
Geonurseonline, 365, 366
George, L.K., 364
Gerdner, L.A., 319
Gerhart, K., 205–206
Geriatric Depression Scale, 135
Gerontological rehabilitation
  abuse or mistreatment, 375
  acquiring disability at an advanced age, 362–367
  advanced practice nurse role, 379–380
  aging issues, 373–378
  aging theories, 359–360
  early-onset disability, 367–371
  normal aging, 360–362
  psychosocial issues, 371–372
  teaching patients, 367
Gerontological rehabilitation nursing (Easton), 367
Gerotranscendence, 360
Gestalt Learning Theory, 128
Gestational diabetes, 275–276
Gharib, S., 104
Giacino, J., 186, 187
Giavedoni, B., 342
Gill, T.M., 365
Gillard, M., 144
Gilligan, C., 329–331
Gilliss, C.L., 348
Gimbel, J., 235
Giordono, B.P., 453
Girard, D., 187
Gitter, A., 342
Giza, C.C., 338
Glaser, D., 148
Glasgow Coma Scale (GCS), 185, 186, 187, 338
Glasgow Outcome Scale, 187
Glass, C.A., 205–206
Glass, T.A., 364
Glendenning, F., 375

Glendinning, C., 351
Global Adult Scales, 400
Global dysphasia, 162
Global positioning systems, 431
Glod, C., 324–329
Glorieux, F.H., 347
Glossopharyngeal nerve, 61, 63
Glucocorticoids, 222
Glueckauf, R. L., 425
Goffman, E., 146
Gold, D.T., 364
Goldstein, L., 95
Gomez, M.J., 147
Goodall, D., 319
Gordon, M., 9, 341
Goshgarian, H.G., 64, 65, 67
Gottschlich, M., 341
Goudas, L.C., 260
Gout, 225–227
Government case management programs, 412
Govoni, A.L., 431
Graham-Eason, C., 27, 28, 32–33
Graham,D.I., 185
Granger, C., 388, 400, 407, 430
Gray, S., 208
Graykoski, J.J., 156, 157, 158, 159
Green, C.F., 285, 286
Greenley, R.N., 345
Gresham, G., 400, 406
Griffith, R., 94
Grimshaw, J., 445
Grol, R., 445–446
Gross, J.C., 95, 372
Grossman, R., 187
Grossman, S., 359
Grosswasser, Z., 187
Grota, P., 75
Grotty, N., 451
Grove, S.K., 434, 437
Grzankowski, J.A., 128
Guardianship, 31, 179
Guideline for prevention and management of pressure ulcers, 101
Guidelines for pulmonary rehabilitation programs (AACVPR), 255
Guidelines for the Practice of Nursing on the Rehabilitation Team (ANA), 458
Guillain-Barré syndrome (GBS), 471
Guzzetta, C.E., 69
Gyldenvand, T., 74

H

Habel, M., 31, 33
Hack, M., 349
Hackbarth, R.M., 337
Hackenberry, M.J., 269
Hadjistavropoulos, T., 272
Hagen-Foley, D.L., 26
Hagen,C., 187, 190
Hagstadius, S., 147
Hales, J.W., 422
Haley, J.A., 388
Haley, S., 407
Hall, J., 348
Hall, K., 400, 406
Hall, Lydia, 5, 6–7
Halm, M.A., 387, 388
Halvey, K., 267–268, 270
Hamilton, B.B., 430
Hammell, K., 147
Hamrick-King, J., 360, 362
Hanak, M., 199
Handicap, defined, 3
Hanel, B.J., 347
Hanks-Bell, M., 267–268, 269, 270, 271
Hardin-Fanning, F., 95, 372
Hardiness theory, *73*
Harlow, R.E., 360
Harris, J.A., 270, 272
Harrison, T.C., 135, 451
Hartke, R.J., 180
Hartley, C.L., 27, 28, 29, 31–32
Harvey, A., 133
Hatton, C., 319
Haussler, P., 387
Havighurst, R.J., 360
Hayes, A., 119
Hayes, E., 144
Hays, S., 72
Health, defined, 71
Health America: Practitioners for 2005, 46
Health belief models, 72
Health care system
  changes and change theory, 451–453
  cost containment, 52
  in crisis, 462
  growth and development of, 51–52
  major milestones, 448–451
  reform, 460
  representatives, 373
Health insurance and service plans, 38–40, 45
Health Insurance Portability and Accountability Act, 44, 48
Health maintenance
  falls and restraints, 74–78

McKennon, S.A., 280
McKinley, W., 198, 199
McKinnis, E.A., 374
McKleskey, E.W., 262
McLennon, S.M., 272, 273
McMahon, S.B., 262
McNeil, J., 45
McPhee, S.J., 242
McQuade, M., 347
McTier, C.L., 268
Mechanick, J.I., 281
Medical model, 3
Medical-surgical nursing: Critical thinking for collaborative care, 263
Medicare Advantage Plans, 35–36
Medicare and Medicaid
 assistive technology, 425
 cap on Part B, 449
 economics and health policy, 36–38, 42–43, 52
 legislation increased demand for rehabilitation, 458
 long-term care financing, 378
 payment systems, 40–42
 set-asides (MSA), 416
 supplemental benefits plans, 40
Medicare Payment Advisory Commission, 408
"Medications to treat arthritis" (Mauk), 222
Medigap insurance, 40
MEDLINE, 442
Medulla oblongata, 60–61
Melillo, K., 130
Melnyk, B.M., 433–435, 438, 441–446
Melnyk's 5 Critical Steps to Evidence-Based Practice, 441
Melvin, M.S., 309
Melzack, R., 260, 263
Memory, 133–134, 173
Menard, R.G., 260
Mendes DeLeon, C.F., 364
Menter, R., 205–206
Merboth, M., 268, 272
Merck Manuals Online Medical Library, 369
Merkel, S., 267
Meta-analyses, 444
Metabolic Arthritis, 225–227
Meyer, C., 374
Meyer, R.A., 261, 262
Meythaler, J.M., 185
Mezey, M., 116, 149, 390
Miacalcin, 217
Miami Project, 206
Michalak, D.R., 28, 31
Midbrain, 60
Mikulic, Mary Ann, 458

Mill, John Stuart, 27
Miller, E., 451
Miller, S.E., 149
Minaire, P., 147
Minaker, K., 362
Mini-Mental State Exam, 116, 129, 133, 136, 314
Minimally conscious state, 186
Minimum Data Set - Post Acute Care (MDS-PAC), 390
Minimum Data Set (MDS), 41, 387, 408
Mink, R.B., 338
Mion, L., 75, 365
Missile injuries, 184
Mitniski, A., 363
Mlcak, R., 341
Mobility and immobility, 109–115
Modified Barthel Index, 199
Modified Facial Action Coding System, 267
Moizo, E., 235
Mokdad, A.H., 43
Molinari, M., 201, 362
Molnar, G., 407
Monahan, F.D., 285–297, 304–306, 309–313, 316
Montagnino, B.A., 350, 351
Montgomery, P., 138, 139
Moore, M.L., 319
Moore, S.M., 431
Moorehead, S., 390, 430
Moorhead, S., 79, 80
Moorhouse, M., 75, 76, 78, 83
Mor, V., 388
Moral development and behavior, 330
Moral dilemmas, distress and uncertainty, 27–29. *See also* Ethical and moral considerations
Moral theories, 329–331
Moretti, M.E., 344
Morgan, A., 338
Morganstein, D., 261
Morganti, B., 201, 362
Morris, H., 94
Morrissey, Alice, 457
Morrissy, R., 342, 343
Mosby Great Performance, 218
Mosby's dictionary of medical, nursing, and health professionals, 56, 57
Mosca, V., 342
Moskowitz, E., 388
Mosqueda, L., 368
Moss, M.M., 215
Motivation (mental), 131–132
Mount, B., 73
Msall, M.E., 430
Multidimensional Acceptance of Loss Scale, 133

Multidisciplinary model, 3
Multiple Sclerosis Foundation, 285, 287, 318
Multiple sclerosis (MS)
 augmentative and alternative communications (AAC) systems, 429
 case studies, 472
 epidemiology, 284–285
 etiology, 285
 management options, 286–287
 nursing process, 287–289
 in older adults, 370
 overview, 284
 pathophysiology, 285–286
 pharmacotherapeutic agents, 287
 symptomatic manifestations, 286
Multipolar neurons, 57
Multistate licensure, 417
Mumma, Christina, 459, 460
Mumma, C.M., 3–4
Munnell, A.H., 359
Murdoch, B., 338
Murison, R., 338
Murphy, K., 341
Murphy, M.P., 135
Muscular distrophy (MD), 345–347
Musculoskeletal and orthopedic disorders
 advanced practice, 233–236
 amputation, 227–230
 arthritis, 218–227
 nursing diagnoses, 230–233
 osteoporosis, 212, 213–218
Muzzolon, F., 235
My Health Directive, 373
Myelodysplasia, 344–345
Myelomeningocele, 344–345
Myers, A., 75
Myocardial infarction (MI), 242

N

Nance, T., 408
Nash, D., 450
Nason, Karen, 463
Nathenson, N., 145
Nathenson, P., 449
National Advisory Committees (NACs), 398
National Agenda for the Prevention of Disability, 46
National Association of People with AIDS, 318
National Association of Subacute/Post Acute Care (NASPAC), 388
National Cancer Institute (NCI), 251, 307, 318

O

Ober, M., 341
Objectivism, 27
Obstructive pulmonary disease, 247, 249, 250–253
Obstructive sleep apnea (OSA), 108
Occipital lobes, 58
O'Connor, P., 148
Oculocephalic reflex, 60
Oculomotor nerve, 61, 62
Oculovestibular reflex, 60
Oddson, B.E., 344
Odegard, P.S.D., 279–280, 280
O'Dell, M., 190
Oder, w., 138
O'Donald, V., 187
O'Donnell, M., 74
Office of Statistics and Programming, 299
Ogle, C., 425
O'Hare, M., 228
O'Hare, T.P., 378
Ohio State University Medical Center, 293
Ojdana, K., 369
Okara, C.A., 43
Old-age and survivors insurance, 44
Olfactory nerve, 61, 62
Olivieri, R.J., 268, 272
Olson, D.A., 425–426
Omaha Classification System, 390
Omery, A., 435–436
O'Neill, P.A., 180
Online journals, 441–442
Oostendorp, R., 133
Open-heart surgical patients, instructions, 248
Operant Conditioning, 127–128
Opportunistic infections (OIs), 293–294, 295
Optic nerve, 61, 62
Oral apraxia, 428
Orbaek, P., 147
Orem, Dorothea E., 5, 8
Orientation (mental), 129–130
O'Rourke, A., 438
ORYX initiative, 396–397
Osteoarthritis (OA), 223–227
Osteogenesis Imperfecta Foundation, 347
Osteomyelitis, 227
Osteoporosis
　client education, 216–217
　diagnosis, 214–216
　disabilities resulting from, 216
　etiology, 213–214
　interventions after diagnosis, 217–218

pathophysiology, 214
prevention strategies, 218
research topics, 218
Ostrander, R.N., 144
Ostwald, S., 364
Ottenbacher, K.J., 348, 350, 406
Ottomanelli, L., 135
Outcome and Assessment Information Set (OASIS), 41, 390–391
Outcome measurement and performance improvement
　accrediting agencies, 396–399
　the future, 410
　key concepts in rehabilitation, 399
　overview, 395
　program evaluation, 408–409
　quality and performance improvement, 409–410
　tools for monitoring outcomes, 400–408
"Overview of neuroanatomy and neurophysiology" (Hickey), 184, 191
Owsley, C., 361
Oxytocin, 60

P

Pachet, A., 208
Packard, A., 272
Paholke, D., 348
Paice, J.A., 267–268, 270, 271
Pain
　assessment and management, 268–271
　clinical manifestations, 263–264
　cultural considerations, 261
　defined, 260
　diagram, 266
　effects on family and society, 260–261
　epidemiology, 260
　etiology, 261
　gender and, 261
　myths about, 272
　nursing interventions, 272
　nursing roles, 271–273
　pathophysiology, 261–262
　pharmacological and nonpharmacological management, 270
　rating scales, 265–269, 272
　stroke patients, 175–176
　theories, 262–263
　variations across lifespan, 264–268
Pain: Current understanding of assessment, management, and treatments (APS), 270

"Pain assessment and management in aging" (Hanks-Bell, et al.), 270
Pain management: Documenting the decision making process (Malek & Olivieri), 272
Painter, C.C., 425
Palliative care, 311–312, 373, 380
Palmer, P.M., 93, 166
Palmer, S., 165
Pang, C.T., 425
Papadakis, M.A., 242
Pape, T., 422
Paralyzed Veterans of America, 102
Paraplegia, 69, 196
Pareto chart, 409
Parietal lobes, 58
Parish nurses, 18, 23–24
Parkinson's Disease Foundation, 289
Parkinson's Disease (PD)
　augmentative and alternative communications (AAC) systems, 429
　drugs for symptomatic control, 290
　epidemiology and incidence, 289
　etiology, 289
　management options, 290–291
　nursing process, 291–292
　overview, 289
　pathophysiology, 289–290
　types, 289
Parsons, L., 238
Partners in care, 390
Passaretti, D., 341
Paterson, C.R., 347
Paterson, J., 130, 138, 147
Pathophysiology. See specific disease or condition
Pathophysiology of hearing and vision, 140, 141
Patient assessment instruments, 41–42
The Patient Care Partnership (AHA), 29
Patient classification systems, 41–42
Patient education
　diabetes, 318
　individualized educational plan, 24–25
　osteoporosis, 216–217
　sex education resources, 118
　stroke, 175
　vocational education, 48
Patient Evaluation and Conference System, 400, 405
Patient rights, 29
Patient Self-Determination Act (1990), 29, 31
Patrick, D., 74
Patrick, L., 363
Patterson, T., 462, 464–465

epidemiology, 249
irritant sources and control measures, 256
management measures, 252–253
nursing process, 253–257
pathophysiology, 250–251
rehabilitation programs, 238
residual effects, 251–252
types, 247, 249
PULSES, 400
Punton, S., 6

Q

Quadriplegic Index of Function, 199, 406
Qualitative research, 439–440
Quality improvement tools, 409
Quality of life issues, 464
Quality of Life Scale, 148, 267
Quality of Social Support instrument, 147
Quantitative research, 438–440
Query, B., 352
Quetsch, J.L., 422
Quigley, P., 390

R

Rader, M., 190
Raja, S.N., 261
Raloxifene (Evista), 217
Ramakerl, R.R., 347, 348
Ramsey, D.J.C., 180, 181
Rancho Los Amigos Levels of Cognitive Function Scale, 129, 187–190, 338
Rancho Los Amigos National Rehabilitation Center, 195
Range of motion, 111–113
Rankin Scale, 168
Rapid eye movement (REM) sleep, 107
Rappaport, M., 187
Ratcliff, G., 370
Rauch, F., 347
Rawl, S., 177
Rawls, John, 27
Receptive dysphasia, 162
Reciprocity as moral principle, 30
"Recommendations for the management of stress and urge urinary incontinence in women," 104
Recovery and rehabilitation, 195
Reding, M.J., 180
Redman, B., 28–29
Redmond, T., 424–425
Rees, T., 361
Reeves, E., 351

Reeves, J., 135, 136
Registered Nurses Association of Ontario (RNAO), 97–98, 106
Registered nurses (RNs), 10
Rehabilitation, Comprehensive Services, and Developmental Disabilities Amendment (1978), 22
Rehabilitation Accreditation Commission (CARF), 388
Rehabilitation Acts, 2, 21–25, 48, 352, 449, 456–458
Rehabilitation and support services in the community, 86–89
Rehabilitation Engineering Research Centers, 423
Rehabilitation history and philosophy, 2–4
Rehabilitation Institute of Chicago, 463
Rehabilitation nursing
ethics defined, 27
focus and core values, 4–5
in the future, 463–465
historical overview, 455–461
legal issues, 31–33, 89
nurses as change agents, 452–453
philosophical worldviews, 5
research validating need for, 25
in the 21st century, 461–463
teams, 3–4, 32
Rehabilitation Nursing: Concepts and Practice - A Core Curriculum (ARN), 459
"Rehabilitation Nursing: Directions for Practice" (course), 459–460
Rehabilitation nursing: Process, application and outcomes, 30
Rehabilitation Nursing and Related Readings (Boucher), 459
Rehabilitation Nursing Certification Board (RNCB), 11, 459, 463
Rehabilitation Nursing Foundation (RNF), 9, 105, 459
Rehabilitation Nursing (Gatens & Hebert), 149, 458
Rehabilitation Nursing in the Home Health Setting (ARN), 461
Rehabilitation Nursing Institute (RNI), 459
Rehabilitation Nursing (Morrissey), 457
Rehabilitation nursing practice, major neurological deficits and common rehabilitation disorders (Rosebrough), 195
Rehabilitation Nursing Research Agenda (RNRA), 9
Rehabilitation Nursing Research (journal), 460
Rehm, R., 348, 350, 351

Reichhardt, G., 362
Reinboth, J., 74
Reinhardt, U.E., 52–53
Reinkensmeyer, D.J., 425
Reintegration within community
barriers, 18–22
care provider issues, 22–23, 24
financial issues, 19, 22
transportation issues, 19, 22
Remington, R., 130, 134, 138, 139
Remote monitoring technologies, 425
Rempher, K.J., 437, 439
Rennick, J.E., 351
Research
evidence-based practice distinguished, 433–435
on human subjects, 32
importance of, 435–436
levels of evidence, 441
locating evidence, 441–442
problem sources, 436–437
quantitative and qualitative designs, 437–440
translating into practice, 445
Resnick, B., 131, 136
Resource Utilization Groups (RUGs), 41
Respiratory disorder (Wilson & Thompson), 255
Respiratory disorders (Wilson & Thompson), 253
Restorative Nursing: A Training Manual for Nursing Assistants (ARN), 461
Restraints, use of, 75, 374–375
Restrictive pulmonary disease, 249, 250, 251, 252, 253
Reticular formation, 61
Reynolds, F., 144
Rheumatoid arthritis (RA), 219–223
Ricci, J.A., 260–261
Ricci-Balich, J.A., 329
Rice, S.A., 339
Richard, R., 341
Richardson, M., 74, 345
Richardson, V., 344
Richie, B.S., 147
Riedel, D., 138, 139
Riegel, B., 148
Riggs, D., 73
Riggs, R., 190
Ringkamp, M., 261
Rintala, D., 145, 147, 148, 151
Ritter, D., 409
Roach, J., 339
Robbins, A., 74
Robinson, G., 339
Robinson-Whelen, S., 145, 151

Index

Notes

Notes

Notes